Homoeopathy

HORSES

'All things are poison. It is the dosage that makes things not a poison'
Paracelsus 1493–1541

Homeopathy *for* HORSES

Tim Couzens

BVetMed, MRCVS, VetMFHom, CertVetAc

KENILWORTH PRESS

First published in Great Britain in 2006 by
Kenilworth Press – an imprint of Quiller Publishing Ltd
Wykey House, Wykey, Shrewsbury, SY4 1JA

ISBN 1-872119-06-9
978-1-872119-06-9 (from January 2007)

British Library Cataloguing in Publication Data
A catalogue record for this book is available from the British Library

Layout by Kenilworth Press
Editorial services and typesetting by Chris Bagshaw

Printed in Great Britain by St Edmundsbury Press Ltd, Bury St Edmunds, Suffolk

Contents

This book is dedicated to my parents
Margaret and Norman Couzens

Acknowledgements

I should like to thank the members of my family and my staff for their help throughout the development, research and writing of this book. I have to add special thanks to Julie, without whose support this book would not have been completed before the end of the current decade, and my children, Caroline, Sophie and Toby, for their patience.

A big thank you also goes to Dee, David and Lesley at Kenilworth Press for their unquestionable support, extraordinary patience and for tolerating (with unerring good humour) the ever-extending deadline.

Finally, many thanks to Tony Pinkus at Ainsworths Homeopathic Pharmacy, London, for his support, help and advice relating to the section on individual remedies, the Materia Medica.

Tim Couzens

Preface

It is not possible for any one single person to hold all the knowledge to write a book such as this. The information it contains has been sourced from many avenues. Much has come from personal experience from treating horses over the last fifteen or so years. Much has come from colleagues through personal contact, from a myriad of conversations, from published articles, from the internet and from existing homeopathic books sourced from around the world. Neither is it possible for any single person to have experienced all the conditions listed, let alone treat them using homeopathy. Where the gaps exist, remedies have been determined, accurately I hope, using both manual and computerised repertorisation. I would like to thank all those who have contributed knowingly or unknowingly to this book.

Tim Couzens
February 2006

Foreword

Veterinary homeopathy has a long history. Dr Samuel Hahnemann, who formulated the system in the early nineteenth century, is known to have treated animals, and his pupil Von Boenninghausen used homeopathy on the animals on his country estate. However, the first veterinary surgeon known to have used homeopathy was Wilhelm Lux. He is also attributed with having invented the use of nosodes and he wrote the first book on veterinary homeopathy, *Zooiasis,* in 1837.

In the United Kingdom the 'father of British homeopathy', James Moore, wrote several books on the treatment of domestic species of animal, among them *The Horse Owner's Veterinary Guide* (1863) and *Horses Ill and Well: Homoeopathic Treatment of Diseases and Injuries,* of which five editions were printed between 1873 and 1885.There then seems to have been a long gap in the publication of such works until George McLeod's *The Homeopathic Treatment of Horses* was released in 1977.

George almost single-handedly kept veterinary homeopathy alive in the UK in the immediate post-war years and, as a co-founder of the British Association of Homeopathic Veterinary Surgeons, played a significant part in its revival. However, the approach to homeopathy evident in his writings was based almost exclusively on pathological symptoms. Equine homeopathy has advanced considerably since then and the need for a more relevant reference work has become ever more pressing. This book is therefore timely.

In this context, perhaps the most important development in equine homeopathy in recent years is the use of constitutional prescribing. Vital to an understanding of this concept is the assessment of the mental and emotional state of the patient, and this is where the major development of this book lies. In the past, horses were viewed as merely sophisticated machines with functions to perform in the service of their owners and, certainly in the medical treatment of their diseases, even with homeopathy, no consideration was made of their mental and emotional state. Modern homeopathy insists that we take these issues into account when prescribing on the deepest level and, while experience and training are necessary to prescribe accurately in this way, the rewards indeed justify the time and effort spent, both in the training of the veterinary homeopath and in the extended consultations necessary. It is at this constitutional level that homeopathy can provide the greatest benefit for its recipient. Careful reading of the relevant chapters of this book will provide a fascinating introduction to this field and hopefully will spur the reader to investigate it more fully.

Tim and I studied homeopathy together at the Faculty of Homeopathy, and we took the examinations for the Veterinary Membership (VetMFHom) together.

Subsequently we followed our separate paths. Tim successfully developed his own style of homeopathy, and concentrated on building up the Holistic Veterinary Medicine Centre in East Sussex; he has written regularly for several magazines, in both the small animal and equine fields. In 1995, I set up my own referral practice, based in and around the Peak District, offering alternative veterinary therapies. At the same time I became involved in teaching homeopathy, primarily to vets and doctors, with the Homeopathic Professionals Teaching Group. Teaching opportunities now regularly take me overseas.

In 2000, Tim and I joined forces when I took up a post in Sussex with him. We exchanged ideas and I'm sure we have learned a great deal from each other. Since that time we have both been engaged in writing books, sharing our individual experiences, but aimed at filling different niches. I have no doubt that this work will perfectly fill the gap which has existed for so long in the homeopathic literature in the English language; an increasing number of veterinary surgeons around the world now practise homeopathy and, for those, the need for a comprehensive equine reference book is at last satisfied.

In addition, while I strongly believe that the homeopathic treatment of horses should remain under the control of a qualified veterinary surgeon, there is much that the informed owner can do to treat minor ailments in their animals. In such cases an understanding of the disease process in operation is vital. Furthermore, for those few horse owners without easy access to a qualified professional, but with an open-minded and co-operative veterinary surgeon on hand, once again this book will be invaluable.

In summary, a comprehensive treatise on equine homeopathy such as this contains something for everyone. For the horse owner unfamiliar with this form of therapy, the first aid remedies can provide a valuable tool in self-help; for the more serious conditions, once a veterinary diagnosis has been made, homeopathy represents a valuable complement or alternative to conventional medicine and, for the aspiring veterinary homeopath, an introduction to the subject in more depth will enable a start to be made; hopefully this will stimulate an interest in further study.

It is a privilege to be requested by Tim to write this foreword, and I look forward to sharing our experiences for a long time yet.

Peter Gregory BVSc VetFFHom CertIAVH MRCVS
Fellow of the Faculty of Homeopathy
Past President of the British Association of Homeopathic Veterinary Surgeons
Partner in the Homeopathic Professionals Teaching Group (HPTG)
Co-author (with John Saxton VetFFHom) of *A Textbook of Veterinary Homeopathy*

Introduction

Homeopathy[1] is a form of complementary medicine based on the principle of 'like cures like'. In contrast to conventional medicine, where drugs are prescribed on allopathic[2] or antipathic[3] principles to fight illness, homeopathic remedies are prescribed on the basis of 'similar to suffering'. In fact the term homeopathy is derived from two Greek words, 'homoios', meaning 'like', and 'pathos', which is translated as suffering.

The Origins of Homeopathy

Homeopathy as we know it today has been practised for over 200 years and was developed by the German scientist and physician Samuel Hahnemann, towards the end of the 18th century. The concept however, was by no means new even in Hahnemann's day. He attributed the original theory to the Greek Hippocrates, the 5th-century physician and 'father of medicine' who, it is claimed, cured a patient dying in the final stages of cholera by using an extract of *Veratrum album*, the white hellebore. In toxic doses this highly poisonous plant causes dehydration, collapse and a potentially fatal gastroenteritis, all symptoms that closely resemble those of cholera. Hippocrates noted that 'by similar things disease is produced, and by similar things administered to the sick, they are healed of their disease' – the principle of 'like cures like' as rediscovered by Samuel Hahnemann.

The Work of Samuel Hahnemann

Samuel Hahnemann was born in Meissen, Germany in 1755, the son of a porcelain painter. Studying medicine in Leipzig and then in both Vienna and Erlangen, he qualified in 1779 and started practising in Dresden. Medicine at this time was founded on dubious practices involving blood letting, along with the use of strong purgatives, emetics and other such drugs, which often did more harm than good.

In 1789 Hahnemann moved to Leipzig, supplementing his income by working as a medical translator. Increasingly, he turned to work of this type as he became disillusioned by the medical practices of the day. Whilst translating one particular medical text in 1790, Cullen's *Materia Medica*, he came across a passage about Cinchona bark in which it was said to cure 'Marsh fever' (better known as malaria), due to its astringent qualities. As a scientist, Hahnemann knew that there were far more powerful astringents that had no benefit at all in treating malaria. Intrigued he investigated further, dosing himself with an extract of cinchona bark (which contains quinine) and noting the effects carefully over the following days.

To his amazement he gradually started to develop the symptoms of malaria one after the other, despite the fact that he did not actually have the disease. Each time he took a dose the symptoms returned and lasted for several hours, eventually disappearing completely when he stopped taking the extract. He rationalised that if an extract of cinchona bark could cause the symptoms of malaria, this was perhaps the way in which the illness was cured by the same medicine. To test his theory, he repeated his experiment on friends, once again observing the same results.

Further experiments followed under strict conditions, on other remedies, some of them involving other popular medicines of the day such as Arsenic and Belladonna (Deadly Nightshade). From this painstaking work he was able to develop 'drug pictures' for each of his remedies by noting the effects on healthy individuals. These effects included the mental (psychological) and physical symptoms the substances produced, as well as more detailed information such as the circumstances in which the symptoms arose, the effect of the weather and even how the symptoms varied with the time of day. These tests he called provings (simply meaning tests), from the German word *prufung*. By careful observation of the symptoms the remedy could produce in a healthy individual he was able to predict which symptoms of illness that remedy could potentially cure in a sick patient. This is the principle or basis of the law of similars; let likes be cured by likes, '*Similia similibus curentur*'.

After six years of testing he published an article detailing the homeopathic principle in a leading medical journal and followed this with a treatise on homeopathy called the *Organon of Rational Medicine* (1810). Over subsequent years he published the results of his systematic provings of potential remedies in his *Materia Medica* (1811–21).

The Dilution Factor

In treating his patients, Hahnemann matched the remedy picture with the disease symptoms and gave the most appropriate medicine, which he termed the 'simillimum'. In many instances, crude doses of his medicines unfortunately produced unpleasant side effects so he started to dilute them in an attempt to minimise this problem. Using diluted remedies, Hahnemann observed that the symptoms of some of his patients seemed to get worse before improving. He termed this effect an 'aggravation' and to prevent this from happening he changed the way in which he diluted his remedies. Rather than using straight serial dilution, his revised method involved diluting a remedy and shaking it vigorously, banging the vial containing the remedy down on a hard surface at each stage of the dilution. Hahnemann is reputed to have used a leather bound bible for the purpose. This method is known homeopathically as succussion and is a critical step in the preparation of homeopathic remedies.

To Hahnemann the diluted medicines certainly provoked less aggravation in his patients but, to his surprise, appeared to work much faster and more effectively. This is in direct contrast of course to conventional medicines, which become less effective when diluted. These new dilutions Hahnemann termed 'potentisations'. The word potency is still used in homeopathy today to describe the strength or dilution of a remedy.

How Remedies are Made

The principles of remedy production as developed by Hahnemann are still used today. Most of the homeopathic remedies we use are made from plant, animal and mineral sources but the sources are now very varied. Sunlight, radiation, magnetism, electricity and modern drugs have been potentised into effective remedies.

Their manufacture is carried out in a very precise and exact way. For homeopathic remedies made from soluble substances such as plant extracts and animal products (such as snake venom), the original base material is dissolved in a mixture of 90 per cent pure alcohol and 10 per cent distilled water and left to stand for between two and four weeks with periodic shaking. After having been strained the liquid produced is termed the mother tincture, and denoted in homeopathy by the suffix Ø. To produce remedies from insoluble substances – minerals, such as calcium phosphate and metals such as silver or iron for example – a process known as trituration is used. This involves repeatedly grinding the original substance using a pestle and mortar with lactose sugar to a point where it becomes soluble in alcohol to produce a mother tincture.

To produce homeopathic potencies, the mother tincture is then serially diluted and succussed at every stage. Two dilution ranges are commonly in use. The decimal potencies, denoted by the suffix x, are produced by dilutions of 1 in 10 dilutions. The centesimal range, denoted by c, uses dilution steps of 1 in 100.

For example, to produce the 6c potency of a remedy, one drop of the mother tincture would be added to 99 drops of an alcohol/water mixture and succussed. One drop of the resulting solution, the 1c potency, would then be added to 99 drops of alcohol/ water mixture and succussed again to produce the 2c potency. The process would need to be repeated a further four times to produce the 6c potency. A few drops of this solution (known as a potentising solution) would then be added to the blank carrier material used for dosing the patient. Normally lactose (milk sugar) tablets, powders, pillules or granules are used for this purpose. Remedies can also be supplied as liquids in which case a few drops of the potentising solution are added to a weak alcohol and water mixture and shaken well.

The Acceptance of Homeopathy

Not surprisingly Hahnemann was regarded with hostility by the medical profession. The apothecaries objected to him preparing his own remedies and his fellow physicians objected to his homeopathic theories and practice, suggesting they were nothing more than utter nonsense. Despite his tireless work he lacked definitive medical evidence of the proof of his methods. In the winter of 1812–13 a typhoid outbreak occurred in Leipzig amongst the remainder of Napoleon's defeated troops. Hahnemann treated 180 cases of which only two died. Again in 1830 an outbreak of cholera was treated by one of his students using the remedy Camphor with dramatic results. The mortality rate in those patients treated conventionally was between 60–70 per cent; in those treated homeopathically it was below ten per cent.

Ultimately cholera was to spread to London and was at its height in 1854 when over 10,000 died in the region of Soho alone. The Royal London Homoeopathic Hospital allocated all its resources to treating the outbreak. Prescriptions were given on the basis of sound homeopathic prescribing – Camphor, Helleborus and Copper were used with great success. So effective was the treatment in fact, that the Board of Health found it necessary to suppress publication of the statistical results on the basis that homeopathic practitioners '...would give an unjustifiable sanction to an empirical practice, alike opposed to the maintenance of truth and the progress of science'.

Despite an increasing interest and mounting evidence for its effectiveness in treating illness in man and animals, homeopathy has always been subject to criticism of this type in one way or another. Without doubt one of the main stumbling blocks to the acceptance of homeopathy has been the dilution factor.

More on Dilution

Hahnemann had found that by diluting his remedies in a specific way they became more potent, and at the same time this removed any toxic or unwanted side effects. On a scientific basis however, progressive dilution soon results in not a single molecule of the original substance remaining, yet the greater the dilution, the more powerful the action of the remedy when correctly prescribed. In fact around the level of the 12c dilution, the limit of Avogadro's number[4] is reached, so that indeed, potencies higher than this contain nothing of the original substance used at the start of the dilution process, yet remain effective.

The key point at this stage is to accept that it is the solvent (alcohol) which carries an, 'energy imprint' from one potency to the next and to understand that it is likely that some kind of electromagnetic effect is involved. This is supported by the observation that the use of a polar solvent is necessary to manufacture homeopathic remedies. Current research involving nuclear magnetic resonance and theories centred around quantum mechanics may yet reveal the mechanism by which homeopathy works. What we do know is that homeopathic remedies work by some form of interaction with the body involving the 'energy' contained in the potentised medicine

The Vital Force

Hahnemann had also given some thought as to how his remedies might work. He proposed that the body must contain some form of subtle energy that responded to the small energetic prompts from the remedies to encourage healing. This energy he termed the 'vital force', a concept that is also recognised in other systems of natural healing. For example, in Chinese medicine it is referred to as *Chi* or *Qi*. In Ayurvedic medicine (an ancient system of healing used in India), the vital force is referred to as *Prana*.

It is this energy that is responsible for maintaining health and harmony within the body. A great many factors can influence the vital force and its role in ensuring equilibrium. These include diet, environment, stress, genetic factors and concurrent administration of conventional drugs. In fact Hahnemann had recognised that health was affected by external influences and was a supporter of healthy eating and good hygiene and was aware of the problems caused by over indulgence and the effects of drinking excess coffee and alcohol. A homeopathic remedy correctly prescribed will support the vital force in fighting ill health and allow the body to heal so that a state of harmony is restored once more.

Acute and Chronic Symptoms and the Concept of Miasms

Symptoms of illness will arise when the vital force is unable to maintain equilibrium. Some problems appear suddenly (such as a respiratory infection or a sprained ligament) causing an acute illness that runs a short course. The body is able to overcome the problem with or without help and the animal recovers. In contrast, in chronic illness such as arthritis the vital force is unable to maintain the balance, despite a number of minor victories or remissions and the symptoms recur and often slowly progress.

Hahnemann believed that many of the chronic health problems seen in people were derived from three fundamental different 'taints'. These he termed infective miasms comprising psora (the itch), sycosis (gonorrhoea) and syphilis. The miasms were inherited through repeated generations within a family, the symptoms of which, if suppressed, would drive chronic disease inward into the body. The outcome of this process would be that an individual could risk the development of more serious disease (such as cancer or epilepsy) if the dormant miasmic trait were triggered by external factors such as stress at any time during life.

Treating animals with well-chosen remedies will sometimes fail for no obvious reason or we might note that the animal's response is poor despite prescribing the correct remedy. The reasoning behind some of these occurrences might be that the miasmic theory has come into play. This may be a single miasm or any combination of psora, sycosis or syphilis. It seems surprising but it appears that Hahnemann's miasmic theory can also be applied to ill health in animals, including horses, and that we can use specific remedies to combat the effects of miasmic traits.

Homeopathic Prescribing – A Brief Outline

This book is divided into sections based principally on body systems. Under each section many of the common problems encountered in horses will be listed along with suggested remedies. A lot of the remedies have been selected solely on the presenting symptoms of the patient, often purely on a pathological basis, an approach that will often yield satisfactory results. Whilst this is a valuable method and one that is easy to apply for the inexperienced, there are a number of other approaches to treating a case that can be useful. Without doubt, the most important of these is the selection of a remedy based on the animal's constitution, an often effective approach which will repeatedly give good results, even in difficult cases.

The remaining information in this introductory section outlines briefly how you can use other ways of prescribing to the patient's advantage.

If in any doubt as to the correct course of action, always seek professional help.

The Importance of Symptoms

The key to using homeopathic remedies successfully is to observe the patent and the patient's symptoms in order to find the correct remedy that will then interact with the vital force and instigate the healing process. Homeopaths group these symptoms into different categories to make the task a little easier.

Local symptoms refer to a particular area of the body or organ system such as the elbow, back, eye, bladder or skin for example.

General symptoms reflect the signs shown by the patient as a whole and might include appetite, thirst, physical appearance, observation on the gait and posture, effects of hot and cold or wet and dry and how the symptoms might vary with the time of year or day.

Mental symptoms reflect the animal's emotional or behavioural state. These might include fear, restlessness, sadness, aggressive behaviour or excitability.
It is also vital to take into account specific characteristics of some of the symptoms. For example where there is a nasal discharge you should note its colour (white, clear, green, yellow), consistency (thin, runny, thick, sticky) and odour if present.

Factors that modify the individual symptoms must also be taken into account. These are termed **modalities** and are divided into two categories.

Aggravations which make the symptoms worse

Ameliorations which ease the symptoms

Examples of **modalities** include the effect of rest or movement, the time of day and the effect of hot or cold and damp or dry. Where a horse is lame, for example, you will need to note if this is better or worse for rest and the effect of the ambient temperature on the degree of lameness, or if the horse resents the affected area being touched because it is painful.

Choosing the Correct Remedy

Selection of the correct remedy is vital in order to enable the body to heal. To do this all the animal's symptoms should be taken together to build up a picture of the animal as an individual. This includes symptoms both past and present, those symptoms that conventional medicine would ignore, strange and peculiar symptoms and those which are common to the particular condition or problem. For example, an anxious, restless, lean, athletic looking horse with sweet itch, with areas of scaling and crusty skin, which rubs intensely so that the skin bleeds, and which feels the cold easily and appears thirsty, will require a remedy encompassing all the symptoms if the case is to be successfully treated.

The best practical approach is to take the history methodically so that all the information can be carefully noted. Depending on the nature of the condition to be treated this will include the following:

Observation of the horse from a distance – first impressions.

General observation to include stance, physical appearance (fat, lean, emaciated), general demeanour (aggressive, fearful, anxious).

Details of the condition to be treated for example, mud fever, chronic cough, lameness, Cushing's syndrome and how long it has been going on for and its periodicity – when does it come and go?

Circumstances or possible trigger factors at the start of the condition, for example loss of a companion, change of yard or a change in diet, effect of vaccination, an accident or injury, access to unsuitable feed. Aim to include relevant circumstances at the present time as well as, for example, the influences of stress and environmental conditions.

Characteristics of each individual symptom. These might include the colour of a nasal discharge, type of cough (dry, wheezy or rattling), type of diarrhoea (watery, soft) and if straining is involved. If the skin is involved this would include the type and appearance of skin lesions – scabs, sores, cracks, crusts, scaling (dandruff), weepy, dry, itchy or bleeding.

Modalities. What makes the symptoms better or worse?

Past health problems of the animal. These will help complete the picture by looking at the sort of symptoms that have been present in the past.

Problems in related animals. This is useful to see if there is a family trait.

Mental symptoms to include, for example, interaction with the owner, reaction to strangers, interaction with other horses and psychological make up – jealous, affectionate, submissive, shy, intelligent, withdrawn, excitable, unreliable, steady, tidy, aristocratic, dominant.

General symptoms – appetite, thirst, likes and dislikes, effect of oestrus, the time of year, the time of day, effect of the weather on the patient as a whole.

The history concludes with an **examination of the patient,** adding notes to the other categories as required. Examine the patient as a whole and each organ system as relevant – ears, eyes, nose, head, mouth, digestive system, respiratory system, urinary system, reproductive system, heart, circulation and lymphatic system, skin, locomotor system (neck, limbs, back, feet) and nervous system.

Levels of Prescribing

Having looked in detail at how to take a history, it is true to say that this approach will not be needed in all cases. A punctured sole for example will simply require a remedy based on the presenting symptoms rather than looking at the animal in its entirety. In contrast, an animal with a chronic cough or sweet itch will require a detailed history to ascertain the correct remedy. The possible ways of prescribing are detailed below.

Constitutional prescribing

This takes into account all the animal's symptoms and then attempts to categorise the patient into one of several distinct types from a list of remedies known as polycrests. These are deep-acting remedies that act on the patient as a whole with a tendency to attempt to cure all the patient's symptoms. Chronic problems nearly always benefit from this approach if it is at all possible to find the animal's constitutional type. It is also a valuable approach to take if another method of prescribing has failed to improve the condition.

Prescribing on the presenting symptom

This is a commonly used approach and requires a less extensive history taking. The prescription is based on local symptoms and the accompanying modalities. You might use this approach to treat a check ligament strain, bruising to the sole or wound to the skin, situations that under normal circumstances would not require a constitutional approach.

Prescribing on the root cause

Regardless of the time period, if a specific incident or illness was the trigger for the condition it is sometimes a good idea to treat this first. Examples might include trauma from a road accident, pathological changes resulting from a wound or symptoms appearing after a specific infection. Prescribing on this basis is usually followed by a further prescription on a constitutional or presenting symptom basis. Past problems can sometimes cause a 'block' on the road to resolving a particular condition, so it is often a good idea to treat these initially.

Prescribing on mental symptoms

It is not always easy to elucidate a horse's character but where this is possible, mental symptoms alone can provide a very effective way of treating illness. Any improvement in the animal's state of mind will tend to help resolve any other problems that might be present. Looking closely at the mental symptoms will often reveal the constitutional remedy.

Prescribing for specific organs

A number of remedies have an affinity for specific organs and can be used alongside other remedies. Examples might include **Solidago** for the kidneys, **Nux vomica** for the liver and **Crataegus** for the heart.

Prescribing using drainage remedies

These are specific remedies used to drain toxins from different organ systems. Examples include **Petroleum** for the skin, **Berberis** for the urinary system and **Chelidonium** for the liver.

Preventative prescribing

Homeopathic remedies can be used in a preventive role both in the possible prevention of specific diseases by the use of nosodes (see page 322) or by preventing predicable problems. Examples of the latter involve using remedies such as **Arnica** before surgery, **Caulophyllum** before foaling and **Calc phos** to ensure the proper growth of bone.

Having worked out the patient's signs and symptoms and having amassed the information and prescribing route, it is not always clear which remedy or remedies might be needed. Employing the use of a materia medica and repertory is the most practical solution to unravelling the information and selecting the best prescription.

Using a Repertory and Materia Medica

The Materia Medica

Since the time of Hahnemann's original *Materia Medica*, which contained his observations on the use of remedies over the period between 1811 and 1821, a great many similar books have been written expanding Hahnemann's original work by adding new remedies and provings. This process continues today with new additions such Aspartame, Coriander and Slate for example. The homeopathic materia medica continues to grow and is constantly evolving.

However, as a basic practical edition to use in conjunction with this book, the *Pocket Manual of Homeopathic Materia Medica and Repertory* by W. Boericke is recommended. The book is essentially laid out as an A–Z of the most common and frequently used remedies including all of those in Hahnemann's original *Materia Medica*. Although the symptomology is human based, the information it contains is easily translated to horses with a little effort and lateral thinking.

For each remedy there is a brief outline of the medicine from a homeopathic perspective followed by a breakdown of its effects on the systems of the body. An indication of what action the remedy will have on an area of the body in real life reveals how the remedy can be employed homeopathically to treat those symptoms. Typically the sections detailed below are found in most books of this type. Where appropriate the equine equivalent is given to help:

- Mind — Psychological and behavioural symptoms
- Head
- Eyes
- Ears
- Nose
- Face
- Mouth
- Throat — Larynx and pharynx
- Stomach
- Abdomen — Small and large intestine

• Stool	Dung
• Urine	Includes the bladder and kidneys
• Male	Stallion and gelding
• Female	Mare
• Respiratory	Lungs, chest, trachea
• Heart	
• Back	Including the neck
• Extremities	Limbs including knee (wrist), fetlock, pastern and coffin joints (finger joints), stifle (human knee) and hock (ankle)
• Sleep	
• Skin	
• Fever	A rise in body temperature
• Modalities	Factors that can make the symptoms better or worse

In short, use the Materia Medica quickly to check if those remedies that you have to mind are suitable and match the symptoms of your patient.

The Repertory

In contrast to the Materia Medica, the repertory approaches the subject of finding the remedy from the opposite perspective. That is by using the patient's symptoms collectively to search for suitable remedies and then narrowing down the choice to a single medicine.

Here we have a book, which in its original form was divided up into sections that are not dissimilar to those above. Older repertories, such as Kent's *Repertory of the Homoeopathic Materia Medica,* use language and section headings which are sometimes archaic and which can make it difficult to locate remedies easily. More modern versions such as the *Homeopathic Medical Repertory* by Robin Murphy are arranged alphabetically, simply from A–Z, commencing with the abdomen through to the wrists. Under each individual section, signs and symptoms are further broken down systematically to a very detailed level including modalities. Under each detailed entry, termed a rubric, will follow a list of graded remedies that have an association with that symptom. A typical entry might appear as:

Extremities (Limbs)	(chapter heading)	
Knees (Stifle joint in horses)	(section heading)	
Sprained ...	(sub heading)	
Stiffness Move on beginning to	(rubric)	*Carbo veg, Causticum, Euphrasia, Lycopodium,* Pulsatilla, **Rhus tox** (Suitable remedies)
At night... (rubric)		

Painful… (rubric)
Rheumatic… (rubric)
Rising from a seat… (rubric)
Sitting while… (rubric)
Walking while… (rubric)
Swelling… (sub heading)
Tearing pain… (sub heading)

The remedies are graded to show how strongly the remedy shows the symptom within its symptom picture. Those remedies listed in **Bold** type are the most prominent, those in *italics* are associated less strongly and those in plain type the least important in relation to the symptom. By taking a selection of the patient's symptoms (which should cover a variety of symptoms across different body systems if possible) the relevant rubrics can be consulted to compile a list of appropriate remedies. By scoring the remedies based on the type classification (those in bold type scoring three points, italic type two points and plain type one point), the remedy or remedies that score the highest should be considered suitable candidates. This is a process referred to as repertorisation. Using a modern computerised repertory such as Macrep, Cara, Isis or Radar, this time consuming process can now be carried out quickly and more reliably than with manual methods. Nevertheless, at the final stage, consulting a materia medica and using past experience and intuition is often the best way to confirm your remedy choice.

Having selected a remedy, the next question is to choose the potency.

Potency and Potency Selection

The question of potency can be confusing, making it difficult to select the best option for the case in hand. The term potency refers to the 'strength' or dilution of the remedy. The two most common potency ranges are the decimal range and the centesimal range. Commonly used decimal potencies include 1x, 3x, and 6x and in the centesimal range frequently used potencies include 6c, 12c, 30c and 200c. Often the suffix c is omitted from the centesimal range so that for example, Arnica 30 is the same as Arnica 30c. The 1M potency is also used from time to time. 1M is equivalent to 1000c. High potencies are considered to be anything above 12c whilst low potencies are normally anything below 6c. Anything between 6c and 12c is considered intermediate.

It is generally accepted that higher potencies have a deeper action and act for a longer duration. This is however, at the expense of breadth of action. In a simple analogy, higher potencies have a narrow target band to hit to achieve an effect, but act with greater force and for longer. In contrast, low potencies act for a shorter duration and have a weaker healing effect whilst having a greater or easier target area to hit. Selecting the potency to use depends on the patient and the nature of the condition to be treated. Unfortunately there are no real hard or fast rules as different homeopaths adopt different approaches but there are some basic guidelines to follow:

Acute conditions often warrant the 30c potency or higher if you are certain that the remedy closely matches the symptoms. If you unsure of the remedy to use, it is far better to use the 6c than no remedy at all. Acute conditions, in general, require frequent dosing; the more acute the symptoms, the more frequently the remedy needs to be given. Lower potencies will need to be given far more frequently in this situation (say up every 15 minutes), than the higher potencies.

Chronic problems often require low potencies if prescribed on a symptomatic basis such as a 6c or 30c or below. Conditions of this type such as degenerative joint disease will often require daily dosing over an extended period of time, possibly for the remainder of the animal's life.

Remedies prescribed on a **constitutional basis** usually require a high potency to act deeply and should be given sparingly. A few doses are often all that are needed.

High potencies are also required for treating **psychological problems** and for conditions that have their root deep in the past, such as a **past illness** or a **particular traumatic episode**.

In this book suitable potencies are suggested for each condition, but may be varied within the context of each individual animal and the symptoms displayed.

If you have now established your remedy, potency and dose, the next step is to observe the effects of the treatment.

Evaluating the Outcome

There are a number of possible outcomes of dosing with a remedy.

No response. This could be due to an:

- **Incorrect prescription.** In this case the remedy does not correlate to the patient's symptoms and the case must be re-evaluated to find a closer match.
- **Correct remedy, wrong potency.** Where the selected remedy is correct, it is possible that the potency is too low to instigate healing and that the patient will require a higher prescription. It is also possible that the potency is too high and that, in effect, it shoots past the target. In this case it is best to try a lower potency.
- **Correct remedy, wrong dosing frequency.** If the correct remedy has been selected it might be possible that the dosing frequency is too low to effect a response. In this case it is worth increasing the frequency of dosing.
- **The action of the remedy is blocked.** This can be due to some past event or illness that will need to be resolved before the remedy will work.

Weak response. The reasons for this are:

- **The potency is too low.** A low potency has breadth of action but has a weaker healing force. In this situation, consider using a higher potency.
- **The dosing frequency is too low.** In this case, increasing the dose frequency may resolve the situation.
- **A close remedy** has been used in which case a related remedy should be selected instead.

The patient's symptoms become worse. This is termed an **aggravation**. In this situation, treatment should be stopped to see the symptoms resolve. If this proves to be the case, the patient will sometimes improve and the condition will resolve. If a resolution is not achieved, treatment should be continued with a higher potency.

Old symptoms appear. This is termed a **recapitulation** and is in effect the unlocking of old symptoms that have been suppressed by previous treatment. This is considered a good sign and treatment should be continued.

New symptoms appear. Treatment with homeopathy can sometimes be likened to peeling the layers from an onion. An initial remedy resolves the symptoms, which are uppermost (on the outermost layer of the onion), only to reveal a new set of symptoms that were hidden on the layer below. Take this into account and re-evaluate the symptoms to see if a more appropriate remedy is required.

The animal's symptoms resolve. When the prescription is correct the patient gets better as the symptoms disappear. Once this stage has been reached, treatment can be stopped and recommenced should the signs return. However, as is often the case, chronic symptoms (especially where there is irreversible pathology) will require remedies to be given on a long-term basis, as a practical cure is not always possible.

Homeopathy and Side Effects

Freedom from side effects is cited as one of the main benefits of homeopathy. In fact if the wrong remedy is given it simply has no effect. It is clear from the list of possible outcomes, however, that some of the results could be mistaken as side effects. Neither aggravations nor the appearance of old symptoms (recapitulation) are side effects. They are short lasting episodes on the road to resolving the condition under treatment.

It is possible to prove a remedy, however, in a similar manner to the way in which Hahnemann proved remedies in the early days of homeopathy. A proving can occur if the animal is particularly sensitive to a specific remedy. This is likely to arise if the remedy is given too often or if treatment is carried on for an extended period of time. If you suspect a proving you should stop treatment immediately, at which time the symptoms should disappear fairly quickly just as they did when Hahnemann conducted his original provings.

How Remedies are Supplied and How to Dose the Patient

Potentised remedies can be supplied in a number of forms:

- Lactose tablets, globules, soft pills or pillules
- Lactose powders

- Sugar (sucrose) granules
- Liquid potency
- Mother tincture, rarely used in horses and diluted in water

Most horse owners will use either hard tablets, the soft pills or powders (which are more expensive). Powders are supplied wrapped individually in small pieces of carefully folded paper. The powder can be tipped straight from the paper into the lower lip of the horse or onto the cut surface of an apple or carrot, which can then be given to the patient. Pills, pillules (which are small round slightly hard balls) and granules (a dose is considered enough to cover the bottle cap) can be similarly tipped onto an apple or carrot. Liquid potencies can be dripped into the horse's lower lip. About ten drops will normally suffice. Liquids are also best suited to mass yard medication as they can be added to a water trough. For the average trough adding about 20–25ml daily will suffice.

Care and Storage of Remedies

As energised medicines, homeopathic remedies need special handling and storage. Given proper care, the remedies will remain viable for many years, but they can be affected by certain factors that can destroy their potency. If this occurs they may become ineffective. There are a few basic rules to follow:

- Do not handle the medicines as this can depotentise them. This applies where the remedy is supplied as tablets, pills or pillules in particular, as opposed to powders, granules or liquid potencies.
- Keep the remedies in darkened glass vials, although for short-term storage, darkened plastic bottles will suffice. Always keep the lid on other than when dispensing the remedy.
- Never return unused remedies back into their container.
- Store the remedies out of strong sunlight and keep at room temperature and away from extremes of temperature.
- Keep away from strong smells, especially camphor, eucalyptus, perfumes and the like.
- Keep well away from sources of electromagnetic radiation such as computers, microwaves, televisions and mobile phones

Interaction with Conventional Medicines

Correctly applied, homeopathy provides an excellent means of allowing the body to heal. Where practical, and with the animal's welfare at heart, it is best to avoid using homeopathy with conventional drugs where possible. Some conventional medications can adversely affect the way in which the remedies work. Drugs particularly to be avoided include steroids. Vaccines too can produce unwarranted effects on the body (see page 322), not only altering the immune system in some cases, but also by changing the way in which the body is able to respond to homeopathic remedies. Antibiotics do not, in general, pose a problem and often will work more effectively in conjunction with some homeopathic remedies.

Other forms of complementary medicine can be used alongside homeopathy with professional guidance and where necessary. Acupuncture, nutraceuticals (supplements) and Bach flower remedies in general work well with homeopathy. Herbal remedies can often provide additional support if well chosen, whilst some of the oils used in aromatherapy can prevent remedies from working effectively if used without care.

Constitutional Remedies and Types

A constitutional homeopathic remedy is one that is matched to the patient as a whole. It encompasses both psychological and physical characteristics and the way in which the patient reacts to disease. In effect, the remedy relates to the mind, body and soul of the patient. Exactly what constitutional remedies cover in their remit is greater than it would initially appear. It includes inherited traits, the effect of life events, and reactions to external stimuli, lifestyle, diet, environment and other modalities. These are remedies that are also classed as polycrests; homeopathic medicines with a wide sphere of action on the body and body systems.

Constitutional prescribing is a very deep and powerful way of treating disease and needs to be used with care, preferably under the guidance of a homeopathic veterinary surgeon. The constitutional approach is one that Samuel Hahnemann frequently mentioned in his writings and greatly encouraged in the homeopathic approach to treating patients. With a little care and observation a great many of the human constitutional types identified by human homeopaths can be seen in horses.

Some Important Constitutional Types

Details of each of the following constitutional remedies are divided into several sections:

- **Remedy name** – The homeopathic name of the remedy and the abbreviation (if any).
- **Common name** – The name by which the remedy is more commonly known.
- **Classification** – The homeopathic classification of the remedy.
- **Preparation** – How the remedy is prepared homeopathically.
- **First impression** – Relates to the initial observation of the patient.
- **Psychological type** – The behavioural characteristics of the patient corresponding to the remedy type.
- **Main health issues** – Relates to the conditions and diseases commonly seen in animals with the corresponding constitutional type.
- **Key pointers** – These are important identifying characteristics which can be tied into the psychological type to help in trying to identify an animal's constitutional remedy.
- **Important indications** – These are the conditions which the remedy can help

treat bearing in mind that the best results are likely to be seen where the remedy is used on a constitutional basis.

- **Related, complementary and incompatible remedies** – The majority of remedies have interactions with other homeopathic remedies, some good, some bad. Some remedies work well (i.e. are complementary) with others, either in conjunction or in sequence with another remedy. Where a related remedy is listed or tagged as 'acute', this indicates that an animal with that particular constitution may benefit from the related remedy when it shows symptoms that appear suddenly, that is to say acutely. Correspondingly, a related remedy labelled as 'chronic' is of benefit in treating symptoms in the patient of a particular constitutional type that have been present over a long period of time. Naturally there are remedies which are incompatible and which do not work well together or which prevent a remedy from acting properly.

THE ARSENICUM HORSE

Remedy name: Arsenicum album, Ars alb
Common name: Arsenic trioxide, White oxide of metallic arsenic
Classification: Mineral: Arsenicums: Polycrest
Preparation: Trituration

First impression

Neat, tidy, compact, well groomed, restless, stylish, thoroughbred type.

Psychological type

The Arsenicum horse appears exceptionally intelligent, well groomed, clean, neat and tidy and is often of an athletic build. Outwardly they often appear worried or anxious. Anxiety is classical Arsenicum trait; the horse is restless (pacing around the box), fidgets around and seems a little uneasy, apprehensive and tense, glancing around to check that everything is as it should be. There are underlying pressures supporting the anxious behaviour. They are sensitive to disorder, confusion and changes in their routine. They are fundamentally insecure and prefer other animals around to give them reassurance. Major changes, such as change of yard, result in considerable stress with anxiety symptoms that will take many weeks to resolve. They can be picky, fastidious, can appear sad, fearful and indifferent, can become vexed and irritable at times and are definitely over-sensitive to pain. Arsenicum horses make neat swift, sometimes jerky, movements. As chilly individuals they feel the cold and will frequently need rugging up, preferring the comfort of a warm stable to the outside, especially if it is cold and wet.

Main health issues

Arsenicum has a very wide sphere of action but problems tend to focus on psychological issues and on the skin, digestive and respiratory systems with an affinity for problems associated with mucous membranes. Arsenicum is a remedy for allergy-based problems such as COPD (respiratory system) and sweet itch (skin). Skin symptoms involve scaling (dandruff) and such an intensity of irritation that the horse will rub itself raw so the skin bleeds. Respiratory symptoms usually encompass a dry cough and wheezing (due to airway constriction). Respiratory infections can also respond where there is a discharge that excoriates (burns) the skin. Digestive symptoms that can respond encompass severe debilitating diarrhoea with weakness leading to collapse.

Key pointers

- Anxious and restless 'nervy animals'
- Fear of being alone
- Chilly-feels the cold
- Thirsty but only for small amounts each time
- Symptoms worse 12pm-2am, around midnight especially
- Sensitivity to disorder and confusion
- Dry, scaly skin, dandruff
- History of sweet itch or COPD

Important indications

- Fever with restlessness or anxiety
- Septicaemia and toxaemia
- Collapse
- As a general tonic after prolonged illness
- Anxiety, restlessness, stereotypic behaviour
- Conjunctivitis with an irritating discharge
- Rhinitis
- COPD, RAO, wheezing, coughing
- Respiratory infections
- Adenovirus, Rhinovirus, Equine flu EHV-1, EHV-4 infections
- Headshaking
- Hydrothorax
- Anaemia especially blood loss anaemia
- Oedema, filled legs
- Stomach ulcers
- Severe watery foul diarrhoea with collapse or weakness

- Severe diarrhoea with blood
- Acute salmonellosis
- Colitis X, Clostridial enterotoxaemia
- Chronic kidney failure
- Pyelonephritis
- Endometritis, pyometria
- CEM
- Sweet itch
- Rain scald
- Seborrhoea
- Alopecia
- Proud flesh especially if infected
- Skin ulcers
- Gangrene
- Pemphigus
- Lice
- Mange
- Vesicular stomatitis virus
- African horse sickness (respiratory and cardiac forms)
- Potomac horse fever
- Horse pox virus
- Equine viral arteritis (EVA)
- Lyme disease

Modalities

Aggravation midnight–2am, exertion, cold, wet weather, by the seaside

Amelioration heat and warmth, company

Remedy interactions

Works well with: Phosphorus, Carbo veg, Rhus tox (especially for skin problems), Thuja, Apis

Incompatible with: Pulsatilla, Graphites, Nux vom

Consider also: Aconite, Hepar sulph, Nit ac, Nux vomica, Phosphorus, Rhus tox, Sulphuric acid, Veratrum album

THE CALC CARB HORSE

Remedy name: Calcium carbonate, Calc carb
Common name: Impure calcium carbonate
Classification: Animal: Molluscs: Polycrest
Preparation: Trituration using the middle layer of the oyster shell

First impression

Heavy horse type, overweight, fat, slow, dull, quiet, lacks interest, excess sweat.

Psychological type

The most striking feature is the lack of interest and lack of response verging on indifference. The Calc carb horse is slow and lacks any great enthusiasm for what is happening around. This is not laziness in itself, but due to very limited capacity for anything that requires effort. This is combined with stubbornness, obstinacy and a number of behavioural issues. These can include fear of specific people, a dislike of being alone, sensitivity to sudden noises, timidity, clumsiness, a tendency to nip if irritated or coerced into activity and dislike of darkened areas, all problems hidden by their 'clam like' unresponsive nature. These are horses that plod in a sluggish manner and are often said to move at the pace of a tortoise. It is an effort to gain any speed and to head in the desired direction. They would rather head back to the stables to rest. This aptly demonstrates their stubborn nature and incapacity for anything energetic mentally or physically. They simply lack stamina. Thankfully not all Calc carb horses fit this picture, for within the remedy we see another type. These are the heavy horses that are strong, sturdy, gentle, reliable and patient. These are hard workers and although they move at a slow pace, they have the capacity for perseverance.

Main health issues

Calcium plays an important part in the metabolism, growth and function of the body. Consequently the actions of the remedy are widespread, encompassing muscle tissue, blood, bone and nerve tissue as well as the respiratory system, eyes, spine and skin. It is a key remedy for joint problems heralded by a combination of stiffness, heat and swelling with the presence of exostoses (the formation of new bone) and where the symptoms are worse in damp, wet weather. Calc carb can also help with tying up, muscular stiffness and muscle weakness, chronic sprains and where the back is weak. Where the skin is concerned we see areas that are thickened or cracked. Respiratory symptoms include enlarged lymph nodes under the chin, the production of thick yellow catarrh and a cough that is worse at night.

Key pointers

- Stubbornness, obstinacy
- Inert, sluggish nature
- Lack of response and interest

- Lack of stamina
- Obesity or appears flabby
- Easy or excessive sweating
- Feels the cold
- Clammy feel to the skin
- Thick, yellow catarrh
- General muscular weakness
- Stiff joints which are worse in damp weather

Important indications

- Joint problems
- Arthritis, DJD
- Osteochondrosis, OCD
- Epiphysitis
- To encourage fracture healing
- Pedal osteitis
- Bone spavin
- Bone cysts
- Curb
- Injuries from overexertion
- Muscle atrophy (wasting)
- Slow-growing horn
- Weak back
- Kissing spines, dorsal spinal disease
- Corneal opacity, clouding
- Cataracts
- Guttural pouch tympany
- Guttural pouch mycosis
- Chronic lymph node enlargement
- Ranula
- Infertility in the mare
- Rigs
- Urolithiasis (bladder stones)

- Deep abscesses
- Skin cysts
- Sinuses and fistulae
- Sweet itch
- Mites
- Fleshy warts
- Hypothyroidism

Modalities

Aggravation exertion of any type, cold weather, wet weather, change of weather from warm to cold, cold water, draughts, full moon, after midnight

Amelioration dry, warm weather

Remedy interactions

Works well with: Belladonna (acute), Rhus tox, Lycopodium, Silica, Pulsatilla

Incompatible with: Nitric acid, Nux vomica, Bryonia

Consider also: Baryt carb, Capsicum, Graphites, Kali carb, Phos, Pulsatilla, Rhus tox, Sanicula, Silica

THE GRAPHITES HORSE

Remedy name: Graphites, Graph
Common name: Black lead, Powdered graphite, Plumbago
Classification: Mineral: Carbons: Polycrest
Preparation: Trituration

First impression

Overweight, obese, poor skin and hooves, can look poorly nourished, dull, restless.

Psychological type

On first impression, the Graphites horse can appear like calc carb but there are major differences. The Graphites horse is just plain lazy all round and does not have the perseverance of the Calc personality. Added to this, the Graphites horse is often described simply as being boring, a state that some homeopaths have described as bland. They are dull and lethargic, slow to act and comprehend, slow to work out what is happening and slow to move. They are slow to learn and unable to undertake new tasks; it is as if they are switched off from the outside world. Their capacity for remembering is not good, added to which they do not have the capacity to make decisions easily. This is a remedy which also lacks confidence resulting in anxious behaviour, restlessness, timidity, apprehension, and anticipatory anxiety. This can extend to impatience and irritability at which stage they would rather be left on their own and will stand apart from the other horses in the field. As decidedly chilly individuals, Graphites animals will feel the cold easily and will need more rugs than the average horse to keep warm when the weather is cold.

Main health issues

Many of the problems of the Graphites horse are focused on the skin and hooves. Skin conditions characteristically include dermatitis where the skin is typically cracked, dry, scaly, often itchy and weepy and which may eventually become thickened given time. The secretion is described as clear and honey like and dries into yellowish crusts which matt into the hair making this remedy one of the most important in treating mud fever. Graphites can also help specifically with other forms of dermatitis affecting the bends of the limbs, around the mouth, around the region of the ears and inside the back legs. Thickened scar tissue comes under its sphere of action and may dissipate under its action and infected wounds that are slow to heal can also respond surprisingly well if the remedy is matched to the constitution. Hoof quality is often poor with flaking and cracks often reflecting past episodes of laminitis.

Key pointers

- Obesity
- Laziness
- Sluggish, slow attitude
- Bland, boring character
- Greedy
- Feels the cold
- Characteristic skin lesions, especially those with weepy, honey coloured secretions
- Cracked thickened skin
- Poor hoof quality

Important indications

- Mud fever
- Mange
- Equine nodular skin disease
- Sweet itch

- Rainscald
- Alopecia
- Skin cysts
- Hyperkeratosis
- Excoriation of the skin (soreness)
- Scrotal dermatitis
- Cracked or sore nipples
- Cracks or sores around the mouth or lip margins
- Fissured skin
- Scar tissue
- To reduce or break down adhesions
- Slow healing wounds especially injuries
- Seedy toe
- Brittle hooves
- Grass crack
- Chronic laminitis
- Conjunctivitis with blepharitis
- Fibrotic myopathy
- Poor libido
- CEM
- Hypothyroidism
- Post-viral syndrome

Modalities

Aggravation cold weather, any form of damp, when over-heated, before midnight, during oestrus

Amelioration warm coverings, fresh air, from rest

Remedy interactions

Works well with: Pulsatilla (acute), Causticum, Hepar sulph, Lycopodium, Sulphur

Incompatible with: Nux vom, Arsenicum album, Aconite

Consider also: Ant crud, Arsenicum album, Calc carb, Calc fluor, Ferrum met, Kali bich, Pulsatilla, Sulphur

THE LACHESIS HORSE

Remedy name: Lachesis, Lach
Common name: Venom of the Bushmaster Snake, Surukuku, *Lachesis muta*
Classification: Animal: Reptiles: Snakes: Polycrest
Preparation: Trituration

First impression

Suspicious, wary, untrustworthy, cautious, anxious, unable to relax.

Psychological type

You are immediately aware of the Lachesis mare as soon as you draw near. She has her eye on you. Equally you need to keep your wits about you and keep a careful eye on her. Exercise care and do not venture too close or you may be the recipient of a very swift kick or a bite, that is at least until she knows you. Even then you cannot be too careful! Lachesis is inherently self-conscious, emotionally charged, suspicious, watchful, wary and misses nothing. She watches carefully. Her eyes are wide open, her gaze intense (staring even) and almost piercing at times. She blinks infrequently.

Possessive by nature and protective of her offspring she can become defensive if her foal is approached. She is jealous, can be mean and spiteful and harbours pent up feelings, all emotions that are released or vented in the form of aggression. She dislikes being touched, especially around the neck and abdomen, finds ill-fitting tack especially uncomfortable and is a noisy (talkative) animal in general. These are all behavioural traits that are intensified in the pre-oestrus period and which diminish once in season. Added to this she is quarrelsome and a problem when kept with other mares, which she is apt to injure by kicking out frequently.

Main health issues

A great many problems centre on behavioural issues such as jealousy and on problems associated with the oestrus cycle. Lachesis is a remedy for the type of aggressive behaviour that is exhibited in the 6 or 7 days prior to oestrus and which manifests as biting and kicking as well as territorial based aggression. It is also a remedy for left-sided ovarian cysts and left-sided ovarian pain. The other main sphere of action is on the blood, linking with the action of the snake's venom on the body following a bite. The venom contains a wide range of enzymes and is an anticoagulant, as well as causing destruction of red blood cells and lowering resistance to infection. Hence the use of the remedy in treating haemorrhages and persistent bleeding, haematomas, deep bruising, septic wounds (especially where the skin takes on a purple colour), other infections (such as cellulitis) and gangrene. Lachesis has a special focus of action on the throat and on the left side of the body.

Key pointers

- Quarrelsome and suspicious nature
- Foxy nature
- Biting and kicking
- Territorial aggression
- Jealousy
- Vengeful
- Highly charged, especially sexually
- Dislike of being touched around the head, neck or abdomen
- History of mareish behaviour, nymphomania
- Left-sided laterality or where symptoms progress from left to right
- Symptoms worse after sleep
- Better for appearance of discharge

Important indications

- Left-sided ovarian pain
- Ovarian cysts, cystic ovaries
- Back pain associated with ovarian dysfunction especially if left-sided
- Sepsis where the skin or wound has a purple hue
- Severe post-operative bleeding
- Bleeding skin wounds where there is dark blood
- Haemorrhage where the blood is dark and fails to clot
- Intraocular haemorrhage
- Recurrent or persistent haematomas
- Iliac thrombosis
- Purpura haemorrhagica
- Cellulitis
- Abscesses
- Infected tooth sockets
- Gangrene
- Snake bites
- Septicaemia or toxaemia
- Lymphangitis

- Myositis
- Quittor
- Severe parotitis
- Pharyngitis
- Laryngeal hemiplegia
- Failure to accept the stallion
- Variocele
- Mismothering
- Mastitis
- Strangles
- Post-viral syndrome

Modalities

Aggravation after sleep (in the morning), on left side, heat of sun, cloudy, oppressive weather, from getting wet, prior to oestrus, tight fitting tack

Amelioration fresh air, onset of oestrus, from exercise

Remedy interactions

Works well with: Hepar sulph, Iodum, Kali bich, Lycopodium, Nitric acid

Incompatible with: Acetic acid, Bufo, Rhus tox

Consider also: Allium cepa, Causticum, Cimicifugia, Croton tig, Hyoscyamus, Lac caninum, Zinc

THE LYCOPODIUM HORSE

Remedy name: Lycopodium, Lycop
Common name: Club moss, also known as Wolf's foot, *Lycopodium clavatum*
Classification: Plant: Ferns: Lycopodiaceae family: Polycrest
Preparation: From a tincture of the spores or whole plant

First impression

Lean (sometimes the ribs are visible), possibly poor muscling to the head and neck and front leg region in comparison to hind quarters, athletic, spare, occasionally emaciated, can be physically weak. Cautious and apprehensive nature. May show aggression in certain situations, especially if cornered.

Psychological type

The Lycopodium horse is highly intelligent and a conscientious performer but underlying this is a lack of confidence that shows as pre-performance nerves, a characteristic trait of the remedy. Despite this they always perform well and are often exceptional performers. There is a general air of uncertainty and apprehension about them, especially in new situations, be that a change of stables, a new route for a ride or a new owner. In fact Lycopodium horses dislike change of any type and rather like an ordered routine, much more so than other horses. They are always better in a group as they feel less vulnerable and will often form a strong bond with one single animal or human. They can become anxious if devoid of human or equine company, they dislike being alone and like to have another animal or human around even if not in close proximity. However, they do not openly welcome strangers and only warm to people once they have known them a while. Outwardly they can appear very submissive and passive but the lack of confidence can show as cowardly behaviour and, if cornered without an escape route, may resort to aggression that may be explosive. Here, there are traits of the less gentle side of Lycopodium, the side that may harbour resentment from ill treatment or from an unpleasant event, and often expressed as malicious and irritable behaviour initiated frequently by very minor problems. They dislike responsibility and will avoid being leader of the pack, as they feel vulnerable in such situations. Prone to boredom, they like to be occupied and may develop stable vices if stressed.

Main health issues

In horses problems are often centred on the digestive system or the liver and very rarely, the urinary system. Appetite can be very variable. Often very greedy horses, they can be picky from time to time. Prone to digestive upsets there is a tendency for loose dung (especially if anxious) and to be gassy or flatulent or even develop colic. Lycopodium is a key remedy for liver disease or liver dysfunction. Many health problems seen with this remedy have a root in the psychological or stress problems which abound. Lack of confidence, obscure fears, spooky behaviour and anticipatory anxiety are prime examples leading to problems such as chronic low-grade colic, stomach ulcers or stereotypic behaviour such as crib biting or wind sucking.

Key pointers

- Highly intelligent but lacks confidence
- Anxious before an event but performs well
- Uneasy with strangers
- Very close bond with another animal or human
- Dislikes being cornered or trapped
- History of digestive problems especially chronic low-grade colic
- Depraved appetite
- Quivering (flapping) like motion of nostrils
- Seborrhoeic (greasy) skin

- Sweats easily
- Headshaking episodes
- History of liver complaints or disease such as hepatitis
- Chilly (feels the cold easily) but feels the heat as well, hates stuffy areas
- Right-sided laterality to symptoms or symptoms proceed from right to left
- Symptoms worse between 4pm and 8pm

Important indications

- Anticipatory anxiety
- Stress related illness
- Lack of confidence
- Some forms of stereotypic behaviour such as crib biting
- Horses difficult to load into horseboxes
- Picky feeders
- Headshaking
- Acute laminitis due to over feeding
- Shivers
- Flatulent colic
- Scabby eczema along the margins of the ears
- Seborrhoeic dermatitis
- Alopecia
- Dandruff
- Mange
- Small, smooth nodular warts
- Sarcoids (smooth and pigmented)
- Melanoma
- Sinusitis
- Neglected pneumonia
- COPD, ROA
- Chronic liver disease
- Oedema due to liver disease or nutritional problems
- Hyperlipaemia
- Haemolytic anaemia

- Stomach ulcers, gastric ulceration
- Chronic peritonitis
- Iliac thrombosis
- Aneurysm
- Urolithiasis, urinary sediment
- Infertility in mares
- CEM
- Variocele
- Poor libido
- Diabetes mellitus

Modalities

Aggravation between 4pm and 8pm, stuffy atmosphere (stables, horseboxes), overexertion, from worry, when idle, right side, right side to left

Amelioration through active movement, removing (or loosening) rugs or other clothing, being occupied

Remedy interactions

Works well with: Natrum phos, Belladonna, Bryonia, Calc carb, Graphites, Lachesis, Phosphorus, Pulsatilla, Sepia, Silica, Iodum, Chelidonium

Incompatible with: Coffea

Consider also: Arg nit, Carbo veg, Chelidonium, Mag mur, Medorrhinum, Sulphur, Thuja, Silica

THE NAT MUR HORSE

Remedy name: Natrum muriaticum, Nat mur
Common name: Sodium chloride, Common salt
Classification: Mineral: Natrums: Polycrest
Preparation: Trituration

First impression

Sad, withdrawn, not happy, stands apart from other horses, lean, can look poorly nourished, scrawny.

Psychological type

The Nat mur horse just looks sad and depressed, rejected even, and demonstrates this trait by simply standing apart from the other animals. They would rather be left on their own and will resist attempts to console and comfort them. In contrast to many other remedies they dislike fuss, cuddles and attention in general. The dull moods, however, can swing in the other direction as shown by behaviour that could be described as excitable from time to time. Strangely though, despite the desire to be left alone, they dislike being ignored completely. There is sensitivity to noise, especially sudden noises, which results in jumpy behaviour, there is a fear of closed-in areas and a tendency to harbour resentment over past problems. They will not forget or forgive the rider who treats them badly. Emotions are often hidden though, and not observed easily; they are in effect, controlled and suppressed. Grief from the loss of a companion, for example, is not expressed and can have consequent effects on health. This seemingly human trait is surprisingly just as much as a problem in horses and needs careful prising from the history.

Main health issues

The health concerns of the Nat mur type horse are closely related to the remedy in life. It comes as no surprise that they are thirsty animals and pass urine frequently. In addition they are hungry and greedy and yet hardly ever gain condition. It was as if their metabolism was working overtime and burning calories at twice the normal rate. In later life this trait is enhanced with gradual weight loss and loss of condition.

Skin problems are common with excessive secretion of grease and oil together with areas of hair loss (alopecia) where it has fallen out. The opposite can also be true with dry patches of skin, lacklustre hair with dandruff like scales. Itching where present tends to derive from red urticarial blotches that are often close to the joints or underside of the body. Hooves are often poor with cracks and flaking. There is a need to be rugged as they feel the cold easily. Respiratory infections are accompanied by discharges that are watery and profuse often like egg white. Coughed-up mucus is always clear. As salt has a relation to fluid retention a frequent finding in horses of this constitution, is filling of the legs. Their dung tends to be dry compared with other horses.

Key pointers

- Depressed, sad appearance
- Stands alone
- Avoids affection
- Sensitivity to sudden noises
- Dislike of closed-in areas
- Thirsty for large amounts
- Good, even excessive appetite but never puts on weight
- Watery eyes and clear nasal discharge
- Excessively greasy, oily skin or dry scaly coat and hair

- Poor hoof quality with flaking
- Filled legs
- Worse between 9am and 11am

Important indications

- Silent or chronic grief and illness arising from this
- Sadness
- Anxiety in irritable animals
- Cataracts
- Blockage of the nasolachrymal duct
- Fly worry
- Headshaking
- Rhinitis with a watery nasal discharge
- Equine flu
- Equine viral arteritis
- Rhinovirus infection
- Adenovirus infection
- Horse pox virus
- Vesicular stomatitis virus
- Post-viral syndrome, equine ME
- Sores and cracks around the mouth
- Bacterial folliculitis
- Infertility in the mare
- Coital exanthema
- CEM
- Chronic renal (kidney) failure
- Excessive panting
- Dry, cracked or flaky hooves
- Alopecia, hair loss, bald patches
- Dandruff
- Seborrhoea
- Emaciation, even with a good appetite

Modalities

Aggravation hot weather, heat in general, stuffy warm stables, noise, by the seaside, for consolation, from exertion, between 9am and 11am

Amelioration in the open air, gentle exercise, from sweating, rest, back being massaged

Remedy interactions

Works well with: Bryonia (acute), Apis, Sepia, Ignatia (Nat mur is the chronic of Ignatia)

Incompatible with: Arsenicum album, Phosphorus, Argentum nitricum

Consider also: Aurum, Ignatia, Natrum carb, Natrum sulph, Pulsatilla, Sepia, Staphysagria

THE NUX VOMICA HORSE

Remedy name: Nux vomica, Nux vom
Common name: Poison nut, *Strychnos nux vomica*
Classification: Plant: Loganiaceae family: Polycrest
Preparation: From tincture and trituration of the seeds

First impression

Lean or normal appearance, tense, alert, sharp, overly sensitive, brisk, fiery.

Psychological type

The Nux vomica horse is invariably male and often suits horses that are put under pressure to perform. Having said this, he is a good performer, precise in his actions, competitive and hard worker but with this there is an underlying tense, irritable, anxious, impatient and short-tempered animal who is often very fired-up and ready to go. If the energy is not vented the frustration is taken out on those around, rider, groom or vet, with a swift kick or bite. He is not sorry and will show no remorse for his actions. Great sensitivity is a key feature, reacting to noise, pain, touch, bright lights and other animals, which he may find irritating and kick out at in a malicious way. Usually greedy they tend to feed frequently but take small amounts each time rather than eating a huge amount in one single go.

Main health issues

Many of the problems resolved with Nux vomica are centred on the digestive system especially various forms of colic, gastric ulcers and a variety of other conditions brought about by over eating, feeding the wrong type of feed or by stress. It is a key remedy for treating liver conditions of any type especially where poisoning is suspected. Nux is considered a good detoxification remedy generally, as well as a good tonic remedy for the digestion where it is upset. There is an action on the muscles relating to cramping, unsteadiness in the gait and lower back pain. Nux is a remedy for the effects of overwork, pressure and cumulative stress. It often works best if given later in the day.

Key pointers

- Irritability
- Short-tempered and impatient
- Fiery nature
- The effects of overwork
- Prone to irregularities of the digestive system including sluggish digestion
- History of spasmodic colic
- History of impacted colic
- Liver problems
- Spasms

Important indications

- Irritable, grumpy nature especially in older horses
- Spasmodic or impacted colic
- Flatulent colic
- Gastric ulceration
- Diarrhoea from dietary causes or changes in feeding
- Slimy diarrhoea with straining
- Constipation with straining
- Meconium retention in the foal
- Acute laminitis originating from dietary problems or toxaemia
- Bowel stasis including post-operatively
- Poisoning (to provide liver support)
- Liver disease including jaundice
- To detoxify the effects of anaesthesia
- Tying up, azoturia-prevention
- Spasm of the lumbar muscles
- Back pain where the horse is irritable
- Cauda equina neuritis

- Paralysis of the bladder
- Wobbler syndrome
- Weakness or partial paralysis of the hindlimbs
- Facial paralysis
- EHV-1 (neurological signs)
- Equine protozoal myeloencephalitis
- Tetanus
- Fever with irritability
- Rhinitis
- Dry cough
- COPD, RAO

Modalities

Aggravation cold air and draughts, early in the morning, if sleep disturbed, after feeding

Amelioration after sleep, in the evening, at rest, from damp, wet weather

Remedy interactions

Works well with: Sulphur, Sepia, Pulsatilla

Incompatible with: Zinc

Consider also: Aurum, Carcinosin, Chamomilla, Ignatia, Lillium tig, Lycopodium, Medorrhinum, Sepia, Strychnine, Sulphur

THE PHOSPHORUS HORSE

Remedy name: Phosphorus, Phos
Common name: Phosphorus
Classification: Mineral: Element: Phosphorus: Polycrest
Preparation: Trituration of red phosphorus

First impression

Slender, athletic, intelligent, nervy, playful, bright eyed, thin skinned.

Psychological type

In contrast to some of the other remedies, Sulphur and Graphites for example, Phosphorus horses are active (even to the extent of being overactive), playful, excitable, bright, fun loving, intelligent but often seem a little anxious or nervous underneath all this. They are very sensitive animals in more ways than one.

There is sensitivity to noises, bright lights, bright colours, touch, effects of the weather, a tendency to start at unfamiliar objects, to be anxious in confined areas and to become excited or apprehensive around crowds, at events and at shows. There is a great desire for affection (which they will actively seek – they love to be groomed and stroked) and for company both human and equine, in fact they hate being alone. However, there is another side to this remedy that may express itself as a sudden outburst akin to a 'temper tantrum' after which they seem sorry. Enthusiasm is abundant for all they undertake, but this can wear off after a while, a trait shared with Tuberculinum, but in the case of Phosphorus it is exhaustion that curtails their intentions. When at a low ebb there is an apparent feeling of indifference and apathy until the energy is rekindled. Phosphorus animals are nearly always thirsty, feel the cold easily, sweat easily when exercised and seek out the benefits of mineral licks more than other animals.

Main health issues

Phosphorus has affinities with bone, nerve tissue, the respiratory tract, mucous membranes, the eyes, liver and the blood so it is in these areas we see the problems that the remedy can address. Where bone is concerned, the remedy can help with conditions arising in young horses where the rate of growth has been too rapid and in older animals where there is evidence of bone weakness, osteomyelitis, exostoses and back pain where the spine is weak. The limbs, particularly the hind limbs may show weakness or paralysis due to nerve degeneration. Phosphorus is a key respiratory remedy helpful where there is a dry, racking cough, pneumonia, yellow-green catarrh or pulmonary-induced haemorrhage (EIPH). Haemorrhage from other areas can also be a problem, with even small skin wounds bleeding excessively. The blood clots slowly and is bright red and watery in character. Not surprisingly the remedy can help with anaemia. Liver problems can also benefit from this remedy where there is liver damage, hepatitis, enlargement, degeneration or jaundice. Digestive symptoms include stomach ulcers and chronic diarrhoea, which can be debilitating and appears to pour out with little discomfort. Cases of diabetes can also benefit.

Key pointers

- Sensitivity both physical and mental
- Excitability particularly due to nervous tension
- Nervy, jumpy or apprehensive before events
- Intelligent, playful
- Jumpy with sudden noises
- Need for affection, friendly, agitated by thunder
- Fine-boned, long-legged, lean, athletic appearance
- Thirsty
- Likes taking short sleeps
- History of EIPH

Important indications

- Excitability
- Great sensitivity generally, 'flighty or easily spooked animals'
- Excitability before an event
- Dry cough, pneumonia, bronchopneumonia
- Respiratory infections where symptoms agree
- Haemorrhage of bright red watery blood
- EIPH, epistaxis (nosebleed)
- Retinal haemorrhage
- Purpura haemorrhagica
- Recurrent haematomas
- Small but persistently bleeding skin wounds
- Petechial haemorrhages
- To limit bleeding after tooth extraction
- Haematuria (blood in the urine)
- Anaemia
- Jaundice, acute hepatitis, chronic liver damage/disease
- Poisoning (liver support)
- Chronic painless diarrhoea
- Diabetes mellitus
- Stomach ulcers
- Hyperlipaemia
- Chronic renal (kidney) failure
- Cataracts
- Moon blindness (chronic cases)
- Vaginal bleeding between oestrus periods
- Mismothering – rejection of the foal
- False rigs
- Osteochondrosis (OCD)
- Osteomyelitis
- Periostitis
- Nerve degeneration

- Muscle wasting/atrophy
- Neuritis
- Paralysis or partial paralysis
- Cauda equina neuritis
- EHV-1 neurological symptoms
- Equine protozoal myeloencephalitis
- Equine infectious anaemia (EIA), respiratory and cardiac forms
- Equine viral arteritis (EVA)
- Babesiasis
- Tyzzer's disease

Modalities

Aggravation cold, before and during a thunderstorm, change of weather, twilight, emotional strain, mental exertion, touch

Amelioration warmth, eating, after rest and sleep, for rubbing or massage, open air

Remedy interactions

Works well with: Arsenicum album, Lycopodium, Silica, Tuberculinum, Carbo veg, Rhus tox

Incompatible with: Causticum

THE PULSATILLA HORSE

Remedy name: Pulsatilla, Puls
Common name: Wind flower, Pasque flower, *Pulsatilla pratensis*
Classification: Plant: Ranunculaceae family: Polycrest
Preparation: From tincture of the whole fresh plant in flower

First impression

Placid, friendly, laid back, affectionate, light-coloured coat, tendency to be obese.

Psychological type

Pulsatilla types are usually sweet natured, gentle, sociable mares but this rule is not hard and fast. A fair number of geldings also have a Pulsatilla constitution. Pulsatilla is often the riding school pony, the popular easy-going mare that everyone loves to ride. They have a cuddly, warm, loving and affectionate nature with a great desire for physical contact and attention; they dislike solitude. There is a motherly feel about them and indeed make excellent mothers. Their sensitive nature is easily hurt and if scolded, their submissive nature shows through. There is practically never ever any aggressive behaviour; it is just not in their nature. Behind this is an individual who is shy, a little coy even, and who takes a few moments to warm to strangers. However, there is another side to the Pulsatilla horse reflecting the fundamental basic changeable, emotional nature of the remedy. This is the side that can show jealousy (but not normally in a malicious way) and irritability; they can be a little touchy from time to time.

Pulsatilla males show many similar traits particularly the lack of aggression and the gentle calm, shy, changeable nature. They are apt to be a little on the excitable side occasionally.

Main health issues

Many of the problems amenable to Pulsatilla are related to the female reproductive system-irregular oestrus cycles, uterine discharges and conditions related to pregnancy and foaling. The typical uterine discharge from a Pulsatilla patient is creamy, yellowish and bland. The same characteristic type of discharge is seen from prepuce (in the male), from the nose in cases of rhinitis and sinusitis and from the eye where conjunctivitis is a problem. Pulsatilla also has affinities with the digestive system (where it can help with flatulent colic and some forms of diarrhoea) and the joints where lameness problems appear to shift from leg to leg.

Key pointers

- General nature, kind, gentle, affectionate, friendly
- Symptoms that change or that shift from side to side or from leg to leg
- Little thirst
- Good appetite
- Bland, creamy discharges
- Prefers to be out in the fresh air
- Dislike of stuffy, airless areas

Important indications

- Catarrhal conjunctivitis with a thick bland yellow discharge
- Rhinitis with a creamy nasal discharge
- Sinusitis
- Guttural pouch empyema or tympany
- Dry cough or rattling mucous type cough with yellow bland expectoration
- Respiratory infections

- COPD, ROA
- Flatulent colic especially from rich feed or over-eating
- Diarrhoea from over-eating
- Parotiditis
- Irregular oestrus cycles and other reproductive disorders
- Infertility in the mare
- Endometritis
- Pyometria
- Prevention of abortion
- Uterine inertia (absence of contractions)
- Retained placenta
- Mareish behaviour
- Orchitis
- Spermatorrhoea (lack of sperm)
- Variocele
- Hydrocele
- Acute cystitis
- Arthritis or DJD especially with shifting lameness
- Strangles
- CEM
- Epizootic lymphangitis
- Grief or pining

Modalities

Aggravation heat, high humidity, over rugging, in the evening

Amelioration in the open air, gentle movement, pressure or lying on painful area

Remedy interactions

Works well with: Graphites, Nux vomica, Silica (chronic), Lycopodium, Argentum nitricum

Incompatible with: Nux moschata

Consider also: Argentum nit, Cimicifugia, Cyclamen, Graphites, Hamamelis, Kali bich, Kali sulph, Merc sol, Natrum sulph, Nux moschata, Phosphorus, Sulphur

THE SEPIA HORSE

Remedy name: Sepia
Common name: Ink from the cuttlefish, *Sepia officinalis*
Classification: Animal: Molluscs: Polycrest
Preparation: Trituration of the ink

First impression

Sad, worn out, overweight and depressed, miserable, dejected.

Psychological profile

Often more suited to mares, the typical Sepia horse has had a hard life that has taken its toll over the years both physically and mentally. Once bright, alert and active, she now appears sad, saggy, sluggish and depressed. This sorry state is partly due to the passage of time and overwork but has been added to in some cases by a modicum of neglect here and there. Everything appears to be a drag and requires effort but surprisingly, once out on a ride the Sepia horse brightens up and actually quite enjoys it. She can be roused out of her depressed miserable state of mind; inherently the Sepia horse is not lazy, just worn out and exhausted. Indifference and apathy is a feature of her personality, especially to those she is closest to. This can be to her own foal, which she may even reject, and to her owner, whom she may shun. She may even resent close affection, becoming irritable, short-tempered and touchy, and would rather be left alone, apart from people and other horses. Strangely, though, they hate being completely alone. Apt to bear grievances they may not forget a past event involving a particular person or animal, which they will not forget in a hurry. Sepia is sometimes referred to as the 'female' Nux vomica.

The dark introverted moods of Sepia mirror the dark black ink of the cuttlefish (which it uses in covering its getaway). The soft body of the cuttlefish resembles the body of the Sepia mare where every thing sags and lacks tone; her back sags as the ligaments have slackened, her muscles are soft and flabby and lack tone and her udder and reproductive organs stretched through the several foals which she has had. Nevertheless the Sepia horse will carry on in a determined fashion, especially if motivated. This is aptly signified by the hard bony core that gives form and support to the body of the cuttlefish.

Main health issues

Many of the conditions associated with Sepia are linked with the female reproductive system and the endocrine system particularly with the oestrus cycle, fertility, pregnancy, foaling and the period following this. It is also a remedy for skin problems including allergy related conditions, seborrhoea and ringworm.

Key pointers

- Worn-out appearance, saggy, sunken
- Sluggish, slow and depressed

- Irregular or lack of oestrus cycles

Important indications

- Mismothering or rejection of offspring
- Mareish behaviour
- Endometritis
- Pyometria
- Prevention of abortion
- Retained placenta
- CEM
- Uterine prolapse
- Spermatorrhoea
- Warts on the tip of the penis
- Seborrhoeic dermatitis, allergies and urticaria
- Alopecia
- Dandruff, scaling
- Ringworm
- Bacterial folliculitis
- Hyperkeratosis
- Vitiligo
- Distorted hooves
- Hypothyroidism
- Lower back pain
- Post-viral syndrome

Modalities

Aggravation damp weather, cold air, before a thunderstorm, dull cloudy weather, in the period before oestrus

Amelioration exercise and stimulation, warmth, after rest, eating

Remedy interactions

Works well with: Nat mur, Phosphorus, Nux vomica, Guaiacum, Sabadilla

Incompatible with: Lachesis, Bryonia

Consider also: Carbo veg, Carcinosin, Causticum, Gelsemium, Ignatia, Lillium tig, Murex, Natrum mur, Nitric acid, Nux vomica, Petroleum, Phos ac, Pulsatilla, Thuja

THE SILICA (SILICEA) HORSE

Remedy name: Silica, Sil
Common name: Silicon dioxide, Pure flint
Classification: mineral: Silicas: Polycrest
Preparation: Trituration of pure precipitated silica

Caution: Silica is a powerful remedy, capable of empowering the body to expel foreign material. As such, it may cause the expulsion of metal screws, wires, plates or other orthopaedic implants, as well as microchips. If in any doubt, seek professional guidance.

First impression

Poor physical structure, poor constitution, weak, quiet, boring.

Psychological type

The Silica horse has many problems, most arising through fundamental inbuilt weaknesses both physical and mental. Although intelligent they are shy and lack confidence. This expresses itself as an apparent lack of inertia, a lack of go, of response, of initiative and determination. They are jumpy with sudden noises, sensitive, sometimes fearful, can appear restless and agitated (especially in unfamiliar situations), and occasionally irritated, leading to misbehaviour if pushed too far. Eventually if over worked or over taxed, the intrinsic weaknesses surface. Psychologically the Silica horse will become quiet, inert, withdrawn, disinterested and depressed. What we see outwardly is a lack of vitality.

Main health issues

Physical problems are abundant and have roots that fundamentally lie in a weak basic structure. Silica is a constituent of connective tissue and some of the other tissues that comprise the basic building blocks and structures of the body – bone, cartilage, tendons, ligaments, skin, hair and hooves as well as blood and blood vessels. It is not surprising that the Silica horse looks poor and often appears thin (even to the point of looking malnourished), feels the cold easily, has a weak immune system, may have swollen glands and lacks stamina. The hooves are often weak, cracked and flaky. There is a tendency to abscesses in the feet, wounds are slow to heal and may become chronic even to the extent that a sinus or fistula may develop. The coat and skin can look poor; a reflection of the poor assimilation of food. Where bone and cartilage are involved, arthritis is a feature with the development of exostoses. Silica has a good reputation in driving foreign material out of the body (such as thorns), in ripening abscesses, in helping to dissolve away scar tissue, in delaying cataracts, in healing eye ulcers and in treating some of the side effects of vaccination.

Key pointers

- Looks poor with a weak constitution
- Lacks drive, determination and confidence
- Poor stamina level, tires easily
- Chilly, needs to be rugged up
- History of problems related to connective tissue such as tendon and ligament injuries, arthritis
- Bone degeneration
- Weak joints
- Poor weak hooves
- Poor skin
- Weakened immune system
- Enlarged lymph nodes, lymphadenitis

Important indications

- Abscesses, fistulae, sinusus and other chronic infections
- Slow healing or infected wounds (where there is little or no pain)
- Scar tissue, prevention and dissolution
- Strictures
- Expulsion of foreign bodies, foreign material
- Illnesses arising after vaccination, vaccinosis
- Guttural pouch empyema or mycosis
- Sinusitis
- Parotitis
- COPD, RAO
- Tooth abscess
- Chronic eye ulcers
- Corneal scarring or opacity
- Cataracts
- Blockage of the nasolachrymal duct
- Osteomyelitis
- Periostitis
- Exostoses

- To encourage fracture healing
- Chronic ligament injuries or sprains
- Splints
- Curb (where there is scar tissue)
- Sidebone
- Pedal osteitis
- Buttress foot
- Quittor
- White line disease
- Thrush
- Gravel
- Seedy toe
- Canker
- Chronic laminitis
- Grass crack, sand crack
- Fibrotic myopathy
- Bacterial folliculitis
- Equine nodular skin disease
- Fibroblastic sarcoids
- Skin ulcers
- Alopecia
- Slow resolving haematoma
- Strangles
- Epizootic lymphangitis
- Post-viral syndrome, equine ME
- Anaemia arising from nutritional causes
- To encourage repair of the bowel lining where damaged
- Chronic pyelonephritis
- Endometritis
- Chronic mastitis
- Spermatorrhoea
- Hydrocele

Modalities

Aggravation cold air, cold weather, dampness, full moon, morning, during oestrus

Amelioration warmth, in the summer, for covering up, for rest

Remedy interactions

Works well with: Fluoric acid, Calc carb, Pulsatilla (Silica is the chronic of Pulsatilla), Thuja, Nat mur

Incompatible with: Merc sol

Consider also: Calc carb, Camphora, Carb an, Fluoricum acidum, Hepar sulph, Kali carb, Merc sol, Natrum carb, Nitric acid, Pulsatilla, Sanicula, Staphysagria, Sulphur

THE SULPHUR HORSE

Remedy name: Sulphur, Sulph
Common name: Sulphur, the element, Sublimated sulphur
Classification: Mineral: Sulphurs: Element: Polycrest
Preparation: Trituration of flowers of sulphur

First impression
Untidy, grubby with poor, unhealthy looking coat and skin, lazy.

Psychological type
The Sulphur horse is usually easy to spot. This is an untidy peevish animal, whose coat and skin look poorly groomed, whose hair is matted in places and caked with mud and dirt. This however, is not only in part due to the constitution, but also as much on the part of the owner, who is quite likely to be of the Sulphur type as well. The general feeling is one of laziness. Sulphur is a slouch and dislikes hard work; indeed there is a lack of perseverance in anything they are asked to undertake. Sulphur leans on the stable wall as he can't be bothered to support himself and would just like to take a nap. If he were human he would sit down at every opportunity. Underlying characteristics are of selfishness, a tendency to sulk, a lack of concern for others, a poor memory, a short temper, irritability and some say a tendency to 'grumble'. There is a dislike of heat, of getting wet and of being washed and groomed. Greed is a problem, which often means that horses of this type are fat and overweight although some Sulphur type horses are lean and long-legged individuals. Sulphur tends to be thirsty.

Main health issues
Sulphur is a remedy of great importance whose main seat of action is on the skin. A wide range of symptoms are covered, including itching and rubbing (often to excess), dry, lustreless hair, scaling and scabs, sores and crusting and a filthy,

dirty, smelly coat and skin. Where the skin exudes a discharge it irritates the surrounding area and makes the skin sore. Often the skin feels hot, almost burning to touch and, if it were possible to see, it would look red and inflamed especially around the eyes, lips, nose, genital areas and bottom. Rugs only make any problems worse as the heat is trapped in. Clipping is resented and grooming results in the loss of great masses of dead hair. Healing can be slow, with wounds taking longer to resolve compared with the average horse with infection becoming a chronic problem in some cases. Sulphur extends its action to the other areas of the body. Respiratory symptoms include foul-smelling mucus from the nose, coughing up of greenish mucus, allergy based problems and pneumonia. Where the legs and back are concerned, the back muscles can be weak and the gait stiff, slovenly and laboured. Heat tends to aggravate the symptoms but cold can also cause problems as this slows the circulation.

Sulphur is a chief anti-psoric remedy (see page 16) and is often referred to as having a centrifugal action, working from the inside out. Able to shift toxins from deep in the body, Sulphur will bring these to the surface. It is often a good remedy to commence with before moving onto other remedies or where there is no clearly indicated medicine. It can also be used as an intercurrent remedy to aid the actions of other remedies.

Key pointers

- General appearance
- Slovenly, lazy attitude
- Untidy coat and skin
- Unhealthy skin
- History of skin problems especially where itching, rubbing, heat and burning are a feature
- Bad odour from the coat
- Dislike of getting wet
- Intolerance of heat
- Greedy and thirsty

Important indications

- Skin conditions in general, often a good remedy to start a case with to 'clear' the way for other remedies
- Illness arising after vaccination
- Sweet itch
- Excoriated skin
- Allergic based skin problems

- Seborrhoea or greasy skin
- Dandruff, scaling
- Hyperkeratosis
- Mud fever
- Bacterial skin infections
- Dirty dingy looking skin and coat, poor hair
- Lice
- Mange
- Thrush
- Headshaking
- COPD, RAO
- Chronic diarrhoea
- Intermittent mild impacted colic
- Smegma
- Dourine
- Post-viral syndrome

Modalities

Aggravation heat, sunshine, having a rug on, cold, damp weather, water, washing, standing around, at rest, 11am, early afternoon, during oestrus

Amelioration dry weather if not too hot, motion, eating

Remedy interactions

Works well with: Aconite, Arsenicum album, Aloe, Nux vomica, Psorinum, Calc carb, Calc phos, Pulsatilla, Belladonna

Incompatible with: none listed

Consider also: Aloe, Ant crud, Argentum nit, Graphites, Lycopodium, Medorrhinum, Mezerium, Nux vomica, Platina, Psorinum, Pulsatilla, Selenium, Symphytum

THE TUBERCULINUM HORSE

Remedy name: Tuberculinum, Tub
Common name: Tubercle bacilli from infected cattle lymph node – Tuberculinum bovinum
Tubercle bacilli from chicken liver or birds – Tuberculinum aviare

Tubercle bacilli from a tubercular abscess – Tuberculinum kock
Classification: Animal: Mammal: Human: Nosode
Preparation: From a glycerine extract of tubercle bacilli

First impression

Narrow-chested, lean, sometimes emaciated or weak if neglected, often light coloured horses, impatient.

Psychological type

The Tuberculinum horse is well known for its obstinate and stubborn nature. Often headstrong and disobedient they are often difficult to control when younger and want to do what they want to do rather than you. Sometimes the behaviour has malicious overtones, even to the point of being destructive or nipping. The general stubborn behaviour is combined with a degree of irritability and impatience often seen as stamping or pawing the ground as if they just want to get on with things. Keen as they are, however, to be first out on the ride and to be leader of the pack, the enthusiasm rapidly wanes as they become bored and fall to the back of the group. Boredom is a typical Tuberculinum trait. They are bored with everyday life and always want something new to do and never seem really content with life. Keen as they are to undertake new things and to go to events, they often are reluctant to travel (that is to say difficult to load) as they hate the stuffy confinement of the horsebox. In the later stages of life they are apt to become dull and a little depressed with a tendency to be lazy with an aversion to work.

Main health issues

Symptoms of ill health are often changeable and can vary from day to day. Weak areas, not surprisingly, are the chest and respiratory system in general as evidenced by slow recovery from respiratory viruses and a tendency to develop coughs and allergy based breathing problems. There are also problems with the immune system as suggested by slow recovery from illness, enlarged lymph nodes (especially those under the jaw) and a tendency to recurrent or stubborn infections. The skin can also present problems, mainly that of severe sweet itch, as can the joints which present with problems such as a wandering or variable lameness which moves around from leg to leg or joint to joint.

Key pointers

- Lean despite eating exceptionally well
- History of COPD and other allergy based respiratory problems
- Chronically enlarged lymph nodes
- Slow recovery from any illness, especially respiratory problems
- Inconsistent and variable or changing symptoms
- Likes to be warm but would rather prefer to be outdoors

- Tires easily
- Lazy, averse to working

Important indications

- Severe sweet itch
- Respiratory conditions, especially unresponsive cases
- Persistent dry coughs
- Bronchopneumonia with much mucus
- COPD, RAO
- Headshaking (where there is pain)
- Teeth grinding
- Post-viral syndrome, equine ME
- Epizootic lymphangitis
- Chronic diarrhoea with weight loss

Modalities

Aggravation for movement, before a storm, damp weather, early morning

Amelioration from being in the open air

Remedy interactions

Works well with: Psorinum, Sulphur, Belladonna, Calc carb, Phosphorus, Hydrastis, Thuja, Pulsatilla

Incompatible with: none listed

Consider also: Bacillinum, Calc phos, Carcinosin, Medorrhinum, Platina, Rhus tox, Sanicicula, Veratrum album

Basic Information – Vital Signs

Here is a quick-reference guide to help you decide if your horse is ill or not by checking vital signs such as temperature, pulse and respiration. If there is any doubt whatsoever that your horse may be ill, seek professional help.

Temperature

Temperature is normally taken per rectum using either a mercury-filled glass thermometer or a digital thermometer. If you are using a glass thermometer ensure that it is shaken down fully before use. Lubricate the thermometer with a little Vaseline first, then insert it into the rectum, carefully making sure that it does not become embedded in faeces and that it is in contact with the rectal wall. Take a reading after one to two minutes (depending on the type of thermometer), repeating the process if you are in any doubt.

Normal average resting temperature for an adult horse is **38 °C (100.4 °F)** although a range of **37.2–38.3 °C (99–101 °F)** is accepted as being within normal limits, depending on environmental factors and effects of exercise, excitement and stress. If your horse's temperature is over **38.8 °C (102 °F)** it would be wise to seek veterinary help.

Respiratory Rate

The respiratory rate can be measured by watching your horse breath and observing the movements of the ribs. Count one inhalation and one exhalation as one breath. Measure the number of breaths over a 30 second period and multiply the result by two.

The rate at which your horse breathes is influenced by exercise, environmental conditions (especially humidity and temperature) as well as pain (such as colic episodes) and illness (for example COPD or respiratory infections). The respiratory rate should never exceed the pulse rate. Rapid or laboured breathing warrants prompt veterinary attention. The normal average rate for healthy adult horse at rest is **between 8 and 15 breaths per minute**.

Pulse Rate

Take the pulse by finding one of the facial arteries located each side under the jawbone where the artery is prominent as it runs over the bone. Use a forefinger to press firmly on the artery and count the number of pulses over a 15 second period. Multiply the result by four to give the pulse rate.

The pulse will vary with exercise but should return to normal quickly. It will also be affected by pain, illness (such as a fever) and stress and is influenced by states of anxiety and excitement.

At rest, the pulse rate of a healthy adult horse should fall within the range of **30–44 beats per minute**. A pulse rate of 50 or over is considered worrying and is a sign of distress on which basis you should seek help. The quality of the pulse can also be used to gauge health and to determine if there are any rhythm disturbances.

For young horses the rate is different:

Foals	70–120
Yearlings	45–60
Two-year-olds	40–50

Capillary Refill Time (CRT)

This is the period of time it takes for blanched mucous membranes to refill with blood and return to the normal salmon pink colour associated with a state of health. To test the CRT lift your horse's upper lip and press your thumb firmly against the mucous membrane of the gum. The white of the blanched gum should return to pink within **two seconds** at most.

If the refill time is longer, then the animal may be in a state of shock, be suffering from blood loss or circulatory (heart) failure.

Mucous Membranes

The colour of the membranes which cover the gums and which line the inside of the nostrils and eyelids are a good indicator of health and of the state of the circulation. In a normal healthy animal the membranes should appear a moist salmon pink colour. Any abnormality necessitates prompt veterinary attention.

- Very pale pink or white membranes could indicate blood loss (haemorrhage), anaemia or fever
- Bright red membranes can suggest toxaemia or shock
- Blue or grey coloured membranes could indicate severe shock, severe respiratory or cardiac problems or other major health problems
- Yellow coloured membranes normally indicate jaundice associated with liver disease.

The Digital Pulse

This is the pulse which can be detected in the palmar digital arteries that supply the feet and can be felt just behind the fetlock (very close to the area of the sesamoid bones), and at the inner, back and outer region of the pastern joint. The rate of the digital pulse relates to the horse's heart rate but the strength of the pulse can indicate a problem. Checking one pulse with that of another foot can help you to decide what is normal.

A strong or bounding digital pulse can be an indicator of laminitis, although this is by no means certain, as a number of other foot problems can also cause an increase in the pulse. These include local inflammation, bruising to the foot, corns and abscesses. Laminitis is likely if the digital pulse is stronger in all four legs. The presence of heat in the hoof will provide an additional indicator of a potential problem.

Gut Sounds

Using a stethoscope or by placing your ear against your horse's abdomen, it is possible to detect the noises made by both the stomach and bowel. You should always be able to detect some gut sounds. The absence of gut sounds altogether is worrying and an indication of colic. Seek immediate veterinary help. A marked increase in the number or intensity of sounds is often less of a problem but nevertheless can be associated with some types of colic.

Dehydration and Thirst

By pinching the skin on the neck of your horse you can tell if your animal is dehydrated. In a healthy, normally hydrated horse, the skin tented by pinching should return to normal in less than one second. The longer the skin remains pinched before returning to its normal flattened condition, the more severe the state of dehydration.

Horses may become dehydrated in hot weather if they drink insufficient water, especially if exercising over extended periods such as during endurance competitions. Horses that are reluctant to drink can be tempted by adding apple juice to the water or by flavouring it with molasses.

Adult horses normally drink around a minimum of **20 litres (4.5 gallons)** of water daily. A significant increase can indicate illness such as kidney disease, Cushing's disease, diabetes or high fever.

The Eye

The eyes enable the horse to see and coordinate its movement accurately and to be spatially aware of the surrounding environment. Clearly the eye must function well for the horse to perform at its best. Other than the eyeball itself, there are a number of vital surrounding structures that are equally important. These include the muscles which control the movement of the eyeball, the conjunctival membranes, the eyelids (which afford protection) and the lachrymal glands that produce tears for lubrication. The eyeball itself is a complex structure. The clear part of the eye is the cornea and is that part which protrudes or bulges forwards. The sclera, also known as the white of the eye, surrounds the eyeball entirely other than at the cornea, and provides protection and structure to the eye as it is composed of tough fibrous tissue. It contains many blood vessels and nerves including a structure known as the uvea.

This comprises the choroid layer (part of which also contains the blue-green reflective layer), the ciliary body and the iris which controls the amount of light reaching the back of the eye. This area consists principally of the retina, which lines the choroid layer and comprises the receptor cells that respond to light and the optic disc (the blind spot) where nerve fibres collect and pass through the sclera to form the optic nerve. Behind the iris sits the lens enclosed in a capsule, in front of which there are two chambers (the anterior and posterior chambers) filled with aqueous humour. The region behind the lens is known as the vitreous body and filled with vitreous humour.

Injuries

Although fairly common, generally injuries to the eye need to be treated with the utmost respect. Injuries are a frequent result of damage by protruding nails or collision with fences or trees, especially in poor light or where the animal has been frightened. If there is any doubt as to the severity of the problem, call in professional help. Cuts may need suturing to avoid distortion to the lids. The following remedies offer excellent first aid treatment for a variety of problems. Details of subsequent problems including conjunctivitis are included under the relevant headings.

Bangs, Blows and Bruising to the Eye and Surrounding Area

Contusions and wounds to the eye

Aconite

Use where shock is evident to calm the horse. Aconite will help limit other changes and reduce the risk of infection.

Dose: *30c potency, three or four doses, five minutes apart*

Arnica

This is the most useful of all remedies where injury is concerned. Arnica will help limit bruising, pain and swelling and may help arrest haemorrhage where the skin is damaged or cut. Arnica will also assist the healing of wounds.

Dose: *200c potency, four doses two hours apart initially then twice daily until healed*

Ledum pal

Ledum is useful where the eye is bloodshot, bruised or contused. Discomfort will be relieved by application of a cold pad to the eye where Ledum is indicated. It is also valuable where there is bleeding

into the front of the eye. Can be alternated with Arnica where appropriate.
Dose: *30c potency, four times daily until symptoms abate*

Symphytum

An important eye remedy particularly where injury is concerned. Assists healing where there is damage to the bony orbit of the eye. Will help reduce pain and discomfort. Injuries to the eye from blunt objects will especially benefit from this remedy.
Dose: *30c potency, four times daily until symptoms abate*

Staphysagria

Administer where there are wounds, cuts or lacerations to the skin of the eyelids and surrounding area. Reduces pain and discomfort.
Dose: *30c potency, four times daily until symptoms abate*

Hypericum

This is the main remedy for pain relief and of additional benefit where there are lacerations to the tissues surrounding the eye. Can be used alongside other remedies where relief of pain is of primary importance.
Dose: *6c potency, four times daily as needed*

Hypericum and Calendula lotion

Use topically to clean any wounds, cuts, lacerations and abrasions. Hypercal lotion will also help stimulate would healing and reduce bruising
Instructions: *Dilute before use adding a teaspoon to a cup of cold boiled water. Bathe affected areas two or three times daily.*

Haemorrhage Into or From the Eye

This is a consequence of severe trauma to the eye and should be treated as an emergency. Check for bleeding into the front chamber of the eye. This will obscure the iris and impair vision. The following remedies can help arrest bleeding and hasten healing.

Arnica

Always administer Arnica in the initial stages to limit bleeding. Specifically indicated where there is retinal haemorrhage.
Dose: *200c potency, four doses two hours apart initially then twice daily until healed*

Phosphorus

A specific where haemorrhage is concerned, notably where the blood is bright red and is intermittent. Also indicated where there is retinal haemorrhage.
Dose: *30c potency, one dose every 15 minutes until bleeding ceases*

Lachesis

Useful where there is intraocular haemorrhage where the blood is dark and remains fluid.
Dose: *30c potency, one dose every 15 minutes until bleeding ceases*

Crotalus horridus

Will limit bleeding from the eye where the blood is dark and remains fluid and will aid absorption of the clot.
Dose: *30c potency, one dose every 15 minutes until bleeding ceases*

Hamamelis

Useful for the effects of ocular trauma in general but of most value in hastening the absorption of clots in the eye.
Dose: *30c potency twice daily until the clot has resorbed*

Sulphuric acid

Specifically indicated where trauma has caused massive bleeding inside the eye along with great swelling of the conjunctival membranes. This swelling is referred to as chemosis.
Dose: *30c potency twice daily until the clot has resorbed*

Corneal Injuries and Abrasions

Damage to the cornea can result in permanent scarring to the eye and impairment of vision or may ultimately lead to ulceration of the corneal surface. Prompt action is always required. Don't forget the value of **Arnica**, **Hypericum, Ledum** and **Aconite** in dealing with injuries to the eye in general and

Euphrasia mother tincture in healing any injury. Consider the following remedies as more specific for corneal damage.

Calendula

A good general remedy for injuries to the eye and in particular to the cornea.
Dose: 30c potency four times daily

Conium maculatum

Useful where pain is evident and out of all proportion to the severity of the damage. The eye reacts to bright light and may water excessively even from the slightest abrasion.
Dose: 6c potency four times daily

Euphrasia mother tincture, Euphrasia Ø

A general remedy to bathe the eyes where sore and inflamed or where the cornea has been damaged. Will help heal any injuries to the eye and reduce the risk of conjunctivitis.
***Instructions:** Dilute before use adding two drops to an eggcupful of cold boiled water. Bathe affected areas two or three times daily*

Cineraria mother tincture Ø or solution

This is a good remedy to help improve the health of the cornea and will assist healing where there is corneal damage.
***Instructions:** Dilute and use as above*

Foreign Bodies

Small pieces of straw, chaff, oat husk or barley awn may occasionally become lodged under one of the eyelids causing damage to the cornea (with possible ulceration) and conjunctivitis. Use appropriate remedies to assist healing after the material has been removed by your veterinary surgeon. Wash out the eye with diluted Euphrasia Mother Tincture to afford extra relief and to help flush away foreign material. The following remedies can provide additional help:

Spigelia

Use where discomfort persists after the foreign body has been removed as indicated by profuse production of tears and frequent closing of the eye. The eyelids appear uncomfortable.
Dose: 6c potency, four times daily

Coccus cacti

Indicated in similar circumstances to Spigelia, but where the symptoms are less pronounced, notably where there is little tear production. The animal may continue to rub the eye although the offending material has been removed.
Dose: 6c potency, four times daily

Conjunctivitis

This is the term applied to inflammation of the conjunctiva, the thin membrane which covers the eye and inner surfaces of the eyelids. Causes include bacterial infection, viral infections (such as influenza), trauma, damage or irritation caused by foreign bodies, allergic-based reactions and rarely abnormalities of the eyelids. Conjunctivitis is more common in dusty dry conditions or where flies are prevalent.

Symptoms

The conjunctivae become congested and inflamed, changing from a normal healthy pink colour to a deeper red colour accompanied by a variable degree of swelling or puffiness of the lids. There is a loss of shine to the cornea as it becomes dull. A discharge is also normally present, which may vary in character from a watery serous type to a more purulent, coloured or gummy variety. Irritation or discomfort may be evident and aggravated by bright light. This often causes the horse to rub or close the eye. Examination is often resented in such cases.

The key to successful treatment of conjunctivitis lies in accurately matching the remedy to the symptoms. Remember **Arnica** or **Calendula** are useful where trauma is the initiating cause and **Ledum pal** would be appropriate where conjunctivitis arises following a scratch or abrasion to the eye.

Aconite

Of most benefit in the early stages. The eye looks dry and red. Inflammation may be evident with accompanying irritation. Useful where conjunctivitis arises after removal of a foreign body or following

injury to the eye. Aconite is also useful where symptoms develop after exposure to cold dry weather. The horse may show a degree of fear or agitation where this remedy is indicated.
Dose: *30c potency hourly until improvement is noted*

Argentum nitricum
Effective in more severe cases where there is a copious purulent discharge. The inner corners of the eyes are especially inflamed with a tendency for material to collect in this area. The lids may be swollen (sometimes called blepharitis) with sticky material crusting along the edges. Severe cases may show corneal changes. Suits animals of an anxious, tense nature.
Dose: *30c potency three times daily*

Arsenicum album
Indicated where the eyelids are particularly puffy and the animal resents bright light. There is a discharge from the eyes that irritates the skin. The animal appears restless and agitated.
Dose: *30c potency three times daily*

Euphrasia
A prominent remedy for conjunctivitis where there is profuse tear production and reaction to bright light (photophobia). The eyes are often sticky and gummy with tacky mucus adherent to the cornea. Symptoms are worse in the evening and aggravated in warm weather. Sometimes these symptoms are accompanied by a watery bland nasal discharge.
Dose: *30c potency three times daily*

Pulsatilla
Conjunctivitis characterised by a thick bland yellow discharge responds to Pulsatilla. The eyelids are inflamed and sore. This form of conjunctivitis is often a sequel to respiratory tract infections. Pulsatilla is suited to affectionate, gentle animals.
Dose: *30c potency three times daily*

Merc sol
Useful in more severe cases where the lids are thickened and swollen and where the conjunctival membranes are intensely inflamed. There is a greenish discharge from the eyes which show a marked degree of redness with congestion of the white of the eye, the sclera. Bright light is resented. Symptoms are worse in the period from sunset to sunrise. Severe cases will show involvement of the cornea as well.
Dose: *30c potency three times daily*

Hepar sulph
Also useful in severe cases where there is a purulent infection with a tacky foul discharge which may stick to the lids and area surrounding the eye. The main guiding symptom to the use of this remedy is sensitivity to the least touch or pain. Indicated where there is pus in the front chamber of the eye (hyopion) and corneal damage.
Dose: *200c potency three times daily*

Kali bich
Conjunctivitis with a thick, yellow, ropy discharge with swollen, puffy lids. Pain or discomfort is absent and there is no photophobia.
Dose: *200c potency three times daily*

Cinnabaris
Indicated specifically where the whole eye appears red, sore and painful.
Dose: *30c potency three times daily*

Graphites
Use Graphites where the main symptom is blepharitis (inflammation of the edges of the eyelids) accompanied by eczema which affects the edges of the eyelids and a generalised conjunctivitis.
Dose: *30c potency three times daily*

Euphrasia mother tincture, Euphrasia Ø
Euphrasia can be used externally in any situation where there is conjunctivitis to help clear the infection. Helps reduce inflammation and heal damaged tissue. Soothe sore inflamed eyes.
Instructions: *Dilute before use adding two drops to an eggcupful of cold boiled water. Bathe two or three times daily*

Hypericum calendula lotion (Hypercal lotion)
Can be used as an alternative to Euphrasia if this is not available.
Instructions: *Dilute before use adding three or four*

drops to an eggcupful of cold boiled water. Bathe two or three times daily

Allergic-based Conjunctivitis

Acute allergic reactions can affect the eyes causing swelling, redness and increased tear production. Prompt homeopathic treatment can bring about relief within a short time.

Apis mel

Swelling or oedema of the eyelids is the most prominent feature where Apis is called for. Pain and discomfort is evident as the eyes sting and burn leading to rubbing. The conjunctival membranes are intensely red and may show considerable puffiness or chemosis almost obscuring the eyeball from vision.
***Dose:** 200c potency hourly until the condition resolves*

Rhus tox

Oedematous swelling of the eyelids is again a notable feature but accompanied by orbital cellulitis which affects the lids. Pain is apparent and the horse will resent examination. There is normally a discharge that is yellowish in colour. Severe cases may show involvement of the iris (iritis) and cornea, which become ulcerated.
***Dose:** 30c potency hourly until the condition resolves*

Keratitis

This can be a sequel to conjunctivitis and is primarily an inflammation of the cornea, which sometimes follows injury or infection. Pain is evident, resulting in almost complete closure of the eye in some cases. A discharge is normally present which may initially be clear, later becoming purulent and discoloured. Progressive cases result in opacity of the cornea with the appearance of grey-white patches or spots, barely visible at first, but later becoming dense and impairing the horse's vision. Small, branched blood vessels may grow in from the periphery of the cornea as the body attempts to heal the area. Where injury is the initiating cause an ulcer may ensue with the risk of possible perforation and loss of the eye.

Thuja

Useful in the early stages where there are a few small opacities on the cornea. There is little discharge but the edges of the lids appear thickened and the sclera (the white of the eye) is inflamed.
***Dose:** 30c potency, four times daily*

Argentum nitricum

Will help where the cornea is almost totally opaque resembling ground glass and accompanied by a profuse purulent discharge from the inner corner of the eye. This area of the eye appear red and swollen and bright light is resented. The cornea shows ulceration in more long standing cases.
***Dose:** 30c potency, four times daily*

Aurum metallicum

Photophobia is most evident where Aurum is needed and aversion to light is extreme, together with sensitivity of the area surrounding the eye. Blood vessel development (vascularisation) of the cornea is also a prominent feature that differentiates this remedy from others in this group. Symptoms are worse in cold weather and from sunset to sunrise. Aurum is also indicated where there is evidence of further damage to the deeper structures of the eye including the retina and choroid layer. Aurum can also be used for treating corneal ulcers where there is marked blood vessel development surrounding the ulcer.
***Dose:** 30c potency, twice daily*

Kali iod

An important remedy indicated where there is keratitis with much swelling of the eyelids (chemosis) and where the conjunctival membranes are intensely red accompanied by profuse watering of the eyes (lachrymation).
***Dose:** 30c potency, four times daily*

Merc sol and Merc corr

Indicated where keratitis is accompanied by a profuse, greenish discharge, which causes skin irritation where it runs down the face and a marked reaction to bright light (photophobia). Severe cases are accompanied by iritis (inflammation of the iris) and pus in the front of the eye. Merc corr suits the more advanced cases where corneal ulceration is

present or where the symptoms are particularly bad.
Dose: *30c potency, four times daily*

Naphthaline

For more acute cases. This remedy has an affinity for the eye and will help where the cornea is totally opaque and the eye appears red and inflamed. May possibly be suitable for allergic-based reactions.
Dose: *30c potency, four times daily*

Apis mel

Indicated in treating cases of keratitis where the most marked symptom is swelling of the lids and conjunctival membranes, so much so that they hide the eyeball from sight. The eye is extremely painful and waters excessively. Touch is resented with the horse becoming fidgety.
Dose: *30c potency, four times daily*

Cineraria mother tincture Ø or solution

This is a good remedy to help improve the health of the cornea. Cineraria will help reduce inflammation and will assist healing where there is corneal damage.
Instructions: *Dilute and use as previously indicated page 67*

Corneal Ulceration

Ulceration of the cornea is a consequence of corneal injury or keratitis. An ulcer will appear initially as a shallow crater like depression in the surface of the cornea. In more advanced cases this will become deeper until the eye perforates resulting in escape of the aqueous humour from the front of the eye. If the ulcer is to heal, blood vessels will grow across the cornea and into the ulcer to provide material for repair. Remedies such as **Argentum nitricum**, **Merc corr** (especially for deep ulcers), **Aurum met**, **Calc carb** and **Hepar sulph** can be used where the symptoms fit. **Euphrasia Ø** can be diluted as previously indicated for bathing the eye.

Conium

Indicated where there is evidence of extreme pain although the ulcer is small and shallow. The horse reacts to bright light and increased production of tears is also present.
Dose: *30c potency twice daily*

Kali bich

The symptoms associated with this remedy contrast to those linked with conium. Useful for deep ulcers and severe inflammation of the eye where there is little or no evidence of pain. A guiding symptom is the additional presence of a yellow, stringy discharge from the eye.
Dose: *30c potency twice daily*

Nitric acid

For cases of corneal ulceration tending towards perforation of the cornea. Also for ulceration associated with iritis which may be recurrent.
Dose: *30c potency three times daily*

Silica

One of the most valuable remedies for more chronic eye problems. Will help heal stubborn ulcers. Indicated where dead corneal tissue is adherent to the ulcer and where corneal perforation is imminent.
Dose: *30c, four times daily until healed*

Cineraria mother tincture Ø or solution

As indicated previously

Corneal Opacity and Scarring

Calc carb

Suited to horses of a heavier build where there are small opaque spots on the cornea with few other symptoms apart from a slight discharge. Ulcers may be present in some instances.
Dose: *30c potency on alternate days for several months*

Silica

Will help dissipate scar tissue and clear any opacity after corneal damage or ulceration has healed.
Dose: *200c potency twice weekly for several months*

Naphthaline

A general remedy for corneal opacities but often works at its best where there is other underlying

pathology such as retinal degeneration or cataract development.
Dose: 6c twice daily

Thiosinaminum
This remedy has a good reputation for dissolving away scar tissue including where the cornea is scarred.
Dose: 6c twice daily

Cineraria Ø or solution
Use the mother tincture externally suitably diluted. Cineraria has a reputation for helping to clear corneal opacities, especially where trauma is an initiating cause. Treatment will need to be continued on a long-term basis.
Instructions: Dilute before use adding two drops to an eggcupful of cold boiled water. Bathe at least once daily when possible

Periodic Ophthalmia Moon Blindness, Iridocyclitis Equine Recurrent Uveitis

This is a recurrent condition affecting the eye, the origin of which is obscure, but likely to be immune mediated and linked with the microfilariae of the parasitic worm *Onchocerca cervicalis*, or more likely with a previous leptospiral infection (see page 292). Even after a full recovery, the condition invariably has a tendency to recur, sometimes in the same eye, sometimes in the other. Normally only one eye is affected, but rarely, the condition will affect both eyes at the same time. Periodic ophthalmia usually affects horses over four years of age. Veterinary help should be sought, as the consequences of this condition can be serious.

Symptoms

Acute pain is most noticeable with closure of the eye, photophobia (light sensitivity), conjunctival congestion (redness), ocular discharge, blepharospasm (spasms of the muscles of the eyelids) and increased production of tears, which may run down the side of the face. As the disease progresses the cornea becomes cloudy and the front of the eye, the anterior chamber, fills with white, occasionally red, blood cells, which collect in the lower half. This situation is sometimes termed hypopyon or pus in the anterior chamber. Other symptoms include contraction of the pupil, which may become unresponsive to light and the accumulation of inflammatory debris on the lens surface.

Long-term problems include damage to the iris which may become adhered to the lens (visible because the pupil assumes a ragged outline), damage to the lens itself leading to cataract development, possible lens luxation, keratopathy (calcification of the cornea), glaucoma (a pressure rise inside the eye) and ultimately loss of vision after repeated attacks. Even during periods between attacks, symptoms of uveitis (pain, photophobia, ocular discharge and pupil constriction) may remain to some degree.

Uveitis

Uveitis can arise independently of immune related problems and occur as a consequence of trauma or damage to the eye or as a result of a systemic bacterial infection that leads to the production of circulating toxins that inflame the uvea. The symptoms are identical to those in moon blindness.

Aconite
Useful only in the very early stages of the condition and where the symptoms appear suddenly. The eye appears acutely red and inflamed. There is an aversion to bright light and increased production of tears.
Dose: 1M potency every 30 minutes over a period of four hours then consider other remedies if the symptoms have not abated

Belladonna
Another remedy for acute stages which can be alternated with Aconite if need be. The eye appears swollen, the conjunctival membranes are extremely red and dry, the eyelids very puffy and photophobia is evident as is blepharospasm and pain.
Dose: 1M potency every 30 minutes until improvement is noted or another remedy is indicated

Merc corr
One of the major remedies for iritis. The eye is

painful and reacts to bright light. There is also a profuse discharge that is greenish in colour. The pupil is unresponsive to light and neither dilates nor contracts. Pus may collect in the front of the eye (termed hypopyon) and adhesions between the iris, lens and cornea may be evident. Symptoms are often worse during the night where mercury is needed.
Dose: *30c potency every two or three hours*

Hepar sulph

Iritis with pus in the front of the eye is a key indication for Hepar sulph. Concurrent symptoms include purulent conjunctivitis, puffy swelling of the conjunctival membranes and fear of touch due to pain in the eye. The eye and the eyelids appear very red and inflamed. In severe cases there may be ulcers on the cornea. The patient is generally irritable and resents examination.
Dose: *200c potency every four hours*

Syphilinum

This is the main remedy for use in cases that repeatedly relapse or which fail to respond to other remedies. Syphilinum can be used alongside other remedies to reinforce their action.
Dose: *1M once daily for three days then once weekly*

Kali iod

A key remedy where the conjunctival membranes are intensely red and injected. There is profuse tear production from the eye and swelling of the lids. Another key point is clouding of the cornea so that it appears like ground glass obscuring the iris from view.
Dose: *30c potency every four hours*

Rhus tox

Indicated where iritis flares up following exposure to damp and cold. The eye appears painful with a profuse yellowish discharge and swollen lids. Pus may be present in the front of the eye. Cellulitis (tissue inflammation) affecting the region of the lids and surrounding tissues is a feature where Rhus tox is needed.
Dose: *30c potency every four hours*

Phosphorus

Useful as a general remedy (especially in chronic cases) to be given in periods between attacks where there are degenerative changes occurring, notably cataract development.
Dose: *200c potency twice weekly*

Other useful remedies

A number of other remedies can also be of use in treating periodic ophthalmia including:

Argentum nitricum 200c

Marked photophobia with purulent discharge, conjunctival membranes very swollen, clouding of the cornea.

Euphrasia 30c

Excessive watering of the eyes which makes the skin sore, swollen eyelids and sticky mucus on the cornea with clouding of the cornea.

Nat mur 30c

Later chronic stages with excess watering (lachrymation) and cataract development.

Bryonia 200c

Acute attacks with extreme pain as most prominent symptom with photophobia, redness. Eye sensitive to the least touch. Eyes gummed up in the mornings but water excessively during the day.

Kali bich 30c

Iritis with a thick, yellow discharge with no photophobia and little pain but with early signs of corneal changes occurring resulting in opacity.

Nitric acid 30

For recurrent iritis with corneal ulceration.

Silica 30c

Will help resolve scar tissue in chronic cases and reduce incidence of adhesions.

Physostigma 6x

As a general remedy where there is glaucoma.

Osmium 6c
For glaucoma accompanied by conjunctivitis and photophobia.

Acute remedies ***Dose:*** *four times daily*
Chronic remedies ***Dose:*** *once or twice daily*

Cataracts

By definition a cataract is an opacity of the lens or the capsule which contains the material which composes the lens itself. Certain types of cataract are present at birth and may vary from small opacities of the lens to complete involvement, rendering vision impossible. Where present, this type of cataract does not progress under normal circumstances. The other form of cataract is the degenerative type. These can arise after injury to the eye, as a result of disease (such as periodic ophthalmia) and general ageing.

Their appearance can only truly be judged by examination using an ophthalmoscope but may appear to resemble a spider's web with radiating lines, progressing to total blindness as the lens becomes completely opaque. The principal remedies to slow the development of cataracts are:

Phosphorus
A general remedy where the lens is uniformly opaque but useful where there is concurrent retinal degeneration. Suited to slender, affectionate animals.
Dose: *200c potency twice weekly*

Calc carb
Indicated where the lens appears misty rather than completely opaque. Calc carb suits animals of a more substantial, heavy stature.
Dose: *200c potency twice weekly*

Calcium fluoride
Another remedy for general use, which can be given alongside other remedies. Effective in slowing cataract development.
Dose: *200c potency twice weekly*

Natrum muriaticum
Useful for slow developing cataracts suiting horses of a lean stature, which exhibit a degree of thirst and reluctance for affection.
Dose: *200c potency twice weekly*

Silica
Cataracts which develop following periodic ophthalmia may respond to this remedy. Silica is also indicated where there may be adhesions between the lens and other structures such as the iris or cornea or where there is scarring of the cornea.
Dose: *200c potency twice weekly*

Cineraria Ø
Use the mother tincture externally suitably diluted. Cineraia has a reputation for helping to clear cataracts and corneal opacities. Treatment will need to be continued on a long-term basis.
Instructions: *Dilute before use adding two drops to an eggcupful of cold boiled water. Bathe at least once daily when possible*

Blockage of the Naso-Lachrymal Ducts

The lachrymal glands, one for each eye, secrete tears that keep the eyes lubricated and moist. The tears drain into tear ducts in the corners of the eyes and travel down the two naso-lachrymal ducts that drain into the nasal cavity.

If the ducts should become blocked, then tears will be unable to drain away, overflowing the lower eyelid and running down the side of the face. This may cause scalding and loss of hair over the affected area. Several remedies can be effective in opening up the ducts over a period of time. Bathing the eye with diluted **Hypercal lotion** will also help both relieve the obstruction and soothe any scalded areas of skin.

Silica
The most useful remedy especially where the lachrymal duct is chronically swollen. Helps to gradually resolve the underlying infection and dissolve away scar tissue.
Dose: *200c potency three times weekly for several months or until the condition resolves*

Thiosinaminum
Gradually dissolves scar tissue and opens up

strictures. Can be used alongside Silica in stubborn cases.
Dose: 6c once daily for as long as required

Natrum muriaticum
Indicated where there is also excessive tear production and where the tears run down and scald the face. A good remedy where there is stricture (narrowing) of the duct.
Dose: 30c potency once daily for four weeks

Eyelid Growths

These principally comprise sarcoids although other types of growth occasionally arise including carcinomas. Consult your vet as to the best treatment option. Where it is surgically difficult or undesirable to remove a sarcoid consider the following remedies:

Thuja
This is the principal remedy for treating sarcoids on or close to the eyelids. Those most likely to respond have a roughened, cauliflower like surface and are prone to bleed occasionally.
Dose: 200c potency three times weekly

Staphysagria
Most suitable for smaller sarcoids that are more nodular in nature.
Dose: 30c potency three times weekly

Nitric acid
Indicated where there is ulceration or bleeding of the eyelid growth.
Dose: 30c potency once daily

Causticum
Useful where the growth has a jagged, rough appearance.
Dose: 30c potency once daily

Sarcoid nosode
This is prepared from potentised sarcoid material and can be used alongside other remedies. Where possible it is best prepared from original material from the horse concerned as this is likely to be the most effective way of using the nosode.
Dose: 30c potency three times weekly

Ptosis

This is drooping of the upper eyelid, in effect a form of paralysis, possibly caused by damage to the oculomotor nerve. Treatment using the following remedies can be effective:

Gelsemium
Useful where the eyelid droops and obscures a large part of the eyeball. Suited to animals of a more nervous nature that seek reassurance from their owners.
Dose: 30c potency three times daily

Causticum
Most useful where the condition arises after exposure to cold. Affected animals are also prone to warts or sarcoids. Causticum is more effective for right-sided paralysis.
Dose: 30c potency three times daily

Other useful remedies include **Spigelia**, **Rhus tox**, **Ledum** (after injury) and **Nitric acid**.

Entropion

This condition is occasionally seen in new-born foals, although rarely it can occur as a result of chronic inflammation of the lids. Either one or both of the eyelids turn inwards so that the eyelashes and hair on the eyelids rub the surface of the cornea. This causes discomfort and inflammation, leading to infection and possible ulceration of the cornea. Where the condition occurs in foals, repeated outward rolling of the lids may effect a cure when combined with using homeopathy. Failing this, it is possible to correct the condition surgically.

Borax
This is the single most useful remedy for the new-born animal and may help avoid surgery. It usually needs to be given for some time to be effective
Dose: 30c potency once daily

Tellurium
Specifically helps where the lids are thickened and roll inwards as a result of chronic conjunctivitis.
Dose: 30c potency twice daily

Periorbital Dermatitis, Periorbital Eczema

This skin condition is localised around the margins of the eye, the skin of the eyelids and orbit region. It may be secondary to an eye problem (for example caused by an eye discharge which irritates the skin) or arise due to self-trauma from rubbing due to an eye irritation. Suitable remedies include (***Dose:*** *two or three times daily*):

Where there is cellulitis or tissue swelling **Rhus tox 30c**

Where the lesions are weepy/sticky with a clear discharge, especially where eyelids are involved **Graphites 30c**

Where the eczema is moist and infected **Merc sol 30c**

Where there are pimples **Hepar sulph 30c**

If scales are present **Sepia 30c**

Where there is scurf or skin is cracked **Petroleum 30c**

Where there are pustules, eyelids involved especially **Tellurium 30c**

Where the eyelids are excoriated (sore) **Ars alb 30c**

Where there are more generalised skin problems and the skin and coat are in poor condition **Sulphur 30c**

The Ear

The ear enables the horse to hear and is vital in maintaining balance. Anatomically it is divided into three distinct parts. The outer ear (the ear flap), which is separated from the second part, the middle ear by the eardrum and the inner ear, which is separated from the middle ear by two membrane covered windows. Three small bones in the middle ear transmit sound to the spiral shaped cochlea in the inner ear and then to the brain by the auditory nerve.

The middle ear is connected to the throat by the Eustachian tube that allows equalisation of pressure between the middle ear and the atmosphere. In the horse and donkey each Eustachian tube has a large outpouching known as the guttural pouch. The inner ear contains those structures responsible for balance, the three semicircular canals (the vestibular apparatus) arranged at right angles to each other.

Ear problems are thankfully few and far between.

Injury

Cuts, nicks and lacerations to the earflap can occasionally occur from accidents during riding. Routine treatment should include **Arnica** to limit the effects of the injury and to reduce bleeding and **Staphysagria** to reduce pain. Topical bathing with **Hypercal lotion** is also beneficial. Fractures to the skull may result in haemorrhage from the ear canal and should be dealt with using appropriate remedies listed under the first aid section, page 325. Rarely blood may appear in the ear canal from guttural pouch problems for which there a number of remedies that may prove useful.

Paralysis of the Earflap, Neural Paralysis

This arises from damage to the facial nerve which controls the muscles of the ear. The ear droops and can no longer be held in an upright position. Other symptoms of facial nerve damage may also be evident such as distortion of the muzzle and dropping of the lower lip. **Causticum 30c** is the principal remedy to use here as detailed in the eye section. Other remedies worthy of consideration include **Curare 30c** and **Gelsemium 30c**.

Eczema

This may arise as part of an overall problem but where there are skin eruptions specifically in this region, the following remedies should prove useful.

Graphites

Most suitable where the eruptions occur around or behind the ears and are sticky or moist, drying to form crusts. The condition may gradually spread away from the ear region to affect other areas of the face.

Dose: *30c potency twice daily*

Tellurium

Eczema affecting specifically the region behind the ears where thick crusts have formed should respond to this remedy. Affected areas are often distinctly circular in shape.

Dose: *30c potency twice daily*

Psorinum

Psorinum should prove useful where there is eczema accompanied by irritation and itching. Affected areas of skin may appear red, raw and produce a mucky discharge that irritates the skin.

Dose: *1M potency, once daily for five days*

Sulphur

Useful where the skin is itchy, dry and red and where the symptoms are worse for heat and on

contact with water. Scaly areas may also be present and the skin generally looks unhealthy.
Dose: *30c potency twice daily*

Incoordination

Loss of balance, vertigo

This is a rare problem which affects the inner ear resulting in disturbance of the vestibular apparatus which governs balance. It is not always easy to treat but the following remedies may help.
Dose: *the selected remedy should be given in the 30c potency three times daily*

Conium

Symptoms worse on moving, shaking the head or when resting.

Agaricus

Unable to keep the head still and symptoms much worse on movement.

Cocculus

Symptoms ease when at rest but are worse on any movement.

Rhus tox

Indicated where the symptoms arise after exposure to damp, cold weather and are worse on first getting up from lying down.

Warts and Sarcoids

Aural flat warts

These occasionally arise on or near to the earflap. **Thuja**, **Nitric acid**, **Causticum**, **Dulcamara** and **Antimonium crudum** are all useful remedies as well as the **Sarcoid nosode**.
Dose: *30c once daily for several weeks*

Aural plaques

These are usually classified as a type of wart and sometimes referred specifically to as flat papillomas growing on the earflap. More of a cosmetic problem, they will often respond well to homeopathic treatment. Suitable remedies include **Dulcamara**, **Causticum**, **Thuja** and **Sepia**. If the affected area is sore **Ruta** is indicated or where the warty area has become roughened or hard **Antimonium crudum** would be a better choice.
Dose: *30c once daily for several weeks*

Conditions of the Guttural Pouches

See page 78

The Respiratory System

Upper Respiratory Tract

This section covers problems relating to the upper respiratory tract, which comprises the nostrils, nasal cavities, sinuses, guttural pouches, pharynx, larynx and windpipe or trachea. Remember that most horses produce small amounts of mucus from the nostrils from time to time, especially after exercise. Abnormal looking discharges especially those that are persistent or pus coloured or associated with a cough warrant veterinary attention.

The Guttural Pouches

The paired guttural pouches are unique to horses and consist of air filled sacs formed from large outpouchings of the two Eustachian tubes that connect the middle ear to the nasopharynx or throat region. The entrance to each of the pouches is closed by a cartilage flap which opens when the horse swallows, equalising pressure in the middle ear, preventing discomfort caused by unequal pressure either side of the ear drum. The anatomical location of the pouches, below the floor of the skull and the top of the nasopharynx, close to important nerves and blood vessels, means that some conditions affecting the guttural pouches can have potentially serious complications.

Empyema
Pus in the Guttural Pouch

An uncommon condition that can arise as a consequence of a neighbouring abscess bursting into the guttural pouch which then fills with pus. Less commonly infections arise from the pharynx or following on from strangles. Streptococcal bacteria are often implicated.

The most obvious symptoms include a bilateral pus-like nasal discharge which may be intermittent in nature and more profuse on the side of the affected pouch. The colour of the discharge can vary but is usually yellow or white and can be foul smelling. The lymph nodes around the throat swell and both swallowing and breathing may be impeded. The area behind the ears and behind the jawbone may show swelling. Drainage of any material in the pouches can be hastened by turning the horse out or by feeding from the floor. Swallowing causes the entrance of the pouches to open and drainage is therefore assisted by gravity.

Hepar sulph
This is the principal remedy to use in the early stages of the condition and where the discharge is thick and has an offensive smell. Where the material is particularly thick and not easily expelled, use the remedy in low potency to loosen the discharge and encourage its expulsion. Higher potencies are indicated where the discharge is more free flowing and will help resorb the material and assist in resolution of the problem.
Dose: *low potency: 6x three times daily until the discharge loosens*
high potency: 1M twice daily until the condition resolves

Pulsatilla
Here the discharge is creamy and yellow or white in colour with little smell. It is bland in nature and usually thick. Horses that respond well to this remedy are quiet and gentle. Good results are obtained with this remedy if it is used in conjunction with Kali mur.
Dose: *200c twice daily until the condition resolves*

Kali mur
This kali salt is beneficial in most chronic cases when the discharge is thick and the submandibular

glands are chronically swollen. Kali mur works well with Pulsatilla.
Dose: *30c three times daily until the condition resolves*

Merc dulcis

Another remedy for chronic cases where the pus is sticky and has an elastic type texture and appearance.
Dose: *30c three times daily until the condition is resolved*

Silica

Silica is most useful where the condition has become more chronic in nature and where the discharge is pale yellow or white in colour. This remedy will also assist the healing of the lining of the guttural pouches and can be used in this context after other remedies such as Hepar sulph have acted with benefit.
Dose: *200c twice daily until the condition resolves*

Calc sulph

Indicated for more chronic conditions, most notably where the discharge is thicker, a deeper yellow and more purulent than where Silica is needed.
Dose: *30c three times daily*

Hippozaeninum

Worth consideration for stubborn cases where other remedies have failed to work. It is likely to be of most value where the discharge from the nostrils remains offensive or glutinous in nature.
Dose: *200c twice daily for seven days*

Streptococcal nosode

This remedy can be used to augment any other chosen remedy.
Dose: *30c twice daily*

Guttural Pouch Tympany
Tympanitis

Young foals can be affected by this condition, which arises due to blockage of the Eustachian tubes. Both pouches become distended with air causing difficulty in breathing and swallowing. Abnormal respiratory sounds similar to snoring may occur in some animals. Externally, a painless swelling is visible in the region of the parotid salivary gland extending towards the throat area. Infection of the pouches is an occasional sequel. Surgical treatment of the condition is often needed in refractory cases. Homeopathic remedies provide a useful first line of treatment.

Calc carb

A remedy normally suited to foals of the heavier breeds where muco-purulent material blocks both Eustachian tubes and the submandibular glands are swollen.
Dose: *30c potency, four times daily*

Pulsatilla

Pulsatilla suits foals of a gentle nature where the catarrh is bland and creamy in character. The external ear may become reddened and swollen.
Dose: *200c potency, twice daily*

Kali mur

Suited to cases where the condition follows chronic catarrhal problems leading to closure of the eustachian tubes and where Pulsatilla fails to work well. The glands about the neck are swollen and some difficulty in breathing is noted.
Dose: *30c potency, four times daily*

Merc dulcis

A general remedy for eustachian catarrh where the material has caused closure of both ducts leading to tympanitis.
Dose: *200c potency, four times daily*

Other indicated remedies include **Kali sulph 30c**, **Silica 30c** and **Petroleum 30c**.

Mycosis
Fungal Infection of the Guttural Pouches

This is a serious condition involving a fungal infection, often by *Aspergillus fumigatus*, of the guttural pouches. Symptoms include a particularly foul smelling nasal discharge, difficulty in swallowing, stiffness of the neck, pain at the base of the ears, paralysis of the larynx and pharynx and more rarely colic and eye problems. The most common symptom, however, is a bilateral nasal haemorrhage unrelated to exercise, caused by erosion of the carotid arteries. Large quantities of blood can be lost leading to possible death. Haemorrhage remedies (see page 98) can be useful while waiting for veterinary help. The following remedies are indicated in the treatment of fungal infections and may complement conventional therapy:

Calc carb

Indicated where the discharge is offensive and yellow in colour and the glands around the neck are swollen. Leaner patients may benefit from Calc sil as an alternative.

***Dose:** 200c, twice daily*

Asafoetida

Foul smelling thin looking purulent material from the nose suggests Asafoetida, a remedy suited to nervous, sensitive animals.

***Dose:** 30c, three times daily*

Aurum

Also indicated where the discharge is foul, purulent, extremely offensive and possibly tinged with blood. The smell of the material from the nose pervades the whole stable and the animal outwardly appears depressed.

***Dose:** 30c, three times daily*

Silica

Will help clear away the infection in stubborn cases and heal the lining of the pouches.

***Dose:** 30c, three times daily*

The Sinuses

Sinusitis and Sinus Empyema

The sinuses are air filled cavities in connection with each other and with the nasal cavity. The maxillary sinuses are associated in particular with the roots of some of the molar teeth. Infection or injury to any of these teeth can lead to inflammation of the sinuses (sinusitis) or collection of pus in the sinus cavities (empyema). Respiratory infections involving the nasal mucosa can also spread to the sinuses, leading to sinusitis.

Mixed bacterial infections are usually involved but often predominantly streptococci are implicated. Symptoms include an intermittent, unilateral nasal discharge that is normally thick and foul smelling, lymphatic swelling on the affected side and swelling and pain over the region of the affected sinus. In the most severe cases the sinuses can become blocked. This may result in abnormal respiratory noises and a discharge from the eye and dullness on percussion of the sinus on the affected side.

Pulsatilla

Most useful where the nasal discharge is bland and a creamy yellow colour and flows more profusely in the morning. Often the discharge will cease in the evening and the nose may appear more blocked. Pulsatilla more often suits mares and animals with a gentle placid disposition.

***Dose:** 30c, twice daily until symptoms resolve*

Hepar sulph

This remedy is suited to more irritable animals and where the discharge is more foul smelling and thick. Cold air will induce coughing and cause the discharge to flow more profusely. In the very early stages of the condition, selecting a low potency may well abort the infection before it reaches a more chronic stage. Higher potencies should be reserved for the later stages where pus has accumulated within the sinuses (empyema).

***Dose:** Low potency: 6x three times daily until the nasal discharge ceases*
High potency: 1M twice daily until the condition resolves

Silica

Silica is indicated for chronic long-standing cases and where there may be damage to the bones of the nasal cavity. It is also useful where the teeth roots may be involved. The typical discharge seen in Silica type cases is thin and white in colour as opposed to yellow. Silica is also valuable where the nose has become obstructed from hardened discharges and in clearing scar tissue from the sinuses following the use of other remedies.

***Dose:** 30c, twice daily until symptoms resolve*

Lycopodium

This remedy is most useful where the discharge is grey in colour and causes the skin around the nostrils to become sore. There is often a more profuse flow from the right nostril, especially in the initial stages of the infection. The nose will often become obstructed later at night, although generally, the amount of discharge may be seen to increase in the early evening.
Dose: 30c, twice daily until symptoms resolve

Kali bich

Another remedy for chronic cases where the discharge is very thick, tough and yellow in character. The nose can appear blocked completely.
Dose: 30c, twice daily until symptoms resolve

Calc sulph

A remedy to use in cases of empyema, where the discharge is whitish-yellow in colour, purulent and contains lumpy material.
Dose: 30c, twice daily until symptoms resolve

Merc sol

Mercury is indicated where the discharge is thick, purulent, greenish in colour and possibly blood streaked. The nature of the discharge is such that it causes the skin around the nostrils to become sore.
Dose: 30c, twice daily until symptoms resolve

Thuja

Reserve this remedy for use in obstinate cases or where other remedies fail to help the situation. Chronic nasal catarrh that is distinctly green in colour and purulent indicates that Thuja may be useful.
Dose: 30c, twice daily until symptoms resolve

Other indicated remedies include **Kali iod 30c** (greenish watery discharge with damage to bones of the nasal cavity) and **Fluoric acid 30c**, **Aurum 30c** and **Asafoetida 30c** where there is destruction of bone or ulceration within the sinuses or nasal cavity. Stubborn cases or where the response to a remedy is poor, **Sycotic co 200c** (*given twice daily for five days*) may allow other remedies to act with benefit.

The Nose

Epistaxis

Epistaxis is another name for nosebleed or nasal haemorrhage and is not uncommon in horses. Normally the haemorrhage affects only one side; bilateral bleeding suggests more serious conditions, such as problems with the guttural pouches or lower respiratory tract. Blood may be present with pus in a small number of cases of sinusitis.

Small unilateral nosebleeds often occur after exercise and should not normally be any great cause for concern unless the problem becomes a very regular occurrence. There are several remedies that can help. Bear in mind that the selection of the remedy should correspond to the character of the blood seen and the underlying circumstances.
In all cases use the 30c potency every 10–15 minutes until the bleeding ceases.
(See also pulmonary haemorrhage)

Aconite

Bright red haemorrhage following exercise or over-exertion.

Arnica

Bright red haemorrhage following trauma to the nasal region.

Phosphorus

Watery bright red blood that does not clot easily. Suited to sensitive lean animals.

Millefolium

Bright red blood that does not clot. Bleeding from the least exertion will often respond to this remedy. Millefolium can also be used for epistaxis associated with trauma, where there is bleeding from the lower respiratory tract or where the temperature of the horse is elevated persistently.

Ipecacuanha

Indicated where there is profuse bleeding of red blood together with laboured breathing. Blood appears from the nose in profuse gushes.

Hamamelis

Useful for passive bleeding where the blood is much darker in colour and does not clot readily.

Coryza and Rhinitis

Inflammation of the nasal mucous membranes is referred to as coryza or rhinitis and can represent the early stages of many respiratory problems, particularly viral infections. Symptoms include a rise in temperature, together with a degree of lethargy. Some horses will sweat. A slight nasal discharge will appear, often clear at first, becoming coloured in later stages. Left without treatment, the condition will progress to a cough or bronchitis as the lower respiratory tract becomes involved. **Aconite** and **Ferrum phos** are the most important remedies in treating initial symptoms of this type.

Allergic reactions due to dust and pollens will also inflame the nasal mucous membranes. In this situation there will be no temperature rise or lethargy. Coryza or rhinitis of this type will often be linked with COPD. Symptoms are a little like 'hay fever' in humans. The remaining remedies listed are those most suited to treating symptoms of this type.

Carefully select the remedy that most closely matches the symptoms.

Use the 30c potency four times daily until the symptoms abate or until another remedy is indicated.

Aconite

Use in the very early stages where the symptoms appear suddenly and the horse is feverish, lethargic, anxious and restless.

Ferrum phos

This is another remedy to use in the early acute stages where there is fever. Anxiety and restlessness are not present where Ferrum phos is indicated.

Allium cepa

Fever is absent but there is a profuse clear watery discharge that makes the nostrils sore. The eyes are also affected and look inflamed. Tears may run down the face. Symptoms are worse in the box and eased when the horse is outside in the fresh air.

Arsenicum album

Again there is a fluent thin watery discharge from the nose which is acrid and makes the skin sore. The eyes burn and the lids appear red and inflamed. Bright light is resented. The animal is restless and anxious. Symptoms are worse in the open air and may occur after becoming chilled when hot.

Natrum muriaticum

Symptoms appear suddenly and include violent sneezing and a nasal discharge that resembles egg white. The horse is thirsty and resents any attention given.

Sabadilla

Check for a copious watery nasal discharge accompanied by increased tear production and redness of the eyes. Sabadilla is suited to symptoms which are allergic based and where there is much snorting.

Nux vomica

Most useful where the symptoms are worse in the morning and better when the horse is outside rather than stabled. Often there is no discharge and the horse snuffles, especially at night. However, the discharge may start during the daytime and become quite fluent.

Euphrasia

The discharge from the nostrils is clear where Euphrasia is indicated, although there may be a mucky, acrid discharge from the eyes. Symptoms are better in the open air, worse in the warmth and contrast with those of Allium cepa.

Pulsatilla

Look for a bland, thick, yellowish coloured discharge that varies in amount from day to day. Symptoms are worse in the heat and in the evening and better for being outside.

Arundo

This remedy is used for allergic-based coryza, characterised by itching of the nose and a nasal discharge that is initially watery, turning later to greenish mucus.

Sanguinaria
Use Sanguinaria where the symptoms of coryza or rhinitis are chronic in nature. The membranes in the nose are congested. Any discharge will be yellow in colour. The larynx will also be involved and may be swollen.

Sycotic co
Consider this nosode in unresponsive cases.
Dose: *with the 200c potency twice daily for five days*

The Larynx

Inflammation of the larynx is normally an extension of any other ongoing respiratory problem, for example flu or strangles. Look for signs that include a harsh cough (which can be induced by palpating the larynx) and a rough snoring sound. In the later stages the larynx can become obstructed due to swelling. This causes laboured breathing
Use the 30c potency hourly for a maximum of six doses until symptoms improve, then consider other remedies if needed.

Aconite
Dose as soon as the symptoms are noted in the early feverish stages of the illness.

Belladonna
Indicated where there are obvious signs of fever, which include a rapid bounding pulse and dilation of the pupils. The horse feels hot and appears restless.

Ferrum phos
This remedy is targeted at the throat region and is used where there is a fever which is less severe than with Aconite or Belladonna, but where the throat is very inflamed and where the glands in the neck are enlarged.

Argentum nit
Use where the larynx is coated in thick mucus and breathing is difficult. There is also a cough.

Rumex
A dry cough will be present where Rumex is needed and can be induced by the slightest pressure on the larynx.

Apis
Apis is the remedy to use where the larynx is badly swollen (or oedematous) and obstructs the breathing. There is a short dry cough. Symptoms are worse for heat and touch. The horse may be distressed.

Laryngeal Hemiplegia Whistling, Roaring

This is the most common condition affecting the larynx and caused by the degeneration of the nerve that supplies the muscles responsible for opening and closing the larynx. The paralysis can be partial or complete and occurs predominantly on the left side. The characteristic symptoms are caused by partial obstruction of the airway. As the air passes through the narrowed larynx on inspiration it causes a whistling or roaring sound. The condition can often be successfully treated homeopathically with one of the following remedies:

Causticum
This is the single most important remedy in treating this condition. Symptoms of laryngeal paralysis may appear slowly and appear worse in clear, fine weather and better when conditions are damp and warm.
Dose: *30c, twice daily*

Lachesis
Suited more to mares with this condition and where symptoms are left sided. The animal resents examination or touch, particularly around the throat.
Dose: *30c, twice daily*

Gelsemium
This is a remedy often associated with general muscle weakness or paralysis. It is a good general remedy to use where other remedies fail to improve the condition.
Dose: *30c, twice daily*

Lower Respiratory Tract

This section covers conditions affecting the lower respiratory tract, which includes the bronchi, lungs and pleura. Respiratory infections are included under the section covering specific diseases.

Bronchitis, Pneumonia and Bronchopneumonia

Bronchitis is inflammation of the bronchi, the larger air passages which carry air to the lungs. Often this problem will lead on to pneumonia, a serious respiratory condition involving inflammation of the lungs. If both the bronchi and lungs are affected, the condition is referred to as bronchopneumonia. Bacteria, mainly Streptococci, occasionally Bordetella or Pasturella, are often involved, although viruses, migrating parasites and foreign material accidentally entering the lungs can also be responsible.

Remember that bacterial respiratory infections are contagious and acquired by inhalation through contact with horses carrying these bacteria or from infected nasal discharges. Where foals are affected, the infection can enter by the navel at birth, with bacteria gaining access to the lungs via the circulation. In such cases abscesses may form in the lungs, causing significant damage and taking months to resolve.

In general foals are more often affected than adult horses, particularly where management is poor and where ventilation is inadequate. Stress has also been implicated. Symptoms include difficulty in breathing, rapid respiration, fever, lack of appetite and depression. A cough or nasal discharge is also sometimes present. In severe cases the nostrils will flare, breathing is laboured and there will be an obvious double respiratory effort (known as heaves).

Always seek veterinary help as pneumonia and related conditions are nearly always serious. Homeopathic remedies can be of immense help in treating these conditions at all stages of their development. You will need to treat most cases with your selected remedy fairly frequently at first, until symptoms improve noticeably. Carry on treatment at a lower dose for at least 48 hours after this to ensure that there is complete resolution of the problem. Where necessary, ensure that the symptoms have not changed markedly as another remedy may be indicated.

If your veterinary surgeon is able to type the bacteria involved, use the appropriate nosode in 30c potency twice daily alongside any other chosen remedies.

Remedies to use in the early stages:

Aconite
Indicated where the symptoms appear suddenly and particularly where the weather has been cold and dry. The horse is restless, often pacing in an anxious fashion. The pulse rate and temperature are elevated. The skin feels dry and hot to the touch.
Dose: *1M, at half-hourly intervals until improvement then re-assess*

Ferrum phos
An excellent remedy in the earliest stages of many respiratory conditions. Differentiated from Aconite by the absence of fear, anxiety and restlessness and from Belladonna by the lack of intense heat and bounding pulse.
Dose: *30c, at half-hourly intervals until improvement then re-assess*

Belladonna
The symptoms where Belladonna is useful are very prominent and arise suddenly. Full bounding pulse with rapid breathing, dilated pupils, a state verging on delirium with agitation, high temperature and burning hot dry skin are characteristic.
Dose: *1M at half-hourly intervals until improvement then re-assess*

Veratrum viride
Indicated where symptoms appear suddenly and where there is marked congestion of the lungs. Breathing is slow and heavy, although the pulse is rapid. Temperature fluctuation at regular intervals is a good indication for this remedy. If a foal is being treated, the standing position will ease the symptoms as opposed to lying down.
Dose: *30c, at half-hourly intervals until improvement then re-assess*

Remedies for more advanced cases:

Kali carb

This remedy is particularly suited to foals and other young stock with acute bronchopneumonia. The condition is markedly worse on the lower right hand side of the chest. Breathing is difficult, sometimes wheezy. There is normally a rattling type cough that is at its worst in the early hours of the morning due to mucus in the chest.

***Dose:** 30c, at half-hourly intervals until improvement then four times daily*

Merc sol

Symptoms responding to mercury are always worse in the evening and at night. Other notable symptoms include excessive sweating, foul breath and reluctance to lie on the right hand side of the chest. Slimy mucus is sometimes coughed up and greenish in colour. Occasionally blood is present as well.

***Dose:** 30c, at half-hourly intervals until improvement then four times daily*

Phosphorus

A very valuable remedy for bronchopneumonia and bronchitis where the respiratory rate is increased and breathing laboured. Phosphorus often suits slender, lean built animals. Additional guiding symptoms to using this remedy include the desire for company, increased thirst and a degree of anxiety together with a dry hard cough. The animal prefers to lie on the right hand side, although the symptoms are worse on this side of the chest.

***Dose:** 30c, at half-hourly intervals until improvement then four times daily*

Ipecacuanha

This remedy is useful for the youngest animals and will help most conditions including bronchitis, pneumonia and bronchopneumonia where the condition either appears suddenly or where symptoms deteriorate rapidly. There is great difficulty in breathing, almost to the point of suffocation. The chest contains much mucus which can be heard rattling in the airways.

***Dose:** 30c, at half-hourly intervals until improvement then four times daily*

Bryonia

Every breath causes pain so the animal is very reluctant to move as this only increases the degree of discomfort. Check for shallow rapid breathing as an indication for Bryonia together with a dry mouth and a dry and hard cough. If water is easily at hand the animal will show increased thirst. Normally used for more advanced cases and particularly in pleuro-pneumonia.

***Dose:** 30c, at half-hourly intervals until improvement then four times daily*

Lycopodium

Indicated for advanced or neglected cases. Useful where the symptoms are accompanied by a fever that peaks between the hours of 4 and 8pm. Rattling sounds can be heard in the chest and the breathing is short and rapid. A characteristic symptom is a fan-like motion of the wings of the nostrils. Affected animals are often irritable.

***Dose:** 30c, at half-hourly intervals until improvement then four times daily*

Chelidonium

Chelidonium can be used for treating right-sided pneumonia in young foals where there is a large amount of mucus in the chest. This is coughed up only with difficulty despite the fact that the cough seems loose.

***Dose:** 30c, at half-hourly intervals until improvement then four times daily*

Remedies for severe or non-responsive cases:

Antimonium tartrate

An important remedy where there are marked symptoms notably extreme difficulty in breathing, approaching a state of suffocation such that the animal has to stand with legs splayed to make breathing as easy as possible. Mucus collects within the chest and can be heard rattling within the airways. Breaths are short and white mucus may be coughed up, but only with difficulty. Symptoms are worse for heat. Affected animals often appear drowsy. Suited to very young or elderly animals.

***Dose:** 200c, at 15 minute intervals until improvement then re-assess*

Ammonium carbonate

Drowsiness is also a feature of this remedy, which shares many symptoms with Antimonium tartrate. Bubbling sounds can be heard within the chest and breathing is slow and laboured. Symptoms are worse for cold. Suited to more elderly animals which are more stout in build or overweight and lazy.
Dose: 200c, at 15 minute intervals until improvement then re-assess

Carbo veg

A remedy for the most severe cases where the animal has reached a comatose state or shows signs of air hunger with the mouth open gasping for air. The body is cold to touch and the mucous membranes are tinged blue.
Dose: 200c, at five-minute intervals until improvement then re-assess

Bacillinum

This is an excellent remedy to use in any non-responsive case especially where there is a lot of mucus present.
Dose: 200c, twice daily for three days then consider other remedies

Remedies indicated where symptoms persist in chronic cases:

Always think of using a constitutional remedy first where possible, in preference to any other remedy.

Arsenicum iodatum

This is probably the most useful remedy to help clear the after effects of bronchitis or pneumonia, particularly where a slight hacking cough remains.
Dose: 6c, twice daily until symptoms have resolved

Pleurisy

The pleura is the lining covering the inside of the chest cavity and the lungs. Where the lining is inflamed, this is referred to as pleurisy, a serious condition normally caused by bacteria. It can arise as a secondary problem to pneumonia, following stress due to transit or exposure to extremes of temperature or following wounds that penetrate the chest cavity.

Symptoms include an increase in the respiratory rate, shallow painful breathing, lethargy, anxious appearance and an increase in temperature. In later stages pus can form inside the chest cavity, collecting at the bottom and impeding expansion of the lungs. This causes markedly laboured breathing. As toxins from the bacterial infection accumulate, the horse's condition deteriorates. During recovery adhesions can form between the lungs and chest walls.

Always seek help, as pleurisy is a serious condition. Homeopathic remedies can help significantly in most cases, especially if administered early on.

Aconite

Always the first remedy to administer when symptoms are first suspected.
Dose: 1M, at 15 minute intervals

Bryonia

The most important remedy for treating pleurisy. The horse is reluctant to move as any change in position causes discomfort. The rib area can also be painful to touch, although sustained pressure from lying down can bring relief. Respiration is increased with obvious difficulty in breathing in.
Dose: 30c, at 15 minute intervals

Squilla maritima

Important in treating pleurisy and broncho-pneumonia where breathing is laboured and painful and accompanied by a particularly violent exhausting cough. Symptoms are slow to develop and are eased when the horse is at rest and worse for movement.
Dose: 30c, at 15 minute intervals

Kali iod

Use this remedy alongside other remedies where pleural effusion occurs and consequently fluid accumulates within the pleural cavity.
Dose: 30c, three times daily

Carbo animalis

Use this remedy in the later stages when the most prominent symptoms have passed but where some evidence of discomfort still remains.
Dose: 6c, twice daily for ten days or until symptoms are clear

The following remedies could also prove useful in treating pleurisy, **Apis mel 30c**, **Kali carb 30c**, **Senega 30c** and **Sulphur 30c**.

Where recovery is slow, think about using **Silica 30c**. This remedy along with **Calc fluor 30c** and **Acetic acid 30c** will also help reduce the chance of adhesions forming.
Dose: *twice daily for several weeks*

Hydrothorax

This is the term applied to the accumulation of fluid on the chest usually as a consequence of pleurisy. Remedies that are likely to prove useful include:

Merc sulph
A specific for hydrothorax where there is marked difficulty in breathing with a rapid respiratory rate.

Apis mel
Use where the symptoms are more intense almost to the point of suffocation.

Apoc cann
Can be used where there is concurrent fluid retention in other parts of the body such as the abdomen and where there are signs of cyanosis.

Arsenicum album
Indicated where the animal is restless and cannot settle.

Kali carb
Where the symptoms include a hard, dry cough, bronchitis or wheezing. The patient is generally irritable.

Dose: *30c four times daily*

Cough

This is a general term and a symptom of numerous conditions that can be broadly divided into the following two categories:

Upper respiratory tract causes:

- Viral infections such as equine influenza virus, rhinovirus and equine herpes virus (EHV-1)
- Bacterial infections such as strangles
- Less commonly, inflammation of the larynx (laryngitis) and pharynx (pharyngitis).

Lower respiratory tract causes:

- Allergic – chronic obstructive pulmonary disease (COPD), recurrent airway obstruction (RAO) and summer pasture associated obstructive pulmonary disease (SPAOPD)
- Bronchitis, pneumonia, broncho-pneumonia and pleurisy
- Less commonly lungworm and chronic chest infections

Treating coughs

Selecting the best remedy

Check under the relevant headings of the individual diseases for more information and remedies. There are a great many cough remedies, so use the list which follows as a basic guide. Remember to try to select the remedy that most closely matches your horse's symptoms.
Dose: *Unless otherwise stated, give the 30c potency two or three times daily until the symptoms have abated*

Bryonia

Keynote: Dry, hard and painful cough triggered by movement.

Cough: Dry, hard and painful. Other guiding symptoms: irritability, increased thirst, horse wants to be left alone, dry mucous membranes.

Worse: For warmth, inside in warm stable, movement, exercise, easterly winds.

Better: For pressure over the chest region.

Arsenicum album

Keynote: Cough with wheezing respiration.

Cough: Asthmatic and wheezy, expectoration of small amounts of watery frothy material and a thin runny discharge from the nose that may make the nostrils sore.

Other guiding symptoms: Restless, chilly (always seeks warmth), scaly flakes in the coat, thirsty for small amounts of water.

Worse: After midnight, in cold wet weather.

Better: For warmth.

Phosphorus

Keynote: Dry cough, little expectoration.

Cough: Dry tickling type of cough, racking or violent and can be exhausting. Coughs up only small amounts of white or rusty coloured mucus.

Other guiding symptoms: Sensitive, anxious animals, jumpy with noises, sensitive to light. Thirsty for large amounts of water.

Worse: Outside in the open air, for going from warm to cold area or vice versa.

Better: In the dark.

Nux vomica

Keynote: Dry cough, irritable nature

Cough: Dry and hacking. Nose blocks up in the stable but clears outside in the fresh air leading to runny mucous discharge.

Other guiding symptoms: Mentally and physically hypersensitive, short-tempered and tense, easily upset.

Worse: In the morning, after feeding, in cold weather.

Better for: Rest and in the evening.

Pulsatilla

Keynote: Changeable symptoms.

Cough: Dry in the evening and at night, loose and catarrhal in the morning with bland, thick, nasal discharge. Coughs up loose mucus in the mornings.

Other guiding symptoms: Gentle nature, drinks little water. May leak urine whilst coughing.

Worse: For warmth, in a warm stable, in the evening and when the horse is lying down and at rest.

Better for: Fresh air and exercise, cool weather.

Causticum

Keynote: Hard cough with difficult expectoration.

Cough: Hard and dry, shakes the whole chest and is triggered when the horse breathes out. Tough mucus collects in the chest. This is difficult to cough up and hence little is seen in the stable.

Other guiding symptoms: Urine may leak out as the horse coughs.

Worse: In dry cold weather.

Better: In damp, wet weather and for warmth.

Rumex

Keynote: Dry, spasmodic cough.

Cough: Dry and spasmodic, often quite severe, triggered by the least amount of exercise. Mucous discharge from the nose.

Other guiding symptoms: Thick mucus in the larynx is coughed up only with difficulty. Lower legs may be itchy.

Worse: Breathing in cool or cold air and at night.

Better: In a warm stable.

Spongia

Keynote: Cough with laboured breathing.

Cough: Chesty, dry cough that sounds like a saw being driven through wood. Laboured breathing, asthmatic sounding in the later stages. Little mucus produced.

Other guiding symptoms: Coughs if touched (especially around the larynx) and sometimes will cough while asleep. Dry mucous membranes. Suited to tense anxious animals.

Worse: At night (near midnight) and on exercise, breathing in and in cold windy weather.

Better: After eating or drinking.

Stannum

Keynote: Cough with loose, slimy mucus.

Cough: Loose type of cough, expelling slimy mucus which is greenish in colour. Can be quite forcible or violent. Cough is sometimes dryer during the night.

Other guiding symptoms: Often starts as a sequel to equine flu. Stannum is useful in more chronic bronchial problems particularly where the horse has become debilitated.

Worse: Early in the morning.

Better: For coughing up mucus.

Drosera

Keynote: Deep, repetitive coughing.

Cough: Deep, spasmodic, irritant cough, usually severe and coming in paroxysms as the coughs follow in quick succession. Yellowish nasal discharge.

Other guiding symptoms: Expectorated material may rarely contain specks of blood.

Worse: At night and especially from midnight to early morning. Lying down.

Better: At rest.

Kali carb

Keynote: Hard, dry, rattling cough

Cough: Rattling type of cough that is dry and hard.

Other guiding symptoms: Little material is coughed up, more often it is swallowed. You may find small round coughed up lumps of mucus in the stable in the morning. Thin yellowish green mucus appears at the nose which crusts around the nostrils but ceases to appear as the nose stuffs up in warm weather.

Worse: At 3am in the morning and in cold weather, from lying down.

Better: The cough is better for warmth and in warm weather and from 6am onwards.

Kali bich

Keynote: Barking sounding cough..

Cough: Hard and hollow sounding, sometimes barking.

Other guiding symptoms: Thick, tough, sticky mucus usually coughed up, yellowish-green in colour, often stringy and in quite large amounts. Horse is sensitive to cold weather.

Worse: At night and in the early morning, in hot weather.

Better: From being covered and hence warm.

Sticta

Keynote: Post-viral cough

Cough: Incessant dry and hacking. Caused by tickling in the trachea.

Other guiding symptoms: Cough originates from the trachea rather than lower down the respiratory tract. Often the type of cough that follows on from equine flu.

Worse: In the evening, during the night and after exercise.

Better: Outside in the open air.

Tuberculium

Keynote: Stubborn cases and stubborn patients

This remedy should be reserved for stubborn cases that fail to respond to more common remedies. Indicated particularly where the cough is dry and hard and where the horse coughs up thick yellow or greenish-yellow mucus. Symptoms are worse in a stuffy warm stable. There is a desire to seek fresh air if stabled.

Worse: For motion, before a storm, damp weather and early in the morning.

Better: In fresh clean air.

Dose: *Give three doses of the 1M potency over a 24-hour period*

Bacillinum

Keynote: Stubborn cases with much rattling catarrh.

Bacillinum works best where there is much catarrh in the respiratory tract giving rise to rattling noises in the chest and where the lungs are congested.

Worse: At night and early in the morning.
Dose: *Give three doses of the 1M potency over a 24-hour period*

Chronic coughs in older horses

The following remedies have proved very useful in treating chronic bronchitic coughs in older animals.

Senega

Chronic long-standing coughs where the mucus is very tough and sticky and therefore difficult to expel. The cough is hard and the horse seems short of breath. Senega helps loosen the catarrh and make expectoration easier. This remedy is also indicated in pleurisy where material collects in the pleural cavity.
Dose: 6c, twice daily on a long-term basis

Baryta carb

Worth trying where the cough is dry and where there is mucus in the chest but the horse lacks the effort to try to expel the material. The cough is eased by being outside in the fresh air but worse for changes in the weather. The lymph nodes are nearly always enlarged where this remedy is needed.
Dose: 6c, twice daily on a long-term basis

Baryta mur

The symptoms are similar to those associated with Baryta carb. However, the mucus, which collects in large amounts, causes rattling in the chest and is coughed up only with difficulty. Dosing with this remedy helps expectoration and eases coughing. Works well where there are associated cardiac problems.
Dose: 6c, twice daily on a long-term basis

Coccus cacti

Coccus cacti will help with coughs where there is thick, tough white mucus which has accumulated in the region at the back of the throat. The mucus is sufficiently thick that it is coughed up only with great difficulty almost causing a suffocating effect. This is also a remedy for chronic bronchitis.
Dose: 30c, twice daily on a long-term basis

Chronic Obstructive Pulmonary Disease (COPD)
Heaves, Equine Asthma, Broken Wind
Recurrent Airway Obstruction (RAO)
Summer Pasture Associated Obstructive Pulmonary Disease (SPAOPD)

COPD and SPAOPD (which occurs during the summer months) have become the most common causes of chronic coughing in the horse. Both conditions are a little like asthma in humans and involve inflammation of the lungs and consequent secretion of mucus that can obstruct the airways. This occurs with a spasm-like constriction of the airways which limits oxygen uptake and makes breathing difficult. More recently however, it has been suggested that the condition be renamed RAO in view of the fact that the underlying nature of this condition is different in horses compared to humans from which the term COPD was originally taken.

The underlying problem in both instances is allergy based, with susceptible horses developing a hypersensitivity reaction to the inhalation of specific allergens. These commonly include fungal spores (*Micropolyspora* and *Aspergillus* species) from hay or straw where COPD is concerned. Plant based allergens, especially pollens such as rapeseed or linseed and those from trees or grasses are implicated in SPAOPD. These conditions can however, sometimes occur in horses that have had viral or bacterial infections. This is likely to happen if management is poor or the horse is returned to work too quickly as the respiratory tract has not had time to recover and is sensitive to potential allergens and pollutants.

Horses under two years of age are rarely affected, with most cases occurring in horses between six and ten years old. Symptoms, which can develop quickly once the horse has been exposed to the underlying allergens, vary with the severity of the disease and can take several forms:

Mild symptoms. This is basically just an intermittent stable cough which occurs when the horse is exposed to hay or straw in the stable environment. If the horse is turned out the cough abates.

Moderate symptoms. This involves a more persistent chronic cough with some difficulty breathing, slightly increased respiratory rate and expiratory effort. Yellow mucus is usually coughed up and there will be a slight nasal discharge.

Severe symptoms. Normally referred to as broken wind, the symptoms are very pronounced. These include a chronic cough (with production of thick yellow mucus and a nasal discharge), increased respiratory rate (up to 15–20 breaths per minute), breathing difficulty (check for flared nostrils), wheezing, expiratory effort with development of the heaves line and crackling noises in the chest due to the development of emphysema. Exercise tolerance is poor.

Management of COPD, RAO and SPAOPD

This is as important as any treatment if the condition is to be controlled successfully. Affected horses should be kept outside for as much time as practical. Remember to groom and to always muck out while your horse is outside. Aim to reduce exposure to hay and straw dust by using substitutes. For bedding consider shredded paper or shavings as alternatives, removing soiled material on a daily basis. This prevents the build up of ammonia which can irritate the respiratory tract.

Dampen down or preferably soak any hay in mild cases, and consider feeding vacuum packed hay or ensiled grass in conjunction with a cubed or pelleted diet in more severe cases. Short crop forage chaffs such as alfalfa and oat straw mixes make good hay substitutes.

Try to keep the stable as dust free as possible by vacuuming on a regular basis, including those stables which share the same airspace. Remember that allergens can travel considerable distances and that affected horses should be stabled as far away as practical from any straw or hay store.

Treating COPD, RAO and SPAOPD

Selecting the most appropriate remedy to treat these conditions is not always easy. Ideally aim to choose a constitutional remedy where possib… likely to achieve the best results. Otherwi… remedy on a symptomatic basis as carefully as… can.

Remember to think of any predisposing or intervening factors that may be implicated in the development of the disease. If the condition has arisen shortly after vaccination consider using: **Thuja 200c** *once daily for five days or if this has no effect try* **Silica 200c** *once daily for five days or* **Antimonium tartrate 30c**. **Potentised vaccine 200c,** *given once daily for five days, is also worth considering.*

Constitutional remedies for COPD, RAO and SPAOPD

Dose: 200c once daily for seven days

Arsenicum album

Suited to thin, lean, neat thoroughbred types.

Attacks are spasmodic and worse at night around midnight. The animal shows signs of restlessness and anxiety. Fear can predominate and there may be a reluctance to lie down as symptoms are eased by standing. Respiration is wheezing in nature.

Pulsatilla

Suited to gentle, sensitive animals, often, but not always, mares.

Symptoms include a dry cough that is worse in the evening and in warmer weather. There is a notable bland yellow nasal discharge that is at its worst in the morning

Nux vomica

Matches the tense, eager and irritable or touchy horse which over reacts to any stimulus. This type of horse is prone to digestive problems and is normally lean in stature.

The cough associated with this remedy is tight and hacking. Symptoms are worse after eating and in the morning.

Lycopodium

Suited to apprehensive horses that lack confidence and which always prefer company human or otherwise. Digestive problems are common, specially flatulence.

Check for a deep, hollow cough with expectoration that is greyer in colour. Symptoms are worse between 4pm and 8pm and often affect the right-hand side of the chest more than the left. The chest is often very wheezy due to an accumulation of catarrh. A characteristic Lycopodium sign is flapping of the outer edge of the nostrils in time with breathing.

Silica

The Silica type matches those animals which have a weaker constitution and which lack both physical and mental capability. Their general resistance to disease is less than most horses but they do have a level of self-will, yet lack confidence in new situations.

Silica suits more chronic cases and is sometimes used after Pulsatilla. Check for a thick nasal discharge or thick lumpy yellow mucus coughed up onto the stable floor or walls. The mucus collects in the airways and leads to noisy rattling breathing.

Sulphur

Outwardly Sulphur types appear robust yet unrefined with a poor coat which looks untidy and which lacks shine. There is a tendency to develop skin problems and a dislike of being groomed or washed. Heat is avoided. Sulphur horses normally have an extremely good appetite.

This is another remedy for chronic cases, although it can be used in cases that are not responding to an indicated remedy. (If this happens give **Sulphur 200c** once daily for five days and then try the original remedy again.) Breathing can appear laboured or difficult with rattling noises due to the mucus that accumulates in the chest. There is a desire for fresh air and symptoms can be worse around 11am in the morning.

Symptomatic remedies

***Dose:** with the 30c potency twice daily as needed*

Antimonium tartrate

Use where there is difficulty breathing accompanied by coarse rattling noises in the chest. This is due to large amounts of mucus which is not easily coughed up. The horse may appear slightly drowsy and irritable if disturbed too much. Suitable for more severe cases and for elderly horses.

Allium cepa

Useful for very mild symptoms where there is nothing more than a clear watery nasal discharge accompanied by sneezing and possibly a discharge from the eyes, which irritates the skin. There is a mild hacking cough worse for breathing in cold air.

Arsenicum iodatum

Matches where the symptoms include a thin watery nasal discharge which makes the nostrils sore or where there is a chronic thick yellow nasal discharge. Sneezing is frequent together with a slight dry hacking cough.

Bacillinum

For severe cases where there are bubbly noises in the chest, difficult breathing and a cough that brings up thick, coloured mucus. Symptoms are worse in the early morning.

Balsamun peruvium

Used for the most chronic cases where there is an extremely thick creamy nasal discharge and loose cough.

Blatta orientalis

Blatta works well where Arsenicum album does not appear to help as much as anticipated and especially where bronchitis has developed as a consequence of COPD/RAO.

Ipecacuanha

An emergency remedy that is often used for severe cases where the horse's symptoms are very pronounced and include wheezing and gasping for air. The chest is full of mucus that is coughed up relatively easily and may hang from the animal's mouth or nostrils.

Lobelia

A good general remedy for COPD/RAO where there is difficulty breathing and evidence of a heaves line developing. It is best used where the symptoms arise due to spasmodic constriction of the airways. Can be used in very elderly horses where emphysema has developed.

Natrum sulph

Symptoms are exacerbated by damp weather or surroundings and include a loose cough with rattling in the chest. You should also look for greenish mucus coughed up onto the stable floor. This remedy is excellent for younger horses that develop COPD after a respiratory infection or pneumonia.

Sabadilla

Sabadilla is used for very minor symptoms that would be similar to hay fever. Look for a watery nasal discharge (which is profuse) accompanied by redness of the eyes and increased tear production.

Sambucus

This remedy is worth trying where the underlying cause is hay or straw dust. Mucus collects in the laryngeal area leading to suffocative explosive bouts of coughing almost as if the animal was going to suffocate.

There are a wide number of other remedies that can be used to help with COPD, RAO and SPAOPD. Check the remedies under the coughs section especially **Spongia**, **Kali carb** and **Kali bich**.

Potentised allergens

Potentised allergens can also be used alongside recommended remedies. Think about using **Hay dust**, **Mixed pollens**, **Rapeseed pollen** or **Linseed pollen** where appropriate, all in the *30c potency given twice daily.*

Some horses exhibit symptoms only during very specific periods of time which may be of short duration. At these times only one or two specific plants may be producing pollen and are responsible for the horse developing signs. In such cases it is possible to use specific potentised pollens to help treat the condition. The following guide is useful in deciding which plants or trees may be implemented in treatment.

Pollen calendar

Feb–Apr	Hazel, Alder
Feb–May	Elm
Apr–May	Birch
Mar–May	Plane
Apr–June	Oak
May–Sept	Grasses
May–June	Mugwort
June–July	Elder, Lime
May–Oct	Nettles
June–Aug	Ragweed
Aug–Nov	Fungal spores

There are also some good combinations of potentised allergens to consider using. R84 Inhalant Allergy Drops from Dr Reckeweg have proved useful. See suppliers list, page 495.

Pulmonary Haemorrhage, Exercise-Induced Pulmonary Haemorrhage (EIPH)

This condition occurs when bleeding occurs into the lung tissue following exercise. EIPH can affect any type or breed of horse. Mechanical stress placed on the delicate tissues of the lung can traumatise the cells causing them to rupture and bleed. It is not known for certain why this happens but any pre-existing respiratory problem is likely to increase the chance of haemorrhage occurring.

The degree of bleeding can vary considerably. Small haemorrhages will go undetected but larger amounts will cause bright red blood to appear at both nostrils and will impair performance. There is no satisfactory conventional treatment but homeopathic remedies can be very useful in preventing and treating the condition.

In all cases dose with the 30c potency every 10–15 minutes until bleeding ceases. In prevention, give a single dose of the 200c potency just before exercising.

Aconite
Use aconite where there is haemorrhage from over exertion and as a preventative in tense anxious horses.

Rhus tox
Haemorrhage occurring after exercise when the horse is at rest. The blood is bright red and the bleeding is worse when the head is lowered.

Phosphorus
Often effective and suited to young, lean, athletic animals with a sensitive nature. The blood tends to be of a bright red watery consistency.

Ferrum metallicum and Ferrum phos (combination)
Best used for younger animals and where the condition is more severe.

Ipecacuanha
Indicated for persistent cases where haemorrhage occurs easily even with very moderate exercise. There is nearly always difficulty in breathing when Ipecac is needed and the blood from the nose appears in small gushes.

Millefolium
This remedy has similar indications to Ipecacuanha and has proved extremely useful in practice.

Melilotus
Use mainly after exercise where bleeding does not stop quickly. Haemorrhage from the nose is normally profuse.

Ficus religiosa
Indicated as a preventative remedy where pulmonary haemorrhage leads to obvious difficulty in breathing.

Erechthites
A specific remedy for haemorrhage from the lungs. Use where the bleeding is profuse and does not stop readily. Erechthites can be differentiated from other remedies by the fact that the heartbeat will be fast and pulse strong and rapid.

For chronic cases there are some remedies that can help tone up and strengthen the nasal blood vessels. The following are worth trying:

Calc fluor and Ferrum phos
Used for younger horses.
Dose: *twice weekly with each remedy in the 30c potency for two to three months*

Baryta carb
Use this remedy to try to strengthen the blood vessels in any age of horse. Older horses will benefit especially.
Dose: *twice weekly with the 30c potency for two to three months*

The Heart and Circulation

Heart and circulatory problems always need thorough investigation to determine the exact nature of any problem and to get an accurate prognosis. Some conditions may not always be very obvious in the early stages as the performance of the horse may be unaffected. Remember that advanced cardiac disease may cause the horse to drop suddenly with risk not only to itself, but to the rider as well.

Homeopathic remedies should be considered as additional support to any advice or treatment that your vet suggests. Selecting an appropriate remedy will depend a lot on the way your horse's heart sounds through a stethoscope and from the character and feel of the pulse. The average pulse rate for an adult horse is between 30 and 44 beats per minute. For very young foals the average is around 80 per minute.

Conditions that affect the heart broadly fall into three categories:

- Murmurs
- Arrhythmias
- Inflammatory conditions which include endocarditis, myocarditis and pericarditis

Murmurs

Distorted or fibrosed (scarred) valves in the heart usually occur as a result of endocarditis and will cause turbulence or interference with the flow of blood leading to abnormal sounds which are called murmurs. Murmurs are classified according to intensity, quality and pitch. Using these details your vet should be able to give you additional information that might help select a suitable remedy. The three main valves that can be affected are the mitral, tricuspid and aortic valves, which can become either narrowed or distorted. Symptoms of valvular murmurs include poor performance, abnormal pulse rate and oedema (swelling), affecting the limbs or brisket due to poor circulation.

Arrhythmias

Disturbances in the rhythm of the heart as opposed to valvular damage, are referred to as arrhythmias. These affect the way the heart beats and cause it to pump the blood inefficiently. The most minor is a dropped beat, often regarded as insignificant, but more serious arrythmias such as atrial fibrillation, can cause significant and worrying problems.

Murmurs and arrythmias – selecting a remedy

The remedies listed provide a general overview of the most commonly used remedies, together with suitable potencies and doses. It is not uncommon to combine cardiac remedies. For example, Cactus and Crataegus are often used together as a general tonic for the heart.

Cactus grandiflorus
Acts best where the mitral valve is affected and where the heart and pulse rate are both increased and forceful as the heart tries to compensate. Cramp-like pains in the heart may cause the horse to halt suddenly.
Dose: *1x potency three times daily*

Crataegus
This remedy is a good general tonic for the heart and excellent for helping with any chronic heart problem. Crataegus also helps improve the circulation and is useful where the legs swell. In contrast to Cactus, the heart muscle is weaker and although the pulse is quicker, it is feeble. This

remedy is said to regulate blood pressure.
Dose: *1x potency three times daily*

Digitalis

Check for a slow pulse and irregular heartbeat. The heart is enlarged as it tries to compensate, yet the heart muscle is weaker. Indicated more for mitral valve problems. The least amount of exercise or exertion sends the pulse racing immediately.
Dose: *6c three times daily*

Lycopus virginicus

A rapid and forceful heartbeat characterises this remedy although the pulse is weaker, irregular or intermittent. Lycopus will help reduce the heart rate and lower the blood pressure. Useful where there is also a dry cough, where a small amount of blood is coughed up.
Dose: *6c three times daily*

Convallaria

Convallaria increases the energy of the heart and helps regulate the heartbeat. It is useful where the heart is enlarged and where the circulation is sluggish. Check for a rapid and irregular pulse.
Dose: *3x potency three times daily*

Strophanthus hispidus

Used to tone the heart especially where the heart muscle is weak and there is a tendency for fluid to collect as a result of poor circulation. The mitral valve is diseased and the pulse rate is increased. Indicated where the lungs are congested and where there may be some difficulty in breathing.
Dose: *6x potency three times daily*

Adonis vernalis

Adonis is mainly used to help remove oedematous fluid from the limbs where the circulation is weakened. Check for a slow, weak pulse. Suited to animals that lack vitality.
Dose: *1x potency three times daily*

Laurocerasus

Used where the mitral valve is damaged and where the mucous membranes are dark (cyanotic) in colour due to poor blood perfusion. The pulse is difficult to feel and feeble in character. Laurocerasus can also be used to stimulate breathing in newborn foals, where the animal is gasping for breath and the membranes are cyanosed.
Dose: *for regular use the 3x potency three times daily*
To revive foals, use the mother tincture Ø, *two drops every five minutes*

Kalmia

Check for a slow, weak pulse together with a stiff, stilted gait. The shoulder region may be especially stiff and pain in the lower back may also be apparent.
Dose: *6x potency three times daily*

Spongia

Used in older horses where there is reduced exercise tolerance accompanied by an increased respiratory rate and some slight difficulty in breathing. The underlying cause is damaged or distorted valves leading to a murmur. Check for a rapid pulse, distended superficial blood vessels and a dry cough for clues to using Spongia.
Dose: *30c twice daily*

Inflammatory Conditions

Endocarditis

Inflammation of the membrane lining the heart chambers is called endocarditis and can be caused by a bacterial infection or much more rarely, parasites. Symptoms include initial fever and poor pulse. The condition ultimately leads to damage to the heart valves. Suitable remedies include:

Aconite

Use in early stages as soon as the condition is diagnosed. The pulse will be full and bounding at this stage and the blood vessels will pulse. The horse will appear anxious.
Dose: *1M potency every 15 minutes for four doses then re-assess*

Naja

This is the most important remedy for helping with acute endocarditis. The pulse is irregular and

gradually slows. The body temperature drops as the heart becomes weaker and weaker. If the animal recovers the heart valves are left damaged.
Dose: *30c, dose at 15 minute intervals.*

Other appropriate remedies which could be given at *15 minute intervals,* include **Cactus grandiflorus 1x**, **Convallaria 3x** and **Adonis vernalis 1x**. Try to choose the remedy that most closely matches your horse's symptoms.

Another useful remedy that can be given alongside those listed is **Calc fluor**, which may help reduce the damage that occurs to the valves.
Use the 30c potency twice daily

Myocarditis

Myocarditis is inflammation of the heart muscle and can occur as a secondary complication to conditions such as strangles or navel ill. The heart muscle becomes damaged leading to a weakening of the heart and compensatory enlargement over time. Affected horses will show exercise intolerance, breathing difficulty and oedema in advanced cases.

Suitable supportive remedies include **Crataegus 1x**, **Adonis vernalis 1x**, **Digitalis 6c** and **Strophanthus hispidus 6x**.
Dose: *three times daily*

Pericarditis

The pericardium is the lining that covers the outside of the heart, enclosing it within a sac. Inflammation of the pericardium, pericarditis, occurs as the result of either a bacterial or viral infection and can arise as a complication in conditions such pneumonia, pleurisy or strangles.

This is a serious condition, initially commencing with a fever and a little later, the collection of fluid within the pericardial sac itself. This interferes with the action of the heart leading to a thin, wiry but fast pulse, pain over the chest wall, reluctance to move, a tendency to hold the front legs in together and muffling of the heart sounds. Long-term consequences include the development of adhesions and chronic heart failure.

In the early stages dose with **Aconite 1M** *every 15 minutes* and re-assess the case after four or five doses. Treatment should then follow with an appropriate remedy:

Spigelia

This is the remedy most often used to help treat pericarditis in the acute stages. Symptoms match closely those of the disease including the reluctance to move, chest pain and weak pulse.
Dose: *30c, dose at 15 minute intervals*

Apis

Will help reduce the amount of fluid in the pericardial sac and relieve the pressure on the heart.
Suggested potency *200c, three times daily*

Spongia

Useful after the acute stages, where symptoms of heart failure are apparent such as a dry cough.
Suggested potency 30c, three times daily

Other remedies to consider include **Colchicum 30c**, **Cantharis 30c** and **Bryonia 30c** in the acute stage and other supportive cardiac remedies later as already listed. **Calc fluor 30c** and **Acetic acid 30c** in combination can be used to help reduce the chances of adhesions forming between the pericardial sac and heart muscle.
Dose: *twice daily alongside other remedies for several months*

The Blood and Blood Vessels

Blood is pumped around the body through a series of blood vessels, comprising arteries, veins and capillaries, by the heart and forms part of a vital transportation system. It carries important nutrients to every area and part of the body as well as removing waste products. It distributes oxygen to the tissues and removes carbon dioxide, delivers hormones to their target areas, regulates fluid and electrolytes, encompasses the body's main defence mechanisms and is involved with temperature regulation. Blood has three fundamental components: red cells (erythrocytes), white cells (leucocytes) and plasma, the fluid in which the cells are suspended.

Conditions Relating to the Blood and Blood Vessels

Haemorrhage

Haemorrhage or bleeding can occur as the result of an injury or as a consequence of surgery. The nature of the bleeding and the type of blood are important in selecting an appropriate remedy, which should be used as an interim measure while waiting for help. Don't forget the importance of first aid techniques such as pressure bandaging to help stop severe bleeding.

The following are general remedies for haemorrhage, which should be used in the 30c potency and given at intervals of between 10 and 20 minutes depending on the urgency of the situation. In fact any potency of the remedy will do in an emergency rather than giving no treatment at all. More specific remedies can be found in other relevant sections within the book.

Aconite
Haemorrhage with bright red blood with accompanying anxiety, restlessness or panic.

Arnica
Best used for bleeding caused by injury. Excellent where mucous membranes are involved or where there is oozing of dark blood. Use routinely before and after surgery to help limit bruising and bleeding.

Carbo veg
Use where there is bleeding associated with collapse. Dark blood oozes or seeps slowly. The limbs, body and tongue appear cold to the touch.

China
Indicated where the animal is collapsed or debilitated and where there has been a steady loss of blood over a long period of time. Dehydration may be evident.

Crotalus horridus
Indicated where the haemorrhage is of very dark blood, almost black, which remains fluid, as clotting does not occur readily. This type of bleeding can be associated with certain types of infection and poisons.

Ferrum phos
Haemorrhage of bright red blood which is profuse and which clots readily.

Hamamelis
Helps where there is bleeding characterised by dark blood that does not clot quickly. The flow is steady with a persistent ooze and often stems from passive venous congestion.

Ipecacuanha
Helps where there is haemorrhage of bright red

blood that comes in gushes or spurts and is persistent. Heavy breathing is another guiding symptom.

Lachesis
Useful where there is passive bleeding of dark, watery blood. The skin surrounding the source of the blood is darkly discoloured with a purple or blue hue. Bleeding of this type can be linked with sepsis or infection.

Melilotus
Best reserved for bright red haemorrhage from the mouth or nose.

Millefolium
Indicated for haemorrhage of bright red blood caused by trauma. A rise in body temperature is a symptom to check for.

Phosphorus
Phosphorus is of most value in treating persistent small capillary haemorrhages, where the blood is bright red and comes in fits and starts.

Strontium carbonate
Best used after surgery where there is slow seepage of blood from the operation site.

Haematomas

This is similar to a blood blister but on a larger scale and is essentially a passive haemorrhage of venous blood which collects under the skin. The most common site for a haematoma to occur in the horse is in the brisket region. Other sites include the flanks, rump area and occasionally the ear. Underlying causes include trauma or from toxins (in mouldy hay for example) which can damage the capillaries causing leakage of blood.
A good remedy combination to use to speed prompt resolution of a haematoma is **Arnica** combined with **Hamamelis** both in **30c potency** and given twice daily. Where there is a recurrent problem dose with either with **Lachesis 200c, Crotalus horridus 200c** or **Phosphorus 200c** three times weekly for one month. If this fails to help consider giving **Secale 200c** twice weekly for one month.

In the rare instances where a haematoma becomes infected, dose with:
Lachesis 200c If the skin is discoloured
Silica 200c If the area is painless
Hepar sulph 1M If the area of infection is sensitive to the least touch
Dose: four times daily until resolved. This may take several weeks

Anaemia

This is a reduction in the number of red blood cells circulating in the blood. Symptoms vary with the underlying cause but can include pale mucous membranes, weakness, increased respiratory rate and poor pulse. Jaundice and the presence of haemoglobin in the urine can be signs of haemolytic anaemia.

There are three main types of anaemia:

Blood loss anaemia

This can be associated with injury, guttural pouch mycosis, parasites and some forms of poisoning such as warfarin. Haemorrhage remedies are all useful in dealing with the underlying cause. **China** is particularly good where the animal has become debilitated and **Crot horr** is useful where warfarin poisoning is the cause.
For either remedy use the 30c potency two or three times daily as needed.
Arsenicum album is a good general remedy to help resolve anaemia after blood loss.
Use the 30c potency once daily for as long as needed.

Anaemia due to bone marrow depression

This can occur as the result of using certain types of drugs, from long-standing infections (which may produce toxins) or from some types of cancer. Iron deficiency, malnutrition and the effects from some poisons can also be included in the list of causes. **Ferrum metallicum** is useful where the cause is iron deficiency or where young animals are affected. **Calc phos** is also useful for young anaemic animals and in any long-standing case of anaemia. **Silica** is indicated where there are nutritional causes.

Plumbum is valuable where poisoning is suspected or where drugs are the cause and especially where there is muscle wasting. Think of using **Merc sol** where the bone marrow has been damaged by toxins.
Use the chosen remedy in the 30c potency twice daily

Haemolytic anaemia

In this form of anaemia the red cells are damaged and destroyed. Underlying causes include some types of infection (although not in the UK), certain poisons and autoimmune disease. The most useful remedies in treating this problem are **TNT**, **Chininum sulph**, **Manganum acetate** and **Lycopodium**.
Use the chosen remedy in the 30c potency three or four times daily

Haemolytic anaemia of the newborn foal, Neonatal isoerythrolysis

This disease occurs mainly in thoroughbreds and affects foals between 12 and 36 hours old. Affected foals inherit red cell antigens from the stallion that the mare does not have. In late pregnancy the mare produces antibodies to these antigens but the foal is not affected, as they do not cross the placental barrier. Although the foal is normal at birth, soon after taking colostrum containing the antibodies (which cross into the foal's circulation), the foal's red blood cells are attacked and damaged or haemolysed to varying degrees. Symptoms include weakness, reluctance to suck, yawning and difficult breathing. Mucous membranes become pale and jaundice can develop as a result of the massive breakdown of the damaged red blood cells.

Treatment is normally by blood transfusion. In the acute phase treat with **TNT** alternating with **Manganum actetate**, both in *30c potency dosing every 30 minutes* to limit damage to the red blood cells. The following remedies can help in the recovery phase:

China
To help with general weakness
Use the 30c potency three times daily

Phosphorus
To assist recovery where jaundice is present
Use the 30c potency once daily for as long as needed

Chelidonium
This remedy is best used alongside Phosphorus to help the liver where there is severe jaundice.
Use the 30c potency once daily for as long as needed

Calc phos and Ferrum metallicum
Acting more on the nutritional side, both these remedies are useful in helping resolve the anaemia.
For each remedy use the 30c potency once daily until the foal has recovered

Oedema

This is the collection of fluid within the tissue spaces and is a little like water logging. Affected areas can become puffy and the swellings pit under pressure. Oedematous fluid can also collect around the heart and within the chest and abdominal cavities. Underlying causes include liver or kidney disease, allergic reactions, circulatory problems, inappropriate feeding and damage to blood vessel walls by toxins. The following are general remedies for oedema, but also check those listed under the section on the heart.

Apis mel
This is the principal remedy for oedema wherever the fluid has collected regardless of cause. It is normally the most effective remedy where the legs have filled.
Dose: *30c potency two or three times daily until the problem has resolved*

Arsenicum album
Suitable where oedematous fluid has collected as the result of allergy based problems including where there is swelling around the eyes or where the legs have filled. Suits animals of an anxious, restless nature.
Dose: *30c potency three times daily*

Apocynum cannabinum
One of the most useful remedies where the skin is affected or where there is fluid within the chest or abdomen due to circulatory problems.
Dose: 6c potency three times daily

Liatris spicata
A general remedy to consider using where there is oedema due to liver, kidney or heart disease.
Dose: 6x potency three times daily

Lycopodium
Useful where fluid has collected due to nutritional or liver problems, particularly in the abdomen (ascites).
Dose: 30c potency twice daily

Urtica urens
Useful where fluid has collected as a result of an allergic reaction.
Dose: 6c potency three times daily

Prunus spinosa
Indicated specifically where the limbs are swollen and an alternative to use if Apis is not effective.
Dose: 6c potency three times daily

Angioneurotic oedema

This is the sudden appearance of subcutaneous oedema (fluid under the skin) due to an acute allergic reaction. It is most likely to occur to horses out at pasture that is in flower. The area most affected is the head (particularly the muzzle and eyelids), although the perineal and vulval areas and udder region can also be affected. There is usually a mild degree of irritation, which shows as headshaking and rubbing. Sometimes just the eyes are involved, which become very puffy with increased tear production and protrusion of the third eyelid.

Apis 200c and **Urtica 200c** are general remedies to think about using in treating this condition. You should also check the following, which are often just as effective where the symptoms match.

Antipyrine
This is a specific remedy for this condition and will help particularly where the eyelids are involved. Check for puffiness of the lids, red conjunctival membranes and increased lachrymation (tear production).
Dose: 6c potency hourly until the signs have cleared

Bovista
Useful where the condition affects large areas and where the allergic reaction is extensive. Look for areas of skin that pit deeply on pressure.
Dose: 30c potency hourly until the symptoms have cleared

Medusa
Indicated where the face is extensively involved with a puffy appearance.
Dose: 200c potency every two hours until the symptoms have cleared

Vespa
This remedy is useful where the membranes of the eye are extremely swollen and where there are swellings over the skin which are itchy.
Dose: 30c potency hourly until the symptoms have cleared

Hepar sulph
Hepar sulph is best suited to chronic cases where the condition is recurrent and affected areas tend to become infected and sensitive to touch.
Dose: 200c potency three times weekly

Proteus
This bowel nosode can often be effective in treating this problem and will help in recurrent cases where it can be used as an intercurrent remedy in cases that are responding poorly.
Dose: 200c twice daily for five days

Verminous Aneurysm and Arteritis Thromboembolic Colic

This condition is caused by migration of parasitic larvae associated with Strongyl worms into the walls of one of the main arteries (and its branches) supplying the intestines. Surprisingly it is not uncommon and leads to inflammation of the artery walls or arteritis. The result is a restriction of blood supply to the bowel causing symptoms of recurrent spasmodic colic in some animals. In rare instances there is secondary infection with bacteria leading to a weakening of the artery wall (an aneurysm) with more pronounced colic symptoms. Abscessation can be a further consequence or the blood vessels can become occluded completely leading to necrosis of the bowel causing thromboembolic colic. These conditions have serious consequences and highlight the importance of regular worming.

Colic symptoms should be treated accordingly but the following remedy can help with acute episodes of thromboembolic colic.

Bothrops lanciolatus
This is the principal remedy for thromboembolic colic as noted from its action on blood vessels. It will help relieve the symptoms of thrombosis and attempt to establish blood flow through the affected vessels. It can be used in conjunction with other colic remedies that focus more on pain.
Dose: 30c every 10–15 minutes

Where arteritis or an aneurysm is suspected consider:

Baryta carb
This remedy acts on the muscular walls of blood vessels and will strengthen arteries particularly where an aneurysm is suspected. It is better suited to younger or very aged animals.
Dose: 30c potency once daily

Lycopodium
Another remedy indicated where an aneurysm is suspected, suiting animals with a lean stature and apprehensive but gentle nature.
Dose: 30c potency once daily

Calc fluor and Acetic acid
This remedy combination will help dissolve away the inflammatory deposits that form on the walls of affected vessels.
Dose: 6c potency of each in combination once daily

Kali iod
This is a general remedy to use where arteritis is suspected.
Dose: 30c potency once daily

Fluoric acid
Use where there is known blood vessel damage especially in older horses.
Dose: 6c potency twice daily

Blood Clots

Rarely blood clots can form in some of the larger blood vessels without any real identifiable cause. The only symptom you may observe will be a swelling in the area or region of the body supplied by the blood vessel concerned. Time is often all that is needed to resolve the problem as the clot shrinks while at the same time the blood may find an alternative route around the site of the obstruction. Several remedies may help the clot to shrink and dissolve away. Ideal remedies to try include:
In the initial stages **Bothrops 200c**
Where there is considerable swelling **Apis 200c**
Where there is swelling and to dissipate the clot **Acetic acid 6c**
To break down the clot long term **Thiosinaminum 6c**
Dose: twice daily

Iliac Thrombosis

A thrombus is a blood clot forming within the circulation leading to thrombosis or the blockage of a blood vessel, in this case the iliac artery or arteries, and occasionally the last section of the aorta or femoral arteries. Parasitic arteritis (caused by larval forms of Strongylus vulgaris) affecting the aorta or iliac arteries is the most common underlying cause in the horse. The condition takes two forms. In the milder version there is only lameness on exercise, with the symptoms abating quickly after rest. In the more severe cases there is hind leg weakness. One of the legs may give way when the horse turns. Pain and anxiety with an increase in pulse and respiratory rate are also evident. The affected leg or legs may feel cold compared to normal. The horse may also sweat but sweat is absent over the skin covering the affected area of the leg.

Remedies to help with iliac thrombosis

Bothrops lanciolatus
This is the most important remedy for this particular condition, helping to reduce the risk of a thrombus formation and in treating the acute phase. In addition to the symptoms already mentioned, trembling is a feature where this remedy is useful.
Dose: *30c potency twice daily as a preventative; 200c potency every ten minutes in the acute phase*

Lachesis
Can be considered as an alternative to Bothrops where more suited constitutionally or where the remedy fails to work.
Dose: *30c potency twice daily as a preventative; 200c potency every 30 minutes in the acute phase*

Vipera
Vipera is best suited to more severe cases where hind limb weakness and cramp like pain is very evident. Where necessary this remedy can be combined with Bothrops.
Dose: *30c potency twice daily as a preventative; 200c potency every 30 minutes in the acute phase*

Secale
This is best used in treating severe cases where cramping muscle pain is very evident and the affected leg feels cold due to impairment of the circulation.
Dose: *200c potency every 15 minutes in the acute phase*

Calc fluor, Acetic acid and Thiosinaminum
This combination can be used in later stages to dissolve away deposits within the iliac arteries to improve the circulation.
Dose: *6c potency of each in combination once daily over several weeks*

Purpura Haemorrhagica

This is a serious non-contagious condition that can be a sequel to an upper respiratory tract infection. The exact cause is unknown but it is suspected that it may arise due to an immunological reaction to streptococcal bacteria, including Strep equi, the cause of strangles. Signs appear suddenly between two and four weeks after an infection and vary in severity. The chief symptoms are extensive oedematous and haemorrhagic swellings under the skin caused by damage to blood vessels. Affected horses are depressed, appear stiff and are reluctant to move. In addition to well-defined areas of oedema (especially on the body, face and muzzle, less so on the upper limbs), there are small haemorrhages on the visible mucous membranes. Where the fluid build up is extensive, there will be difficulty eating and breathing and the legs may exude serum. Bacterial infection can complicate matters.

Treatment should be combined with conventional medicines to improve the chances of survival and carefully selected according to the symptoms.

Remedies to reduce oedema

Apis
An important remedy to use in the earliest stages to reduce oedema and swelling regardless of location.
Dose: *200c hourly until symptoms improve then three times daily*

Bovista
Another remedy to reduce oedematous swellings where large areas are affected and suitable where there are haemorrhages still visible on the mucous membranes.
Dose: *200c hourly until symptoms improve then three times daily*

Medusa
Use specifically where swelling around the face and muzzle is very marked.
Dose: *200c hourly until symptoms improve then three times daily*

Remedies to limit haemorrhage and its consequences

Phosphorus

Indicated where small haemorrhages on mucous membranes are particularly prominent.
Dose: 200c three times daily

Sulphuric acid

A good alternative, particularly if the animal is in a more debilitated or weakened state.
Dose: 30c three times daily

Crotalus horridus

This is the prime remedy for treating this condition and should be used as soon as the condition is diagnosed as the remedy picture matches closely the signs of this disease even where there are secondary bacterial complications.
Dose: 200c hourly until symptoms improve, then three times daily

Other snake venom remedies are also useful. **Lachesis 30c** is a good second choice where there is a poor response to Crotalus and where symptoms are more marked on the left-hand side and where the throat area is very swollen. **Bothrops 30c** is also worth considering.

Remedies to help with recovery

Hamamelis

This will help reduce haemorrhagic swellings in the later stages of the disease.
Dose: 30c twice daily

Arnica 30c is also useful, especially where there are secondary bacterial complications and difficulty in moving due to muscular soreness. **Sulphuric acid 30c** is also useful in resolving the after effects of haemorrhage. These remedies can be given twice daily.

The Lymphatic System

This is a complex network of fine vessels, which runs throughout the whole body. These contain lymphatic fluid, or lymph, which gradually drains towards the heart with the flow assisted by natural massage as muscles and tendons contract. Some of the vessels contain valves preventing back flow of lymph and at various points there are lymphatic glands, which help to filter the fluid, and which play a part in the immune system.

The lymphatic system functions to drain excess fluid from the body, particularly the limbs, so that they do not swell. This is the fluid which surrounds the cells of the body and which bathes them. When the flow of fluid into the lymphatic system is blocked, the tissues will become swollen or waterlogged, a condition referred to as oedema, characterised by swelling which pits upon pressure. There is a fine fluid balance within the body between water within the spaces between the cells, the blood and the lymphatic system. Any imbalance results in oedema. Factors that influence this include levels of protein, sodium and potassium within the blood, toxins or allergic reactions that can affect the permeability of the walls of the blood vessels (causing excess leakage of fluid and proteins). The level of exercise, concurrent disease (especially liver and heart problems and conditions such as lymphangitis and purpura haemorrhagica) and incorrect feeding can also be influencing factors.

Filled Legs

This is a very common condition of horses (often Heavy Hunters) that are stabled overnight and is really more of a management problem rather than an illness. Overfeeding and too little exercise predispose to the problem as this disturbs the balance of proteins and electrolytes within the blood. The legs swell, as excess fluid is not removed against the pull of gravity, causing normally prominent structures, such as tendons to become ill defined. Normally the fluid will quickly disappear on exercise. Where the condition remains a problem, attend to the underlying causes in addition to using any remedies. Keeping the legs bandaged can help.

Apis

This is the most helpful remedy and will assist in removing excess fluid quickly.
Dose: *30c or 200c, two or three doses, 30 minutes apart when needed*

Arsenicum album

This can be used as a constitutional remedy in thoroughbreds that are prone to the condition.
Dose: *30c or 200 c, two or three doses, 30 minutes apart when needed*
Where the fluid is slow to clear it is worth considering cardiac remedies such as **Digitalis 6x** or **Strophanthus 6x** to help.

Lymphangitis

Inflammation of the lymphatic vessels is known as lymphangitis and normally arises as a result of an infection from a wound. Swelling of the lower limbs is the most obvious feature, starting at the top of the leg and extending down to the coronary band. This condition can become chronic with the legs remaining filled, in contrast to the previous condition. In the most severe cases, the inflammation can spread to the surrounding tissues leading to seepage of fluid through the skin and the development of sores. Lymphangitis is a painful condition and usually most horses will be reluctant to weight bear on affected limbs.

In the very early stages **Aconite** (*1M potency*

every 30 minutes for four doses) is useful, followed by **Belladonna** (*1M potency given every 30 minutes*) where there is fever and an elevated pulse rate. Other remedies to follow with include:

Bothrops lanciolatus

Useful where the symptoms are not too advanced and where there is little swelling. The lymphatic vessels in the leg are very prominent.
Dose: 30c three times daily until symptoms resolve

Apis mel

This is the prime remedy for helping to remove fluid when the leg is starting to swell and there is pitting oedema.
Dose: 30c three times daily until symptoms resolve

Bovista

This is a good remedy to use either where Apis fails to work or where fluid is just starting to seep through the skin.
Dose: 30c three times daily until symptoms resolve

Bufo

Bufo is specifically indicated for lymphangitis caused by infection. Affected horses stand apart from others in the herd and movement is difficult with a degree of staggering. Check for exudation of sticky fluid from the skin.
Dose: 200c three times daily

Crot horr

The most severe cases should respond to Crot horr, where there is not only considerable swelling and great discomfort, but seepage of fluid through the skin as well. The skin over the affected areas will be discoloured. An alternative remedy is Lachesis, which has also proved useful.
Dose: 200c three times daily until symptoms resolve

Manganum aceticum

Indicated where there is a secondary cellulitis as surrounding tissues are affected. Check for fluid seepage through the skin, which is infected, and suppurating.
Dose: 30c three times daily until symptoms resolve

Rhus tox

This is an alternative to Manganum aceticum as a treatment for cellulitis. The horse is stiff but the discomfort eases on movement.
Dose: 200c three times daily until symptoms resolve

Sporadic Lymphangitis

Monday morning disease

This non-contagious form of lymphangitis normally occurs in horses that have been overfed and kept in with restricted exercise for a few days. Typically the disease would arise in working horses stabled over the weekend. The lymphatic vessels on the inside of the leg are very visible and the leg will be hot and swollen. Lymph nodes are enlarged. The horse will stop feeding and exhibit thirst along with patchy sweating. Constipation is also a common feature. Look for small wounds and ulcers on the leg, entry points for infection.

Consider using **Aconite** and **Belladonna** in the very early stages and **Apis** or **Bovista** where the symptoms fit in later stages when the acute symptoms have subsided. The most valuable interim remedy to use is:

Bryonia

Use Bryonia after either Aconite or Belladonna. Symptoms which fit this remedy include hot swollen limbs, increased thirst, constipation and reluctance to move. Irritability can also be a feature.
Dose: 200c three times daily until symptoms resolve

Ulcerative Lymphangitis

This is a mildly contagious form of lymphangitis caused by a variety of bacteria including *Corynebacterium pseudotuberculosis*, streptococci and staphylococci. It arises most frequently in horses kept in poor, unhygienic conditions or where overcrowding occurs and follows wounding or cracked heels. One of the first signs is swelling and pain around the pastern or fetlock joints. Nodules then develop in the tissues, following the course of the lymphatic vessels, especially around the fetlock region. These can grow quite large and burst, releasing creamy green pus. Affected areas then ulcerate. Local lymphatic vessels enlarge and become thickened with some of these areas eventually ulcerating. Affected areas will slowly heal, but more nodules and ulcers can occur over a period of several months.

In addition to your selected remedy, the **nosode** of the appropriate bacteria can be used as well.
Dose: *30c potency twice daily for five days*

Arnica
Use as soon as the condition is diagnosed to limit the course of the illness, prior to nodules bursting and discharging pus.
Dose: *200c potency three times daily*

Merc sol
This is the main remedy to use where the nodules have burst and are discharging green pus or where there are deep ragged ulcers that bleed easily when touched.
Dose: *30c three times daily*

Anthracinum
Useful where there is no response to Merc sol, or where crops of discharging nodules keep appearing.
Dose: *30c twice daily*

Hepar sulph
Again, useful where the nodules have burst and ulcerated and where there is discharge of putrid material. Affected areas are very painful and sensitive to touch, standing this remedy apart from the others. Hepar sulph is also useful in the early stages before the infection causes suppuration of the glands if the affected region is sensitive to the slightest touch.
Dose: *200c potency three times daily*

Other useful remedies include **Muriaticum acid 30c** to help heal limb ulcers, **Kali iod 30c** to prevent more nodules appearing and **Silica 30c** to help remove scar tissue and open up the lymphatics if the condition has become chronic.

Lymphadenitis

Inflammation of the lymph nodes is referred to as lymphadenitis and occurs as the result of an infection (such as strangles) or as a consequence of lymphangitis. The enlarged lymph nodes are painful during the acute phase and can be palpated easily. Where they are chronically enlarged, they are often smaller and painless. Local swelling can occur as swollen glands can impede the passage of lymphatic fluid. In the early stages of infection, **Aconite** and **Belladonna** can be useful, remembering **Apis** where there is swelling and heat. In rare cases the lymph nodes can be cancerous and become larger than normal.

Hepar sulph
This is another remedy for situations where the lymph nodes become acutely inflamed and infected. The glands are very tender to touch and the horse may be irritable.
Dose: *200c potency twice daily*

Merc sol
Mercury attacks the lymphatic system and is used homeopathically to treat problems including acute lymphadenitis where the glands are inflamed and the horse appears weak and sweats easily.
Dose: *200c potency three times daily until the symptoms resolve*

Phytolacca
This is an important general remedy for slightly less acute cases where the glands are enlarged, inflamed, painful on palpation and hot. Phytolacca is particularly useful where the glands around the throat are involved and where associated discomfort extends around the neck region making the neck stiff.
Dose: *30c potency three times daily*

Silica
Chronic enlargement of the lymph nodes will often respond to Silica which works best when the glands are painless and indurated or hardened.
Dose: *30c potency twice daily*

Calc fluor

Like Silica, this remedy is useful in treating chronically enlarged glands, working best where the glands are extremely hard and non-pliable.
Dose: *30c potency twice daily*

Other remedies which could be used twice daily, include **Baryta mur** or **Baryta carb 30c** for chronic enlargement of the lymph nodes around the neck in older animals, **Calc carb 30c** where the constitutional type fits (heavy, slow horses) and the glands around the neck are enlarged and **Iodum 30c** where glandular enlargement is accompanied by emaciation. **Scrophularia 6c**, **Conium 6c** and **Cistus canadensis 6c** are indicated where the glands are hardened, chronically enlarged and possibly cancerous.

The Digestive System

This section covers the whole of the digestive system including the mouth, salivary glands and teeth, stomach, small and large intestine and includes important conditions such as colic and diarrhoea.

The Mouth

Teeth

Abscess

True dental disease in the horse is rare although it is possible for teeth roots to become infected in rare instances leading to an abscess. Signs to look out for are swelling on the side of the face or a discharging wound near the lower jaw. Occasionally a nasal discharge may be seen. You will need to call your vet for advice but the following remedies can be used as an interim treatment:

Hepar sulph 200c Where there is pain and sensitivity over the affected area or tooth

Merc sol 200c Where the tooth is decayed or damaged

Silica 200 In chronic cases where little or no pain is evident

Fluoric acid 30c Add where there is a persistent sinus of fistula present

Dose: *twice daily*

Teeth extraction

This mainly applies to the wolf teeth, which are small vestigial teeth with small roots. These can cause problems with the bit and are often easily removed. Cheek teeth can be removed with more difficulty under anaesthetic. Remedies to help include:

Arnica
This will help with bruising and limit tissue damage and bleeding.
Dose: *200c twice daily starting the day before the work is carried out and continuing for five days afterwards*

Phosphorus
This will help stop any bleeding after the teeth have been removed where the blood is bright red in colour.
Dose: *30c three times daily*

Lachesis
This is useful where there is continual oozing of dark blood or where the tooth sockets have become infected afterwards.
Dose: *30c three times daily*

Calendula
For slow healing wounds after dental work has been carried out.
Dose: *6c three times daily*

Hypericum
Where there is pain evident. Can be used routinely in all cases
Dose: *30c three times daily*

Facial paralysis

See Nervous system page 229

Stomatitis and Ulceration of the Mouth Mouth Ulcers

Stomatitis is inflammation of the mouth and results from infection, trauma or ingestion of poisons which lead to areas of ulceration. The presence of ulcers otherwise indicates a poor general state of health and a weakened immune system. It is not a common condition in the horse. Vesicular stomatitis is seen in horses in North and South America and is viral in origin. This particular condition is a notifiable disease in the UK. See page 281.

The following remedies can be used in the *30c potency three times daily* to help resolve ulcers within the mouth:

Merc sol
Use where the mouth is sore and there is drooling of sticky, thick saliva.

Merc cyanatus
Indicated where the membranes inside the mouth are ulcerated and look intensely red and sore.

Kali Chlor
For very severe cases where the whole of the mouth is involved and looks red with dark looking ulcers and salivation. Best used for stomatitis arising from toxins or poisons.

Rhus tox
Use Rhus tox where the tongue is affected and the corners of the mouth are ulcerated or cracked.

Nitric acid
Helps where there are sore ulcerated areas on the roof of the mouth or on the margins of the membranes of the mouth and skin of the lips.

Nux vomica
Use where there are many small, ulcerated areas.

Borax
For small, ulcerated areas where the animal is sensitive to noise or is easily frightened.

Syphilinum
Suitable for unresponsive or refractory cases.

Cracks and Sores Around the Mouth

Conditions which affect the mouth can also affect the skin locally as well as the lips. Trauma, infection or badly fitted tack can also cause problems leading to inflammation and discomfort. The following remedies are useful and can be used in the *30c potency twice daily until the symptoms are clear.*

Nat mur where there are small vesicles around the mouth or where the corners are cracked, ulcerated and dry.

Graphites where there are weepy, sticky sores or where there are crusty scabs.

Nitric acid indicated where there are sores at the junction of the lips and mucous membranes that tend to bleed.

Rhus tox for ulcerated sores at the corners of the mouth or sores around the chin region.

Kreosotum for sores which discharge and excoriate (inflame) the surrounding skin.

Merc sol is useful where there are green, sticky infected areas, which have a bad odour.

Petroleum where the skin is dry cracked and rough. You may also see thick hard greenish scabs. The area around the nostrils may also be affected.

The Salivary Glands

There are three paired salivary glands located on either side of the face, the most important of which are the parotid glands. These lie in the area between the back of the jaw and the bottom of the ear.

Parotiditis

This is inflammation of the parotid salivary gland and is a condition that usually occurs in animals kept at grass and is believed to have an allergic basis. Affected animals look as if they have mumps. Parotiditis will resolve on its own if the animal is kept in but homeopathic remedies can help shorten the recovery time.

Pulsatilla
Use in the initial acute stages as soon as the condition is diagnosed.
Dose: *200c potency twice daily until the condition resolves*

Cistus canadensis
Generally useful where the condition is slow to resolve and the gland feels hard to the touch.
Dose: *30c potency twice daily*

Parotitis

Conditions such as strangles or trauma can lead to severe inflammation of the parotid salivary gland or parotitis. Often only one gland is affected which then becomes hard, swollen and painful. In the initial stages **Belladonna** is a useful remedy (*30c potency given at hourly intervals*) if fever is present, followed by one of the remedies listed. In the later stages the gland may remain hard even after successful treatment. Think about using remedies such as **Bromum**, **Calc fluor** or **Silica** (*6c potency twice daily for several weeks*) to help at this stage.

Merc sol
Indicated where the gland on the right side is affected. The whole region around the gland is painful to touch including the throat area. The horse swallows frequently. Symptoms are worse at night.
Dose: *30c three times daily*

Rhus tox
A good general remedy but worth using especially where the left gland is involved. Again the affected region is sensitive to touch. Check for difficulty opening the mouth and symptoms extending to the region around the eye.
Dose: *200c three times daily*

Phytolacca
This is a good second choice general remedy where the parotid gland is inflamed, hot and swollen. Look at the eye on the same side as the affected gland and check for excess tear production as a useful pointer.
Dose: *200c three times daily*

Lachesis
Lachesis is best reserved for severe, septic infections, where there is considerable pain in the area around the gland. Touch is resented.
Dose: *200c three times daily*

Ranula

This is a cyst-like swelling that can occur under the tongue due to blockage of one of the salivary ducts. It often responds well to homeopathic treatment. Use the selected remedy in the *30c potency three times daily for ten days*

Thuja is the main remedy to consider.

Calc carb for more heavily built horses.

Ambra grisea Use in more nervous, shy horses that are likely to become excited when examined.

The Pharynx or Throat

The pharynx is the area at the back of the mouth and is divided into two parts. The oropharynx, behind the tongue leading to the oesophagus, and the nasopharynx leading to the trachea.

Pharyngitis

Inflammation of the pharynx is termed pharyngitis. The cause is normally an infection and includes such diseases as strangles and viral infections. Symptoms include initial fever and lethargy followed by difficulty feeding and swallowing. Lymph nodes around the throat swell and can cause narrowing of the pharynx. **Aconite** and **Belladonna** are useful in the early acute stages. *Use the1M potency given every 30 minutes for four or five doses*

Ferrum phos
This is a good alternative to either Belladonna or Aconite and is best used in the early stages before there are marked symptoms. Indications for this remedy include fever with the absence of the anxiety associated with Aconite and the lack of intensity linked with Belladonna.
Dose: *30c every 30 minutes for four or five doses*

Apis mel

Indicated where the throat is swollen and constricted causing difficulty breathing. The horse will refuse to drink. If the horse is stabled there will be a desire for fresh air.
Dose: 200c three times daily

Phytolacca

This is best used in the later stages or where the condition has become chronic. Check for enlarged lymph nodes around the throat, difficulty swallowing and in turning the head.
Dose: 30c three times daily

Lachesis

Lachesis works best for severe infections where symptoms start on the left-hand side. The throat is extremely painful and the slightest touch is resented.
Dose: 200c three times daily

Merc sol

There are symptoms which stand this remedy apart from the others, namely constant swallowing, increased salivation, sweating and the presence of ulcers in the throat. You may also notice a bad smell from the mouth.
Dose: 200c three times daily

Lac caninum

This is another remedy where the throat is sensitive to touch and where swallowing is difficult. The neck is stiff and there is also difficulty in moving the tongue. You may also hear a slight cough associated with the discomfort in the throat area.
Dose: 200c three times daily

Other useful remedies worth considering include **Nux vomica 30c** where there is sneezing, desire for warmth and irritability, **Lycopodium 30c** for symptoms confined to the right-hand side of the throat and **Dulcamara 30c** where the problem starts after damp, cold weather. *Dose: three times daily*

Oesophageal obstruction and dilatation (choke)

Obstruction occurs as a consequence of food impacting in the oesophagus causing the horse to stand with its neck extended with food and saliva dribbling from the nostrils. Dilation follows from repeated episodes of oesophageal obstruction and predisposes the horse to yet more attacks. The following remedies are worth trying on a preventative basis in horses that are prone to attacks: Either **Cajuputum**, **Condurango**, **Asafoetida**, **Baryta carb**, **Alumina** or **Baptisia** given in the 6*x potency twice daily on a long term basis.* Remember the importance of giving **Aconite 1M** to affected horses when impacted to help calm the situation.

The Stomach

Gastric Ulceration

This condition has become recognised more recently in horses and reflects changes in the way we feed horses and the degree of stress that we place them under. Gastric ulceration is most likely to occur in horses undergoing training which induces high stress levels. Removal of the stress factor inevitably leads to recovery. Most horses with the condition do not show symptoms. Where present however, these can include loss of general condition, weight loss, anaemia, low blood protein levels and signs of mild colic and sweating after feeding.

Where gastric ulceration is suspected the following should help recovery. Try to carefully match the remedy on the basis of the psychological make up of the horse as the underlying constitution often underlies the condition.

Lycopodium

This needs to be used on a constitutional basis where possible. Horses that respond are intelligent and respond badly to stress and changes in daily routine. Before being asked to perform they will show symptoms of anticipatory anxiety but will always perform to the best of their ability. They are prone to minor digestive upsets and flatulence. Symptoms are always worse between 4 and 8pm.
Dose: 30c twice daily for two weeks; follow with higher potencies if necessary

Argentum nitricum

This remedy suits horses with an apprehensive

nature, which are prone to panic at times. They hate confined spaces and are difficult to load. Their movements are often quick and hurried. Anticipation is also a feature that can induce loose droppings or flatulence. Mild colic attacks are often accompanied by some gas production.
Dose: *30c twice daily for two weeks*

Dys co

This is one of the bowel nosodes and is another anticipatory type remedy linked with the development of ulcers. It suits horses of a tense, nervous nature that are rather shy, fearful and lack confidence, yet are conscientious. The tension inevitably leads to bowel problems including general digestive disturbances such as loose droppings passed before a competition.
Dose: *30c once daily for seven days*

Arsenicum album

This remedy is most suited to the refined thoroughbred type where hidden tension affects the stomach, leading to the development of ulcers. Colic symptoms occur soon after feeding and cause the horse to become restless and pace the box. There is an increase in thirst but only small amounts are drunk at any one time.
Dose: *30c twice daily for two weeks*

Nux vomica

Tense, lean, irritable and impulsive horses often respond to Nux vomica. This type usually tends to be precise and accurate, aiming for perfection. Animals of this character are usually stallions or geldings and are likely to have a history of recurrent digestive symptoms. Symptoms of gastric ulceration can arise some time after feeding and may include tenderness of the abdominal walls and sudden desire to pass droppings.
Dose: *30c twice daily for two weeks*

Anacardium

Anacardium is suited to horses of an anxious, suspicious nature, which are prone to be lazy and which have occasionally an unpleasant side to their character. In contrast to other remedies, eating relieves any symptoms of colic. Food is normally consumed very rapidly compared to other horses.
Dose: *30c twice daily for two weeks*

Phosphorus

Sensitive, affectionate animals respond well to this remedy, notably those that are jumpy with sudden noises. A keynote to the use of Phosphorus is an increase in thirst.
Dose: *30c twice daily for two weeks*

If you are unable to pick a constitutional approach, the following remedies are more generally useful and should be given in the *30c potency twice daily for about ten days*:

Hydrastis as a specific remedy for stomach ulcers, **Ornithogalum umbellatum** as a general remedy for long term problems and where pain and gas are evident and **Kali bich** where there is absence of thirst. This last remedy is also suitable for chronic cases. **Atropinum** can also be used to help with ulcers in horses that show periods of excitable or manic behaviour.

The Small and Large Intestine

Colic

There can be few horse owners who are not aware of the symptoms and potential complications associated with colic. Such is the case that veterinary help should be sought as soon as the symptoms are noticed, however minor. Homeopathic remedies can help a great deal, but should really be considered as a first aid measure while you are waiting for help to arrive.

Colic is in fact a very general term given to abdominal pain; it is not a diagnosis or specific disease. Not all colic symptoms originate from the digestive system. For example, ovarian pain can cause colic like signs in some mares and cystitis can also produce symptoms of abdominal discomfort.

Broadly, digestive based colic can be divided up into a number of different types. Try to take note of the symptoms and then match these as closely as you can to the list of remedies. All of these have keynotes to help identify a suitable remedy quickly.

Aconite (*1M potency given every 15 minutes*) or **Bach Flower Rescue Remedy** (*four or five drops* *every 15 minutes*) can help a lot in calming any horse in the earliest stages of any colic attack.

Spasmodic colic

This the most frequently encountered form of colic and is caused by the muscles within the walls of the intestines going into a state of hypermotility or spasm. The most common cause is damage to the walls of the intestine by migrating parasitic larvae. This is likely to occur in horses where a proper worming program has not been instigated. Less frequently encountered triggers include behavioural problems (excitement, stress or fear induced colic), inappropriate physical activity or environmental factors (such as chilling) and dietary problems such as feeding or drinking straight after strenuous exercise.

Look for symptoms such as sweating, elevation of the pulse rate (up to 70 per minute), lying down and rolling, turning round and looking at the flank, kicking at the abdomen and in more severe cases becoming cast. Relatively few droppings are passed. Gut sounds are noisy and gassy but may also be absent altogether. Symptoms come and go quickly and can be quite intense one minute and absent the next.

Colic due to impaction or constipation

Impaction of the intestine is most likely to occur at the relatively narrow part of the large intestine, the pelvic flexure. Older horses are more prone to this type as their teeth may be poor and they cannot break up their feed sufficiently. Otherwise, the underlying cause is likely to be solely dietary. Ingestion of large quantities of poor grass, straw bedding or other indigestible feed are frequent causes. Less frequently impaction can be due to accumulations of ingested sand which form masses in the gut known as sand enteroliths.

Signs are less dramatic than with spasmodic colic as pain symptoms are less pronounced and gradual in onset and may persist for some days. Affected horses often look off colour and will lie down, moving with obvious discomfort. Some horses will roll and look round at their flanks. Gut sounds are minimal or absent and appetite is poor. The pulse rate is moderately elevated to between 40 and 50 per minute. Dung is passed but is normally very small in quantity and appears dry or hard.

Flatulent and tympanic colic

Milder forms of this type of colic arise from fermentation of food within the bowel leading to gas build up within the stomach or intestines. Causes include ingestion of unsuitable foods such as grass cuttings or apples or just sudden changes in concentrate diet. In contrast to spasmodic colic, symptoms of pain are continuous. The pulse can rise to 80 per minute. Gut sounds are reduced and the bowels are distended.

Severe forms of tympanic colic (often requiring surgery) can arise as a consequence of acute obstruction of either the small or large intestine. Other serious problems such as a twisted bowel (known as volvulus) and intersussusception (where the bowel telescopes in on itself) can also cause this severe form of colic. Abdominal pain is intense and continuous, with affected horses rolling and sweating profusely. Gut sounds are absent and the bowels gradually become distended with gas. The pulse rate is high (between 80 and 100 per minute) and the mucous membranes will appear dark as the horse becomes toxic. In the later stages the stomach may fill with fluid and the horse may regurgitate some of this through the nose.

Thromboembolic colic

This form of colic arises due to partial or complete obstruction of the blood supply to part of the bowel. The underlying cause is thromboemboli produced by verminous arteritis and is a consequence of poor worm control (see the section on blood and blood vessels). Signs vary with the degree of blockage ranging from mild spasmodic colic (see above) to complete death of part of the intestine with rupture, resulting in death of the horse.

Main Colic Remedies

These are the most important and most often prescribed remedies. The actual dose depends on the severity of the symptoms:

Mild symptoms: 30c every 30–60 minutes
Severe symptoms: 200c every ten minutes
Remember that these remedies should be used as an interim measure while waiting for professional help.

Belladonna

Keynotes: severe to violent colic, great pain
Look for profuse sweating and a high pulse rate (over 80 per minute). The abdomen looks distended and is tender to touch. Mucous membranes deep red in colour. There are signs of distress and the horse may kick out if approached.

Rhus tox or Dulcamara

Keynotes: colic from getting wet or chilled
Symptoms of mild colic which improve on moving about and which are worse for resting. Check for noisy gut sounds and some gas in the bowel. These signs ease as the horse moves around. Warmth also helps relieve the symptoms.

Nux vomica

Keynotes: colic from over eating, dietary changes or from cold weather, colic from impaction, constipation
A good general remedy for spasmodic and flatulent colic as well as impaction. Suits greedy animals. Look for irritability, a tense anxious expression or extreme sensitivity. Symptoms occur after eating and can include some degree of gas build up. Any dung passed is small in quantity, dry and passed with difficulty. Straining is a common feature. Symptoms are better for resting and worse for movement.

Colocynthis

Keynotes: spasmodic colic, colic after drinking water
This is one of the main colic remedies and will help with reducing the intensity of the spasms. Symptoms are relieved by the horse arching its back or by pressing up hard against the stable wall.

Dioscorea

Keynotes: flatulent colic with symptoms better for stretching
Where Dioscorea is needed the symptoms are eased by the horse stretching out. This is in fact the opposite of Colocynthis where the symptoms are better when the horse bends and tucks itself up. Rumbling noises can be heard from the bowels and large quantities of gas are passed.

Mag phos

Keynotes: flatulent colic, tympanic colic
The horse is uncomfortable due to gas build up in the bowel but the symptoms are eased by the horse tucking itself up. Passing the gas does not appear to help relieve the symptoms but gentle walking does reduce the degree of discomfort.

Lycopodium

Keynotes: flatulent colic from fermentation of food, colic from anticipation before an event
Symptoms can appear after feeding and particularly after over eating where the food starts to ferment. Gas gradually collects causing the abdomen to become uncomfortable and tight so that touch is resented. Very little dung is passed. Typically signs of colic are likely to be worse between 4 and 8pm and eased by walking the horse gently. Passing the gas helps improve the symptoms.

Chamomilla

Keynotes: colic with anger, impatience or irritability, flatulent colic
Horses needing Chamomilla are mentally irritable and difficult to handle. They are also very vocal, whining relentlessly. Chamomilla works best for mild flatulent colic accompanied by the characteristic behavioural symptoms.

Colchicum

Keynotes: tympanic colic with much distension
This remedy is indicated where the colon is grossly distended with gas to the extent that the horse is unable to move without great discomfort. Gut sounds are excessively loud and noisy.

Plumbum

Keynotes: colic due to impaction, constipation
The symptoms suiting Plumbum are typified by very tight abdominal muscles. The horse is very tucked up and obtains relief by stretching. The colon may be impacted with dung. When dung is passed it is very dark in colour and in very hard lumps. It is passed only after considerable urging.

Alumina
Keynotes: colic due to impaction with severe straining. Colic due to constipation or sand enteroliths

Check for very dry crumbly dung as an indication for this remedy. Symptoms are often left sided and the horse may turn around to look at this side. Painful straining is obvious as the horse tries to pass the dry dung.

Bryonia
Keynotes: colic due to impaction, symptoms made worse by movement, with much thirst
The horse will be unwilling to move where Bryonia is indicated as the discomfort intensifies on slightest movement. Affected horses are irritable and thirsty. Any dung seen is hard, dry and larger in diameter than normal.

Carbo veg
Keynotes: flatulent colic with weakness, colic arising from poor or sluggish digestion
This is a remedy to use in more severe cases of flatulent colic where the horse has become weakened. The back will be arched with pain and the abdomen is greatly distended with gas. This is passed in large quantities along with small amounts of mucus easing the symptoms considerably. The animal appears cold but is better in the fresh air.

China
Keynotes: tympanic or flatulent colic due to dehydration, post-surgical colic
Indicated where there is considerable gas build up and pain, causing the horse to appear tucked up. Touch is resented but symptoms are eased by gentle walking in the open air.

Opium
Keynotes: Severe colic due to impaction or obstruction, recurrent obstructive colic
This remedy is for more severe cases where the horse is down, depressed and takes little interest in surroundings. Straining is normally absent, but may be observed when the pain intensifies. Any dung seen is hard and black. This remedy is worth considering for recurrent cases and constipation where no straining at all is observed.

Bothrops
Keynotes: thromboembolic colic
This is the most important remedy for this particular condition, helping to reduce the risk of a thrombus formation in horses prone to this condition and in treating the acute symptoms. Nervous trembling is often a feature where Bothrops is indicated. Lachesis is sometimes considered a useful alternative. Other colic remedies can be used alongside Bothrops to ease the symptoms of pain.

Minor Colic Remedies

Sulphur
Colic after drinking. Colic due to intermittent impaction with very large piles of hard dung passed.

Pulsatilla
Flatulent colic after eating rich food, usually in the evening, with rumbling noises

Staphysagria
Colic arising from anger, resentment or frustration

Cuprum metallicum
Spasmodic colic with intermittent violent spasms

Raphanus
Tympanic colic with great abdominal distension due to gas that continues to build up despite treatment.

Zinc
Flatulent colic from over eating or eating too quickly. Horse appears tucked up.

Argentum nitricum
Flatulent colic from anticipatory anxiety or from claustrophobia.

Podophyllum
Mild rumbling colic accompanied by diarrhoea.

Paraffinum
Can be used for mild impaction type colic in foals

where intermittent straining is seen. Symptoms recur every few days.

Grass Sickness

The exact cause of grass sickness is not known although the disease was first identified over 100 years ago. Current research is looking at the possibility of some type of bacterial involvement, possibly clostridia, which may produce some form of neurotoxic factor which affects the control of the bowel. The disease rarely occurs in younger horses and is more common in summer and in certain regions, e.g. in the UK it is seen mainly in Scotland and the South. Horses out at pasture are almost exclusively affected. The UK has the highest incidence in the world.

Grass sickness is a serious condition which is difficult to treat and often results in the horse being destroyed. The sooner the signs are recognised and treated, the greater the chance of survival of the animal. Symptoms can mimic other conditions making diagnosis difficult. Cases can be divided into three main types:

Acute

Check for restlessness, colic and distension of the abdomen. Also look for trouble swallowing, drooling of saliva, food material appearing at the nose (often as a greenish discharge), patchy sweating, trembling and muscle tremors (especially in the forelimbs), difficulty passing urine, bowel stasis, constipation and lethargy.

Sub-acute

The symptoms are very similar to acute cases but less pronounced. Additional signs include loss of weight, particularly around the muscles of the hind limbs, pawing at the ground, restlessness and tendency to lie down. Small amounts of soft dung may be passed.

Chronic

This is categorised by chronic and severe weight loss and accompanying weakness. Food is chewed slowly and swallowed with difficulty. Mucus collects around the nostrils. There may also be bouts of abdominal pain with sweating.

Dedicated nursing care is vital in attempting to treat grass sickness. The following remedies provide valuable additional help:

Gelsemium

This is the most useful remedy to try since it covers the majority of the symptoms of grass sickness.
Dose: *200c. For acute cases dose every two hours. In sub-acute cases dose three times daily. In chronic cases give the remedy twice daily*
The best way of approaching difficult cases is to try to combine Gelsemium with one additional remedy fitting the more localised symptoms from the list of remaining remedies.

Nux moschata

This remedy is most useful where the bowels are grossly distended due to paralysis. Passage of a little soft dung is another additional pointer.
Dose: *200c twice daily*

Plumbum

Indicated particularly where the limb muscles are wasted. It may also have some influence on the paralysis of the bowel.
Dose: *200c twice daily*

Alumen

Alumen may be helpful where difficulty in swallowing fluids is pronounced. It will also help with muscle weakness.
Dose: *200c twice daily*

Cocculus

Cocculus is also worth considering where there is great difficulty in swallowing food. This remedy also covers within its symptom picture muscle trembling and abdominal distension.
Dose: *200c twice daily*

Zinc

Consider using zinc as an additional remedy where muscle trembling and twitching is a prominent feature. This remedy will also help where there are colic symptoms with noisy bowel sounds and distension of the abdomen together with general weakness and lethargy. ***Dose:*** *200c twice daily*

Phosphorus

Indicated where regurgitation of food is prominent and where there is general muscle weakness.
Dose: *200c twice daily*

Other remedies which are worth looking at include **Thallium 6c** indicated for tremors and muscle atrophy and **Phosphoric acid 6c** for progressive weakness and emaciation as the disease reaches its later stages. ***Dose:*** *three times daily*

Diarrhoea or Enteritis in Adult Horses

There are a number of underlying reasons why horses develop diarrhoea resulting in severe acute, less acute or chronic problems. Minor cases of diarrhoea in adult horses will often start to clear up within a day, particularly where dietary changes are the underlying cause. In these situations feeding hay and water is often sufficient. Severe, acute diarrhoea, any cases lasting longer than 24 hours or so, and diarrhoea in foals all need veterinary help.

Diarrhoea in foals

See The Foal, page 163

Severe, acute diarrhoea and colitis (Rudiosa disease), Colitis X

These conditions need urgent veterinary attention. Use the remedies as an interim measure to help back up any conventional treatment. Underlying causes of acute diarrhoea include infection with Salmonella (see page 288) or Clostridial (see page 290) bacteria, the overuse of antibiotics and poisoning. Colitis or Rudiosa disease is normally only seen in adult horses and involves inflammation of the large intestine. The result is diarrhoea often containing mucus and blood and damage to the lining of the gut allowing toxins and bacteria to gain access to the bloodstream eventually leading to a state of toxic shock. This acute and potentially fatal condition is known as Colitis X.

Symptoms are acute and pronounced and include fever (although the temperature may be subnormal in colitis X), increased pulse and respiratory rate, weakness, lack of appetite, abdominal pain and discolouration of the mucous membranes. Diarrhoea may not always be present in the initial, acute stages of these diseases, but can be explosive and watery, sometimes haemorrhagic (depending on the cause), leading to dehydration. Septicaemia leading to death is a distinct possibility. Where antibiotics are the cause, symptoms may appear suddenly a few days after administration and can lead to severe diarrhoea and dehydration.

Remedies to use in the very early stages of acute diarrhoea/colitis

Initially aim to use remedies that can help with the symptoms of any fever, before any more dramatic symptoms appear. The aim of doing this is to reduce the severity of the illness. If bacteria are involved the appropriate nosode can be used as well. *Give one dose every 15–20 minutes.*

The following remedies should be given in the 1M potency every 15–20 minutes:

Aconite

Use in the very early stages where there is an element of fear and anxiety together with fever and very few other signs. The abdomen may be painful to touch and the horse is extremely restless.

Belladonna

Indicated where the pulse is extremely strong and bounding, mucous membranes are discoloured, congested and red. The horse appears distressed. Small quantities of fluid diarrhoea may be passed. If the pupils are dilated as well, this is a good clue to using Belladonna. Abdominal pain is often present but the pain comes and goes in spasms.

Baptisia

This is a remedy for septicaemia and is likely to be most useful where diarrhoea is already evident and where this is putrid and offensive in nature and passed with a little gas. The horse will appear confused and drowsy. Fever symptoms are less pronounced than with other remedies. Mucous membranes are often a dark dusky colour where Baptisia is helpful.

Pyrogen

Pyrogen is another remedy indicated in septicaemia, especially where there is extreme restlessness and the horse cannot remain still. Any diarrhoea seen is offensive. Although the fever may not be as high as with other remedies, the pulse rate will be raised out of all proportion to the temperature.

Remedies to use in treating severe or acute diarrhoea/colitis

Use the 200c potency every 20–30 minutes.
The first three remedies are the most important. The signs of distress and weakness that are associated with these medicines are pronounced in their symptom pictures.

Veratrum album

Keynote: Profuse diarrhoea and weakness, cold skin
Use Veratrum where there is violent diarrhoea and purging with pain preceding any diarrhoea. Check for cold sweating. The skin will feel cold and tacky and the animal appears weak with a feeble pulse. The diarrhoea is watery, frequent, passed with some force but with little straining. Blood may be present. Loss of condition is evident with sunken features.

Cuprum

Keynote: Severe diarrhoea with colic and cramping
Cuprum should help where there is severe diarrhoea, with blood, accompanied by straining and weakness. The abdomen is tender and painful to touch. Colic is evident as well as cramping pains. The horse will appear unsteady on its legs and the jaws may be forcibly clenched together.

Camphor

Keynote: Severe diarrhoea with prostration, exhaustion and collapse
Signs of weakness are prominent where Camphor is needed and where collapse is evident. The skin feels cold to the touch. Diarrhoea is profuse, dark in colour and passed with little effort.

Arsenicum album

Keynote: Severe diarrhoea with emaciation and weakness, diarrhoea from excessive water intake, restlessness
This is an important remedy where the diarrhoea is watery, possibly tinged with blood and offensive in nature and where the horse is weakened or exhausted and has lost condition quickly. The diarrhoea makes the area around the back legs and anal region very sore where the skin has been contaminated. Other vital guiding symptoms include intense restlessness, anxiety or fear and thirst for small quantities of water. Symptoms intensify during the night, especially around midnight.

Carbo veg

Keynote: Diarrhoea from bad food, foul diarrhoea with weakness and coldness
Think of using Carbo veg where diarrhoea originates from consumption of bad or stale feed and where the dung is foul. Mucus and blood may also be present. Signs can be quite severe and the animal feels cold to the touch and in a weakened state.

Other than using these remedies it is worth bearing in mind that the following remedies are also extremely useful:

China

Keynote: Dehydration and debility, severe watery diarrhoea
China can be used to help with the effects of dehydration and associated weakness in any case but is also a diarrhoea remedy in its own right helping where the dung is profuse and watery in nature with some bloating of the abdomen.

Ipecac

Keynote: Straining with severe watery, frothy diarrhoea containing shreds of bowel lining and bright red blood
Ipecac can help where the diarrhoea is severe and characteristically is passed with slimy mucus, bright red blood and shreds of intestinal lining. Severe straining accompanies each passage of diarrhoea with signs of abdominal pain as the horse stretches out each time something is passed.

Aloe

Keynote: Diarrhoea involving a mixture of watery and solid material with gas, drug-induced diarrhoea, Colitis X
Useful where the diarrhoea is jelly-like or lumpy and

contains blood or is a mixture of watery and lumpy material interspersed with gas. Sometimes the horse may be unaware that anything has been passed. Violent straining can accompany each bowel movement and there may be bleeding from the rectum in some cases. Check also for rumbling, gurgling noises from the abdomen as well as bloating. Aloe is a useful remedy for antibiotic induced diarrhoea where it should be combined with the use of probiotics to help restore the levels of natural bacteria in the bowel.

Merc sol and Merc corr

Keynote: Slimy diarrhoea with mucus, some blood and prominent straining, Colitis X
Straining is the main feature associated with these remedies. The dung is slimy in character and tinged with blood. Discomfort continues even after material has been passed. Symptoms are worse during the hours of darkness. The horse will appear sweaty. Merc corr has the more violent and pronounced symptoms of the two remedies.

Remedies for less acute diarrhoea/colitis cases

Unless otherwise noted, dose using the 30c potency between two and four times daily depending on the severity of the condition.

Colchicum

Keynote: Watery diarrhoea accompanied by abdominal distension from gas, weakness
Colchicum is useful where there is watery diarrhoea with some mucus present and where there are traces of blood. Straining is slight. The horse will appear weak. Gaseous distension of the abdomen is a good pointer to selecting this remedy. Diarrhoea arising in the autumn should also respond well to this remedy.

Crot tiglium

Keynote: Copious watery diarrhoea expelled with force
The forcible degree with which the diarrhoea is shot out differentiates this remedy from others. The consistency is always watery with loud gurgling sounds from the bowels. A large volume of diarrhoea is passed each time.

Nux vomica

Keynote: Diarrhoea from changes in feeding or from over-eating
Nux vomica is useful for diarrhoea arising from changes in diet or pasture or from over feeding. The dung will be slimy and passed in small quantities with some straining evident. The discomfort ceases after the dung has been passed. Irritability and over sensitivity are clues to using this remedy.

Dulcamara

Keynote: Diarrhoea from getting damp and cold
This is the main remedy for diarrhoea arising after getting wet or when the weather becomes cold and damp, typically in the autumn. The diarrhoea is characteristically green and watery.

Bryonia

Keynote: Diarrhoea from hot weather
Increased thirst and a dry mouth are clues to using Bryonia, which is an ideal remedy to use where diarrhoea seems to occur in hot weather.

Aconite

Keynote: Diarrhoea from becoming chilled or after a fright
Green watery diarrhoea originating after a chill, a fright or stressful situation suggests Aconite.
Use the 1M potency hourly until the problem resolves

Antimonium crudum

Keynote: Diarrhoea from becoming overheated
This is also a useful remedy for diarrhoea which alternates with hard dung or where there is a mixture of hard and watery material together. Suited to more elderly horses.

Gambogia

Keynote: watery diarrhoea which appears suddenly
Look for sudden onset diarrhoea with loud rumbling noises and forceful stools. Gambogia is more suited to elderly horses.

Elaterium

Keynote: Forceful watery diarrhoea
Useful where there is watery diarrhoea that squirts out and is expelled forcibly.

Gelsemium
Keynote: Diarrhoea from emotional excitement or fright
Look out for soft dung or more watery diarrhoea that is passed without the horse being aware. Trembling or a general appearance of weakness are useful indicators.

Argentum nitricum
Keynote: Diarrhoea from excitement
Indicated where the diarrhoea is watery, appears like chopped spinach and is accompanied by much gas. Affected horses appear agitated.

Pulsatilla
Keynote: Diarrhoea from overeating fruit or feed which is too rich
Look for diarrhoea that is changeable in nature and predominantly watery, often containing mucus. The character of the stool varies and symptoms are inconsistent from day to day. Absence of thirst is a pointer.

Phosphoric acid
Keynote: Diarrhoea associated with grief or pining, useful during recovery generally
Check for painless watery diarrhoea that is passed almost unnoticed along with gas. Phos ac is a good general remedy that can be used during recovery from debility and exhaustion caused by prolonged or severe diarrhoea.

Chronic diarrhoea in adult horses

There are several important causes, which need specific remedies to help.

Diarrhoea caused by infection with strongyles

Damage to the bowel by parasites is probably the most common cause of chronic diarrhoea in the horse. Strongyle worms are often implicated, with those horses under five predominantly affected during the spring and winter. Protracted cases will lead to weight loss, emaciation and filling of the limbs due to low blood albumin levels. Worms may be seen in the dung.

In addition to using either conventional worming treatment or homeopathic remedies, the following remedies should be of help:

Cina
This is the principal remedy for diarrhoea resulting from worms and especially suited to younger animals. The diarrhoea is typically mucoid in character and may lead to itching of the anal region so the horse rubs this area. A degree of irritability is a clear indication that this remedy is needed.
Dose: 200c twice daily

Acetic acid
Look for watery dung (particularly in the morning), progressive emaciation and weight loss where Acetic acid is needed. Ascites, fluid in the abdomen, can also be a feature. An increase in thirst is also another key feature, accompanied by the frequent passage of large quantities of clear urine.
Dose: 200c twice daily

Abrotanum
This is another remedy to use where there is wasting associated with worms and diarrhoea. Weight loss continues despite a good appetite. Over a period of time the abdomen becomes distended as the condition progresses.
Dose: 30c twice daily

Iodum
The symptoms associated with Iodum are very similar to those of Abrotanum. Appetite is increased yet there is weight loss and emaciation. Thirst is also increased. Check for general weakness, dislike of heat and exhaustion on the least exercise. Loose dung may alternate with diarrhoea.
Dose: 30c twice daily

Diarrhoea caused by infection with coccidia – coccidiosis

See infectious diseases page 296

Diarrhoea due to chronic Salmonella infection

See infectious diseases page 288

Diarrhoea due to malabsorption type syndromes

This covers a selection of diseases that result in weight loss (despite eating well), chronic diarrhoea, emaciation, muscle wasting with the development of subcutaneous oedema in advanced cases. Good remedies to think about using include **Abrotanum 30c, Acetic acid 30c** and **Iodum 30c**.

Additional remedies for chronic diarrhoea include:

Gaertner-Bach

This bowel nosode is one of the main remedies for general malnutrition where there is emaciation and chronic diarrhoea. The digestive system is weak with a tendency to pick up heavy worm burdens.
Dose: *30c twice daily*

Silica

Indicated in animals with a weak constitution and where the lining of the bowel has been damaged leading to poor absorption of food. Silica may help repair the lining of the bowel in some circumstances and assist the absorption of nutrients.
Dose: *30c twice daily*

Nat mur

This is a remedy for chronic diarrhoea together with weight loss, increased thirst and increased appetite. Try to use Nat mur on a constitutional basis where possible. It is suited to horses that are prone to appearing depressed, withdrawn, and which reject affection.
Dose: *30c twice daily*

Podophyllum

This is an excellent remedy for chronic diarrhoea where the dung is watery, passed with little effort and in considerable quantities. The diarrhoea may contain jelly-like mucus. Symptoms are worse in the morning and in hot weather.
Dose: *30c three times daily*

Phosphorus

Indicated in chronic diarrhoea in lean, athletic, sensitive horses. The dung is watery and passed in large amounts often along with gas. The nature of the diarrhoea leads to a degree of debility and weakness. Increased thirst is usually a feature.
Dose: *30c three times daily*

Sulphur

Sulphur matches horses which appear untidy and where the coat is out of condition. The type of diarrhoea that responds is worse in the morning and leads to soreness around the rectum. Sulphur is also the main remedy to use where diarrhoea arises in association with conventional (suppressive) treatment of a skin condition.
Dose: *30c twice daily*

Other causes of chronic diarrhoea

It is not always possible to isolate a definite cause but you should consider the possibility of poisoning, diarrhoea induced by drugs or diarrhoea caused by moulds or mycotoxins. Each case needs to be assessed individually and symptoms carefully matched to an appropriate remedy.

Internal Abscesses

Abscesses can arise within the abdominal cavity following abdominal surgery or other surgical procedures such as castration. Other causes include external penetrating wounds to the abdominal wall, tears to the rectum and or penetration of the gut wall from a foreign body. Internal abscesses are most commonly seen in foals, but can occur in horses of any age. Symptoms to be aware of include periodic bouts of fever and colic, poor appetite and gradual weight loss. Treatment is difficult but remedies to consider which may help include:

Hepar sulph

In high potency, this remedy will help abort the abscess when given over a period of time. Guiding symptoms include symptoms of abdominal pain, irritability and a desire to seek heat.
Dose: *200c daily over a period of several weeks*

Silica

This is an excellent remedy for chronic abscesses and suited to horses of a weaker constitution. There is a desire for heat as with Hepar sulph, but the absence of pain differentiates these two remedies from one another. Silica will help reabsorb the abscess material and significantly reduce the chances of scar formation and adhesions.
Dose: 200c daily over a period of several weeks

Peritonitis

Peritonitis is an inflammation of the peritoneum, the membrane which lines the abdominal cavity. It is not a common problem, but can arise as a complication following abdominal surgery (especially for colic) or more rarely spontaneously. Symptoms include abdominal pain, increased pulse rate and dehydration. Urgent conventional care can be augmented by using some of the following remedies:

Aconite

This should be given as soon as the problem is suspected. Aconite will also serve to allay any fear.
Dose: 1M every 10–20 minutes as needed

Belladonna

Belladonna will help where there is a high fever, rapid and forceful pulse rate and congested mucous membranes. It can be used alongside other remedies.
Dose: 1M every 30 minutes as needed

Apis

Indicated where there is fluid present in the abdominal cavity and the slightest pressure on the abdominal wall is resented. The horse appears agitated and hot.
Dose: 200c every 20 minutes as needed

Bryonia

This is an important remedy for acute peritonitis and indicated where the slightest movement induces abdominal pain. Consequently the animal is unwilling to move as symptoms are eased by resting. Other pointers include increased thirst and a degree of irritability.
Dose: 200c every 30 minutes as needed

Lycopodium

This is the main remedy to conside becomes chronic in nature and whe of the digestive system is impaired.
Dose: 30c once daily

Other remedies worth consideration include **Merc corr 30c**, **Merc dulcis 30c**, **Lachesis 30c**, **Cantharis 30c** and **Colocynthis 30c**

Lack of Appetite, Anorexia

Poor appetite is not a definite condition, but rather a symptom of another problem and will ultimately affect an animal's condition and performance. Any underlying disease or health problems should be investigated first and attention paid to other areas such as feed type, ease of access and the condition of the teeth. Poor appetite can also be a problem following surgery. Use the following remedies to help improve appetite where the underlying cause has been identified and treated.
Unless otherwise stated use the 30c potency twice daily for seven to ten days.

Nux vomica

Useful as a general tonic to the digestion. It is especially good after abdominal surgery and digestive upsets.

Iris versicolor

Used to help improve appetite following severe diarrhoea or flatulent colic.

Alfalfa

A good general tonic for the digestion and the appetite in particular. Helpful where malnutrition has been a problem. Use the 6x potency three times daily.

Chin arsenicosum

Indicated where there is overall weakness accompanied by lack of appetite. It acts as a general tonic and should be used in the 6x potency twice daily.

Lycopodium

Useful where the digestive system is weak or where

ulent colic has been a problem. Often useful where only small amounts of feed are taken at any one time.

Ant crudum

Excellent for loss of appetite accompanied by bloating of the abdomen and where the horse is of an irritable nature and resents attention.

Arsenicum album

Indicated after prolonged illness and where the animal appears in poor condition. Acts as a general overall tonic improving appetite at the same time.

Vitamin B12

This is a general remedy for improving the appetite. The ideal potency to use is 12x, which should be given twice daily.

Worms

The majority of horse owners are aware of the problems that worms can cause such that regular worming is an important and vital aspect of health care. All horses will have worms which potentially can cause serious damage to the bowel leading to digestive problems (such as colic) or damage to the associated blood vessels leading to problems with the circulation. Other symptoms associated with heavy worm burdens include loss of condition or weight, poor appetite, diarrhoea, anaemia and filling of the legs. There are several types of worms that affect horses:

Small strongyles This type of worm can cause severe damage to the gut wall leading to weight loss and chronic diarrhoea.

Large strongyles (bloodworms) These migrate into the blood vessel walls from the bowel and can lead to colic, debility and diarrhoea.

Pinworms These live in the large intestine and damage the bowel wall. They also lay eggs around the anus that can lead to itching and rubbing of the tail area.

Tapeworms Tapeworms can cause weight loss and chronic diarrhoea as well as colic.

Ascarid worms These can migrate from the bowel to the liver and lungs. Foals are most at risk from ascarids which can impact the bowel.

Bots These attach themselves to the stomach lining after the eggs have been swallowed as the horse grooms itself.

Modern conventional wormers are very effective and their value should not be underestimated. They should be used regularly in combination with good pasture management together with homeopathic support where appropriate.

Homeopathy and worms

Used correctly, homeopathic remedies can be a valuable adjunct to conventional approaches to worming. They can:

Be used to support a weak constitution. Some horses seem more prone to worm infestations than others. This could be due to a weak constitution so that in effect, the natural resistance to worms is not good. Constitutional prescribing can be used to improve the overall level of general health and ability to resist worms. *Refer to section on constitutional remedies.*

Be used specifically to help eliminate worms. Remedies that act against worms can be used alongside conventional wormers if need be. If your horse reacts badly to routine wormers or you wish to avoid using chemicals, then it is possible to carry out a worming programme using a combination of remedies, supported by constitutional prescribing. The main proviso to doing this is that regular worm egg counts need to be undertaken on the dung to monitor the efficiency of the treatment. If the number of eggs per gram rises above 800, then there is no doubt that you should use conventional treatment. To be realistically effective, aim for a level of around 200 eggs per gram. Monitor the worm egg count every six weeks to ensure that you know the level of infestation. Remember also that correct pasture management is vitally important if you are to achieve any level of success. Always use conventional worming programmes if you are in any doubt about your horse's health.

Remedies and worms

The following remedies can be used to help eliminate worms:

Strongyles – strongylosis
Cina 6x
Kamala 6x
Chelone 1x

Tapeworms
Filix mas 3x
Granatum 3x

Pinworms
Cina 6x

Ascarids – threadworms
Cina 6x
Chenopodium 3c
Chelone 1x
Abrotanum 6c
Santoninum 6c
Teucrium marum 6c
Natrum phos 6x

Using remedies on a practical basis

Determine your horse's constitutional remedy.
Dose: *using the 1M potency once weekly for three weeks.* It would not be wise to repeat this dose without professional help.
Use a combination of remedies to try and help eliminate worms. **Cina 6x**, **Chelone 1x**, **Granatum 3x** and **Filix mas 3x** seem to work well together. Add **Nat phos 6x** if you are treating an animal less than one year old.
Dose: *twice daily for three weeks. Repeat this combination every 8–12 weeks*

Combine with good pasture management.

Pick up any droppings in your field each day to remove eggs and larvae. Harrow the field in dry weather to break up and spread out the droppings so that the worm eggs will be destroyed by sunlight. Do not overstock the grazing – try to avoid more than one horse per acre. Rest the pasture if possible from time to time. A minimum of five months is needed to be effective in assisting control. Rotating the grazing with cattle and sheep can also help. Remember to keep the stable and its fittings as clean as possible.

Other useful worm remedies

Cina 30c
This is useful where heavy worm infestations have caused emaciation and weakness. Cina is a good general remedy for worm related problems.
Dose: *twice daily as long as needed*

Calc carb 200c
This remedy can be used where tapeworms are a persistent problem.
Dose: *twice weekly for eight weeks*

Gaertner-Bach 200c
This is one of the bowel nosodes and can be an extremely valuable remedy where the horse becomes persistently infested with worms. It is also indicted where there is chronic diarrhoea or emaciation associated with worms and especially suited to younger animals.
Dose: *three times weekly for three weeks*

The Liver

The liver is one of the most important organs as it performs a wide range of functions vital to good health. Its importance is often underestimated. In fact, liver disease is not often diagnosed in the horse but is almost certainly more of a problem than realised. This is mainly due to the fact that the liver can regenerate to some considerable extent and is therefore able to cope quite well until the reserve capacity is used up. At this point disease symptoms will appear, normally reflecting the role the liver plays within the body. Liver disease will often respond well to homeopathic remedies. In Eastern medicine the liver is linked to the muscles, tendons and eyes and is associated with the emotion of anger. The remedies listed will also help with problems in these areas by acting on the liver.

The Role of the Liver

The work of the liver can be divided up into five main areas, metabolism, storage, manufacture, detoxification and excretion. The liver is involved in carbohydrate metabolism and in the maintenance of normal blood glucose levels. It also stores glycogen which is broken down in the liver to glucose when an extra energy source is needed. In addition to carbohydrate metabolism, the liver also plays a part in protein metabolism, manufacturing blood proteins, carrier proteins, lipoproteins and clotting factors. It is also involved in the breakdown of some proteins and the conversion of ammonia into urea, which is then excreted by the kidneys. In addition the liver is also involved with fat metabolism. Cholesterol and other fats are made by the liver and used either as an energy source or to make the structural parts of new cells.

The liver also produces bile, which is needed for fat digestion and absorption. Bile stimulates the process of digestion and plays a part in the absorption of the fat-soluble vitamins. The liver is also involved in the storage of vitamins A, D, K, B12 and folate.

Another important role is in detoxification. This involves the breakdown not only of some of the body's own substances such as redundant hormones, but also the breakdown and excretion of many drugs. The liver also removes toxins absorbed from the bowel before they reach the general circulation and has cells that will remove circulating debris such as damaged cells, bacteria and endotoxins from the blood.

Liver Disease

Signs of liver disease become apparent when the liver can no longer fulfil its functions. In the horse, liver disease takes two forms. Primary liver disease which occurs as a result of a problem with the liver itself and secondary liver disease which occurs when the liver is damaged as a result of another condition. There are two principal conditions that arise as a consequence of liver disease.

Hepatitis or Liver Damage

Hepatitis simply refers to inflammation of the liver cells, which can arise from a variety of causes.

Jaundice

Jaundice, often thought of as a disease, is in fact a symptom, and results from the inability of the liver to excrete bile, leading to a build up of bile pigments imparting the characteristic yellow colour to the mucous membranes, sclera (the white of the eye) and skin. There are three basic types of jaundice:

Haemolytic jaundice

This is caused by damage to red blood cells and the breakdown of the haemoglobin that is released when the cells are destroyed. This type of jaundice is sometimes seen in the newborn foal and has an immunological basis (page 100). Haemolytic jaundice can also arise as a result of certain viral, bacterial or parasitic infections in which toxins produced by these organisms damage the red blood cells releasing haemoglobin.

Obstructive jaundice

In this instance the flow of bile from the liver to the duodenum is blocked often by blockage of the bile duct itself. The backlog of bile enters the blood stream and leads to the development of jaundice as bile pigment is deposited in the tissues of the body.

Jaundice as a consequence of hepatitis

Here the liver cells are damaged, allowing bile pigment to gain access to the blood via the lymph channels. There are many different causes of hepatitis.

Primary Liver Disease

This occurs either as an acute condition or in a more chronic form.

Acute liver disease or hepatitis

Causes of acute liver disease or hepatitis include viral infections such as Equine Infectious Anaemia (page 282) and infections such as Leptospirosis (page 292), Babesiasis (page 293) and Tyzzer's disease (page 160), poisoning by chemicals or heavy metals (such as arsenic or lead, page 317) and by damage caused by plant toxins. Other causes involve obstruction of the bile duct (for example by tumours, by bot larvae or by impaction with ascarid worms), obstruction of the small or large intestine and as a consequence of a metabolic condition referred to as hyperlipaemia.

Symptoms of acute liver disease can include a sudden change in appetite, weight loss, diarrhoea, abdominal pain, jaundice, oedema, odd or abnormal behaviour and dark coloured urine.

Chronic Liver Disease

In chronic liver disease, the damage to the liver occurs over an extended period of time. Often symptoms will appear acutely as the ability of the liver to function is suddenly exceeded. This form is by far the most common in horses and is most often caused by Ragwort poisoning (page 315).

Symptoms of chronic liver disease typically include depression, depraved or abnormal appetite, head pressing and other neurological symptoms, leading to an odd gait or stance. As the disease progresses weight loss becomes apparent, jaundice develops and the dung will become loose and sometimes pale in colour. Oedema can also be a feature as fluid collects around the brisket region. Some animals will also develop photosensitisation, with white areas of the skin reacting to sunlight. This leads to inflammation and blistering of the skin.

Secondary Liver Disease

Endotoxins (toxins produced within the body) are largely responsible for secondary liver disease. Conditions such as septicaemia and some acute digestive tract problems will result in the production of endotoxins, which will damage the liver cells.

Liver remedies

Homeopathy has a good reputation in supporting the functioning of the liver and in assisting recovery where it is not damaged beyond hope. Try to match one of the remedies as closely to the symptoms as you can, bearing in mind the cause of the problem and other characteristics such as temperament of the animal.

Dose: *For acute liver disease use the 200c potency up to four times daily. For chronic liver disease use the 30c potency once daily*

Nux vomica

Keynotes: General liver remedy, poisoning, digestive problems

This is a good general liver remedy and especially

useful where poisoning is suspected as it helps detoxify the liver. It is also useful where signs of colic are present or where there are other symptoms involving the digestive system. Animals with gait abnormalities may also respond particularly where the gait appears unsteady or uncertain. A clue to using Nux vomica is a degree of irritability or a tendency to show anger as well being tense with an increased sensitivity to noise, wind and light. Nux vomica is also a good remedy to use in the later stages of laminitis where the liver needs detoxifying.

Lycopodium

Keynotes: Wasting and flatulence, chronic liver disease, oedema
Lycopodium is another major liver remedy and useful where there is either wasting or poor appetite. It is therefore of most use in chronic cases. Animals that respond well are keen to always have company as they dislike being left on their own and are often apprehensive in nature. Digestive disturbances, particularly with flatulence, are a clue to using this remedy. It is also the remedy to use where liver disease underlies the accumulation of fluid in the body (oedema).

Phosphorus

Keynotes: Acute hepatitis, jaundice, gait abnormalities and eye problems, hyperlipaemia
Horses with acute liver disease will often benefit from Phosphorus. It is indicated in cases of poisoning where the liver is acutely damaged. Phosphorus will also help where jaundice and liver enlargement is present. It is also a remedy to consider using where there are concurrent eye symptoms, hind limb weakness or suspected hyperlipaemia. Clues to using this remedy include increased thirst, weakness of the back legs, a lean athletic stature and haemorrhages due to a failure of the liver to produce clotting factors. Other clues include a liking for salt licks, a craving for affection and a dislike of being left alone.

Chelidonium

Keynotes: Jaundice, muscle weakness and stiffness
This is a prominent liver remedy for both acute and chronic cases. It is useful where there is jaundice and loss of muscle power and with muscle stiffness. The dung may also appear to have an odd clay like or yellow taint. An excellent guiding symptom is pain over or near the right shoulder region often showing as a slight lameness or recurrent lameness. Check the tongue for a yellow coating. This is often present where Chelidonium is needed.

Berberis vulgaris

Keynotes: Liver disease and back pain
This is an ideal remedy to use in more robust older horses with liver disease and acts as a general liver tonic. It suits horses with a reduced level of stamina, lethargy or with concurrent back pain in the lumbar region. It is also one of the remedies to consider where build up of toxins in the liver has caused laminitis.

Chionanthus

Keynotes: Jaundice
This lesser known but powerful liver remedy can help where jaundice is present, where the urine is very dark and where the liver is enlarged. Chionanthus will also help where there is pain around the region of the liver and possibly where there is oedema.

Carduus marianus

Keynotes: Liver enlargement, jaundice, chronic hepatitis
This is primarily a remedy for jaundice but works especially where the urine is a bright yellow colour. A clue is left sided abdominal pain. Carduus is an excellent remedy for chronic hepatitis. This remedy combines well with Taraxacum in draining away liver toxins.

Merc dulc

Keynotes: Chronic hepatitis, catarrhal jaundice, cirrhosis
This is remedy for chronic liver disease, especially where scarring (cirrhosis) is present leading to jaundice. It is a specific for catarrhal jaundice, where the action of the liver has become clogged due to catarrh. Some horses may show gastrointestinal symptoms as well, such as loose green dung. Merc dulc is a suitable remedy for helping with ragwort poisoning.

Merc sol

Keynotes: Jaundice, sweaty skin, slimy soft dung, ascites
Merc sol is a remedy for treating liver disease where there are also skin symptoms, especially where the skin is greasy, oily and the horse sweats easily. In severe cases where there is jaundice, there may be swelling of the lower limbs and loose, slimy dung. Another pointer in some cases is the accumulation of fluid in the abdomen (ascites).

Natrum sulph

Keynotes: Symptoms worse for damp weather, hepatitis
This is a prominent liver remedy for treating inflammation of the liver (hepatitis) where the symptoms are specifically worse in wet, damp weather and where there is pain around the region of the liver, flatulence as well as jaundice in more severe cases.

Taraxacum

Keynotes: Enlarged liver with marked neck pain
Indicated where the neck is stiff and the joints or muscles are sore. The liver may be enlarged together with obvious jaundice. In lower potency Taraxacum combines well with Carduus to provide general support for the liver and to assist the removal of toxins. The suggested potency for both these remedies when used in this way is *4x, given twice daily.*

Ptelea

Keynotes: Removal of toxins
Ptelia is known as a liver drainage remedy and will help remove toxins from the liver. It can also be used to help stimulate the appetite where the appetite is poor.

Specific liver conditions

Liver abscess

Liver abscesses are rare but can result from bacterial invasion of the liver. Symptoms of overt liver disease may not appear until there is extensive liver damage. However, other signs will become apparent which can include weight loss, poor appetite and bouts of fever. The outlook is often poor.

Hepar sulph 30c

This is the principal remedy to try to help abort the suppuration. It needs to be given over an extended period of time.
Dose: twice daily

Other indicated remedies include **Merc sol 30c**, **Merc corr 30c**, **Silica 30c** and **Lycopodium 30c**

Equine Hyperlipaemia

In this condition there is a disorder in the way that fats (lipids) are metabolised within the body leading to signs of liver failure as it becomes infiltrated with high levels of fats known as triglycerides. The kidneys can also be affected by infiltration with fats leading to signs of kidney failure as well. Ponies (especially Shetland ponies) and donkeys are most likely to be affected, with a definite bias to female animals rather than males. There are a number of predisposing factors which include obesity, starvation (enforced or as a consequence of illness), stressful situations (such as changes in diet, bad weather and transportation, other diseases (such as Cushing's disease, laminitis, colic and diarrhoea), pregnancy and lactation.

The main presenting symptoms are a drop in appetite, lethargy and dullness followed by signs indicative of liver failure, specifically jaundice, swelling of the liver, weight loss, diarrhoea, oedema (affecting the underside of the abdomen), skin symptoms, impaction of the gut, incoordination (ataxia), muscle twitching, head pressing and possibly other behavioural abnormalities. In the most severe cases the animal will exhibit convulsions and will lapse into a coma in the final stages of the illness. Those animals with the added problem of kidney failure will show other signs that may include an increase in thirst and urination and congested mucous membranes. A high proportion of cases fail to recover from this condition.

Careful and specific management combined with homeopathic treatment can offer some hope of recovery.

Homeopathic treatment of equine hyperlipaemia

Dose: 30c four times daily

As specific liver remedies for this condition **Phosphorus, Carduus, Lycopodium**

With swelling of the liver **Carduus, Lycopodium, Nat sulph, Chionanthus**

Jaundice **Phosphorus, Chionanthus**

Ataxia **Phosphorus**

With skin symptoms **Sepia, Sulphur**

With diarrhoea **Merc sol, Nux vom, Podophyllum**

Head pressing **Helleborus**

Muscle twitching **Agaricus**

Convulsions **Agaricus, Nux vomica**

The Urinary System

This section covers the urinary system and conditions affecting the kidneys, bladder and urethra. Urinary tract disease is not often diagnosed in the horse in comparison with other animals. This is probably because the symptoms are either less obvious or not easily recognised. Prompt homeopathic treatment can often help in both acute and chronic situations.

An ideal way to approach urinary problems is to divide the urinary system into two main sections. The first covers conditions affecting the kidneys, which often reflect on their role in controlling the water and electrolyte balance of the body. Symptoms that arise can often have far reaching effects on other areas or organs of the body. The second section covers diseases affecting the bladder and urethra. These manifest as changes in the flow or appearance of urine.

Normal horse urine is opaque with a little turbidity (cloudiness) especially near the end of urination. Clear urine is not normal. Mares in season normally squirt out small amounts of urine that is darker and thicker than normal. Other than this, most adult animals will urinate between four and six times per day. Horses normally pass urine at rest, often when put back into their stable and when there is clean bedding. If you look at your horse passing urine you will see the characteristic stance in which the back legs are moved apart and the body is leant forward a little. Changes in this normal routine, in the frequency of urination or the character of the urine should alert you to a problem.

The Kidneys

Kidney Disease

Kidney disease is rare in horses and not easy to detect. Symptoms may not appear until disease is advanced due to the fact that the kidneys have a reserve capacity. Up to 75 per cent of the functional tissue of kidneys can be damaged before any signs of disease are apparent. Whatever the cause, kidney disease will lead to kidney damage and symptoms of either acute or chronic kidney failure, encompassing conditions referred to as nephrosis (destruction of kidney tissue) and nephritis (inflammation of the kidneys).

Acute Renal Failure

There are several important causes of acute renal failure. These include fluid loss arising from haemorrhage and diarrhoea as well as septicaemia and endotoxaemia. Toxic damage to the kidneys from some drugs can also result in acute renal disease. Those drugs implicated include certain types of antibiotic (such as aminoglycosides and sulphonamides) and non-steroidal anti-inflammatories such as phenylbutazone. Plant poisons have also been involved in kidney damage (such as acorn poisoning) as well as damage from heavy metals (including lead, arsenic or mercury) and from pigments such as myoglobin, which can be released from muscle tissue during azoturia (tying up). Damage or blockage of either the bladder or urethra can also result in kidney damage caused by the back pressure of urine. Acute kidney damage can occur in foals in association with *Actinobacillus (Shigella) equuli* infection, otherwise known as sleepy foal disease (see page 158).

Specific symptoms include a reduction in the output of urine, which will appear concentrated, dark in colour and may contain blood. You may also see the horse straining to pass urine. The kidneys become swollen and there will be tenderness over the lumbar spine in the region overlying the kidneys, possibly with symptoms of general abdominal pain and an odd stance. There may also be a fever present as well as signs of shock (increased pulse and bright red mucous membranes), lethargy and inappetance.

In general, the most obvious symptoms of acute renal failure are related to the primary underlying cause such as toxaemia or diarrhoea. These conditions will need treating in their own right so that prompt treatment will improve your horse's chance of survival. Remember the value of dosing with **Aconite** (*1M potency given every 15–20 minutes*) in the early stages of acute renal failure until symptoms indicate the use of another remedy. Other fever remedies should also help in the early stages. Remedies to consider include **Belladonna** and **Pyrogen**. The *1M potency* is ideal and should be given *every 10–15 minutes*. Other useful remedies especially where there is diarrhoea include **China 30c** which is useful where there is dehydration, **Carbo veg 30c** where there is collapse and the animal is cold and **Phosphoric acid 30c** where there is debility and an associated increase in the production of urine.
Dose: 30c as often as needed

Remedies for acute renal failure

Apis mel

Pain over the kidney region is the main indication for this remedy due to swelling of the kidneys. Where Apis is needed there is little production of urine. The urine is dark in colour and contains high levels of protein and cell debris and may be passed with some discomfort. The horse may appear agitated.
Dose: 200c three times daily

Cantharis

Pain is also present over the back where Cantharis is needed, but the pains come and go causing the horse to keep changing position to minimise the discomfort. The area over the kidneys is tender to touch. Urine is passed in small amounts with some discomfort and may contain blood cells.
Dose: 200c three times daily

Terebinthina

Indicated where the kidneys are inflamed and where the urine contains large amounts of blood together with protein and has a smoky colour. The urine may also have a sweet odour and is passed with some amount of straining and discomfort.
Dose: 30c three times daily

Eucalyptus

This less well-known remedy is indicated in acute nephritis where the urine contains blood and large numbers of white blood cells. Discomfort is apparent as urine is passed.
Dose: 30c three times daily

Merc corr

The key indicator to the use of this remedy is the appearance of the urine which contains both blood and shreds of mucus. There is very marked discomfort on passing urine and obvious straining. Heavy metal poisoning may respond to this remedy.
Dose: 30c three times daily

Colchicum

This is an ideal remedy to use in acute situations where signs include little urine output and where the urine is dark, contains blood and a high level of protein. Pain is evident in the lumbar region and the horse is disinclined to move.
Dose: 30c four times daily

Eel serum

This remedy is indicated where there is little output of urine and the level of urea (a waste product excreted by the kidneys) in the blood is very high. The urine contains high levels of albumin (a protein) and red blood cells. There may also be concurrent heart disease.
Dose: 30c three times daily

Merc sol

Merc sol is useful in acute situations where toxins have led to acute kidney damage. The urine contains protein, blood and is only passed in small amounts. Sweating is a prominent feature differentiating this remedy from others.
Dose: 30c three times daily

Other useful remedies

Dose: 30c three times daily

Kali chlor where there is ulceration of the mucous membranes within the mouth.

Nux vomica is useful as a general remedy where poisoning is involved.

Chronic Renal Failure

This condition is rarely seen and is most likely to occur in older horses as a result of ageing. Acute kidney disease can lead onto **chronic renal disease** but there are also a number of other specific underlying causes. These include conditions affecting the glomeruli, the parts of the kidney that filter out the urine, which can become damaged. Tumours and kidney stones can also lead to chronic kidney disease.

The main symptoms are poor appetite and weight loss. The urine becomes dilute and is passed in increased quantities due to poor kidney function. There will also be an increase in thirst (although this is often difficult to gauge in horses), some degree of lethargy and depression as well as bad breath and possibly ulceration within the mouth. In severe cases, fluid may collect under the brisket area due to leakage of protein out through the kidneys. The urine may contain protein and cell debris. Anaemia can also be a feature.

Remedies for chronic renal failure

Arsenicum album

Look out for thirst for small quantities of water, general unthrifty appearance and dry flaky coat. Most animals that will respond to this remedy exhibit symptoms of restlessness and anxiety and even prostration in later stages. Affected animals are easily exhausted.
Dose: 30c once or twice daily

Phosphorus

Phosphorus suits lean athletic looking animals. Notable symptoms indicating this remedy include sensitivity to noise, thirst for large amounts of water, albumen and cell debris in the urine, loose dung and possibly the collection of fluid in the brisket region. Most horses that respond well to Phosphorus are of a friendly if not flighty, nervous disposition.
Dose: 30c once or twice daily

Natrum muriaticum

Suited to less friendly animals who shun attention and are more insular in nature. They tend to be greedy by nature but have a lean build. Check for thirst for large quantities of water and an increase in urination which is sometimes slow to start. Skin problems may also be apparent. Look for areas of hair thinning and patches of greasy skin. The eyes may appear very watery or runny. Horses that respond to Nat mur often have a craving for salt licks.
Dose: 30c once daily

Berberis vulgaris

Most chronic cases will benefit from this remedy. Pain over the lumbar region is the most prominent symptom together with lethargy or a reduction in stamina. Some discomfort is evident during urination and the urine will contain some sediment. Variable thirst is also a symptom associated with this remedy. Berberis is a useful remedy where azoturia is the underlying cause.
Dose: 30c once daily

Lespidiza

This is a less well-known remedy that is a good general remedy for chronic renal disease. It can be used alongside any other remedies.
Dose: 6x once or twice daily

Other useful remedies

Dose: 30c twice daily

Apis mel useful where there is fluid build up in the brisket area.

Benzoic acid indicated where the urine has pungent repulsive odour.

Solidago as a general kidney remedy indicated where the urine is clear but where there is pain over the kidney region.

Alfalfa to generally assist kidney function, helping to lower urea levels. Indicated where there is increased urination.

Plumbum where there is marked evidence of muscle wasting together with anaemia and unsteady movements.

Pyelonephritis

This is an infection affecting the pelvis of the kidney and is most common in mares after foaling. Infection ascends up the urinary tract although bacteria can also gain access through the blood from an infection at another site in the body or from septicaemia. Foals with an infected navel can develop pyelonephritis as a result of the infection spreading by the blood route. Symptoms can be acute or chronic.

The acute signs can resemble cystitis and include the presence of blood and pus in the urine accompanied by a fluctuating temperature, abdominal pain and a reduction in urinary output. In chronic situations, the symptoms develop more slowly and can include weight loss, lethargy and oedema of the lower limbs and stomach region. Anaemia may also be present as well as the symptoms generally associated with chronic kidney disease. Often the kidney damage which results is not reversible. For this reason the outlook can be very poor. Homeopathic remedies can help if treatment is started early on.

Pyrogen

This is an ideal remedy to use in acute feverish cases and where infection is blood borne. In these situations there is usually evidence of the primary source of infection as well. Straining to pass urine is a characteristic as well as the presence of a high fever (which may fluctuate up and down) and malaise.
Dose: 1M hourly until symptoms abate

Cantharis

This is one of the best known urinary remedies and is useful in acute cases where the symptoms appear suddenly and are intense. The urine contains a large amount of blood and is passed in small amounts and with obvious discomfort. Prompt use of this remedy can limit damage to the kidneys by preventing any infection ascending to the kidneys.
Dose: 200c hourly until symptoms abate

Hepar sulph

Hepar sulph is indicated where there is a low fever or where blood and most notably pus are present in the urine. Straining or discomfort during urination is usually a feature. Affected animals are also sensitive to cold and resent touch over the back region close to the kidneys. Weight loss may also be apparent as well as an increase in thirst.
Dose: 200c three times daily

Arsenicum album

High levels of protein together with pus, blood and debris in the urine indicate Arsenicum, especially where little urine is passed and the horse appears restless. In later stages if the situation becomes chronic, Arsenicum is indicated where there is anaemia, increased thirst and general ill thrift. It is also useful where infection remains at a low level despite treatment with antibiotics.
Dose: 30c twice daily

Merc corr

Very painful urination and the presence of much blood and greenish pus act as pointers to this remedy. Typically urine continues to dribble after the end of urination. Sweating is also a good indicator in cases where this remedy will help.
Dose: 200c three times daily

Terebinthina

The main indicator for this remedy is the presence of oedema in addition to the other symptoms associated with pyelonephritis. The urine appears slimy with blood and is passed with a degree of straining. Affected animals appear stiff and uncomfortable.
Dose: 200c three times daily

Silica

Chronic cases are suited to Silica. Again there is blood and pus in the urine but to a lesser degree than with Hepar sulph. Thirst and urine output are usually increased. There is discomfort on urination.
Dose: 30c twice daily over several weeks

Ocimum canum

This lesser known remedy is useful where the urine has a very offensive smell and contains large

amounts of urine and pus. The urine appears thick. Pain over the right kidney area is a useful pointer.
Dose: 30c three times daily

Methylene Blue
This remedy could prove useful where a large amount of pus is present in the urine, which takes on a greenish colour.
Dose: 3x three times daily

The Bladder and Urethra

The bladder stores the urine that is produced by the kidneys, expanding as it fills with urine. When full, the bladder will empty to the outside, the urine passing through the urethra. Conditions involving this portion of urinary tract are not common and show mainly as changes in the way urine is passed.

Cystitis

Cystitis, or inflammation of the bladder, is more likely to arise in mares as the urethra is relatively short and empties into the vagina, which can itself can harbour infection. In male animals the urethra is much longer and narrower, so the risk of infection is much less. The main cause is a bacterial infection arising as a result of changes affecting the passage of urine or trauma to the bladder lining. These include bladder stones, bladder cancer, paralysis of the bladder and concurrent disease (such as metritis in mares). Cystitis can also arise as a result of veterinary investigations involving either catheterisation of the bladder or endoscopy of the reproductive tract. Symptoms of cystitis can be both acute and chronic

Symptoms of acute cases to look out for include frequent urination (with only small amounts of urine passed each time), evidence of pain during urination including straining to pass urine (even though urine may just have been passed) and the presence of blood in the urine. Chronic cases tend to show less severe symptoms and in addition will include dribbling of urine, urine scald to the skin of the surrounding area and evidence of dry crusty material around the vulval area.

There are several useful remedies that can be used to treat cystitis successfully but it is always important to try and determine the underlying cause and use appropriate remedies to help. A few animals with cystitis may run a fever. If this is the case **Aconite 1M** is useful in the initial stages.

Cantharis
This is the best known of all the homoeopathic remedies used in the treatment of acute cystitis and certainly one of the most effective. Pain is one of the key elements in selecting Cantharis as the correct remedy, so much so that the horse may appear to have symptoms of colic rather than cystitis. Urine is only passed with much discomfort and with frequent urging even after urine has been passed. Blood in the urine is often a feature.
Dose: 30c hourly until symptoms abate

Terebinthina
The symptoms associated with this remedy are similar to those of Cantharis except that the urine has a very pungent smell, contains large amounts of blood and is very cloudy.
Dose: 30c hourly until symptoms abate

Staphysagria
The main indication for this remedy is cystitis arising after physical trauma, particularly where investigations of either the urinary or reproductive tract have been carried out and after bladder surgery. Signs of straining and discomfort are evident but not as pronounced as with Cantharis but affected animals may show signs of irritability.
Dose: 30c four times daily until symptoms abate

Pulsatilla
Pulsatilla is more suited to treating cystitis in mares where the key symptom is dribbling of urine in between bouts of straining. This is particularly so when the animal moves. Again the familiar symptoms of cystitis are present; discomfort, frequent urination with only a little urine passed each time and blood in the urine. The signs are less pronounced than with Cantharis and so this remedy may be useful in treating chronic cases.
Dose: 30c twice daily until symptoms abate

Sepia
This is another remedy more suited to chronic cases

and particularly in mares. One of the main points to selection of this remedy is the grumpy offhand nature of the patient. Urination is often slow and the urine may contain gravel-like material or sediment.
Dose: 30c twice daily until symptoms abate

Copaiva and Solidago

These less well-known remedies are useful as a follow-up to some of the other remedies when the most severe and obvious symptoms have passed. Copaiva acts mainly on mucous membranes and will help heal the bladder lining and Solidago will help cleanse the urinary tract.
Dose: 6c twice daily

Sarsaparilla

Useful where discomfort is most apparent after urine has been passed and dribbles out while the horse stands. An ideal remedy for more chronic cases.
Dose: 30c twice daily

Equisetum

This is another remedy for more chronic cases where large amounts of urine are passed each time rather than the smaller quantities characteristic of other remedies.
Dose: 30c twice daily

Other useful remedies

Dulcamara 30c Cystitis arising from changes in weather especially in damp cold conditions

Arnica 30c Where cystitis develops after direct trauma to the abdomen such as after a fall

Causticum 30c Where cystitis develops due to retention of urine in the bladder, most notably after surgical operations

Chimaphila 30c Where the urine contains large amounts of thick mucus usually with blood

Urethritis

Inflammation of the urethra is known as urethritis and is most likely to arise in stallions as a result of injury to the penis or in other male animals from an ascending bacterial infection. Symptoms can appear very similar in nature to those resembling obstruction of the urethra leading to pain and reluctance to cover a mare in stallions. Suitable remedies include **Arnica** in the first instance to cover the effects of trauma followed by one of the following used in *200c potency three times daily* until the symptoms clear:

Argentum nitricum

This is the most important remedy for the treatment of urethritis, especially where there is some dribbling of urine and the urethra is inflamed and appears uncomfortable.

Apis

A good remedy for urethritis where the passage of urine is uncomfortable causing the animal to become restless, fidgety and irritable.

Cantharis

Where there is an ascending infection and the symptoms resemble those of cystitis.

Staphysagria

Where there has been trauma involved leading to symptoms similar to cystitis.

Stubborn cases may respond to **Sycotic co 200c**, **Medorrhinum 200c**, **Thlaspi bursa pastoris 30c**, **Sycotic co 30c** or **Thuja 200c**.
Dose: twice daily for five days

Urolithiasis (Urinary Calculi)

This relates to the presence of stones in the urinary system. In the horse the most common site for these to form is the bladder, although they can also occur in the urethra. Several factors are involved in the formation of stones including the pH of the urine, diet and water intake leading to precipitation of material dissolved in the urine to form stones. Most of the gravel and stones which form are composed of calcium carbonate although phosphate, magnesium and ammonium can also be present.

Bladder Stones, Cystic Calculi Vesical Calculi, Urinary Gravel

Symptoms of bladder stones include symptoms very similar to those of cystitis which is usually present as a secondary problem. Signs not unlike those of mild colic causing the horse to walk with a stiffened gait may also be present as well as dribbling of urine which can contain blood. Treatment is usually surgical to remove the calculi. The following remedies may be useful in preventing recurrence.

Remedies specific to the composition of the calculi

Dose: once daily on a long-term basis

Calc carb 6x indicated where the stones are composed of calcium carbonate

Phos ac 6x where the stones contain phosphate

Mag phos 6x where the stones contain magnesium

Ammon carb 6x where the stones contain ammonium

Non-specific remedies for urolithiais

Hydrangea 3x a good general remedy but will also help where there is an increase in the frequency of urination or where it takes longer than usual to start to pass urine.

Urtica 6c useful in eliminating the material that forms the basis of the crystals and stones.

Lycopodium 6c another general remedy useful where the urine contains sediment.

Berberis 30c a useful remedy to help cleanse the urinary tract indicated especially where there is concurrent back pain in the lumbar region.

Urethral calculi

Stones which form in the bladder can pass down into the urethra leading to complete or partial obstruction to the flow of urine. This is most likely to occur in males where the urethra is narrower. Clinical signs include colic, frequent attempts to try to pass urine, restlessness and agitation. If the situation is left untreated the bladder gradually distends and can rupture. Surgery to remove the offending calculi is the only course of action. In the short term while awaiting help the following may bring some relief:

Pareira brava
Indicated where there is constant urging to pass urine with only small amounts passed sometimes followed by dribbling. The urethra is inflamed and the bladder distended.
Dose: 30c every 15 minutes

Thlaspi bursa pastoris
Helps where the symptoms are similar to the previous remedy but more specifically the urine contains blood. This is also a useful remedy for chronic cystitis where the stones contain phosphate.
Dose: 30c every 15 minutes in urethral blockage, once daily for chronic cystitis

Sarsparilla
Pointers to the selection of this remedy include some straining to pass urine which appears as a weak stream, dribbling of urine, blood in the urine and distension of the bladder. Useful in less acute cases.
Dose: 30c three times daily

Stricture of the Bladder or Urethra

This can arise post-operatively and can be minimised or possibly removed by using the following combination of remedies all in *6c potency given twice daily* over a period of several weeks: **Silica**, **Thiosinaminum** and **Calc fluor.**

Paralysis of the Bladder

There are a number of conditions which can lead to damage or disease of the nerves which supply the bladder leading to paralysis. The success of treatment will ultimately be linked to the nature of the underlying cause. The list includes damage to the lower lumbar vertebrae, pelvis or coccygeal region, the presence of spinal tumours, infection with Equine herpes virus 1 (EHV-1) and Cauda equina neuritis.

As a result of becoming paralysed the bladder does not empty and gradually becomes distended with urine. The signs to look out for include dribbling of urine, either constantly or intermittently, dribbling or spurting of urine during exercise or coughing, urine scald, secondary cystitis and possible hind limb weakness. Where injury is concerned remember the value of giving both **Arnica 30c** and **Hypericum 30c** (which is a specific remedy for nerve damage) as first aid remedies. **Bellis 30c** is another useful remedy where injury to the pelvis is involved. If cystitis is present you will also need to treat these symptoms.

Useful remedies for paralysis which should be given in the *30c potency twice daily include*:

Causticum
This is one of the principal remedies for bladder paralysis where the symptoms appear slowly over a period of time. Dribbling of urine is particularly noticeable during movement or if the animal coughs. Also indicated in paralysis arising after surgery to the bladder.

Gelsemium
Gelsemium is another excellent remedy for weakness of the bladder especially where there is general muscular weakness as well.

Opium
For loss of contractile power in the bladder particularly after an accident or where shock is involved.

Nux vomica
Indicated where there is concurrent hind limb weakness as well, resulting in dragging of one or both limbs. If signs of cystitis are also present but not marked, then Nux vomica may also be of value in clearing the symptoms.

Conium
For paralysis accompanied by other neurological symptoms, particularly where the hind limbs appear to be affected, resulting in an uneven gait.

Incontinence

This is a rare occurrence in horses and most likely to be associated with some of the conditions previously listed. If there is no immediate cause then **Causticum 30c** is one of the main remedies to think of using. Additional remedies worth consideration are **Lycopodium 30c**, **Sepia 30c**, **Arsenicum album 30c** and **Pulsatilla 30c**.

Haematuria

The presence of blood in the urine is referred to as haematuria and is actually a clinical symptom rather than a diagnosis. There are numerous causes, which include some of the conditions listed previously such as cystitis or the presence of calculi. There are also several other causes. The list would include trauma to the bladder region, the side effects of some drugs (including non-steroidal anti-inflammatories), the effects of ingesting some poisonous plants, the presence of a tumour in the bladder, concurrent liver disease or bleeding induced by exercise.

Non-specific homeopathic treatment for haematuria will help to resolve the immediate symptoms but the underlying cause should still be sought and dealt with.
Dose: between once and four times daily depending on the severity of the condition with the remedy that most closely matches the symptoms and cause

Arnica 200c Where the cause is injury and blood is dark in colour

Hamamelis 30c Where there is continued haematuria following injury where the blood is dark.

Millefolium 30c Where the cause is unknown and the blood is bright red

Erigeron 30c Where there is persistent chronic haematuria

Phosphorus 30c Where the urine contains watery blood

Ipecac 30c Where the urine contains very large amounts of blood

Thlaspi bursa pastoris 6c From the presence of urinary calculi

Anilinum 30c From tumours in the urinary tract

The Reproductive System

This section of the book covers both the female and male reproductive systems and suggests remedies to deal with common problems. The problems associated with breeding, pregnancy and parturition (foaling) are also included.

The Mare

The Female Reproductive Tract and Normal Oestrus Cycle

The reproductive organs of the mare consist of two ovaries, the fallopian tubes that connect the ovaries to the uterus, the cervix and vagina which opens to the vulva, which is the external opening of the genital tract. Most people familiar with the mare will be aware of the oestrus cycle and the behavioural and physical changes that normally occur. The nature of the cycle classes the mare as a seasonally polyoestrus animal, meaning the mare will repeatedly come into season during specific times of the year as influenced by a number of important factors. These include the climate, state of general health and nutrition and the most important of all, daylight length, which is normally determined by the season of the year. In the Northern Hemisphere the period of cyclical activity occurs over the spring and summer months although where problems arise, some mares may show activity outside these normal periods. The period of the year where no sexual activity takes place is known as anoestrus.

As the daylight length increases in the spring, the ovaries become active initiating a sequence of events that are controlled by hormonal activity. Within the ovaries follicles start to develop each containing an egg. Following the release of the first egg from an ovarian follicle, the cycle will generally settle down to a regular pattern marking the transition from anoestrus to regular cycles. The normal cycle of the mare lasts around 21 days on average, and can be divided into two distinct phases. The first is the **oestrus** or follicular phase, which lasts between five and seven days. The second is the **dioestrus** or luteal phase that lasts usually between 14 or 15 days.

During the period of oestrus, ovarian follicles release the hormone oestrogen which causes a number of changes to occur. The mare will show increased sexual receptivity and a number of significant behavioural changes. These include winking (eversion of the lips if the vulva to show the clitoris), raising of the tail, excessive urination, squatting (as if going to urinate), kicking or striking out and squealing with the ears pushed back. At the same time, both the cervix and vagina will become relaxed which occurs concurrently with an increase in the secretions produced by the uterus, cervix and vagina together with an increase in the amount of fluid present within these tissues. In the last 24–48 hours before the end of oestrus, ovulation occurs and an egg is released from one of the follicles.

During the dioestrus period, the ruptured follicle develops into a corpus luteum which produces another hormone known as progesterone. This has a number of effects including assisting in closure of the cervix, preparation of the reproductive tract for pregnancy and to stop sexual behaviour so that any further advances from a stallion are rejected. If the mare is not mated or conception does not occur, then the mare will return to oestrus after a period of 14–15 days. Oestrus will occur regularly in most mares throughout the breeding season. As daylight length shortens in the autumn, the cycle will normally cease and the mare will enter the period known as anoestrus until the following spring.

Abnormalities of the Cycle and Infertility

A proportion of mares will show abnormal cycles, that is that the pattern deviates from the normal regular cycle in some way. This can occur for a number of reasons leading to infertility, which in seasonally polyoestrus animals such as the mare, can be a major problem. The most common abnormalities of the cycle, which interfere with breeding, are listed together with the main remedies to help deal with these problems. As always seek professional help where necessary to establish an accurate diagnosis.

Prolonged oestrus

Normally oestrus lasts between five and seven days except in the spring period where it may last longer and can be as long as several weeks. This can cause problems early on in the breeding season and is most likely to occur in mares in poor condition and in young mares. Often the condition will correct itself after a period of time.

Prolonged dioestrus

In this instance the dioestrus period lasts longer than the regular 14–15 days, in some cases as long as several weeks or even months. The cause is normally persistence of the corpus luteum, which continues to produce progesterone. This occurs as a result of the failure of the uterus to release substances known as prostagandins. Prolonged dioestrus can also occur as a result of embryonic death in a pregnant mare.

Prolonged anoestrus

Anoestrus means that there are no oestrus cycles and no oestrus, a situation which is normal over the winter period. However, this state can continue into the spring and into the breeding season so that the mare cannot be bred. Stress is a major factor in animals that show prolonged anoestrus periods. Factors such as poor environment, bad weather, poor nutrition, heavy worm burdens and poor body condition can lead to persistent anoestrus periods. It is imperative that these underlying causes are attended to in conjunction with any other treatment well before the breeding period.

Suboestrus or dioestrus ovulation

This term refers to a lack of visible behavioural oestrus in cycling mares. The underlying causes are very similar to those that apply to periods of prolonged anoestrus.

Main Remedies for Irregular Oestrus Cycles and Infertility

Aim to treat this problem on a constitutional basis where possible. The following remedies are the most important.
***Dose** with the 200c potency once daily for 5 days then once weekly for 4 weeks*

Pulsatilla
Pulsatilla is suited to mares with a mellow, gentle temperament and which have good mothering abilities and a sensitive nature. This is an ideal remedy to help with anoestrus problems.

Sepia
For sullen touchy mares that avoid company.

Platina
For haughty headstrong mares which are apt to kick out or bite.

Lilium tigrinum
For mares of an anxious irritable fidgety nature that may have symptoms of nymphomania as well.

Lachesis
For mare that dislike being touched or which show jealousy. They are apt to bite or kick.

Calc carb
Suited to stubborn or heavy breeds particularly, Calc carb can help establish the cycle where oestrus is prolonged.

Lycopodium
The typical Lycopodium mare is lean and lacks confidence, dislikes being alone and will often become attached to one other particular horse. Lycopodium will help where the period of oestrus lasts too long. Pain over the right ovarian region is a good pointer to this remedy.

Nat mur
This remedy is suited best to animals that tend to be sullen and which tend to isolate themselves from the others. Mares with prolonged anoestrus or irregular cycles will benefit from this remedy.

Other Homeopathic Remedies for Irregular Cycles and Infertility

***Dose** using the 30c potency twice daily for five days initially and then 200c once weekly for four weeks*

Kali carb
Suited best to mares with an irritable temperament or those that are moody or touchy, Kali carb is worth consideration where anoestrus, suboestrus or prolonged dioestrus is a problem. Any pain in the lumbar region of the back or down the back legs is a useful indicator to the use of this remedy.

Luna
Acts as a general remedy for infertility and is a good choice if no other remedy is clearly indicated.

Folliculinum
This remedy can be used where a state of suboestrus is suspected where the mare cycles but shows no external signs as such or where a state of anoestrus persists.

Sabina
This remedy is indicated where there is accompanying back pain, particularly around the area of the pelvis.

Senecio aureus
This is a general remedy that may help with periods of anoestrus suiting mares with an irritable and nervous temperament.

Gossypium
A good remedy to use in cases of prolonged anoestrus where other indicated remedies fail to act.

Infertility with Normal Cycles

For mares, which persistently fail to become pregnant despite cycling normally, consider the following: **Progesterone 12c** together with **LHRH 12c** (Lutenising hormone releasing hormone)
***Dose:** twice daily for five to seven days prior to mating*

Behavioural Problems and Pregnancy

Where the stallion is refused and the mare is aggressive use: **Platina 200c** *twice daily for seven days* prior to serving with the stallion.

If the mare is in a state of excitement and difficult to control or aggressive use **Lachesis 200c** *twice daily for seven days* prior to serving with the stallion.

Where the mare is particularly nervous or anxious consider **Ignatia 200c** *twice daily for seven days* prior to serving with the stallion.

Cystic Ovaries, Ovarian cysts

True cystic ovaries as such do not exist in the mare but it is thought that follicular over-development can occur in some instances. This can lead to irregularities in the oestrus cycle or changes in behaviour. Often the condition will resolve itself. Cysts can also arise as the result of ovarian tumours which, can in turn, give rise to symptoms of abdominal colic, weight loss and possibly fluid in the abdomen.

The best way of dealing with these problems is to match the symptoms to the most suitable remedy.
***Dose:** 30c twice daily until symptoms resolve*

Apis mel
This is the principal remedy to consider especially if there are no signs of oestrus and there are symptoms that include back pain over the region of the ovaries and general restlessness. Abdominal discomfort can also be a sign. This remedy should be considered in cases where fluid collects in the abdomen as the result of a tumour.

Lachesis
Indications for this remedy include left-sided ovarian discomfort. Lachesis suits mares with an unreliable, suspicious temperament and which are apt to kick out or bite.

Lilium tigrinum

This remedy is most helpful where there are signs of ovarian pain which appear to extend down to the legs. Affected mares are restless, anxious and often hurried in nature.

Colocynthis

Useful where ovarian discomfort is extreme and causes the mare to become restless. The back is arched due to the pain. This position helps ease the discomfort.

Palladium

An important ovarian remedy, especially where the symptoms are more right-sided. There is usually some evidence of lower back pain as well.

Thuja

Indicated where there is intense left ovarian pain. Animals which have a history, which includes the appearance of warts or sarcoids, should respond well to this remedy.

Medorrhinum

This remedy is worth considering where other remedies fail to act. Ovarian pain is more evident on the left side with this remedy.

Also worth consideration:

Platina where there are also signs of nymphomania

Bovista where there is intolerance of tight-fitting tack

Iodum for thin anxious restless mares

Lycopodium best used constitutionally where the ovarian pain is markedly right-sided

Ovarian Haematomas

Haemorrhage can occur within the ovary as a result of excessive bleeding following ovulation. On examination these may feel like cysts. Although common, they can persist for several weeks they do not, however, cause an changes to the regular ovarian cycle. Ideal remedies to encourage resolution include **Arnica** and **Hamamelis**. Use both in the *30c potency twice daily* until the symptoms resolve.

Vaginal Bleeding between Oestrus Periods

This is not a common problem and normally the mare remains well. There are several remedies that can help put a stop to the bleeding.
Dose: *using the 30c potency twice daily for five days*

Sabina

Where the bleeding is worse for movement and bright red in colour. Signs of nymphomania may be present as well.

Phosphorus

Indicated where there is only a small quantity of watery blood present.

Ipecac

Where there is much bright red blood that appears in sudden gushes.

Secale

Where there is constant oozing of watery blood.

Nitric acid

This remedy is best used in persistent cases where the flow of blood is bright red.

Endometritis and Infertility

This term refers to inflammation of the endometrium, which forms the lining to the uterus, and occurs as a result of infection by bacteria and yeasts. The condition can be acute or chronic and is a major cause of infertility. There are numerous causes which include foaling, breeding, poor conformation and as a result of veterinary investigations. In the majority of mares, the body's own defence mechanisms will effectively remove any contamination so that infection does not become established. If the immune system is weakened or the anatomy of the region is changed there is an increased risk of contamination.

The most common symptoms include a coloured vaginal discharge, although this may not be present in all cases. Veterinary examination will usually reveal other signs including the presence of fluid within the uterus, thickening of the uterus and swelling in the region of the cervix. Treatment should include correcting any underlying defects as well as any other treatment that is needed. Homeopathic remedies can be of use in both acute and chronic cases.

In acute cases prompt treatment with **Aconite** and **Belladonna** may allay the symptoms before they progress any further. **Pyrogen** is indicated if there is a fever.
Dose: hourly using the 1M potency of these remedies until symptoms resolve or until another remedy is indicated

Remedies for endometritis

Dose: 30c twice daily until symptoms resolve

Pulsatilla
Indicated where the vaginal discharge is bland, thick and is yellow or creamy in colour. Pulsatilla works to its best advantage in mares that have a gentle nature. They often have light coloured coats.

Sepia
A yellow, greenish discharge with a degree of irritation suggests Sepia. This remedy will work best in mares with a sullen somewhat sad irritable nature. They will often have darker coloured coats.

Caulophyllum
Indicated where there is a degree of exhaustion and where the discharge is dark, almost chocolate like in colour.

Arsenicum album
A thin watery vaginal discharge that irritates the skin characterises Arsenicum. Affected animals are restless and thirsty for small amounts of water.

Hydrastis
A general remedy which helps where the discharge is sticky in nature and which irritates the skin leading to discomfort.

Sabina
This less well-known remedy has an affinity for the uterus and works where the vaginal discharge is offensive in nature.

Medorrhinum
This is a powerful remedy indicated where there is a profuse, chronic, dark and foul smelling discharge. Concurrent symptoms can include increased thirst and ovarian pain which is worse on the left side. The mare will be restless and fidgety.

Silica
Silica is suited to mares which have a weakened constitution and which have sensitive, yielding nature. They are over sensitive and can be nervous and excitable. The typical type of discharge that responds to Silica tends to be milky in nature.

Secale
Secale is effective where the vaginal discharge is brown and offensive in nature and works best where the animal is in generally poor condition.

Nosodes
It is also possible to use the appropriate **nosode** alongside any of the remedies mentioned depending on the organism involved. Nosodes that might prove useful include *Streptococcus zooepidemicis, E. coli, Klebsiella aerogenes, Staph aureus* and *Pseudomonas aeruginosa.*
Dose: with the 30c potency twice daily

Pyometra

Pyometra is different from endometritis in that pus collects inside the uterus which then becomes enlarged and distended as a consequence. The cause of this condition is uncertain but is thought to be due to adhesions within the cervix which interfere with the drainage of fluid. Symptoms can be hard to spot but sometimes include a mucky uterine discharge. Other signs such as septicaemia and lethargy are rare. Treatment consists of establishing drainage of the material through the cervix.

Appropriate remedies include those mentioned under endometritis. Additional remedies to break down any adhesions include **Graphites**, **Silica**, **Calc fluor** and **Thiosinaminum**.
Dose: 30c potency once daily

Other useful remedies include:

Calc sulph

This remedy should be considered once drainage has been established and where the discharge is yellow and thick to assist resolution of the problem.
Dose: 200c potency three times daily until symptoms resolve

Hepar sulph

Hepar sulph should prove useful where the discharge is purulent and has a very offensive smell.
Dose: 1M potency three times daily until symptoms resolve

Fraxinus americana

An ideal remedy to use in the treatment of pyometra if no other remedy seems appropriate.
Dose: 200c potency three times daily until symptoms resolve

Pyrogenium

Indicated where there is fever, depression and a purulent, foul vaginal discharge.
Dose: 1M potency two hourly until symptoms resolve

Abortion

Pregnancy in the mare lasts on average 340 days. Loss of a foal before 300 days gestation is termed abortion. The causes are varied and include:

Infections

Viral: EHV-1 virus (Equine herpes virus 1), Equine viral arteritis (EVA)

Bacteria: *Streptococcus zooepidemicus, E. coli, Klebsiella* and rarely *Salmonella abortus equi*

Fungi: Aspergillus and Mucor species

Other organisms: Leptospirosis, Protozoa

Non-infectious: Twinning, twisting of umbilical cord, trauma, shock

Treatment of abortion from a homeopathic perspective is largely either preventive or symptomatic.

Preventative measures involve using the appropriate **nosode** in anticipation of a known problem. Dose with the appropriate nosode in *30c potency twice daily for five days* at the start of pregnancy and repeat this procedure again after three and six months of gestation.

Symptomatic treatment involves using the best-indicated remedy for the situation.

The following remedies should be used in the 200c potency every two hours:
Arnica where trauma is involved

Baptisia where shock is involved

Bellis perennis where trauma to the pelvic region is involved

Aconite best given for shock and in the early stages of any infection

China off should be given where there is blood loss and weakness

The following remedies should be used in the 1M potency hourly:
Pyrogen where there is fever resulting from infection or sepsis

Baptisia where there is fever from infection and the mare appears confused and dull

The following remedies should be given in the 6c potency once daily from the start of pregnancy:
Viburnum opulus a general remedy to help prevent abortion

Sepia where the character of the mare is sad and sluggish

Pulsatilla for gentle, friendly mares

Kali carb where there is weakness and irritability

Helionas where there is back pain

Sabina where abortion occurs in the first four months of pregnancy

Caulophyllum useful for repeated abortion or where debility is a feature

Foaling and Associated Problems

Foaling or parturition is divided up into three distinct phases. The **first stage** is often difficult to detect and occurs some hours before the foal is delivered. This stage involves a number of signs which lead up to stage two. Signs to check for include colic-like symptoms with the mare becoming uneasy, pacing the box and looking around at her flank and swishing her tail. You may also see sweating (especially behind the ears and elbows and on the flanks and neck) and pawing at the ground. The hormone oxytocin, which is released from the pituitary gland, is responsible for initiating the uterine contractions and for stimulating milk production from the mammary glands. In some cases milk may even spurt out from the glands.

Avoid as much interference at this stage as possible. If the mare seems particularly agitated dose using **Aconite 1M** every 15 minutes until things appear calmer.

Near the end of stage one, the cervix opens ready for **stage two** which starts with the breaking of the waters. As the muscles of the uterus contract the foal moves into the birth canal and the mare will probably lie on her side. The contractions at this point are forceful and after a short while the white amniotic membrane covering the foal will appear between the lips of the vulva. If the foal is in the correct position, the forefeet will appear followed by the nose. The amniotic membrane will rupture and following stronger contractions, the body and hips will follow. After the mare has completed delivery she will probably rest. The whole of stage two should last no longer than one hour and normally takes little more than 20–30 minutes. It is imperative to seek help if you suspect any difficulties or that the foal is not presenting correctly.

There are several remedies which can also be used routinely to help prevent problems arising and to speed recovery.

Dose: *using the 30c potency twice daily, starting two or three days before the foal is due. During the actual delivery of the foal, the remedies can be given every five to ten minutes if need be*

Arnica will help minimise trauma, bruising and reduce the risk of haemorrhage.

Bellis can be used in a similar way to Arnica and is particularly indicated where there is much bruising to the abdominal walls and to the walls of the uterus.

Caulopyllum is one of the most important remedies in regard to strengthening weak or irregular contractions.

Causticum will help stimulate contractions if they cease completely (termed uterine inertia).

Calc phos can be used to tone the muscles of the womb and should be used in the period leading up to foaling.

Secale another alternative remedy to consider in cases of uterine inertia

Pulsatilla also has a reputation where there is insufficient tone in the uterine muscles to deliver the foal. It is best used on a constitutional basis.

The **third stage** commences after delivery of the foal and involves the expulsion of the afterbirth or placenta and involution (shrinking) of the uterus. Gradually the placenta separates from the uterus and as the mare stands, the placenta will protrude from the vulva. The uterus continues to reduce in size and eventually, about 30 minutes after foaling, the placenta will separate completely and drop to the ground.

Complications Following Foaling

Bruising

This is a common occurrence and can involve the vagina and the area of the vulva and anus known as the perineum. **Arnica 200c** or **Bellis 200c** can be given twice daily for five days to help resolve any problems.

Lacerations

During delivery, lacerations can occur to the perineal area. Injuries of this type are often the result of the foal's feet damaging or stretching the tissues. Always check to see if the damaged tissues will need suturing. A combination of **Arnica 30c** and **Hypericum 30c** should be given three times daily for the following ten days to encourage healing. Where lacerated areas are slow to heal, dose with **Calendula 30c** twice daily until the areas are healed completely. Where infection is involved dose with **Hepar sulph 200c** instead.

Haematoma

A haematoma is a blood-filled sac. The most common site for this problem to arise is in the wall of the vagina. Rupture will result in considerable bleeding and can be fatal. Ideal remedies to use to allow resolution include **Arnica 30c** and **Hamamelis 30c**, which should be given *twice daily for ten days. For persistent haematomas use* ***Secale 30c*** *given three times daily until the problem is resolved.*

Retained placenta

Although not a common problem, if the placenta has not separated within two to three hours after foaling, seek emergency help to avoid the risk of infection. There is a considerable risk of toxic metritis developing and subsequent problems such as laminitis. Remedies which can be used at this time to encourage expulsion include:

Sabina which has a special action on the uterus and is particularly indicated in cases where the placenta is retained. Some bleeding with clots of blood is a useful pointer.

Caulophyllum is worth consideration where the mare is exhausted and the contractions in general have been weak.

Sepia which can be used on a constitutional basis.

Pulsatilla can also be used on a similar basis.
Suggested dose 200c every ten minutes for six doses

Toxic metritis

This condition arises as a consequence of retention of the placenta and in essence constitutes an emergency situation. Remedies to use while waiting for help include:

Secale
An important remedy to use where there is an offensive, dark brown coloured discharge.
Dose: 200c every 10–15 minutes

Pyrogen
Indicated where there is overwhelming infection accompanied by a foul discharge. The mare will be restless and agitated with a high temperature although the pulse may be slow in comparison to Belladonna.
Dose: 1M every 10–15 minutes

Belladonna
Indicated in cases where there is a high fever, bounding pulse and risk of peritonitis.
Dose: 1M every 10–15 minutes

Echinacea 30x, **Crot horr 200c**, **Veratrum viride 200c** and **Baptisia 1M** are also worth consideration.

Post-Partum Haemorrhage

Bleeding can arise from the lining of the uterus, from a ruptured haematoma or from a torn artery. The latter is far more serious and normally involves the utero-ovarian artery which travels across one of the main ligaments which suspends the uterus, the broad ligament. Haemorrhage can also occur in conjunction with prolapse of the uterus or with torsion (twisting) of the uterus.

Bleeding from the uterus is not common in mares and is rarely serious. Normally after foaling, the uterus will contain some blood-tinged fluid as a matter of course. The haemorrhage from a ruptured haematoma or from a torn artery is serious and can prove potentially fatal as the mare may simply bleed to death. Signs to look out for include symptoms resembling colic, increased pulse and respiratory rate, sweating, rolling and trembling. A few mares will appear nothing more than vaguely depressed so it is wise to check the colour of the mucous membranes or the gums. Pale or white membranes will confirm any suspicions.

Treatment of post-partum haemorrhage is often difficult but a number of homeopathic remedies can help. Remember the benefit of giving **Arnica 30c** beforehand as a preventative remedy.

Erigeron is the principal remedy for major haemorrhage from a ruptured blood vessel

Ipecac is indicated where the haemorrhage is profuse, bright red in colour and comes and goes in gushes

Phosphorus will help where the blood is bright in colour but watery in nature

Nitric acid helps where there is bright red blood and a persistent flow

Sabina is useful where the blood is fluid with clots present

Millefolium can help where the blood is bright red and fluid and originates from the wall of the uterus

Ustilago helps where there has been a degree of uterine inertia beforehand or where the slightest movement causes further bleeding

Secale where there is dark coloured blood where the bleeding does not stop

Platina for persistent bleeding with large clots

Trillium where the blood gushes out on the least movement

Dose: with the 200c potency every 10–20 minutes depending on the severity of the problem

Where an animal has collapsed try giving **Carbo veg 200c** and **Veratrum album 200c** alternately every ten minutes.

During recovery there are a number of indicated remedies to help in the recovery phase. **China 30c** is indicated for blood loss and weakness, **Acetic acid 30c** will help with the anaemia resulting from blood loss after foaling, **Strontia 30c** with the after effects of haemorrhages in general, **Phosphoric acid 6c** for debility and **Arsenicum album 6c**, **Ferrum metallicum 6c**, **Ferrum arsenate 6c**, **Silica 6c** and **Phosphorus 6c** will help with anaemia in general.

Dose: using the 30c potency twice daily until the symptoms resolve

Uterine Prolapse

This is most likely to happen straight after the birth of the foal but can sometimes occur a few days later. Uterine prolapse is an emergency situation and will warrant emergency veterinary treatment. Think of using **Aconite 1M** for shock, **Arnica 200c** for the injury and trauma aspect and **Opium 1M** if the mare appears very fearful and keeps straining. Where there is continual straining and the uterus is very congested (swollen) think of using **Lilium tigrinum 200c**, dosing every five to ten minutes, to assist return of the uterus to its correct position. After the uterus has been replaced an ideal remedy to hasten resolution is **Sepia 30c**. *Use the 30c potency three times daily for ten days*

Weakness

Foaling can prove exhausting for some mares, which will be weakened by the experience. Remedies to help include:

Arnica as a general remedy

Gelsemium where the mare appears dull or where there is trembling

Kali carb is also an excellent remedy to use in general, particularly where there is back pain or the back legs appear weak

Use the 30c potency three times daily for ten days

Bleeding from the Umbilical Stump in Newborn Foals

If the umbilical cord is allowed to part naturally, (which should occur at a point about 3cm from the abdominal wall of the foal), the blood vessels within the cord should retract and seal themselves naturally preventing bleeding. In a few instances this fails to occur and the cord will bleed, sometimes profusely. To help stop the bleeding consider **Erigeron 30c**. *Dose: every 2–3 minutes until the bleeding stops*

Mismothering

It is the mare's natural instinctive behaviour to bond with the foal and allow it to suckle. In a few mares the maternal instincts are such that the mare will not approach the foal or even resents the foal attempting to feed. Remedies to help here include:

Pulsatilla for timid placid mares which appear shy of the foal initially

Platina for mares with a haughty, arrogant attitude, which may try to injure the foal

Sepia for mares which appear sad or sullen and which try to avoid the attentions of the foal

Lachesis where the mare appears suspicious of the

foal and may try to injure it

Lilium tigrinum where the mare appears agitated or anxious

Luna where there is a history of infertility or nymphomania

Use the 200c potency twice daily until the foal is accepted

Cramping

This is caused by uterine contractions that occur after the delivery of the foal and will give the appearance of mild colic. The purpose of these contractions is to ensure that the placenta is expelled and that the uterus shrinks in size. If the contractions appear to cause distress to the mare consider giving **Chamomilla 30c** *every two hours until the mare settles.* If the spasm seen unduly painful try giving **Cuprum met 30c** *hourly until the spasms seem to ease.*

Colic

Cramping pains which continue longer than about 12 hours suggest colic. Check in the section for colic for the most suitable remedy.

Eclampsia (Hypocalcaemia)

This condition which is also referred to as hypocalcaemia, is an infrequent occurrence in the mares, either in late pregnancy or in early lactation. Heavier breeds seem more prone to the condition as well as mares lactating heavily on rich pastures. Stress and overwork may also play a factor in some cases. The underlying cause is incorrect feeding particularly in relation to supplying sufficient levels of calcium, magnesium and Phosphorus during pregnancy and lactation. Symptoms can resemble colic, those seen with a torn ovarian artery or even tetanus, so an exact diagnosis is needed. Signs include unsteady movements or stilted gait, thrashing of the limbs, muscle twitching, stiffness of the back legs, and increased respiratory rate and sweating.

Suspected eclampsia constitutes an emergency if the mare is not to go into a coma and die.

Prevention is the best way of dealing with the problem. Dosing the mare with **Calc phos 30c** three times weekly during pregnancy and once daily during lactation will help.

Where symptoms are apparent dose with:

Calc phos 30c and **Mag phos 30c** every five minutes and where there is:

An unsteady gait dose with **Agaricus 200c** every five minutes

Violent thrashing give **Belladonna 200c** every five minutes

If the limbs or the body go into a state of contorted spasm dose with **Cicuta 30c** every five minutes

Where there are muscle twitchings dose with **Cuprum met 200c** every hour

Mastitis

Mastitis is not often seen in the mare but can occur during lactation and in the period afterwards when milk production has ceased. This is known as the dry period. The mammary glands will become swollen and painful to touch. Often the area is hot and in severe cases the swelling will extend to the area behind the glands and along the underside of the abdomen. This may cause the mare to move awkwardly and appear stiff. Appetite may be affected and the milk will usually change in appearance or consistency. Mastitis often responds well to homeopathy but where practical it is advisable to strip out the udder as well. In the early stages consider giving two or three doses of Aconite 1M about 30 minutes apart. If trauma is involved consider **Arnica 200c** instead.

Apis

Keynote: Swelling
This remedy is indicated where there is heat and considerable swelling of the glands and surrounding area. Touch is resented, as the area is very painful
Dose: *200c three times daily*

Belladonna

Keynote: Heat
Belladonna works well in very acute cases where the

mammary glands are acutely swollen and very hot to touch. Skin over the region will take on a reddish hue. Both pulse and respiratory rate will be elevated and the temperature will be raised.
Dose: 1M potency four times daily

Bryonia

Keynote: Better for pressure
Another remedy for acute cases but especially where the udder feels hard and indurated. Pressure on the affected area will give relief from the discomfort. Due to the pain the mare will often lie down.
Dose: 200c three times daily

Hepar sulph

Keynote: Suppuration
The glands will be very painful to the least touch and the milk will appear thickened with a pus-like consistency. Affected animals will seem irritable.
Dose: 200c three times daily

Phytolacca

Keynote: Glandular swellings
This is a good general remedy for both acute and chronic cases. In acute cases the milk will show clots and the glands will appear hard and lumpy. In chronic cases the glands will appear hardened, indurated with hard lumpy masses palpable and slightly sensitive to touch.
Dose: Acute cases – 200c three times daily
Chronic cases – 30c twice daily

Lac caninum

Keynote: Pain on least movement
Pain is very evident where this remedy is needed such that the mare will refuse to move and will seem very depressed. The mammary glands will appear swollen. Lac caninum will also help dry up the milk. This is a key remedy for mastitis of traumatic origin.
Dose: 200c three times daily

Lachesis

Keynote: Aggression
The main clue to using this remedy is the colour of the skin over the affected glands that will appear to have a blue discoloration. The left gland is usually the worse of the two where this remedy is needed. Affected mares will generally be of a suspicious and aggressive nature and may kick out as the glands are examined.
Dose: 200c three times daily

Silica

Keynote: Harp lumps
Silica is best reserved for chronic cases where there has been scarring leaving hard knotty lumps in the glands.
Dose: 30c potency once daily for a number of weeks

Conium

Can be used where there are numerous small hard nodules palpable in the gland.
Dose: 6c potency once daily for a number of weeks

Problems with Lactation (Milk Production), Inadequate Milk Supply

The following remedies can help increase the production of milk where it is insufficient.
Dose: three times daily.

Urtica 200c A good general remedy to use initially

Alfalfa 6x Best used where the mare is in poor condition. Will also improve the quality of the milk

Medusa 30c As an alternative to Urtica

Agnus castus 6c Where the mare appears depressed

Zincum met 30c Where the udder is painful

Calc carb 200c Use constitutionally

Calc phos 200c Use constitutionally

Pulsatilla 200c Use constitutionally

Where the mammary glands are under developed as well consider these remedies to help:
Iodum 30c, **Conium 30c**, **Sabal serrulata 30c**, **Kali iod 30c**
Dose: twice daily

Excess Milk Production

To dry up the milk

These remedies can be used to dry up the milk where production continues after a foal has been

weaned or where milk appears in non-pregnant animals due to hormonal problems.
***Dose:** three times daily*

Urtica 3x This is the main remedy to consider

Lac caninum 30c Use where the udder is very enlarged and painful

Cyclamen 6x Where the problem is due to hormonal problems, or following oestrus

Bryonia 30c For irritable, thirsty mares

Pulsatilla 30c Use constitutionally

Calc carb 30c Use constitutionally

Sore, Painful or Cracked Nipples

This can occasionally be a problem. The mare will show discomfort when the foal suckles. Apply **Calendula cream** twice daily where possible along with one of the following remedies:

Graphites A good general remedy to use where the nipples are sore, cracked or blistered

Castor equi Use where the nipples are ulcerated or cracked

Petroleum Indicated where the nipples are very cracked and sore with itching as well

Phytolacca Indicated where the nipples are extremely painful. Small ulcers may be present

Helionus Useful where the glands are very full and sensitive to the least touch

***Dose:** 30c once or twice daily until the condition improves*

Mareish Behaviour

A number of mares exhibit changes in behaviour in the period leading up to oestrus, which can include difficulty in handling or riding, aggression or rearing up. The symptoms bear some similarity to PMT and tend to disappear as the mare comes into season. You will however, need to differentiate this type of behaviour from the behavioural changes observed during a normal oestrus period. In this case the mare will often refuse to move freely, show excessive tail twitching and pass small volumes of urine repeatedly.

The signs associated with typical mareish behaviour occur in the period preceding oestrus and are related to fluctuations in hormonal levels. During this period progesterone levels start to fall and levels of oestrogen start to rise in preparation for ovulation. Although the changes in hormone levels will affect behaviour, there are often physical changes as well.

Some mares will become unpredictable both in their behaviour and in their performance. Some will show symptoms of back pain and will resent being saddled, others will not jump and a few will show colic-like symptoms. For the most part the majority of signs are behavioural. These include impatience, irritability, sensitivity to touch, aggression, rearing, non co-operation and destructive tendencies such as box chewing or kicking.

This condition often responds well to homeopathy when the most appropriate remedy is selected.
***Dose:** using the 200c potency once daily until the symptoms resolve*

Lachesis

Keynote: Suspicion
This remedy suits mares that tend to kick out and which show signs of aggression particularly when touched or examined around the hindquarters or abdomen. Mares matching Lachesis are often suspicious in nature and exhibit jealousy. There is a tendency to nip and kick at stable walls.

Pulsatilla

Keynote: Changeable
Pulsatilla suits mares of an altogether more gentle nature and those which are affectionate. Clues to using this remedy include dislike of heat and little thirst compared with other horses. In the pre-season period they often become touchy and sensitive to any changes in routine. Back pain is often a feature that manifests as difficulty in riding the animal.

Platina

Keynote: Haughty
Arrogance is one of the key features of Platina, together with a tendency to be rather headstrong and difficult to control. Sometimes mares needing this

remedy become almost hysterical and may become dangerous to approach. Signs often include violent behaviour such as kicking out with definite intent to injure.

Sepia

Keynote: Sullen and saggy
This remedy suits sullen animals that become more withdrawn as oestrus approaches and those which could be termed grumpy. They also become disinclined to work and will only perform well if pushed. Back pain can also be a feature as well as stiffness in the back legs. They will also show indifference to those that they are closest to. They often have a saggy, worn out look.

Hyoscyamus

Keynote: Aggression
This is another suspicious remedy but in addition mares which respond to this remedy show definite aggressive tendencies in the pre-oestrus period and behaviour which could be called hysterical at times. This manifests as difficulty in handling. Animals which respond well are also rather noisy.

Cimicifugia

Keynote: Intolerance of pain
Mares which exhibit pain in the region of the ovaries and around the pelvis and hindquarters in the period leading up to oestrus often respond to this remedy. They will also show stiffness in the region of the neck and lower back. Mentally they appear agitated or sometimes depressed.

Also consider

Lilium tigrinum for mares that appear hurried all the time

Luna where other remedies fail to act

Nymphomania

Opinion varies as to the cause of this type of excessive sexual behaviour in mares but it may well be linked with follicular cysts in the ovaries. The mare will cycle regularly but will become difficult to handle during the period she is on heat showing some of the symptoms associated with mareish behaviour. An appropriate remedy should be given for a few days in the period leading up to this time and over the period she is on heat.
Use the 200c potency and dose twice daily

Platina if the mare is haughty, headstrong or strong willed

Lachesis is there is sensitivity to touch, suspicion and aggression

Lilium tigrinum often best suits younger mares showing this type of behaviour for the first time

Murex with markedly excessive sexual excitement and possibly aggression

Origanum as an alternative to Murex

Hyoscyamus where there is marked degree of aggression

Ustilago maydis where the behaviour is very pronounced or fails to respond to other remedies

Coital Exanthema

Equine herpes virus 3, EHV-3, Spots

This venereal condition is caused by the Equine herpes virus 3, EHV-3, and affects the penis and prepuce in the male and the vulva, vaginal membranes (mucosa) and perineal area in the mare. The first signs are watery blisters or papules that then develop into pustular lesions followed by the appearance of small deep circular ulcers that are about 0.5cm and 2cm in diameter and surrounded by a zone of reddened tissue. Later these may develop yellowish scabs on top. The prepuce can sometimes become swollen in the male as can the vulva in the mare. This can happen some days after infection from the stallion has taken place. Infections often go unobserved and are resolved within about two weeks unless secondary bacterial infection complicates matters. In rare cases EHV-3 can cause lesions to appear on the lips, nostrils and conjunctival membranes of the eye.

This condition is self-limiting but mating should be avoided until all the lesions have cleared. Remedies that will hasten resolution include:

Nat mur 30c
Nat mur should be given at the earliest stage when the blisters or papules are present.
Dose: three times daily

Arsenicum hydrogenisatum 30c
This little known remedy is a specific to consider at the stage where both pustules and ulcers cover the prepuce in abundance.
Dose: three times daily

Merc sol 30c
This remedy should be used at the stage where ulcers are present and scabs are starting to form in both the mare and stallion.
Dose: three times daily

Nitric acid 30c
Use as an alternative to Merc sol, especially in the mare, but also where the ulcers are more stubborn in clearing and may appear painful along with a slight discharge.
Dose: three times daily

Rhus tox 30c
Useful where there is swelling of the prepuce in the male and vulva in the mare.
Dose: three times daily

Hepar sulph 200c
Hepar is another remedy to help treat the condition at the stage when ulcers are present. The lesions are sensitive to touch or may bleed slightly where this remedy is indicated. This remedy should also be used where secondary bacterial infection is present.
Dose: twice daily

Calc sulph 30c
Will help resolve the final stage where yellow scabs are present, overlying the healing ulcers. Calc sulph is also worth consideration where a thick preputial discharge is present due to secondary bacterial infection in the stallion or where a similar vaginal discharge is present in the mare.
Dose: three times daily

Borax 30c
This is the remedy of choice to use in the rare cases where there are lesions on the lips and nostrils.
Dose: three times daily

The Stallion

The basic reproductive anatomy of the stallion consists of the penis, which lies within the sheath, the testes which are situated within the scrotum, the epididymus, spermatic cord (which contains the vas deferens, blood vessels, lymphatic vessels, nerves and muscle fibres) and a number of glands known as the accessory glands. The control of the reproductive organs and reproductive behaviour is under the influence of the nervous system and a number of hormones.

The Testes

During most of gestation the testes develop and lie near the kidneys, passing into the scrotum in the last few weeks of pregnancy. After birth the testes continue to grow in size within the scrotum and attain maximum size around three years of age. The function of the testes is to produce sperm which are stored and then mature within the epididymus. During ejaculation the sperm leave the epididymus and enter a tube called the vas deferens or deferent duct. This connects to the pelvic portion of the urethra which serves as a passageway for both semen and urine. There are a number of conditions of the testes that can cause problems.

Testicular trauma and Orchitis

Trauma to the testicular region is normally the result of a direct blow or from injury resulting in lacerations to the area. Both conditions will often result in haemorrhage into the tissues of the testes resulting in subsequent loss of fertility. First aid treatment should be implemented as soon as possible. Dose with **Arnica 200c** and **Hamamelis 200c** *every 15 minutes* while waiting for professional help.

Orchitis is a term that applies to inflammation of either one or both testes and which can result in the horse becoming sterile. Trauma is a common cause although infection should also be considered.

Symptoms include obvious pain and swelling of the scrotum. Initial treatment should involve **Arnica 200c** followed by:

Spongia tosta

This is the most important remedy and particularly indicated where the horse appears anxious and where there is considerable swelling involving the testes and spermatic cord. Pain is an obvious feature.
Dose: 30c every 30 minutes

Pulsatilla

Suits animals of a more gentle nature and should be used where the pain appears to extend to the abdomen. The presence of a urethral discharge, which is yellowish in colour, should confirm the use of the remedy.
Dose: 200c four times daily

Rhododendron

Inflammation of the left testicle with considerable swelling suggests the use of this remedy. It is also an ideal remedy to use where the condition has become chronic in nature.
Dose: 200c four times daily

Testicular Degeneration

Testicular atrophy

There are a number of causes which underlie this condition including trauma, infection, damage to blood vessels supplying the testes and some types of medication. It can also arise as a result of ageing. The end result is a loss of fertility. Depending on the cause the condition may be reversible.

Suggested remedies to help include **Kali iod**, **Iodum**, **Sabal serrulata** (where there is also loss of libido), **Argentum nitricum** (where the animal is especially nervous), **Aurum** (where there is pain), **Thuja** (for very chronic cases) and **Capsicum**.
Use the 30c potency once daily for several weeks

Rigs or Cryptorchidism

Undescended testicles

Sometimes also referred to as a ridgeling, a horse is considered a rig or cryptorchid if either one or both testes have not descended into the scrotum. Surgery is normally the best option. Remedies that are reputed to aid the decent of the testicles include **Clematis**, which is the most important in respect of this problem. **Calc carb**, **Tuberculinum** and **Aurum** are also worth considering.
Use the 200c potency once daily for seven days

False rigs

This term is applied to horses that have been castrated which still retain stallion like behaviour. Observed behaviour can include rounding up of mares, attraction to mares in season, erection and in rare cases ejaculation. Remedies which may help tone down this behaviour include **Murex**, **Ustilago**, **Staphysagria**, **Phosphorus** and **Cantharis**.
Use the 1M potency repeating the dose as needed

Spermatorrhoea

This term essentially relates to stallions that have a low sperm count. Remedies which are reputed to help with this problem include:

Pulsatilla for stallions with a more gentle nature

Platina for animals with an aggressive nature

Cantharis which suits over sexed animals

Sepia for irritable animals

Silica which suits those animals with poor conformation
Use the 30c potency and dose twice daily for two weeks prior to the stallion serving the mare

The Scrotum

The scrotum protects the testicles and associated structures including part of the spermatic cord. It is also involved in the thermoregulation of the testes, which is vital to the production of sperm as this needs to take place at a lower temperature than the core temperature of the body.

The scrotum is subject to trauma which can occur during mating and result in lacerations, bruising and secondary infection. First aid treatment should include **Arnica** for general trauma, **Hypericum** where there are lacerations or puncture wounds (**Hypericum** will also protect against tetanus), **Apis** where there is oedematous swelling and **Hamamelis** where there is haemorrhage and or pain.
Use the 200c potency three times daily as needed

Scrotal dermatitis

The most common form of dermatitis is contact dermatitis, which affects the scrotum locally resulting in inflammation and discomfort. Causes include contact with irritant chemicals (which can include fly deterrents, shampoos and disinfectants), contact with and scalding by an accumulation of manure, reactions to fly bites and infection with the microfilariae associated with *Onchocerca cervicalis*. Ideal remedies to use include:

Rhus tox
Ideally suited in situations where the skin of the scrotum is swollen and puffy and where there is intense irritation.

Graphites
Helps where the skin is weepy and sticky.

Crot tig
Can help where there is intense itching with oozing, and skin vesicles.

Cantharis
Indicated where there is much agitation due to the intensity of the inflammation. The skin appears puffy and reddened.
Use the 30c potency four times daily until the symptoms subside

Varicocele

Varicocele refers to a condition that affects the blood vessels of the pampiniform plexus (a tortuous mass of blood vessels associated with the testes), which can become distended. Diagnosis can be made by palpation of the neck of the scrotum, checking for any thickening of the tissues. Depending on the severity of the condition there may be no obvious symptoms and no reflection on breeding performance. In severe cases thrombosis of the vessels can occur, resulting in discomfort and a possible reduction in breeding potential. Remedies that may help include **Hamamelis**, **Pulsatilla**, **Aesculus hippocastanum**, **Lachesis** and **Lycopodium**. **Bothrops** is useful specifically if thrombosis is suspected.
Use the 30c potency three times daily for seven days

Hydrocele

Accumulation of fluid within the tissue layers of the structures contained within the scrotum is referred to as hydrocele. This can arise as a consequence of local inflammation or from fluid which has collected in the abdomen draining into the scrotal region. The most obvious choice of remedy to help with this condition is **Apis**. Other indicated remedies include **Graphites** (in horses with a heavy build), **Iodum** (for animals with a leaner build), **Pulsatilla** (suited to those with a gentle nature), **Rhododendron** (specifically indicated for this condition) and **Silica** (in subjects with a poor conformation).
Use the 200c potency three times daily for seven days

The Urethra

The urethra extends from the bladder to the penis and transports both urine and semen. In the stallion the urethra secretes mucus into the urine and seminal fluid. There are relatively few conditions that can affect this part of the horse's anatomy.

Trauma

The urethra can be subject to trauma during breeding or from an injury such as a kick. It can also be damaged during investigative procedures such as catheterisation or endoscopy. Calculi which have passed down from the bladder can also become lodged in the urethra leading to tissue damage to the walls. These will need to be removed by surgery.

Arnica 200c should be given three times daily at the first signs of any damage followed by **Calendula 30c** given twice daily will facilitate healing of any injuries. One of the consequences of urethral trauma is the formation of scar tissue which can result in stricture of the urethra. Surgical intervention to remove calculi will also result in likely scar or excess granulation tissue.

Urethral strictures

The formation of scar or granulation tissue can restrict the diameter of the urethra. Since scar tissue is inelastic in nature, there is a tendency for it to tear during breeding, resulting in haemorrhage which will mix with the semen. Urethral problems of this nature are normally dealt with surgically. To limit the formation of scar tissue the following three remedies can be used:

Silica 30 once every three days

Graphites 30c once every three days

Thiosinaminum 6c once every three days

Where inelastic scar tissue results in haemorrhage or where there is excessive granulation tissue consider using:

Nitric acid 30c twice daily where there is bright red blood

Sabina 30c twice daily where there are clots

Urethritis

This term refers to inflammation of the urethra and is an uncommon condition arising as a result of cystitis, local injury or direct bacterial infection. Suitable remedies are listed under urethritis in the urinary system (see page 136).

The Penis

The penis is a complex structure that allows copulation to take place. Normally the penis is not visible as it is contained within the prepuce. This can make examination extremely difficult unless performed under sedation. The majority of horses will let the penis drop during the passage of urine allowing a cursory glance. The inability of the penis to protrude beyond the prepuce is termed phimosis.

Phimosis

This condition can be either congenital (present at birth) or occur as the result of inflammation of the prepuce. This can occur as a consequence of an injury or an infection. Phimosis can also occur due to changes to the penis including growths or other lesions arising on the penis.

Congenital phimosis normally resolves naturally several weeks after birth. Where injury or infection is involved, the prepuce will become swollen, preventing the penis from protruding so that it is trapped inside. Initially think of using **Arnica 200c** where injury is involved, giving three or four doses over the course of an hour or so combined with local application of ice packs. **Apis 200c** is useful to help reduce preputial oedema by giving a dose every hour until the swelling is reduced. Where Apis appears ineffective **Vespa 30c** can be considered a good alternative. Other remedies that may help, particularly where infection is involved, include **Cinnabaris**, **Cannabis sativa**, **Merc sol, Sabina** and **Nitric acid**.
Use the 200c potency and dose hourly

Paraphimosis

Inability of the penis to retract back into the prepuce is termed paraphimosis and is essentially the opposite of phimosis. Trauma to the prepuce is the most likely initiating cause resulting in swelling of the prepuce which prevents the penis returning back into the prepuce. However, paraphimosis can occur following prolapse (paralysis) of the penis and after castration where the prepuce may swell.

First aid remedies such as **Arnica** and **Apis** or **Vespa** should be the first line of treatment whilst awaiting veterinary help.
Dose: *30c every 15 minutes*

Paralysis/prolapse of the penis

The majority of horses will drop the penis partly at least when they pass urine, after which it will be withdrawn back into the prepuce. In some situations the penis will hang out of the sheath as the horse is unable to retract it. This can occur in horses which are exhausted, debilitated (as the result of another underlying condition), which have spinal or nerve damage and as a consequence of the use of some types of tranquillisers. Paralysis can also arise as a result of trauma such as a kick or accidental whip injury.

Often the condition will resolve naturally especially if any underlying problems are treated. However, during the time the penis is prolapsed it is in danger of sustaining bruising and other trauma that will result in the tissues of the penis swelling. Some of the tissues are also susceptible to drying and cracking. This only serves to add to the problem of tissue swelling which can eventually lead to paraphimosis.

Initial treatment should involve cold water hosing and most importantly support of the prolapsed penis. **Arnica 200c** should be given where trauma is involved and **Apis 200c** or **Vespa 30c** to help prevent any immediate swelling given every 10–15 minutes. If the condition is not treated promptly or does not resolve quickly, then the penis will swell considerably (a condition referred to as priapism) leading to the possibility of gangrene developing in both the penis and prepuce. Local tissue damage occurs, as well as damage to the nerves and muscles supplying the area so that the condition can become irreversible.

Additional remedies, which may help prevent this situation from arising, include the following, which can be given in *30c potency three or four times daily:*

Secale where there is likelihood of gangrene developing

Hypericum where nerve damage is suspected

Bellis perennis as an additional remedy to use where trauma and swelling is involved

Phosphoric acid where debility is involved

In addition to help resolve the actual paralysis consider **Causticum, Conium** or **Gelsemium**.

Priapism

This condition is a form of penile paralysis where the penis is constantly erect in the absence of sexual stimulation. The underlying reason why this occurs is not known, but one of the known initiating factors is the administration of phenothiazine type tranquillisers such as ACP. If the condition does not resolve, both the penis and prepuce become swollen. The remedies most likely to help treat this condition are **Lyssin 200c** or **Cantharis 200c**.
Dose: *every 30 minutes whilst waiting for veterinary help*

Smegma

The foul smelling greyish black substance that collects mainly around the end of the penis and around the end of the prepuce (in the folds of skin) is called smegma. This is composed of a mixture of oily sebaceous secretions mixed with dead cells and with dirt. In some situations where hygiene is poor, the build up of smegma can lead to a low-grade infection termed balanoposthitis. Along with ensuring that the penis and prepuce are cleaned with warm water with the addition of Calendula mother tincture (1 teaspoon to 1 pint of water) at regular intervals, the following remedies are helpful in resolving the condition:

Cinnabaris where the prepuce is swollen as well

Merc sol where there is a greenish coloured preputial discharge and there are signs of irritation

Nitric acid where the smegma has a particularly offensive smell

Rhus tox where there is marked irritation of the penis and prepuce

Thuja for chronic stubborn cases

Medorrhinum where the symptoms coincide with a low sperm count

Sabina where there are warts or papillomas present as well

Syphilinum if there are ulcers present on the penis or prepuce

Use the 30c potency and dose three times daily for a few days

Penile warts or papillomas and other growths of the penis and prepuce

It is unusual for warts or papillomas to develop on the penis or prepuce but they are, however, benign in nature. Treatment using homeopathic remedies is often successful in resolving this problem.

Thuja The main remedy to consider in all cases and especially useful where the lesions are near the tip of the penis

Sabina Can be considered another good general remedy especially where there is some slight local irritation as well

Cinnabaris Where the lesions bleed very easily or are present on the prepuce

Nitric acid Where they have a cauliflower like appearance or bleed considerably

Psorinum Where there is a considerable amount of smegma present as well

Sepia Can be useful in irritable horses where the lesions are near the tip of the penis

Natrum sulph As an alternative general remedy where there is a general tendency to have warts
Dose with the 200c potency three times weekly

Other types of growth can also be found on the penis or prepuce. These include melanomas and sarcoids which are dealt with under the skin section (see page 263).

Poor libido

The following remedies may help with stallions that have a low sex drive or are reluctant to mount the mare

Agnus castus is a good general remedy to use in most situations

Ginseng is another good general remedy

Kali brom where there is general weakness as well

Graphites is useful in animals with a heavier build

Lycopodium can be used in stallions that have an apprehensive nature

Dose: *using the 200c potency twice daily for five days prior to serving the mare*

The Foal

This section of the book covers conditions that occur in the foal in the period from birth to weaning which takes place at around four to five months of age. Broadly the problems encountered fall into three main categories. Those that are infectious, those that are developmental and finally those that have an immunological basis. A few of the conditions are described elsewhere in the book and are not included within this section.

Foals should be seen standing within one hour of birth and sucking within around three hours although it is accepted that some thoroughbred foals are known to take much longer than this. This period is critical, as it is vital that the foal receives colostrum from the mare as soon as possible. Colostrum contains the antibodies needed to protect the foal from infection and can only be absorbed from the small intestine during the first 12 hours of life. The earlier the foal sucks, the more efficient the transfer is likely to be. Immunity gained in this way lasts about six weeks and is replaced by active immunity gained by the foal's own immune system challenging infection. It is during this period of changeover, at six weeks, that the foal is most vulnerable to disease.

Infectious Conditions

Septicaemia

Sleepy Foal Disease, Sleeper, Shigellosis, *Actinobacillus (Shigella) Equuli* infection

This condition is an acute form of septicaemia caused by an organism known as *Actinobacillus equi*, which is present naturally in many adult horses. *Actinobacillus equi* targets the brain, adrenal glands and the kidneys (causing nephritis and uraemia). Once infected, susceptible foals become ill extremely quickly and may die, even if treated promptly. Those that survive may develop kidney microabscesses and joint ill.

Initially there are signs of a fever followed by lethargy and failure to suck. Diarrhoea accompanied by colic symptoms may follow. Convulsions are common in many cases. Damage to the kidneys results in a rise in the urea level in the blood (uraemia) as the kidneys start to fail. The end stage nears as the foal enters into a coma state from which it can be aroused briefly – the 'sleepy foal'. Death commonly ensues from septicaemia within 24 hours of the initial infection.

Treating Sleepy Foal Disease

Dose: *every 30 minutes unless otherwise indicated*

Initially at the very earliest stage **Aconite 1M** every 15 minutes, follow with other remedies if the symptoms progress:

For septicaemia **Pyrogen 1M**, **Echinacea 30x**, **Ars alb 200c**

If convulsions develop **Belladonna 200c** (with violent fits and high temperature), **Kali brom 200c** (especially where there is uraemia), **Stramonium 200c**, **Ars alb 200c**, **Bufo 200c** (if entering coma stage)

Where there is uraemia **Urtica 200c**, **Terebinth 200c**

For diarrhoea with colic **Colocynthis 200c**, **Nux vom 200c**

At the coma stage **Opium 1M** (main remedy), **Bufo 200c**, **Ars alb 200c** (if cold)

Septicaemia in Foals Arising from Other Causes

Septicaemia can also occur as a result of a number of other bacterial infections, paricularly by *E. coli, Streptococcus, Klebsiella* and *Salmonella*. The period of most risk is between the second and fourth day after birth. The lungs, joints, umbilicus, pleura, peritoneum, brain, and liver can all be targeted by a variety of different bacteria.

The most obvious initial signs are raised temperature, lethargy and reluctance to feed. As the illness progresses body temperature may rise to 41°C or 106°F with a rise both in the pulse and respiratory rate. Dehydration, a subnormal temperature and collapse follow with convulsions in the later stages. Pneumonia and joint swelling may also occur.

Remedies for septicaemia

***Dose:** every 30 minutes with 30c potency unless otherwise indicated*

Specific for septicaemia, animal is restlessness, breath smells foul or bad-smelling diarrhoea **Pyrogen 1M**

As a general remedy **Echinacea 30x**

With haemorrhage, tissue swelling, skin abscesses **Anthracinum**

With exhaustion, restlessness, very high temperature **Arsenicum album**

With offensive discharges and weakness **Baptisia 1M**

If cellulitis is present and skin is purple or black **Lachesis**

Where there is pneumonia or hepatitis **Phosphorus**

With lymphangitis **Crot horr**

With increased thirst **Sulphur**

With toxaemia **Tarent cubensis**

With convulsions **Belladonna 1M**

Shaker Foal Syndrome, Forage Poisoning, Botulism

This condition is caused by a bacterial infection with an anaerobic spore-forming organism known as *Clostridium botulinum* that multiplies in decaying animal or plant material when the correct humidity and temperature are present. The actual symptoms of botulism are caused by the toxin produced when the spores multiply. Horses are very susceptible to botulism, with infection resulting from ingestion of contaminated vacuum-packed hay or silage.

In foals (which may be as young as two months old), the symptoms can appear quickly with the intensity of the signs related to the dose of the ingested toxin. As the toxin interferes with the transmission of nerve impulses, the clinical signs reflect this. Affected foals will show an inability to swallow, loss of muscle tone in the tail and eyelids, dilated pupils, muscle weakness with tremors, progressing to a state of collapse from which the foal is unable to rise.

Aconite 1M

Indicated in the very initial stages only.
***Dose:** give three doses 15–20 minutes apart then follow with the most appropriate remedy*

Gelsemium 200c

Principal remedy to consider covering all the symptoms.
***Dose:** every 20–30 minutes*

Causticum 200c

Best considered where Gelsemium fails to act.
***Dose:** every 20–30 minutes*

Stramonium 200c

Stramonium acts best where the muscle tremors are pronounced and the pupils are widely dilated.
***Dose:** every 20–30 minutes*

Opium 1M

Use in later stages where the foal is weak and is nearing a state of collapse and is unaware of its surroundings.
***Dose:** every 20–30 minutes*

China 30c
Indicated in the later stages of he condition where the foal is collapsed and the limbs show signs of a pronounced tremor.
***Dose:** every 20–30 minutes*

Botulinum 30c
The nosode can be used alongside any of the other remedies.
***Dose:** every 20–30 minutes*

Joint Ill/Septic Polyarthritis

See page 185

Navel Ill
Umbilical Abscesses

Infection of the navel following birth is termed navel ill and may be first apparent at about one week of age. The affected area will be swollen and painful and the navel visibly enlarged. Where possible the abscess should be drained and treated appropriately. In a number of cases the infection may become systemic leading to septicaemia in which case the foal will appear depressed, fail to feed and will have a raised temperature. In such cases the infection enters the blood stream and is spread to other sites in the body and is most likely to settle in the joints or in bone leading to the risk of septic polyarthritis or septic arthritis.

Homeopathic remedies

In the absence of septicaemia **Hepar sulph 200c** and **Abrotanum 30c**
***Dose:** two-hourly until improvement*

Where the infection is slow to resolve and there is little pain **Silica 200c**
***Dose:** twice daily for ten days*

Where discomfort remains in the umbilical region once the infection has cleared **Calc phos 30c**
***Dose:** twice daily for ten days*

Where there is septicaemia **Pyrogen 1M**
***Dose:** every 30 minutes until improvement is seen*

See also **Septic polyarthritis** page 185

Tyzzer's Disease

Tyzzer's disease is rare and occurs sporadically in foals aged between two and six weeks of age and is caused by a spore-producing bacillus called *Bacillus piliformis*. The factors underlying the reason for infection are rare but are believed to involve ingestion of spores present in bedding or droppings. Symptoms appear rapidly and encompass acute hepatitis. In its most extreme form affected foals will be found dead. Where the infection is less acute, the foal will appear to exhibit a fever, appear depressed or collapsed and may be jaundiced. Convulsions follow, progressing to a coma and death.

Homeopathic remedies

Main remedy to consider **Aconite 1M**
***Dose:** every ten minutes*

If symptoms continue to progress **Phosphorus 30c** and **Hepar sulph 30c**
***Dose:** every ten minutes*

Where there is a high fever or convulsions add **Belladonna 1M**
***Dose:** every 15 minutes*

Respiratory Tract Infections in Foals

Foals and yearlings in yards and studs are especially prone to respiratory infections especially where the animals on the site are prone to frequent changes. There are a variety of underlying causes including viruses (Influenza virus, Equine herpes virus, Rhinovirus and Adenovirus), bacteria (*C. equi, E. coli*, Staphylococci) with secondary bacterial infection with Streptococci also occurring in some cases. Occasionally parasites can also be implicated. Respiratory problems in foals are divided into upper and lower respiratory tract problems.

Upper respiratory tract problems

Initial symptoms involve a nasal discharge which may be watery at first, progressing to a profuse, mucky discharge. A fever ensues with a dry cough and difficulty breathing as pneumonia with the risk of bronchopneumonia develops. If treated quickly, most foals recover. However, there is a risk of permanent lung damage or the formation of abscesses within the lung.

Lower respiratory tract problems

Problems here can arise as a consequence of upper respiratory tract conditions, although stress and poor conditions can also be implicated. Symptoms of pneumonia are evident with a rise in temperature and accompanying lethargy and failure to suck from the mare. The typical cough is harsh and moist, possibly with rattling or wheezing present in the chest and a blue tinge to the tongue and membranes of the mouth.

Homeopathic treatment of respiratory infections in the foal

Remedies for the early stages

Aconite 1M
Use Aconite in the very early stages of infection or where the symptoms appear suddenly with a fever present. Affected foals will appear restless or anxious. Chest symptoms tend to be worse on the left side.
Dose: every 15 minutes

Bryonia 30c
Bryonia is suited to cases where the symptoms appear more slowly and where breathing becomes progressively more difficult. Fever is present with the temperature climbing progressively as the infection progresses over a few days. A dry cough is also present which is worse or triggered when the foal is disturbed. Affected foals tend to hide away, have an increased thirst and resent being handled. Symptoms are worse on the right-hand side of the chest.
Dose: every hour

Ferrum phos 30c
Ferrum phos is another remedy to consider where symptoms appear over a few days with the development of a high fever. The keynote for this remedy is the absence of symptoms other than an irritating, painful cough that appears better at night.
Dose: every 15 minutes

Phosphorus 30c
Symptoms develop quickly where Phosphorus is needed but with less pace than with Aconite. There will be a dry cough with obvious difficulty breathing to the extent that the neck may be extended to ease the symptoms. Symptoms are worse on the right-hand side of the chest.
Dose: every hour

Tuberculinum 200c
This is an excellent remedy to use in any foal with a respiratory infection especially those that are not responding to other remedies.
Dose: give three doses over 24 hours

Remedies for later more advanced stages:

Hepar sulph 30c
The chief guiding symptom is a thick, mucky nasal discharge that develops from a runny discharge over a day or two. A dry cough follows which is worse when the foal moves around, eventually becoming a rattling cough with a degree of wheezing and difficulty breathing.
Dose: every hour

Kali bich 30c
Indicated where there is a thick, yellowish nasal discharge that has a foul odour and which obstructs the nasal passages. This is accompanied by a hacking cough that may produce thick yellow mucus.
Dose: every hour

Lycopodium 30c
Lycopodium is suited to more advanced cases where there is a dry cough which is worse between 4 and 8pm. The foal will appear weak with noisy breathing and laboured respiration with flaring of the nostrils. The airways will be clogged with yellow mucus that is not loosened by coughing. Symptoms are worse on the right-hand side of the chest.
Dose: every hour

Pulsatilla 30c
Where Pulsatilla is needed, the cough is loose with the foal producing yellow, moist, cream-like mucus. There is a desire for company and to seek human affection. Being in the open air eases the symptoms in contrast to being in a stable.
***Dose:** every hour*

Antimonium tartrate 30c
This remedy is best used where the symptoms include weakness (possibly collapse), a blue tinge of the mucous membranes and tongue, great difficulty breathing, a weak moist cough and obvious rattling of mucus in the chest. Where the foal is lying on its side, symptoms will be eased if it is propped up onto its brisket.
***Dose:** every 30 minutes*

Ipecacuanha 30c
Ipecac is indicated where the foal appears to be suffocating as the airways are clogged with so much mucus. Accompanying symptoms include wheezing and great difficulty breathing.
***Dose:** every 30 minutes*

Carbo veg 30c
Carbo veg is reserved for advanced cases where the foal is weak and collapsed or nearing a coma. The body feels cold and membranes are blue. The airways are laden with mucus and rattling sounds can be heard from the chest.
***Dose:** every 15 minutes*

Laurocerasus 1x
Worth consideration where the foal is failing to make any progress and appears in a pathetic state but is not collapsed. The breathing may be jerky interspersed with sudden gasps for breath. The mucous membranes are cyanosed (a purple colour rather than pink).
***Dose:** every 15 minutes*

Remedies for the recovery stages

Use these remedies to clear any remaining symptoms that are left once the signs of pneumonia have abated.

Stannum 30c
Indicated for prolonged weakness following a respiratory infection. Affected foals will appear dull and lethargic despite the fact that the chest and upper airways are now clear.
***Dose:** three times daily*

Senega 30c
For persistent coughs where the airways are clogged with mucus which is thick and not easily loosened by coughing.
***Dose:** three times daily*

Where there are abscesses within the lungs
Consider **Calc carb 30c**, **Hepar sulph 30c**, **Calc sulph 30c** or **Phos 30c** *twice daily*

Rhodococcus equi Infection *Corynebacterium equi* Infection

This condition is rare in foals and only occurs sporadically in the UK appearing more commonly in dry, hot countries. Foals between the ages of one and four months are affected with changes in the lungs well advanced before any visible clinical signs are present. The organism is found in the droppings of normal horses as well as some of the lymph nodes in the abdomen. It is also thought to survive in the soil. The route of infection is unclear but thought to be by inhalation or ingestion.

The first signs will be of a mild, chronic cough, progressing to bronchopneumonia and general ill thrift. Later symptoms encompass persistent fever, difficulty breathing, a mucky nasal discharge, abdominal pain and the formation of abscesses in the lungs. Diarrhoea is an occasional finding due to abscesses appearing in the lymph nodes linked with the bowel. The outlook can be poor with death occurring in seven to ten days. Conventional and homeopathic treatment can be used together and will only be of benefit if the condition is diagnosed early enough.

Homeopathic treatment

Initially where infection is suspected but no symptoms **Aconite 1M**

***Dose:** hourly until use of another remedy is apparent or symptoms abate*
Then dose with single dose of **Tuberculinum 200c** *then follow with*

Where there is bronchopneumonia **Ant tart 30c, Kali bich 30c** and **Kali sulph 30c** in combination
***Dose:** hourly*

With mucky nasal discharge **Hepar sulph 30c, Kali bich 30c**
***Dose:** hourly*

Treatment of lung or bowel abscesses **Hepar sulph 30c, Calc sulph** 30c
***Dose:** four times daily*

Diarrhoea

Diarrhoea in foals is a common finding, especially up to the age of five months and is a routine finding at least once in most animals before weaning. There are a variety of causes – nutritional, viral, bacterial and parasitic.

Nutritional causes

Change in the composition of the milk, the so-called 'foal heat scour' causing mild diarrhoea.
Excessive milk consumption causing persistent or recurrent diarrhoea.

Treatment

In conjunction with reducing or restricting milk intake along with oral rehydration:
Aethusa cynapium 30c, Natrum carb 30c and **China 30c** in combination.
***Dose:** four times daily*

Coprophagia

Ingestion of faecal material – common in foals between two and five weeks of age causing diarrhoea if contaminated with pathogenic bacteria

Consumption of bedding or foreign material leading to diarrhoea

Treatment

Veratrum album 30c or **Merc sol 30c** where coprophagia is the cause
Nux vomica 30c, Podophyllum 30c from other dietary causes
***Dose:** four times daily*

Viral causes

A problem which appears to be on the increase.
Rotavirus infection causing watery diarrhoea with abdominal pain, fever and teeth grinding
Adenovirus infection and **Coronavirus** infection can also cause diarrhoea

Treatment

Podophyllum 30c with teeth grinding
Elaterium 30c for forceful, squirty diarrhoea with abdominal pain
Crot tig 30c with watery forceful diarrhoea with straining, possibly with mucus
***Dose:** four times daily*

Bacterial causes

The following bacteria have been implicated:
E.coli which causes a mild diarrhoea which may develop into a serious problem leading to dehydration

Salmonella which causes more serious problems including fever with an increase in pulse and respiratory rate, abdominal pain and dehydration caused through passage of severe, foul, watery diarrhoea containing blood and mucus. Mucous membranes will become reddened. See infectious disease page 288

Campylobacter causing mild diarrhoea with colic

Rhodococcus equi the alimentary (bowel) form of this disease which may occur alongside respiratory symptoms causing diarrhoea with abdominal pain and weight loss

Clostridial diarrhoea caused by *Clostridium perfringens* type B or type C. This is a serious condition that can lead rapidly to the death of the foal. Symptoms in less acute cases include bloody diarrhoea and fever with a rapid heart rate.

Treatment

Match the symptoms as closely as possible to the remedy. *Dose: every one to two hours* depending on severity of the symptoms unless otherwise indicated.

Podophyllum 30c Profuse watery yellow diarrhoea may appear explosively

Ars alb 30c Acute foul smelling watery diarrhoea with blood, foal appears weak and anxious

Merc sol 30c Bloody diarrhoea with mucus and marked straining

Rhus tox 30c Yellow mushy diarrhoea with blood streaks

Verat alb 30c Profuse watery forcibly expelled diarrhoea with blood, foul smelling leading to exhaustion, chilling and collapse

Gambogia 30c Sudden bouts of watery diarrhoea preceded by straining

Elaterium 30c Diarrhoea which forcefully squirts out (no blood or mucus), may appear frothy

Colocynthis 30c Diarrhoea with colic

Colchicum 30c Diarrhoea, nearly all mucus, abdomen distended with gas

Phosphorus 30c Very watery diarrhoea containing some mucus in lumps, foal has a marked thirst

Aloe 30c Acute diarrhoea with gas producing a spluttery diarrhoea

Nux vomica 30c Slimy diarrhoea with some blood and marked straining without effect. Abdominal pain present as key symptom

Phos ac 30c Profuse diarrhoea which is watery leading to dehydration and weakness

China 30c Add in any case where dehydration is present also indicated for painless yellow diarrhoea

Carbo veg 200c Severe offensive diarrhoea with collapse, nearing death.
Dose: every 15–20 minutes

Nosodes can be added where appropriate such as **E.coli 30c**, **Salmonella 30c**

Parasitic causes

Diarrhoea can arise as a consequence of infection with Strongyle worms and Coccidia. Suitable remedies can be found in the above lists.

Gastroduodenal Ulceration

Ulceration of the stomach and duodenum is linked with stress and with the use of non-steroidal anti-inflammatory drugs such as phenylbutazone, although infectious causes may be involved in some way.

Foals aged between 1 and 120 days may be affected showing signs of varying degrees. Some will show virtually no symptoms. At the other end of the scale the worst cases will show abdominal pain, cessation of feeding and depression with peritonitis due to perforation of the stomach or duodenum.

Homeopathic treatment

Dose: three times daily

As a general remedy **Uranium nitrate 30c** or **Ornithogalum 6x**

Where stress is a factor **Arg nit 30c**

For abdominal pain which is worse after feeding **Kali bich 30c**

For more severe pain **Colcocynthis 30c**

As remedies to help heal the mucosal surface **Symphytum 6c**, **Calendula 6c**

Where there is peritonitis **Pyrogen 200c**, **Belladonna 200c**

Developmental Disorders
Meconium Retention or Impaction

The meconium is the first dung and normally starts to pass within four hours of birth and is cleared through completely by about the fourth day. If the meconium is retained the foal will show symptoms of colic often within the period between birth and the third day. The cause of this is not known but the symptoms are easily spotted. These include straining, lying in odd positions and abdominal pain. Affected foals do not seem very ill and will continue to suck.

Suitable remedies

Dose: *every one to two hours until the meconium is passed*

With straining **Nux vom 30c**

With weakness **Gelsemium 30c**

Protracted cases no straining try **Opium 200c**

To ease pain try **Colocynthis 30c**

Neonatal Maladjustment Syndrome (NMS), Wanderers, Barkers, Dummies, Dummy Foals, Convulsive Foals

This condition is most often seen in thoroughbred foals and develops within the first 24 hours of life with many foals appearing normal initially. In some cases NMS may appear in as little time as one hour after birth. The exact cause is uncertain but basically is thought to stem from either a haemorrhage within the brain or from swelling (oedema) around the cells of the brain. Fluctuations in blood pressure and low oxygen concentrations in the blood (hypoxia) are also thought to be involved, resulting from a difficult birth or from damage to the chest area interfering with the heart and circulation.

The signs are variable and may include all or some of the following:

- Loss of the sucking reflex and ability to nurse
- Inability to stand
- Convulsions with a rise in body temperature and sweating
- Coma episodes with a fall in body temperature
- Violent galloping movements of the limbs
- Extension of the head and neck with limbs extended and tail held upright (opisthotonus); increased extensor tone
- Hypersensitivity to touch, exaggerated response to handling
- Aimless wandering
- Grinding of the teeth
- Sneezing
- Vocalisation or 'barking' or grunting
- Haemorrhages into the retina and sclera
- Blindness with pressing against walls
- Unequal pupil sizes

With good nursing and support many foals will make a complete recovery, particularly if special attention is paid to preventing further trauma, to feeding and to maintaining of body temperature. The symptoms of NMS may last only a few hours or may take as long as a month to disappear completely. Recovery follows an established sequence progressing from the coma stage to standing, then the return of auditory and visual senses followed by the ability to suck.

Treating NMS

The variable signs associated with this condition lend themselves to treatment with homeopathic remedies which can be used alongside conventional drugs where needed. Broadly taking the symptoms as detailed above, the following remedies will be useful.

Dose: *200c three or four times daily, changing the remedy as the symptoms change*

In all suspect cases immediately after birth dose with a single dose of Arnica 200c and Opium 200c follow with:

- Weakness, failure to suck **Phos ac** or **Gelsemium** (if weak), **Carbo veg** (if cold)
- Convulsions **Belladonna** (violent, with rise in temperature), **Stramonium** (with limb paddling/galloping), **Bufo** (alternating with coma episodes), **Hyoscyamus** (with 'barking'), **Zinc** (if no other remedy fits the picture)
- Coma episodes **Aconite** (to assist recovery generally), **Opium** (preceded by periods of

'delirium'), **Carbo veg** (with a fall in body temperature)

- Opisthotonus **Cicuta** (main remedy to consider), **Belladonna**, **Hyoscyamus**, **Nux vom**, **Strychnine**
- Hypersensitivity **Strychnine** (with extreme hypersensitivity), **Ignatia** (with muscle spasms/twitches), **Coffea** (with mild symptoms), **Zinc**
- Aimless wandering **Thuja**, Stramonium (with 'barking')
- Vocalisation or 'barking' **Stramonium**, **Hyoscyamus**
- Grinding of the teeth **Belladonna**, **Hyoscyamus**, **Bufo**
- Retinal haemorrhage **Phosphorus**
- Blindness with pressing against walls **Helleborus**
- Unequal pupil size **Opium**, **Laburnum** (with convulsions)

Immunological Disorders

Haemolytic anaemia of the newborn foal Neonatal isoerythrolysis

See page 100 (blood section)

The Locomotor or Musculoskeletal System Part One

This section covers conditions relating to those parts of the body concerned with movement and gait. As the name suggests, it encompasses both the skeleton and the muscles with the addition of other vital structures such as peripheral nerves, ligaments, tendons, bursae and joints.

Broadly divided into two sections, the first covers the basic general structure and function of the essential anatomical components of the system together with details of more general conditions involving these areas. The majority of the remedies listed are common to many of the conditions in this section of the book as a whole. To avoid unnecessary repetition, less detailed reference will be made to these key remedies in the second section. This part of the book outlines more specific conditions relating to the forelimb and hindlimb and also includes the spine (back) and the foot, which are covered separately.

General Structures and Related Conditions

Bone

Bone is a type of rigid connective tissue that makes up the majority of the skeleton. Its fundamental structure consists of cells within a matrix that is made up of collagen fibres, responsible for the resilience of bone, and an inorganic component which accounts for about ⅔ of the weight of bone. It is this part which gives bone its strength and rigidity comprising around 85 per cent calcium phosphate, ten per cent calcium carbonate with smaller quantities of calcium and magnesium fluoride.

The are two types of bone, spongy or cancellous bone which contains cavities filled with bone marrow, and the more compact or dense bone which appears solid. With very few exceptions, both types of bone are present in every bone to varying degrees. In a typical long bone such as the femur, the shaft (or diaphysis) is chiefly composed of compact bone with a central cavity (containing bone marrow) and each end (known as the epiphysis) composed of spongy bone covered by a thin layer of compact bone.

During bone growth, a specific region of the epiphysis produces new cartilage, which then becomes bone in all but two areas. The first is over the ends of the bone where the cartilage becomes articular (or joint) cartilage. The second is at the junction of the epiphysis and diaphysis where it forms the epiphyseal or growth plate. It is this area which is involved in the condition known as epiphysitis. The region between the growth plate and the diaphysis (shaft) in known as the metaphysis and together with the epiphysis, forms an area anatomically responsible for some of the growth disorders seen in foals. Except over the joint surfaces, each bone is covered by a special tough connective tissue layer known as the periosteum.

It is likely that the mineral composition and the strength of bone during growth can be influenced favourably by some homeopathic remedies. To ensure good bone growth and strength a foal of lean stature should be dosed with **Calc phos 30c**, three times weekly. Animals of a heavier build, breed or stature would be better suited to **Calc carb 30c**.

Conditions Affecting Bone

Osteomyelitis

This term refers to infection and the inflammation of bone caused by bacterial infection. The area involved can be relatively localised but in more severe cases, it can involve the bone marrow and periosteum as well. The most common initiating cause is a penetrating wound which introduces infection locally. The areas most at risk are those regions with little muscle covering, such as the cannon bones.

Symptoms include swelling at the site of injury with the appearance of a small sinus through which pus exudes in varying degrees. Pain is usually evident, although in many cases, the horse will not show signs of lameness. Suggested remedies to help include:

Aconite 1M
Aconite is best given at the very earliest stages when osteomyelitis is suspected and before the condition has had a chance to develop.
Dose: *Every 30 minutes for the first two hours then one dose every hour until symptoms abate or another remedy is needed*

Gunpowder 3x
This is the remedy of choice to use if Aconite fails to contain the condition. It is indicated where there is an active septic osteomyelitis and in cases which are proving difficult to resolve even with the use of antibiotics.
Dose: *four times daily until symptoms resolve*

Silica 200c
This remedy is of most value in later stages where pus is actively draining from a sinus on the surface of the skin and in also in very stubborn cases.
Dose: *three times daily until symptoms resolve*

Phosphorus 200c
This is a good general remedy to assist resolution by improving the health of bone and is best used alongside cases where Silica is required.
Dose: *one daily*

Hypercal lotion
Where there is a sinus present discharging pus, daily cleaning with diluted hypercal lotion will help.

Periostitis

This term refers to inflammation of the thin, tough layer that covers bone, the periosteum. There are two basic causes. The first is direct blunt trauma from a blow or kick. This is most likely to occur at sites where there is little protection from other tissues such as muscle. The metacarpal and metatarsal (cannon) bones are at most risk here. Periostitis can also arise as a result of the periosteum lifting away from the underlying bone. This is either usually from a tendon or a ligament attachment pulling the periosteum away. This can be acutely traumatic in nature or by the far more subtle effect of repeated damage to an area which can then result in the periosteum lifting gradually, little by little. The familiar and common problem of splints (see page 196) is a classic example of the latter.

The lifting or damage to the periosteum results in inflammation and pain which will cause varying degrees of lameness depending on the cause, severity and location. In the acute phase there will be soft tissue swelling over the affected area which will be painful to touch, although the horse may not be lame. This swelling will be far more easily noticeable where the metacarpal and metatarsal bones are involved. In response to the damage to the periosteum, the underlying tissue starts to form new bone, which has an irregular or rough outline. Once the inflammation has subsided, the new periosteal bone will start to remodel resulting in bony lumps with a much smoother contour known as exostoses.

Initial treatment, particularly where direct trauma is involved should consist of **Arnica 200c**, *one dose hourly for three or four hours* followed by:

Asafoetida 6c
Indicated where the affected area is very painful to the touch and where there is a marked degree of swelling.
Dose: *three times daily*

Ruta 30c
This remedy acts specifically on the periosteum and is indicated in any situation where the periosteum has been bruised or subject to trauma. Ruta will help minimise the risk of exostoses developing as well as

being of benefit to more chronic cases.
Dose: *once daily until the reaction has settled down*

Phytolacca 30c
This remedy is specifically indicated where the periosteum has lifted as a result of being pulled away by a tendon attachment. It is a good general remedy for conditions relating to the periosteum.
Dose: *three times daily until signs of pain subside*

Mezereum 30c
This is a specific remedy for periostitis and exostoses where pain and lameness is apparent. Some past history of skin problems is an additional guide to the use of this remedy.
Dose: *once daily*

Silica 30c
This is a good remedy in general for diseases affecting bone. It is of most use in cases of long standing and where exostoses have developed. Silica is best suited to helping animals with a poor basic physical make up and which are timid, quiet and submissive in nature. Flaky or brittle hooves are an additional indicator to the use of this remedy.
Dose: *once daily*

Calc fluor 30c
This is a valuable remedy, which is specifically indicated in minimising the development of exostoses. Where already formed it may act to help to reduce the size of the lesions if used over a period of many months.
Dose: *once daily*

Phosphorus 30c
Phosphorus will help more constitutionally in longer drawn out cases in animals with a lean slender build and which appear anxious and over sensitive. The presence of exostoses is a guide towards the use of this remedy.
Dose: *once daily*

Manganum aceticum 30c
This less well known remedy will help in protracted cases where the periosteum has become chronically inflamed and where there are also signs of pain associated with the problem.
Dose: *once daily*

Ruta ointment
Wherever there is a periosteal reaction, twice daily application of Ruta ointment will help to settle the problem down.

Exostoses and Osteophytes

Bone spurs

These are hard bony lumps which form as a result of disturbance or damage to the periosteal layer of bone or as a result of damage or degeneration of joint cartilage. A reaction occurs in the tissue layer under the periosteum or cartilage resulting in the formation of new bone. Once all the inflammation has died down, the periosteal new bone undergoes remodelling to form the smooth bony lumps known as exostoses or osteophytes.

Prevention

There are a number of remedies that can be used to help prevent or minimise reactions in the periostium.

Ruta 30c
This remedy should be given at the earliest opportunity to help prevent a reaction in the periosteum flaring up.
Dose: *twice daily for seven to ten days following suspected trauma or reaction occurring, then once daily for the following three weeks*
In long-term cases to slow the development of further bony reaction, dose three times weekly with the 200c potency

Symphytum 6c
Symphytum can be used as a routine remedy where the periosteum has been damaged. It is especially useful where periosteal pain is evident.
Dose: *twice daily for four weeks*

Kali bich 30c
Indicated where the cannon bone is involved and the overlying skin is obviously damaged and the underlying soft tissues inflamed.
Dose: *twice daily for seven to ten days following the initial trauma, then once daily for the following three weeks*

Lactic acidum 30c
This less well-known remedy should be considered in cases where there is a long-standing problem with periostitis which is unresponsive to other remedies.
Dose: *once daily*

Ruta ointment
This should be routinely applied twice daily to the affected area to further aid in preventing problems arising.

Treatment

These remedies are useful where exostoses are already present to reduce further development, inflammation and discomfort. **Ruta 200c** should be considered along with:

Calc fluor 30c
This is the most ideal remedy to select for problems arising either near the carpal (knee) joint or near the tarsal (hock) joint.
Dose: *once daily on alternate days on long-term basis*

Hecla lava 6c
Hecla is a good routine remedy to give in any situation where exostoses are evident, especially where sizeable.
Dose: *once daily*

Silica 30c
Silica is another valuable remedy to consider where exostoses are present. It is best used for younger animals or those that have a weaker general constitution.
Dose: *once daily*

Merc sol 30c
The chief indication to the use of this remedy is where periostitis and subsequent exostoses are accompanied by necrosis (decay) of bone is the local area. Local swelling and pain is a consistent feature.
Dose: *twice daily for ten days then once daily*

Fractures

A fracture is a break in a bone. The break can be simple and consist of just two pieces in contrast to a comminuted fracture which has more fragments and is of a much more serious nature. The location and nature of the fracture as well as any secondary complications will determine the eventual outcome. Fractures once thought of as irreparable can now be treated with success.

Urgent veterinary intervention and appropriate first aid are of paramount importance. Do not forget the importance of using **Aconite 1M** for shock and **Arnica 200c** to help with the initial injury. If the fracture involves a joint which then becomes very oedematous (swollen), dose with **Bovista 200c**, three times daily, to reduce the swelling.

To promote good fracture healing, there are a number of remedies that will help. Treatment should be continued until the fracture is healed completely.

Calc phos 30c
As a constituent of bone, calcium phosphate in homeopathic potency will help support bone metabolism and ensure that the fracture heals well. This remedy in general is suited to patients with a lean build.
Dose: *one tablet on alternate days*

Calc carb 30c
Calcium carbonate is also a constituent of bone and can be used in horses with stout build in preference to Calc phos.
Dose: *one tablet on alternate days*

Ruta grav 30c
Dosing with Ruta will help prevent non-union of the fracture.
Dose: *one tablet on alternate days*

Symphytum 6c
Symphytum is the herb Comfrey in homeopathic potency. The colloquial name for this herbal remedy is knitbone and in fact in its homeopathic form it has a similar effect in promoting the healing of fractures. It is specifically indicated in assisting the healing of non-union fractures.
Dose: *once daily*

Eupat perf 30c
This is an ideal remedy to use where there is bone pain originating from the fracture site and can be used in all situations to help make the animal feel more comfortable.
Dose: *once or twice daily depending on the degree of pain*

Silica 30c
Silica will also help with bone metabolism and its use should be considered in horses that have a poor conformation and bone structure.
Dose: *one tablet on alternate days*

Calendula 30c
The addition of Calendula to the treatment regime will promote healing in general both of the fracture and of the surrounding tissues.
Dose: *once or twice daily*

Ligaments

Ligaments join bone to bone and are constructed from very strong and inelastic connective tissue. There are two types. Those which are located on the outside of a joint or within the fibrous joint capsule itself, and those which are located actually inside the joint. Both function to hold joints together and to allow joint movement.

Conditions Affecting Ligaments

Sprains or tears
Desmitis or inflammation of a ligament

Ligament injuries or sprains are common, leading to inflammation and pain. Damage can occur to varying degrees ranging from a partial tear involving only a few fibres to a complete rupture. The clinical signs and eventual prognosis will vary accordingly. Initial treatment following a suspected injury should consist of **Arnica 200c** and **Ruta 200c** both given *three times daily for five days* and then followed by:

Ruta 30c
This lower potency should be used over an extended period of time until the ligament has healed completely. This often takes several weeks. Ruta is the principal remedy to use where there is inflammation of any ligament.
Dose: *once daily*

Rhus tox 30c
Indicated along with Ruta where signs of stiffness or lameness are apparent following rest. These symptoms ease with movement.
Dose: *once daily*

Bryonia 30c
Indicated in very acute sprains where there is continued severe pain, worse for the slightest motion and where the animal avoids moving as much as possible to minimise the pain.
Dose: *three times daily*

Silica 30c
Silica should be reserved for chronic cases where the affected ligament has become thickened or where healing has been particularly slow.
Dose: *once daily for several weeks*

Natrum carb 6c
This is a remedy for ongoing problems where a ligament repeatedly suffers from weakness leading to recurrent lameness. It is particularly indicated where the hock is involved.
Dose: *once daily over a long-term period*

Ledum pal 6c
Ledum can be used in a similar situation to Natrum carb and is helpful with recurring sprains. It is specifically indicated where the hock is involved.
Dose: *once daily over a long-term period*

Sympytum 6c
This is a good general remedy to assist healing of any damaged ligament.
Dose: *once daily over a long-term period*

Other useful remedies include:

Nat mur 6c
Where there are repeated sprains involving the fetlock, pastern or coffin joints.

Calc carb 6c
Chronic sprains from over-exertion.

Strontium 6c
For weak joints following repeated sprains, especially suits the fetlock and hock joints.
Dose: twice daily

Tendons

The tissues which surround each bundle of muscle fibres combine to form the strong fibrous tissue known as tendon. Tendons function to attach muscle to bone and at the point of insertion their fibres are interwoven with those of the periosteum. Known for their great strength, tendons also have a degree of elasticity and the ability to store energy when stretched. To function efficiently, tendons need to be able to move freely over adjacent structures. To allow this to happen there are a number of other structures which help. These include bursae, small sacs of fluid which cushion a tendon as it travels over a bony structures and tendon sheaths which will surround a tendon as it changes direction over a joint. Tendons are subject to a number of common problems.

Conditions Affecting Tendons

Tendonitis, Tendosynovitis and Bowed tendons, Tendon strains

The superficial digital and deep digital flexor tendons of the forelimb are the most commonly involved. The superficial digital flexor tendon is more likely to be injured, particularly in the middle region where the area of the cross section is the smallest. The tendons in the hind limb can also be affected but much less frequently so.

Tendonitis is the term applied to inflammation of a tendon where the tendon sheath is not included. In contrast, tendosynovitis involves the inflammation of any area of tendon covered by a tendon sheath. The most common cause of both conditions is trauma resulting in a strain to the affected area. The symptoms will vary with the extent of the damage. Minor strains will result in slight swelling of the area and a little heat but no apparent lameness if the correct treatment is instigated and the animal rested. If the strain is more severe or an original (minor) injury is not given the opportunity to heal, the symptoms will become more obvious. Both swelling and heat will become more apparent together with a degree of lameness.

The visible swelling is classically referred to as a 'bowed' tendon. Depending on the site of the swelling, these are classed as:

High bow if the affected area is just below the carpal (knee) joint.

Middle bow if the middle third of the metacarpal (cannon) bone is involved.

Low bow if the lower third of the cannon in involved.

The initial injury causes the fibres of the tendon to tear and separate, leading to both swelling and haemorrhage into the affected tissues and then into the surrounding uninjured areas. This has the effects of weakening the damaged tendon further by the release of enzymes which break down the tissues composing the tendon. Further complications ensue as the blood flow to the area is disrupted leading to additional damage.

After the initial damage phase, healing starts and new collagen fibres are produced to replace those which have been damaged. Scar tissue also forms during the healing process causing adhesions and areas of fibrosis which will have the effect of limiting tendon elasticity and range of movement. The healing process takes some considerable time.

Treatment of tendon injuries

Acute (severe) strains
Initially aim to reduce the swelling as soon as possible over the first 48 hours following appropriate veterinary advice. Dose with:

Arnica 200c, **Ledum 200c** and **Hamamelis 200c** every two to three hours for the first 48 hours (to help limit the effects of the injury) and then

Apis 200c three times daily where swelling and heat are still in evidence. Massage the area to help reduce the swelling and assist flexibility.

Once the swelling has subsided dose with

Rhus tox 1M once daily for seven days to help reduce the pain associated with the injury and

Ruta 200c twice daily for seven days to initiate healing adding

Phytolacca 30c once daily can be added if a tendon insertion is involved
Externally apply:

A combination of **Arnica** and **Ruta** lotion three times daily

Less severe or subacute tendon injuries

Follow any advice given by your veterinary surgeon. Dose with:

Arnica 30c combined with **Ruta 30c** three times daily for 10–14 days.

Externally apply:
A combination of **Arnica** and **Ruta** lotion twice daily.

Healing phase

This is a prolonged phase and takes several weeks during which time the damaged tendon repairs and undergoes a degree of remodelling. External warmth should be applied to encourage blood flow to the area whilst cold applications should be used if the tendon becomes inflamed. Exercise should be limited to avoid excess formation of scar tissue and trauma to the weakened tissue. Dose with:

Ruta 30c, single dose on alternate days to encourage continued healing and to reduce swelling.

Calc fluor 30c, to help minimise the risk of adhesions. *Dose: once daily*

Silica 30c, to also help minimise the chance of adhesions forming and to help break down any adhesions already present.

Where there are adhesions or where the tendon has become thickened consider:

Graphites 30c can be used to help break down existing adhesions. *Dose: once daily*

Proteus 30c, a bowel nosode which is an excellent choice in helping to reduce the thickened, fibrosed scar tissue which can form where the tendon has become chronically thickened.
Externally apply:
Ruta lotion or **Ruta** ointment once daily.

Where healing is slow, blood supply to the area can be improved by using remedies which will improve the circulation in general. The following remedies are suitable:

Crataegus 6x as a general tonic for the circulation.

Secale 30c is indicated where there has been damage or compromise to the local blood supply near the injury.

Xanthloyium 6c can be used to improve the circulation to lower parts of the limbs.

Other useful remedies

Dose: twice daily

Calc phos 6x can be added to speed up the general healing process where healing is slow

Causticum 30c where tendon contracture is a problem

Calc carb 30c Indicated in chronic tendon injuries

Strontium carb 6c for chronic sprains leading to joint weakness

Tendon Rupture or Breakdown

This is the most serious of all tendon injuries and occurs when the tissues of the tendon are completely torn apart. First aid treatment should be given using **Arnica 200c**, **Ledum 200c**, **Hamamelis 200c** and **Apis 200c**. These remedies should be given in rotation, with 20 minutes between each dose together with the application of ice packs to reduce haemorrhage and reduce inflammation and pain. Repair of the damaged tendon may be possible. Remedies indicated under the healing phase section are indicated during recovery.

Tendon Lacerations

Lacerations or cuts to the flexor tendons are considered serious and often need surgical intervention to clean the area and remove damaged tissue. Surgical repair is often possible. First aid treatment and remedies to be given during healing can be used as outlined previously. **Hypericum 30c** and **Rhus tox 30c** are indicated three times daily, where much pain is evident.

Tendon Sheaths and Tenosynovitis

Depending on the location, a tendon sheath may cover all or part of a tendon. These sac-like structures are lined with synovial membrane which secretes synovial fluid, providing lubrication for the tendon as it moves through the sheath. Inflammation of the tendon sheath is called tenosynovitis and results in an accumulation of synovial fluid within the sheath which appears externally as a swelling. Windgalls and thoroughpin are the most frequently encountered examples. Lameness is rarely evident.

Remedies which will help treat tenosynovitis:

Apis 200c is the principal remedy to consider. *Dose twice daily* until the swelling is reduced, then once weekly to prevent recurrence.

Bryonia 30c is a useful alternative especially where lameness is evident. ***Dose:*** *twice daily as above*

Bursae and Bursitis

Bursae are also sacs lined with synovial membrane and which contain synovial fluid. They act to cushion muscles or tendons as they pass over bony prominences. Bursal inflammation is known as bursitis and occurs in specific areas which are anatomically defined. These bursae are known as true bursae as they are present in all horses. Inflammation will result in swelling of the bursa involved with or without lameness. Examples include bicipital bursitis, cunean bursitis and trochanteric bursitis.

In contrast, false or acquired bursae, arise due to repetitive low-grade trauma and may become fibrosed (thickened) and firm to the touch. This type of bursa is likely to remain. Capped hock, capped elbow and hygroma (a bursal swelling over the knee) are common examples. Bursae of this type rarely cause lameness and are more of a cosmetic problem.

Remedies for bursitis

Arnica 30c is the main remedy to consider for newly acquired bursae where trauma is the initiating cause.
Dose: *twice daily for ten days followed by the next appropriate remedy*

Bellis perennis 30c can be considered as an alternative remedy to Arnica and is also indicated where repeated trauma to an area is the cause leading to the development of a false bursa.
Dose: *twice daily until the situation improves followed by dosing once daily to prevent recurrence*

Apis mel 30c is the principal remedy to consider in treating inflammation of true bursa (bursitis). Apis will also help in reducing the fluid present in false or acquired bursae.
Dose: *twice daily until the problem resolves*

Bryonia 30c in indicated in treating true bursae where bursitis leads to lameness. Inflamed areas feel hot to the touch. Symptoms are better for rest and are worse for exercise. Even the slightest movement leads to discomfort.
Dose: *twice daily until the problem resolves*

Ruta 30c can help in treating true bursae where a tendon is involved. A good example is bicipital bursitis.
Dose: *twice daily until the problem resolves*

Rhus tox 30c where acute symptoms arise (both pain and stiffness) and are caused by overuse but are eased by continued movement or stretching.
Dose: *three times daily until the symptoms abate*

Sanguinaria 30c is a specific remedy for bursitis affecting the shoulder joint. Discomfort is usually worse at night but eased for moving the limb very gently.
Dose: *twice daily until symptoms abate*

Silica 200c will help resolve acquired bursae where the problem has been present for some time. This remedy will help reduce fibrosis and break down

some of the scar tissue present. Treatment will need to be continued for some time.
Dose: three times weekly for several months

Muscles

Muscle is a very specialised tissue which allows the body to move as a whole and allows parts of the body to move with respect to each other. The muscle cells or fibres are grouped in bundles and have a good blood supply to provide the oxygen and nutrients they need to function efficiently and also to remove the waste products of muscle metabolism. There are several types of muscle but it is striated or skeletal muscle which composes the muscles concerned with movement and which is attached to bones by tendons. Muscles can also be attached to ligaments, cartilage, fascia (a sheet of fibrous tissue) and skin.

Muscle is closely associated with synovial membrane. This tissue forms sacs similar to the synovial membranes linked with joints and forms the bursae which reduce friction between muscles or tendons and underlying bony structures. It also forms the synovial sheaths which are associated with and which surround tendons.

Muscle Strains

A muscle strain occurs when a muscle is overstretched. Initially there will inflammation, heat in the affected area and some degree of swelling. These signs are accompanied by pain which will manifest itself as lameness. The exact muscle or muscles affected can be detected by careful manipulation or the application of pressure to the muscle in question. Following the initial inflammation, healing starts, followed by repair to the damaged area.

Rest followed by controlled exercise is vitally important in allowing the injured muscle to heal properly. Other treatments such as ultrasound can help heal along with the following remedies:

Arnica 200c should be used as soon as possible after the injury. If the injuries involve the muscles close to the pelvic area or some of the deeper muscles of the body, use **Bellis perennis 200c** as an alternative.
Dose: twice daily for five days together with:

Hamamelis 200c to help reduce the swelling and to absorb any bleeding that has occurred into the muscle.

Follow this with
Rhus tox 6c which should be used routinely during the healing phase to help relieve stiffness and discomfort.

Where the healing process appear slow consider the following as additional remedies:
Conium 30c where the limbs appear heavy

Calendula 6c to assist healing in general.

Sulphuric acid 6c to help with the after effects originating from the original injury.
Dose: twice daily

Myositis

Myositis is the term applied to inflammation of muscle and occurs immediately after the initial injury where trauma is the cause. Myositis can also be caused by bacterial or viral infection and by the injection of irritating drugs into a muscle.

Arnica 200c and **Rhus tox 6c** are the principal remedies to use where trauma is the underlying cause. *Dose as above.*

Where infection is involved, either Streptococci or Clostridial bacteria are involved and normally gain entry after an injury involving muscle tissue. Use **Aconite 1M** initially giving three doses over a period of one hour followed by:

Hepar sulph 200c where pus is present and the wound is extremely painful even to the least touch

Anthracinum 200c where the muscle is starting to decompose and where the tissue is very swollen.

Pyrogen 1M where there is a fever and foul discharge from the wound

Lachesis 200c where the overlying skin is blue or black in colour and cellulitis is present

Carbo veg 200c where the muscle shows signs of gangrene

Dose: four times daily

In cases where myositis has been caused by injection of irritant drugs, dose initially with **Ledum 30c** giving *four doses over the period of one hour* followed by **Silica 200c** *three times daily* until the reaction resolves.

Muscle Weakness

Muscles may weaken due to a number of causes. Nerve damage or paralysis, poor nutrition, over use, exhaustion, ongoing illness or disease and ageing are the most likely reasons. Symptoms present as hind limb or fore limb weakness or both. Remedies which may help include:

Arnica Following over-use in healthy animals.

Baryta carb Weakness due to old age.

Conium Progressive weakness sometimes with trembling, can be old age.

Gelsemium Weakness after even slight exercise, loss of power, trembling.

Arsenicum album Weakness after the least exertion.

Carbo veg Muscle weakness with signs of collapse.

Kali carb Weak hind limbs after foaling.

Picric acid With generalised lethargy or with spinal cord degeneration.

Plumbum With muscle wasting (atrophy) as well.

Phosphorus Due to nerve degeneration.

Dose: 30c potency once or twice daily depending on severity of the symptoms

Muscle Atrophy

Atrophy is the term applied to wasting, degeneration or reduction in size of an area of the body. Where muscle is concerned, there are several underlying reasons why this might occur. Lack of use is a common cause. This might arise following lameness where the leg is not used properly for a while. Muscle atrophy can also occur as a result of nerve damage, damage to the muscles blood supply, poor nutrition, ageing and lastly due to direct trauma to the muscle tissue.

An underlying cause will need to be identified and dealt with before deciding what action to take. Remedies which might be considered in helping to reverse any muscle atrophy include:

Plumbum 30c is the principal remedy to consider especially where there has been nerve damage to the affected region.

Calc carb 30c should be considered in heavy breeds.

Phosphorus 30c is ideally suited to leaner more athletic builds.

Dose: twice daily

For older animals showing general signs of muscle wasting due to old age dose with:
Hydrastis 6c and **Abrotanum 30c** *once daily* with each remedy as a good general combination or

Acetic acid 30c where there is muscle wasting accompanied by tissue swelling (oedema). ***Dose:*** *twice daily*

Muscle Spasm or Cramp

This is a constant state of muscle contraction which can result in considerable pain or discomfort. Muscle spasm may be seen in conditions such as metabolic problems, after injury (especially to the spine), epilepsy, with some forms of poisoning and in infectious diseases such as tetanus. Indicated remedies will be found in relevant sections. The most important to consider are:

Strychnine Indicated in violent spasms or jerking often with considerable pain.

Nux vomica Spasm of the muscles of the lumbar spine.

Berberis Helpful with spasm of the back muscles in general.

Mag phos Cramps and spasms of limb muscles with general muscle weakness and spasms associated with some metabolic causes.

Belladonna For violent spasms associated with epilepsy.

Hyoscyamus For muscle spasms where the animal shows irritability, anger or delirium. Can help with some forms of poisoning and epilepsy.

Stramonium For partial spasms with trembling or twitching.

Cuprum met For muscle jerking or twitching and cramps or spasms in hind limbs.

Cicuta Spasms and cramping of the muscles of the neck. The neck may be bent back to one side.

Dose: 30 or 200c, two or three times daily depending on nature and severity of symptoms

Specific Conditions Affecting Muscle Tissue

Fibrotic myopathy

In response to exercise, small injuries to muscle tissue will occur and will provide a stimulus for regeneration and strengthening of the muscle. In this way it will be better able to resist further injury. More severe injuries will however, cause damage that results in scar tissue developing rather than healing taking place. As scar or fibrous tissue is inflexible, the action of the muscle will become limited eventually affecting the horse's gait.

The most frequently affected animals are those which perform strenuous exercise or those which are prone to slip and slide on the ground causing muscle trauma. The most often affected groups of muscles are those in the back legs, which form the muscle mass to the back of the femur. Several different muscles are involved so over a period of time adhesions will develop between them, limiting movement. In some cases the tissue scarring can become ossified (meaning to develop into bony like tissue) which leads to a hard defined mass appearing in the muscle tissue. Although strenuous exercise is the main cause of fibrotic myopathy, some types of drug given by intramuscular injection can also cause muscle scarring.

Affected muscles may feel firm or hard but do not show signs of pain or discomfort. As the gait of the horse is affected, the leg will show a shortened stride with limited flexion of the hock and stifle. This causes the hoof to 'slap' the ground as the forward part of the stride is shortened and the backward movement is lengthened. The effect of the condition on the horse's gait is best seen at a walk.

Remedies to help with fibrotic myopathy

Proteus 200c *Once weekly*

Graphites 30c *Give a single dose every three days*

Silica 30c *Give a single dose every three days*

Thiosinaminum 30c *Give a single dose every three days*

Given over a long period, these remedies can be used together to help break down the scar tissue that develops as a result of this condition. Also consider **Calc fluor 30c.** This remedy can be added and used where ossification of muscle tissue is occurring. **Acetic acid 30c** is also worth consideration.
Dose: once every three days

Azoturia
Monday morning disease
Tying up
Set fast/Setfast
Exertional rhabdomyolysis
Atypical myoglobinuria
Paralytic myoglobinuria

This is a condition affecting the muscles, leading to a variable degree of muscle damage, pain and stiffness. The exact cause is not known, although, incorrect training, management and feeding prior to exercise can predispose horses to this condition. Traditionally azoturia was seen in heavy horses on high carbohydrate diets, put back to work after several days resting usually after a weekend. It is also seen in other circumstances, notably in fit horses after rest days and in endurance horses during rest breaks. Mares and highly strung animals appear more susceptible with some animals prone to repeated attacks.

The signs and symptoms can vary considerably from slight stiffness with reluctance to turn and shortening of gait (tying up) to complete reluctance to move accompanied by sweating, elevated temperature and respiratory rate, extreme muscle pain and production of dark, coffee coloured urine referred to as myoglobinuria (exertional rhabdomyolysis/ paralytic myoglobinuria).

The muscles of the back and hindquarters are normally affected and become hard, painful and firm to the touch, although the neck muscles may also be affected. Quivering or trembling of the hind limbs may be noted in some horses. In severe cases, damaged muscle cells release a pigment called myoglobin that is excreted through the kidneys causing the urine to become very dark, almost beer like. In some instances myoglobin can damage the kidneys leading to further complications. In all instances, even if the symptoms of azoturia are very mild, work should stop immediately as continued exercise will cause further muscle damage.

Suggested remedies

Acute remedies

Use in the very early stages.

Aconite 1M
Use early in the initial stages where there are signs of fever and sweating accompanied by fear, anxiety and a tendency to panic.
Dose: *every 15 minutes until symptoms abate*

Belladonna 1M
Also useful in the initial stages where is a degree of excitement and urgency. The animal appears fearful and tense. Concomitant symptoms include dilated pupils, a full rapid throbbing pulse, profuse sweating and a general feeling of heat radiating from the body.
Dose: *every 15 minutes. Alternate with Aconite if necessary*

Specific remedies

Consider using these remedies when the acute symptoms have eased or in less severe episodes.

Aesculus hippocastanum 30c
One of the most useful remedies in less severe case or where intense signs have abated. Aesculus matches many of the symptoms seen in mild cases of azoturia. The urine is hot and darkly discoloured. The hind limbs appear heavy and are obviously painful. Lumbar pain is also evident. Symptoms are eased when the affected area is cooled.
Dose: *every two or three hours until symptoms abate*

Berberis vulgaris 30c
Berberis is also one of the most important remedies, particularly where the symptoms are quite severe. Indicated where the pain is most intense around the region of the kidneys and seems to radiate to the hip and thigh region. Movement is difficult and the horse almost appears paralysed.
Dose: *every two or three hours until symptoms abate*

Actea racemosa or Cimicifuga racemosa 30c
This remedy (which goes under either of two names), has muscular soreness as a keynote feature and is best reserved for treating cases where recovery appears slow. Areas which respond well, include the larger muscles of the body notably those in the hind limbs as well as the muscles of the neck and back. Movement is difficult as the limbs appear as if weighted down and seem sore. Cold appears to make the symptoms worse whilst warmth eases the signs.
Dose: *30c three times daily until symptoms abate*

Bryonia 1M
Indicated where all the symptoms are worse for the least motion and for warmth and ease with rest or when the animal is cooled down. Thirst is a feature together with a degree of irritability. The urine is dark in colour and of similar appearance to beer.
Dose: *every two or three hours until symptoms abate*

Rhus tox 1M
Symptoms are opposite to those of Bryonia and improve with movement and are aggravated by rest. The back is painful and the hind limbs appear extremely stiff and almost paralysed. Trembling is usually a feature, especially after overwork.
Dose: *Two or three doses, one hour apart should be sufficient to ease symptoms*

Other useful remedies

These remedies are useful in helping to prevent the condition from occurring or as additional remedies in treating azoturia.

Arnica 200c
Useful where the condition arises after overuse or over exertion. Pain is evident in the back and hind limbs. Least movement is resented, as is touch or examination. Animals prone to developing this condition can be dosed prior to an event,
Dose: *three times daily in susceptible animals or single dose before riding as prevention*

Bellis perennis 200c
Similar to Arnica and useful after over-exertion. Bellis acts more specifically on the muscles of the back and pelvic region and especially where the deeper muscles are affected. Additional pointers to Bellis include dark urine and pain particularly over the pelvic area.
Dose: *three times daily in susceptible animals or single dose before riding as prevention*

Nux vomica 1M
Best used on a constitutional basis where possible and may be used in a preventative role. Suits horses of a tense, irritable nature. Pain is normally evident over the lumbar area and worse for touch. Particular points to check for include unsteady gait, stiffness, trembling and a degree of weakness after over-use.
Dose: *once daily for three days prior to an event*

Chelidonium 30c
Chelidonium is a prominent liver remedy and has a preventative role in the treatment of azoturia. Influences the muscles hind limbs and pelvic region. Used best in combination with Berberis 30c.
Dose: *once daily for ten days prior to an event*

Cuprum metallicum 1M
Cuprum is a good general remedy for preventing azoturia where the muscles of the hind legs are specifically affected and where the condition only occurs periodically.
Dose: *once weekly*

Benzoicum acidum 30c
Indicated in the later stages where the urine remains darkened with a pungent odour. May help in limiting kidney damage where this is suspected.
Dose: *twice daily until the animal improves*

Calc carb 30c
This remedy is best used constitutionally and where the symptoms arise during damp, wet weather.
Dose: *two or three times daily in a preventive role as needed*

Joints

Joints allow movement and principally connect bones and allow them to move in relation to each other. The fundamental structure of all the joints connected with movement, that is those joints which compose the limbs, is the same. Cartilage referred to as articular cartilage covers the end of the bones and the whole joint is surrounded by a dense fibrous capsule known as the joint capsule. The inside of the capsule is covered in a layer known as the synovial membrane which envelops all the structures except articular cartilage. Its purpose to provide lubrication and to aid this function it produces synovial fluid as a lubricant. The joint capsule and various ligaments around each joint ensure that the joint remains stable and also help to limit its range of movement.

Conditions Affecting Joints

Chronic arthritis
Degenerative joint disease (DJD)
Degenerative arthritis
Osteoarthritis

This is the most common chronic, long-term condition to affect the joints and occurs when the cartilage surface covering the ends of the bones is damaged. Sometimes this will occur as a secondary change, as a result of inflammation of some of the other joint structures, such as the joint capsule or synovial membrane. As the condition progresses, new bone may form changing the contours of the joint and causing additional inflammation and pain.

Symptoms can arise naturally as a result of ageing, although trauma (such as a severe sprain), infection (see septic arthritis) or poor conformation can also lead to joint damage and consequent arthritis.

The symptoms are familiar. Lameness in varying degrees is common, together with a variety of other symptoms, which can include stiffness, joint swelling, joint enlargement, heat, pain, limited range of movement and occasionally cracking noises. The weather commonly affects the symptoms you might see. Cold, wet weather will normally make symptoms much worse whilst symptoms will often ease in warm, dry weather, although this is not always the case.

The most frequently affected joints include those of the lower limbs, the fetlock, pastern and coffin joints as well as the hock and knee. Upper limb joints, the elbow, shoulder, stifle and hip, are much less likely to develop symptoms of arthritis.

Remedies for arthritis or DJD

Symptoms of arthritis will often respond well to homeopathic treatment although the remedies need to be chosen with care to achieve good results. There are a fair number of remedies to select from. For ease of use they have been divided into three groups. The most often used remedies are listed first followed by those are often useful but prescribed less frequently. Keynotes are given for each of these remedies together with the joints which respond most favourably. The final group briefly mentions some of the other remedies that are useful from time to time.

Major joint remedies

Rhus tox

Keynotes: Worse in cold, damp weather, for rest, on first movement, at night, if overworked
Better for continued movement, changing position, dry warmth, stretching
Target joints: All joints, including the shoulder
This is by far the most often used remedy and is certainly the one most often cited as being useful in treating arthritis. Rhus tox will only work well where the symptoms closely match those associated with the remedy. Characteristically this remedy will be of benefit where the symptoms are worse in cold, damp weather and better for warm dry weather. Symptoms are also worse for any period of rest and on first movement but will ease with continued movement to a point. However, exercise may well cause problems if prolonged, leading to further stiffness after rest. Stretching or flexing of the limbs prior to moving off after a period of rest may also be a symptom. Restlessness, typically in the evening, may also be observed in some cases as the pains in the joint cause the animal to shift around trying to get comfortable. Symptoms can be worse at night.
***Dose:** 6c twice daily, or 30c once daily, or 1M three times weekly*

Bryonia alba

Keynotes: Worse for least movement and exercise, for touch, in warm weather, jarring of joints
Better for rest, pressure on affected part, cold
Notable aversion to being examined
Target joints: All joints
The symptoms associated with Bryonia are largely the opposite of Rhus tox. Painful joints are eased by cold weather and are worse in warm weather. Movement is difficult as the animal will be reluctant to use the joint, any movement making the symptoms worse, whereas rest eases the discomfort. Pressure on affected joints will also ease any discomfort. This may be seen as the animal lying down with the affected joint tucked under the body or leaning with the affected leg against the stable wall so the weight of the body puts pressure on the joint. Bryonia will also help where the joints are swollen, hot and painful to touch. Horses that respond especially well, have a tendency to sweat easily, are often thirsty and may have an irritable nature. This often makes proper examination of the horse that requires Bryonia difficult.
***Dose:** 6c twice daily, or 30c once daily, or 1M three times weekly*

Ruta grav

Keynotes: Worse for lying down, cold and damp weather, at night
Better for movement, warmth
Exostoses, periosteal reaction
Target joints: Fetlock, coffin, pastern, knees, hock
Ruta is often used alongside Rhus tox with which it shares some symptoms including those of restless, shifting movements of the legs as the animal tries to get comfortable. This remedy is especially applicable where there are signs of bony changes in the joints (exostoses) as a result of degenerative

changes.
Ruta is particularly suited where the knee, fetlock, pastern or coffin joints are involved. The symptoms of stiffness associated with this remedy are less ameliorated by warmth when compared with Rhus tox.
Dose: 30c once daily, or 200c three times weekly

Calc carb

Keynotes: Worse in cold, damp weather, for exertion, full moon
Better in dry weather, warmth
Target joints: Fetlock, coffin, pastern, knees, hock
One of the main features of this remedy is that symptoms of joint pain and stiffness are much worse in cold, damp weather and in this respect match those of Rhus tox. Similarly, warm, dry weather eases the symptoms. However, the animal that will respond well to Calc carb will sweat easily on the least exercise and will be overweight and sluggish in nature. Symptoms are often worse around the time of the full moon. Calc carb is especially useful where the stifle joint is involved and in heavy horse breeds.
Dose: 6c twice daily, or 30c once daily, or 1M three times weekly

Causticum

Keynotes: Worse in clear fine weather, in dry cold wind
Better for warmth and in damp, wet weather
Suits older or prematurely aged animals
Advanced stages of joint degeneration
Target joints: All joints
Causticum is one of the remedies indicated for more chronic arthritic problems where this is accompanied by loss of strength and advanced bony changes to the joints. Older animals often respond well, especially those that appear unsteady on their legs and have a pottery gait and appear older than they really are. Joint pains may cause the animal to become restless at night. Symptoms are worse in good weather and ease when the weather is damp or wet.
Dose: 30c once or twice daily

Pulsatilla

Keynotes: Worse for heat, first movement, in the evening
Better for gentle motion, in the open air, for pressure
Shifting lameness from joint to joint
Target joints: Stifle, hips, knees
Pulsatilla targets the stifle and hip joints or where the lameness shifts from joint to joint or from leg to leg causing the animal to become restless. Symptoms ease with gentle movement but are worse for warmth. Pressure on the affected area gives some relief of the discomfort, a symptom shared with Bryonia. In contrast horses responding to Bryonia are irritable and thirsty; those likely to respond to Pulsatilla drink very little and are more placid in character.
Dose: 30c daily, or 200c three times weekly

Calc fluor

Keynotes: Worse for changes in weather
Better for warmth
Exostoses, bony changes
Target joints: Fetlock, pastern, coffin, shoulder, hips
This is one of the major remedies where there are joint deformities resulting as consequence of ongoing arthritic changes. Calc fluor is specifically indicated where there is synovitis of the stifle joint or where the fetlock, pastern and coffin joints are involved. Symptoms are worse for changes in the weather and better for warmth.
Dose: 30c daily, or 200c three times weekly

Ledum

Keynotes: Worse for heat and at night
Better in cold weather
Cracking in joints
Target joints: Fetlock, pastern, coffin, hock
Arthritic joints that respond well to Ledum appear less painful in cold weather. Discomfort is also reduced if a cold compress is applied locally and for cold hosing. In contrast symptoms aggravated by hot weather or local application of a warm compress. Affected limbs appear painful to the extent that very little weight can be put onto the foot. This is due to the joint pains that shoot up the leg as the horse tries to weight bear. Where an affected joint is swollen, there is absence of any heat. Ledum is a useful remedy where joint pains appear to persist after a previous injury, or where lameness results from repeated low-level joint trauma or concussion.
Dose: 30c daily

Minor joint remedies

Actea spicata

Keynotes: Worse for slight exertion, change of temperature, cold
Joint swelling, heat
Target joints: Knee (especially), hock, fetlock, pastern, coffin
This less well-known remedy targets specifically the smaller joints (the fetlock, pastern and coffin joints) and the more complex joints of the body, the carpal (knee) and metacarpal joints and the hock and metatarsal joints. Affected joints are swollen and hot. The swelling is aggravated by movement. Ideally this remedy is suited to treating more recent cases rather than long-standing conditions.
***Dose:** 30c three times daily until improvement, then 6c once daily if needed on a long-term basis*

Caulophyllum

Keynotes: Worse for motion
Stiffness
Target joints: Fetlock, pastern and coffin specifically, knees
Caulophyllum is suited to treating degenerative joint changes affecting the fetlock, pastern and coffin joints where stiffness is a key feature. Symptoms are worse for motion, which only leads to further discomfort.
***Dose:** 6c once or twice daily*

Kali carb

Keynotes: Worse at night and in cold, damp weather
Better for warmth and for moving about
Exostoses, weak back legs
Target joints: Stifle specifically, but also hips, fetlock, pastern and coffin
One of the clues to using this remedy is general weak nature of the patient as a whole as well as intolerance of cold weather and a degree of irritability. Animals which respond well will also show signs of back pain and a heaviness in their movement, sometimes showing jerky movements. Bony enlargements (exostoses) may also be present.
***Dose:** 30c once daily*

Chelidonium

Keynotes: Worse for motion and for touch, changes in the weather
Better for local pressure
Lethargy and general stiffness
Target joints: Right shoulder joint specifically, but useful for generalised joint stiffness
Chelidonium is a well-known liver remedy but is also extremely useful as a supportive remedy in treating DJD. Horses that seem to respond best will show signs of lethargy and will not be performing to the best of their ability.
***Dose:** 30c once daily*

Berberis vulgaris

Keynotes: Worse for motion and changes in weather
Pain moving from joint to joint, sudden twinges of pain, variable lameness
Target joints: Mainly the fetlock, pastern and coffin joints, hips and stifle
Berberis is also a remedy that is associated with treating the liver. The joint pain associated with this remedy comes in twinges and is by nature spasmodic causing variable and intermittent lameness as the pain moves from joint to joint. A history of urinary or lower (lumbar) back problems would be additional pointers. Affected horses often tire easily and have poor endurance abilities.
***Dose:** 30c once daily*

Manganum aceticum

Keynotes: Worse in cold weather
Better for resting
Chronic DJD with stiffness and tendency to stumble easily
Muscles and joints are sore when touched
Pains shift from joint to joint
Inflammation of the periosteum
Target joints: Stifle and hocks especially
Manganum is suited to treating chronic arthritis where the lameness shifts from joint to joint or where the muscles or joints appear tender when touched. A notable feature of this remedy is a tendency to stumble when moving either forwards or backwards. The horse's gait may also be altered with the back feet slapping against the ground in an unusual fashion. Manganum symptoms are worse in cold wet weather and better for resting.
***Dose:** 6c once or twice daily*

Angustura vera

Keynotes: Cracking joints with general stiffness
Target joints: All joints but stifles especially
Based on the simple keynote of cracking joints, this remedy has proved successful in treating many cases of arthritis when the only other symptom is generalised stiffness.
Dose: 6c twice daily

Colchicum

Keynotes: Swollen joints with heat
Extremely sensitive to the slightest touch or movement
Target joints: All joints
Colchicum acts on the periosteum and synovial membranes specifically and is indicted in chronic cases where the affected joints show persistent swelling, heat and sensitivity to both examination and to the least movement of the joint.
Dose: 30c once daily

Benzoic acid

Keynotes: Cracking joints and joint deformity
Target joints: Any cracking joints. Knee joints especially
This remedy will help where cracking noises can be heard from the joints. It also will help in cases where there is joint enlargement and deformity. Benzoic acid is especially useful in treating chronic swollen knees where the joints are enlarged and where there is some limitation in movement.
Dose: 30c once daily

Hekla/Heckla lava

Keynotes: Exostoses, bony spurs, arthritic nodosities, periostitis
Target joints: Any affected joint
Hekla is one of the main remedies to bear in mind when dealing with arthritic joints that have evidence of bony spurs, nosodities (bony lumps) or exostoses. These form as a consequence of arthritic changes and consist of new bone formed as a result of the degenerative changes or stresses placed upon affected joints. Hekla is often used alongside other remedies where appropriate.
Dose: 30c once daily

Harpagophytum

Keynotes: Arthritis with bony degeneration in older horses
Target joints: Any joints but especially the stifle and the hip
More familiar in its herbal version Devil's claw, this is a good general remedy for older horses with DJD where there is bony degeneration and exostoses.
Dose: 6x twice daily

Other useful remedies

These remedies are less commonly prescribed in treating joint problems but none the less can be equally as effective in treating arthritic symptoms when accurately prescribed.

Dose: where indicated: 6c potency twice daily, or 30c potency once daily, or 1M once weekly

Rhododendron 6c General stiffness worse before storm, affecting the shoulder, elbow and fetlock joints particularly. Rhododendron has similar modalities to Rhus tox.

Salicylicum acid 30c Arthritis of the stifle and elbow joints where the joints are swollen and painful.

Tylophora indica 1M Lameness originating from arthritic changes in the fetlock, pastern and coffin joints can respond, where the symptoms are worse in cold weather and for exercise.

Symphytum 6c Indicated as an additional remedy in treating arthritic joints where the periosteum is inflamed and painful. Symphytum can be used in a more general way to help stimulate healing of damaged joints.

Argentum metallicum 30c Improves blood flow to the cartilage of damaged joints. Best used early on as an additional remedy where either cartilage or other surrounding connective tissues are inflamed.

Shark cartilage 6c Acts as a general remedy for arthritis and in particular may improve the health of articular cartilage by improving blood supply.

Bamboo gum 6x Acts in a similar fashion to Shark cartilage to improve the health of cartilage.

Abrotanum 30c Lameness and stiffness in aged

horses where there is a degree of emaciation. Knee and hock joints respond particularly well.

Aesculus hippocastanum 30c where there is general stiffness and discomfort around the pelvis and hip area.

Formica rufa 6c Acts best where there are signs of chronic stiffness, mainly affecting the hind limbs. Other signs to check for include hind limb weakness and restlessness causing the horse to keep shifting the weight from one back leg to another. Formica can also help where arthritic symptoms wander from joint to joint and where joints swell suddenly with obvious heat and pain.

Radium bromide 30c Indicated where there is chronic joint pain accompanied by restlessness. Symptoms are eased by movement and are worse on first movement. This remedy is most suited to problems affecting the stifles and hocks.

Homarus 1M This little known remedy is a specific for treating bone spavin.

Lithium carb 30c Lithium is of most value in dealing with arthritis accompanied by bony nodosities affecting the hock particularly as well as the fetlock, coffin and pastern joints to a lesser extent. Lithium is also a good remedy for helping with bone spavin.

Guaiacum 30c The principal indication for this remedy is in helping with very stiff almost immovable joints where there is a very restricted range of movement. Additional signs include bony nodosities and contracted muscles and tendons.

Kali iod 6c Indicated for arthritis where there is considerable joint swelling or where the periosteum is thickened. Affected joints are extremely painful and the horse will show marked lameness. Suited in particular to the knee joints.

Dulcamara 6c Think of using this remedy for symptoms that appear specifically in the autumn when the days are warm and the nights cold. Any joint may be affected. Symptoms include general stiffness which is worse in damp weather and eased by warmth.

Silica 30c Silica is useful supportive remedy where the basic structure of a joint is badly damaged by arthritic changes and where there is a degree of calcification or exostoses present.

Mineral 6x Is a non-specific remedy that appears helpful in some arthritic horses.

Acute Joint Pain and Swelling

In contrast to the remedies used to treat chronic joint pain and stiffness, the homeopathic management of the acutely swollen joint requires short-term use of a number of remedies to deal with the immediate problem, followed by a more long-term prescription where appropriate. Acute symptoms usually arise as a result of trauma but can be a consequence of infection leading to septic arthritis, both conditions causing acute lameness and joint swelling.

Remedies for acute symptoms where trauma is the cause

Arnica

Keynotes: Trauma
This is the first remedy to use where trauma is involved. Touch or even the slightest movement of the affected joint is resented.
Dose: 200c three times daily followed by another indicated remedy where appropriate

Apis mel

Keynotes: Worse for heat, movement, red hot, swollen joints
This remedy is best suited to acute symptoms where a joint suddenly puffs up and is hot to the touch and visibly swollen. The affected joint may even have a rosy or shiny hue and the pain is such that the horse will be unwilling to move. However, cold hosing affords some relief and seems to ease the symptoms.
Dose: 200c three times daily until symptoms abate. Follow with an appropriate remedy where indicated

Kalmia

Keynotes: Acute lameness with cracking noises
Kalmia is one of the least well-known remedies but is useful where there is acute swelling of a joint accompanied by cracking noises as the joint moves. Affected joints will appear red, hot and swollen and the animal resents the least movement of the joint.

This remedy acts best on the shoulder joint and joints of the hind limb.
Dose: *30c every two hours until symptoms abate*

Rhus tox, **Bryonia** or **Ledum** may be needed as acute remedies where the symptoms agree.
Use the 200c potency and dose three times daily until the symptoms abate or another remedy is indicated

Septic Arthritis

Septic Polyarthritis
Joint Ill, Joint Infection

Joint infection is most common in foals (usually under one month of age with those which fail to receive colostrum at most risk). More than one joint is usually affected. This condition is usually referred to as 'joint ill' and can originate from a blood-borne infection originating elsewhere in the body. Common sources include respiratory or gut infections or sepsis (infection) involving the umbilicus.

Adult horses can suffer from septic arthritis involving a specific single joint. The source of the infection is most likely to be a penetrating wound to the joint. Bear in mind that **Ledum** is a useful remedy to use at this stage.

The condition results in severe lameness with enlargement of the joint capsule with obvious heat and pain. Other signs can include a raised temperature and lethargy. Prompt treatment is required in order to avoid damage to the joint. It would be unwise to rely on homeopathic treatment alone in this situation. Use of appropriate remedies can help immensely while waiting for professional help. Infections which have been present for several days will undoubtedly result in long-term degenerative changes to the joints.

Remedies for septic arthritis and joint ill

Aconite
Keynotes: Infection
Aconite is best used where there is a risk of infection developing. To be used to its best advantage, it needs to be given early on, before more definitive symptoms have developed. Symptoms where Aconite is needed develop suddenly and quickly.
Dose: *1M every 30 minutes until symptoms abate or another remedy is indicated*

Belladonna
Keynotes: Swollen joints with fever
Indicated where the affected joint or joints are very swollen. The skin over the joint will have a red hue and is painful to the slightest touch. Any motion is resented. Affected animals will also have raised temperature and show signs of lethargy.
Dose: *1M every one to two hours until symptoms abate*

Pyrogen
Keynotes: Sepsis
Use Pyrogen where joint ill develops concurrently with infection originating from either a gut condition or respiratory infection. A fever will be present causing the animal to sweat and the pulse rate will be high. A key feature is marked restlessness with the animal constantly shifting position.
Dose: *1M every one to two hours until symptoms abate*

Hepar sulph
Keynote: Sensitivity to touch
This remedy is best used in the later stages of ongoing sepsis where infection remains in the joint or joints, which remain swollen and painful. The joints are painful to the slightest or least touch.
Dose: *200c three times daily as needed*

Other remedies such as **Silica 30c** or **Calc sulph 30c** may be needed in treating adult animals where joint infection leads to a chronic discharging abscess developing which then becomes a fistula or sinus (see page 245).

Where the umbilicus is the source of the original infection, **Abrotanum 30c** (*three times daily*) can be given as an additional remedy.

Joint luxation and subluxation
Displacement, Dislocation

Luxation refers to the displacement of the bones that make up a joint in relation to one another. Injuries of this nature are serious and thankfully rare but will cause marked lameness. Occurring normally only after considerable trauma, there is usually extensive damage to the surrounding tissues. Treatment should be given promptly and aimed at minimising the trauma. Realignment of displaced bones normally requires anaesthesia. The long-term consequences of this type of injury can also respond.

Subluxation refers to the partial displacement of the bones that compose a joint. Again this is rare but is sometimes seen in younger horses where the pastern joint can be involved.

Suggested remedies

Acute injuries – *use 200c three times daily for seven to ten days*

Arnica Use in all cases as soon as possible to minimise the trauma

Bryonia Indicated where the horse is unable to put the limb to the ground and any movement is painful

Ruta To help minimise damage to surrounding ligaments and tendons

Rhus tox During recovery where the limb is stiff after rest and the lameness improves with movement

For long-term problems – *use 30c once daily*

Petroleum For chronic problems where cracking noises form the joints are apparent

Calc carb In general for old injuries where there is residual weakness in the limbs

Ruta Use where there is residual lameness in the knees and stifle

Natrum carb Indicated where there is residual weakness in the hocks

Strontium carb Also for weakness of the hock where there is persistent swelling of the joint

Developmental disorders

Developmental orthopaedic disease (DOD)

DOD comprises a group of growth or developmental disorders that affect the musculoskeletal system of young growing horses. Within the group are 5 separate conditions; Osteochondrosis and related problems, Growth plate problems, Angular limb deformities, Contracted tendons and Wobbler syndrome.

Osteochondrosis
Osteochondritis dissecans (OCD)
Subchondral bone cysts

Osteochondritis dissecans (OCD) and subchondral bone cysts are both consequences of osteochron-drosis, a condition seen in young growing horses showing intermittent lameness.

Several factors, acting either alone or in combination, underlie the development of osteochondrosis. These produce changes in actively growing cartilage or bone which may remain undetected until the affected area is subjected to physical stress. Such biomechanical stresses may interfere with or prevent the normal conversion of cartilage into bone by interfering with the blood supply or act by weakening the supporting bone that underlies the joint cartilage. Weak areas of cartilage lead to deficits in the cartilage surface, essentially lesions typical of osteochondrosis. Where concussive forces act on these areas, subchondral bone cysts form in contrast to areas where shearing forces predominate. In these areas the forces cause the cartilage to separate from the underlying bone either forming a flap or to detach completely forming a free floating piece of cartilage, lesions typical of OCD.

One of the most important factors in the development of osteochondrosis is nutrition. Nutritional problems include imbalances in the levels of calcium, Phosphorus, zinc and copper in the diet, excess carbohydrate levels leading to an accelerated growth rate and similarly obesity resulting from feeding a high-energy diet. Genetic factors also play a part. Some foals are simply genetically programmed to grow far too quickly so that their body weight exceeds that which the growing skeleton can support. There is also a degree of joint susceptibility, periods during growth when certain joints are vulnerable to damage. Finally trauma can be considered a factor. This induces biomechanical joint stress caused by poor conformation (leading to uneven or abnormal forces upon a joint), restricted exercise (causing weak joints to develop) and sudden management changes leading to an increase in exercise levels.

OCD tends to occur in specific joints, usually the stifle, hock, fetlock and shoulder. The condition is normally clinically evident as a variable lameness within the first 2 years of life. Joint swelling together with obvious pain may also be seen in some cases.

Subchondral bone cysts are literally holes in the bone close to the surface of a joint sometimes linked to the surface by a narrow tract. They can form in any joint but are more likely to appear in the stifle joint, where the end of the femur is affected and in the third metacarpal bone. Depending on the exact location, the cyst may or may not cause lameness, which in fact, may resolve given time. Lameness is often not apparent until the horse is subjected to more strenuous exercise.

Remedies for OCD and subchondral bone cysts

Homeopathy can play both a preventative role in treating animals likely to be at risk of OCD and bone cysts, as well as helping those with diagnosed lesions. Treatment needs to be carried out along with careful attention to the composition of the feed. This needs to be balanced to contain the ideal quantity and ratio of minerals to ensure that cartilage forms properly and that the ideal growth rate is not exceeded. Management is equally as important; time and rest are the most important aspects, allowing the lesions to heal. Surgery is indicated in some cases.

Calc phos 6x

Calc phos will help regulate bone and cartilage growth and enable the body to utilise effectively the minerals supplied in the diet.
Dose: twice daily

Calc carb 6x

This remedy is an alternative to Calc phos and should be given in preference to those animals of the heavier breeds or where an animal is considered overweight.
Dose: twice daily

Phosphorus 6x

Suited to animals of a thin and lean stature and of flighty temperament, Phosphorus will ensure the correct utilisation of Phosphorus by avoiding a relative calcium deficiency caused by excessive Phosphorus in the diet. This will help to guarantee that the bone underlying the joint cartilage form correctly and is sufficiently strong to support the overlying cartilage reducing the risk of bone cysts.
Dose: *twice daily*

Zinc met 6c

Excessive zinc in the diet can induce a relative deficiency of copper which is a vital component of the diet needed for the proper formation of bone. Zinc in homeopathic potency will ensure that the copper in the diet can be utilised properly by regulating zinc levels.
Dose: *once daily*

Cuprum met 6x

In a similar way, dosing with cuprum in low potency will help the proper utilisation of copper that is needed by an enzyme which helps with the formation of bone.
Dose: *twice daily*

Argentum metallicum 6c

Silver is a remedy whose action is centred on the structures that compose joints with particular focus on bone and cartilage. Its action in homeopathic potency is to improve the blood flow to these structures so that sufficient nutrients are supplied ensuring that they form properly. This is an excellent preventative remedy for OCD and bone cysts and one which can also be used in treatment of the condition.
Dose: *twice daily*

Shark cartilage 30c

One of the properties of shark cartilage is to inhibit the growth of blood vessels in actively growing tissue. Used in homeopathic potency it appears to help to repair damaged cartilage (probably by encouraging a good blood supply to the damaged

cartilage) and to ease some of the pain and discomfort associated with OCD.
Dose: *once daily*

Ruta grav 6c
Ruta is a good general remedy to use where there has been damage to joint cartilage. It will help prevent arthritic lesions developing and can be given alongside other remedies.
Dose: *twice daily*

Growth plate disorders Epiphysitis (physitis) or Physeal dysplasia

This is a growth disorder affecting the growth plates of the long bones most frequently seen in the radius at the level of the carpal joint or just above the fetlock involving the lower growth plate of the cannon bone. There are a number of predisposing factors including poor diet, trauma and rapid growth. Animals at risk can be dosed with **Calc phos 30c** three times weekly but attention should also be made to correcting any dietary imbalances. **Calc carb 30c** can be used to effect in heavier animals instead. Lameness is rare in cases of epiphysitis but pain may be apparent at the level of the affected growth plate or you may see slight swelling just above the knee and with some heat. The gait in affected animals is sometimes described as choppy. Dosing with **Eupatorium perf 30c** twice daily will help alleviate any discomfort.

Angular deformities Carpus valgus Carpus varus

Angular deformities of the limbs can occur in newborn or growing foals as a result of poor conformation or poor development. One side of a growth plate develops faster than the other side due to a problem with the growth of either the metaphysis or epiphysis. The result of this is that the limb deviates to one side or the other, away from the side that grows the fastest. Where the joints of the limb appear to angle inwards and the limb below angles outwards, the condition is referred to as valgus. In varus, the opposite occurs with the joints appearing to deviate outwards and the limb below inwards. The most commonly affected joints are the carpus (where valgus is more likely to be seen) and the fetlock (where varus is more likely) and lower end of the tibia (which is more prone to valgus).

There are a number of causes of which trauma is one of the most important. Injury can result in uneven pressure on the growth plate leading to the death of some of the cartilage cells. The consequence of this is that at this point of greatest damage, the growth of new bone ceases, and the limb starts to lengthen faster on one side than the other with the resulting deviation. Other factors known to be implicated in some cases, include developmental abnormalities of the carpal bones, partial and incomplete growth of the splint bones and nutrition. The latter is poorly understood and involves the complex relationship between calcium, Phosphorus, vitamins A & D, zinc and copper.

Treatment

Rest is of prime importance, as any activity will only serve to increase the trauma on the affected joints. Confinement to a loosebox is the best option. Trimming of the feet (or foot balancing) is also recommended as this can help correct the stresses placed upon the joints. A combination of these two options is often all that is required to help correct the deviation in uncomplicated cases. Homeopathy has a role to play here and can help immensely. More severe cases will require surgery.

Suggested remedies

Calc phos 6x
This remedy should be given routinely in all cases to tackle the problem nutritionally and structurally.
Dose: *twice daily*

Symphytum 6c
Routine use of Symphytum will minimise the effects of any trauma on the growth plate.
Dose: *twice daily*

Argentum metallicum 6c
Another remedy which can be used regularly to help improve the blood flow to the areas of the growth plates and cartilage damaged by trauma.
Dose: *twice daily*

Contracted tendons
Flexural limb deformities

This condition occurs in both the newborn and growing foal. Where newborn foals are concerned the condition will often resolve in a few days. In older animals, deformity occurs due to uneven muscle and tendon development in relation to the growth of bone in the affected limb. Affected foals appear up on their toes and upright in the leg with the fetlock appearing above the foot. In the most severe cases the knee appears flexed with knuckling over at the fetlock joint.

Suggested remedies

Calc phos 6x
This remedy should be given routinely in all cases to tackle the problem nutritionally and structurally in regard to the development of bone.
Dose: *twice daily*

Causticum 30c
This is the principle remedy to consider where the tendons are contracted helping to relieve the contraction and to straighten the limb.
Dose: *2 or 3 times daily*

Colchicum 30c
Consider Colchicum as an alternative to Causticum and especially where the affected leg or legs appear painful or swollen.
Dose: *2 or 3 times daily*

Wobbler syndrome

See page 227

The Locomotor or Musculoskeletal System Part Two

This second section on the locomotor system covers individual conditions and links in with the first where more specific details of the remedies are provided to avoid repetition. Additional information on suitable remedies is included where appropriate. The content is organised anatomically starting with the neck, forelimb (working form the shoulder downwards), back and pelvis, hindlimb (from the hip downwards) and finally a section specifically relating to the foot and the hooves. For each condition only the most prominent remedies are listed. As others may fit the picture it is always best to refer back to Part 1 under the relevant sections. Needless to say it is important to observe proper management of all the conditions listed alongside any homeopathic remedies used. This might include, (where appropriate), rest, rehabilitation, physiotherapy, chiropractic, osteopathy, acupuncture, hydrotherapy, exercise, ultrasound, laser therapy and shoeing amongst others.

The Neck

The main anatomical structures of the neck comprise the 7 cervical vertebrae (the first of the 5 different types of vertebrae comprising the spinal column), the substantial nuchal ligament (which takes the weight of the head) and its laminae that attach to the individual vertebrae and the associated musculature, nerves and blood vessels. Problems with the neck are rare and are mostly associated with injury or the use of improper tack or riding technique. Useful remedies include:

Injury **Arnica 30c**, **Ruta grav 30c** (especially where ligaments are involved)

Stiffness **Rhus tox 30c**, **Chelidonium 30c**, **Bryonia 30c**, **Causticum 30c**, **Rhododendron 6c**, **Lachnantes 30c**

Spasm/rigidity **Cicuta 30c**, **Cimicifugia 6c**, **Strychnine 30c**

Lameness originating from the neck **Aesculus 30c**, **Hypericum 30c**

Specific Conditions

Wobbler syndrome
See Nervous System page 227

The Forelimb

Forelimb problems are more common than those of the hindlimb, with the foot more often involved in comparison to other parts of the limb. Anatomically the area is divided into the shoulder, upper arm (the humerus), forearm (radius, ulna and elbow joint), carpus (knee), metacarpus (cannon bone), fetlock joint, pastern and coffin joints. The foot and associated structures are detailed under a separate heading.

The Shoulder and Shoulder Joint Shoulder Blade Scapulohumeral Joint

This region comprises the shoulder blade and the shoulder joint. This joint is of the ball and socket type formed by the shoulder blade (scapula) and the humerus and allows a wide range of movement, especially flexion and extension. Sideways movement (adduction and abduction) is limited.

Specific Conditions of the Shoulder and Shoulder Joint

Fractures

The most likely cause of a fracture in this area is trauma, particularly from a fall or poor landing after a jump. The degree of lameness and prognosis depends on the exact site of the fracture. Fractures to the shoulder blade itself are rare as it is well protected by muscle tissue. Where the break involves the scapular spine, the outlook is good and with rest and appropriate remedies. The fracture is likely to heal and the horse will go sound. Other areas of the shoulder blade carry a less favourable outlook with the possibility of surgery as an option, especially if the area known as the point of the shoulder is involved. Some fractures of the shoulder joint carry the risk of nerve damage.

Suggested remedies

Arnica 30c, **Ruta grav 30c**, **Calc phos 6c**, **Calc carb 6c**, **Symphytum 6c**, **Hypericum 30c** (where nerve damage is suspected).

See Fractures page 170.

Torn or ruptured muscles

The forelimb has no bony attachment to the rest of the skeleton (unlike the hindlimb), being held in place by muscles and ligaments, an arrangement that allows great flexibility and speed in movement. Some of the muscles are prone to injury (usually from jumping) and can result in extreme pain and guarded prognosis.

Suggested remedies

Arnica 200c, **Rhus tox 200c**, **Bellis 200c**, **Calendula 30c**

Lacticum acidum 30c This could be a useful remedy in the later stages if residual pain persists.

Dose: twice daily

Sweeny, Suprascapular Nerve Paralysis

See Nervous System page 230

Bicipital bursitis, Intertubercular bursitis

The bicipital bursa is a small sac which is lined with synovial membrane and which contains synovial fluid and sits between the tendon of the biceps and a groove in the top of the humerus. Its function is to cushion the tendon as it passed over the bone. Inflammation of the bursa (bursitis) can occur from trauma and occasionally from infection and results in local pain over the area. Lameness can be severe but will usually resolve with treatment and rest; however,. some horses may continue to show long-term problems.

Suggested remedies

Acute cases

Arnica 30c, **Bryonia 30c**, **Apis 30c**, **Ruta grav 30c**, **Rhus tox 30c**

Chronic cases

Sanguinaria 6c, **Calf fluor 30c**, **Silica 30c**, **Ruta grav 30c**

See Bursitis page 174

Dislocation of the shoulder joint Scapulohumeral luxation

This problem will only arise after considerable trauma to the area with the result that the humerus will be displaced either in an inward (medial) or outward (lateral) direction. Severe lameness will be apparent and the area will be extremely painful. If joint damage is minimal, then the dislocation can be reduced under anaesthetic.

Acute remedies **Arnica 200c**, **Bryonia 200c**, **Ruta 200c**, **Rhus tox 200c**

For acute pain **Hypericum 30c**, **Chamomilla 30c** (with anger or irritability)

For long-term consequences **Ruta 30c**, **Calc carb 30c**, **Natrum carb 30c**, **Strontium carb 6c**, **Petroleum 6c**

Arthritis of the shoulder joint

This can occur as a result of local trauma to the area (such as a direct blow, dislocation or fractures), as the result of an infection (particularly navel ill in young foals), as a complication of an intra-articular drug injection or as a consequence of osteochrondrosis dissecans (OCD).

The symptoms associated with arthritis of the shoulder joint can be quite variable. Initially the horse may be quite lame, holding the head to the affected side as the limb is moved forward at the same time avoiding flexing the joint. Subsequently the horse may become chronically lame.

Suggested remedies

Initially **Arnica 200c**, **Bryonia 200c**, **Rhus tox 200c**

Long-term – principally **Rhus tox 30c**, **Ruta grav 30c**, **Bryonia 30c**, **Calc carb 30c**, **Causticum 30c**, **Chelidonium 30c**, **Phytolacca 30c**

Consider **Ferrum phos 6c**, **Ferrum met 6c**, **Sanguinaria 6c**, **Dulcamara 30c**, **Ledum 30c**, **Colchicum 30c**

Where there are bony changes **Calc fluor 30c**, **Heckla lava 30c**, **Silica 30c**

OCD

See page 186

The Upper Arm/Humerus

This area comprises the humerus, the large bone of the upper arm and the bulky muscles which surround it. Many of the major muscles of this area are supplied by one of the most important nerves in the body, the radial nerve.

Specific Conditions of the Upper Arm

Fracture of the humerus

Fractures of the humerus are rare as the muscles in this region protect the bone well, nevertheless a kick or awkward fall may result in the bone fracturing.

Helpful remedies have already been detailed (see Fractures page 170) but remember the importance of **Hypericum 30c** if there is associated radial nerve damage. Humeral fractures are serious and the outlook is not favourable.

Radial nerve paralysis

See page 230

The Forearm
Radius and Ulna
Elbow (Humeroradial Joint)

The two principal bones of this region are the radius and ulna which, together with the humerus, comprise the elbow or humeroradial joint. This is a simple hinge type joint that allows extension and flexion.

Specific Conditions of the Forearm

Fractures of the radius and ulna

Fractures of these bones are rare and most likely to arise as a result of severe trauma, particularly road traffic accidents. The ulna is most likely to break in the part known as the olecranon process, anatomically at the point of the elbow. Affected horses (most likely to be foals) will be unable to flex the elbow or will be unable to bear weight on the limb. Visibly the elbow joint will appear to be dropped. There is nearly always some degree of radial nerve damage present as well. This type of fracture carries a good prognosis in comparison to other types of fracture in this region, which are difficult to repair with no guaranteed outcome.

Useful remedies have already been detailed (see Fractures page 170) but remember the importance of **Hypericum 30c** if there is associated radial nerve damage.

Capped elbow, Hygroma of the elbow Bursitis of the point of the elbow Olecranon bursitis, Shoe boil

This condition is caused by trauma to the area known as the point of the elbow and results in the formation of an acquired (false) bursa over the olecranon process. The most likely cause is the shoe on the foot of the affected leg hitting the olecranon during movement or more frequently hitting the region when the horse is lying down.

Characteristically a swelling appears over the point of the elbow that may contain fluid. In more chronic cases the swelling consists largely of fibrous tissue. Lameness is rarely present and then only mildly.

Suggested remedies

See Bursitis page174

Acute cases

Initially for trauma or newly acquired lesion **Arnica 200c**

Where fluid is present **Apis 200c**, **Bovista 200c**

Where there is pain, heat or lameness **Bryonia 200c**

Where the bone is bruised **Ruta 30c**

Chronic cases

(To reduce scar tissue) **Silica 30c**, **Calc fluor 30c**, **Thiosinaminum 6c**, **Proteus 30c**

Fracture of the olecranon

Fracture of the olecranon process of the ulna can occur spontaneously but is more likely to occur as a result of local trauma, often a kick or a fall, and occasionally as a result of a collision with a vehicle. Typically the horse will stand with the elbow in a dropped position with the joiny partly flexed and unable to weight bear. Movement of the affected leg is extremely difficult and painful. Grating noises (crepitus) may be apparent. Box rest (around 6 weeks) is sometimes all that is needed to allow the fracture to heal if the fragments of bone are not displaced. Where the fragments are displaced, surgical treatment is the only viable option. In either instance, homeopathy can greatly assist promoting the fracture to heal quickly and soundly.

See Fractures page 170

Arthritis of the elbow joint

This is a rare problem normally arising through age related wear and tear, occasionally through trauma. Remedies are prescribed by closely matching the symptoms of the patient to those associated with the most commonly prescribed remedies. See Arthritis page 179

Strain/Sprain of superior check ligament Strain of radial check ligament

Also sometimes termed the radial head of the superficial flexor tendon, this ligament forms part of the check apparatus that also incorporates several other structures. Collectively these aid in supporting the forelimb and form part of the more general stay apparatus which supports the limb, the fetlock, and helps to prevent over-extension of the fetlock, pastern and coffin joints. The stay apparatus also helps reduce the effects of concussion on the limb and joints.

Symptoms vary with the degree of damage to the ligament but include changes to the gait and signs of lameness which may only become apparent after the horse has been ridden for a while. Local swelling may be evident in the synovial sheath surrounding the ligament.

Suggested remedies

Acute cases

Arnica 200c, **Ruta 200c**

Chronic cases

Rhus tox 6c, **Ruta 30c**, **Silica 30c**, **Calc carb 30c**, **Sympytum 6c**

See Sprains page 171

The Carpus, The Carpal Joint
The Knee Joint

The carpal joint or knee is a complex joint consisting of three individual joints and two rows of bones. The first of these rows comprises (working from the inside of the joint to the outside), the radial, intermediate, ulnar and accessory carpal bones. These bones form a joint with the radius (the radiocarpal joint) above and the second row of bones, the first, second, third and fourth carpal bones, below (the intercarpal joint). This second row forms another joint with the second, third and fourth metacarpal bones. The third metacarpal bone is also known as the cannon bone. The second and fourth metacarpals are poorly developed and are commonly known as the splint bones.

Specific Conditions of the Carpus

Fracture of the carpal bones

The bones most commonly involved are the third and the radial carpal bone and to a lesser extent the intermediate. The cause is invariably trauma caused by over extension of the leg as this places great stresses on the individual bones. Symptoms include heat, pain and lameness. The accessory carpal bone is also subject to fracture (being in a prominent position) most often as a result of local external trauma.

Suggested remedies

See Fractures page 170

Hygroma of the carpus

This is an acquired bursitis or swelling over the front of the carpal joint which can involve the tendon sheath of the one of the extensor muscles as well. The cause is traumatic (as there is not normally a subcutaneous bursa at this point), often as the result of a fall onto a hard surface or repeated knocking against the stable wall as a consequence of pawing at the ground. The hygroma appears as an evenly distributed swelling over the front of the joint, differentiating this condition from herniation of the synovial membrane of the radiocarpal and intercarpal joints. These conditions usually cause irregular swellings which do not cover the front of the joint uniformly.

Affected horses are rarely lame and the swelling itself is painless when touched. Flexion of the joint may be limited slightly due to the size of the swelling. In long-standing cases the tissues may become fibrosed or scarred with adhesions to surrounding tissues forming.

Suggested remedies

See Bursitis 174

Acute cases
Initially for trauma or newly acquired lesion **Arnica 200c**

Where fluid is present **Apis 200c**, **Bovista 200c**

Damage from repeated low-level trauma **Bellis 30c**

Chronic cases
In chronic cases the knee will remain permanently swollen and the swelling will be partly composed of fibrous scar tissue. In this situation dose with **Silica 30c** and **Calc fluor 30c**, giving one dose of each on alternate days over a period of several months to try and breakdown the scar tissue. **Thiosinaminum 30c** or **Graphites 30c** can also be added. *Give one dose daily.*

Carpitis

This term is applied to both acute and chronic inflammation of the carpal joint involving one or several of the bones comprising the joint. The initiating cause is trauma, concussion or more often over-extension of the joint. In acute cases the joint will be painful to touch or to flex and the horse will be lame. Joint swelling will also be evident and is often the only symptom present in chronic cases. Arthritis can occur as a consequence of carpitis.

Suggested remedies

Acute cases
Initially **Arnica 200c**, **Ruta grav 200c**

Where there is heat, swelling and lameness **Apis 200c, Bryonia 200c**

Chronic cases
Caulophyllum 6c, Rhus tox 6c, Chelidonium 30c

Arthritis of the carpus
DJD of the carpal joint
DJD of the knee

Arthritic changes (also referred to as DJD) in the knee affects all the associated structures; joint cartilage and associated bones, ligaments, synovial membrane and joint capsule. Repeated trauma over a period of time is the usual initiating cause as the forces to which the carpal bones are subjected to can be enormous. Signs and symptoms include a varying degree of lameness, limited joint flexion, reduced production of joint fluid, degeneration of joint cartilage, joint swelling and pain. As the condition progresses the joint capsule can become thickened and invariably cartilage degeneration leads to the formation of bony lumps known as exostoses or osteophytes which further inhibit the range of joint movement and cause pain.

In addition to helping the condition homeopathically, corrective shoeing and the use of shock absorbing pads should be employed where appropriate.

Suggested remedies

Initially after injury, acute cases, flare ups **Arnica 200c, Ledum 200c, Bryonia 30c** (least movement painful), **Ruta grav 200c, Rhus tox 200c**

For chronic cases **Actea spic 6c** (with swelling), **Caulophyllum 6c, Chelidonium 30c, Rhus tox 6c, Ledum 30c, Calc carb 30c, Bryonia 30c**

Lesser known remedies **Viola odorata 6c** (right knee only), **Stannum 6c** (where there is weakness leading to stumbling), **Kali iod 30c** (for severe pain with thickened joint), **Guaiacum 6c** (extreme stiffness)

Chronic low-level soreness/pain **Eupat perf 30c**

Where there are exostoses or osteophytes **Calc fluor 30c, Heckla lava 6c, Ruta grav 30c, Silica 6c** (where there is marked bone degeneration), **Benz ac 6c** (with cracking joints), **Calc carb 30c**

To slow cartilage degeneration **Argentum metallicum 30c, Shark cartilage 6c, Bamboo gum 6c**

Carpal tunnel syndrome

This condition is not dissimilar to carpal tunnel syndrome in humans and involves pressure or swelling within the confines of the carpal tunnel or canal. Inflammation of the flexor tendons, check ligament or fracture of the accessory carpal bone are all known precipitating factors leading to swelling and pressure on both the blood and nerve supply to the lower limb. The presenting symptom is intermittent lameness with swelling of the tendon sheaths and carpal canal.

Where there is tendonitis **Ruta grav 30c**

Where ligaments are involved (desmitis) **Ruta grav 30c**

Where the swelling affects the nerves **Hypericum 30c**

With swelling of tendon sheaths **Apis mel 30c**

With reduced circulation to lower limb **Secale 30c, Xanthoxylum 6c**

With lameness or stiffness **Causticum 30c, Calc phos 6c**

For pain **Viola odorata 6c, Caulophyllum 6c**

The Metacarpus

The metacarpal bones

There are three metacarpal bones of which the largest is the third, often referred to as the cannon bone. Structurally this is a strong bone which forms a joint with the third row of carpal bones at the knee and forms the fetlock joint with first phalanx and the two small sesamoid bones sited at the back of the joint. The poorly developed second (medial/inside) and (lateral/outside) fourth metacarpals flank the third and articulate with the carpal bones of the knee. These are known better as the splint bones that commonly cause problems in young horses.

Each splint bone is joined to the third metacarpal

by a ligament known as the ment which undergoes ossification as the horse ages. The inside splint degree support to the knee joint whilst the outer splint plays a less important role. Both splints are stronger and are more firmly attached to the top of cannon bone. This is at the point where they are required to bear weight from the knee joint. The lower ends of the splints are thinner and somewhat flexible to allow some movement in association with the suspensory ligament.

• Splints and splint bone fractures

Splints are common and can result in nothing more than a slight blemish on a horse's leg through to causing severe and problematical lameness. The term correctly applied, refers to the appearance of bony lumps on the splint bones representing new bone (exostoses) formed in response to inflammation of the periosteum, the thin outer layer covering all bones. In younger horses, where the majority of splint problems arise, the periosteum is thicker and more likely to react to injury or stress. More current thinking now suggests that splints also arise from fractures of the splint bones which occur in many cases, at a microscopic level. This again disturbs the periosteum leading to what is essentially bony callous, a reaction not dissimilar to that seen in response to a normal fracture. Splints may form for one of several reasons.

• Trauma

Traumatic splint injuries occur as a result of direct trauma to the splint bones, which are covered by little protective soft tissue. Splints of this type are most often seen in young horses and usually involve the inner splint, rather than the outer one. Problems occur, as the movement in young horses can sometimes be uncoordinated causing them to knock themselves easily. Kicks from other horses can similarly damage the outer splint bone. The resultant trauma, either fractures the splint bone, or causes the periosteum to become inflamed (periostitis). Always check for wounds where trauma is involved. Infection can delay healing and cause long-term problems.

• Injury to the interosseous ligament

Concussive trauma or poor conformation can lead to stress and consequent inflammation of the interosseous ligament. The ligament may also tear if the stress forces are sufficient. The resulting periostitis will lead to the formation of new bone and the formation of exostoses.

• Injuries to the suspensory ligament

The suspensory ligament is closely associated with the lower portions of the splint bones and is joined to them by tough connective tissue. Stresses placed on the suspensory ligament or injury to this area can result in disturbance to the interosseous ligament or fracture of the splint bone.

Signs and symptoms

These vary with the nature of the problem. Lameness may be minimal on one extreme, or the horse may be acutely lame. Swelling and pain may be apparent at the site of the problem although this may subside consequently if the splint is not recent. The formation of new bone in response to periostitis or as a result of splint bone fracture (forming a callous) is a common outcome. This results in the formation of a bony lump or exostosis easily visible on examination of the leg.

Treating splints using homeopathic remedies

Initially where trauma is involved **Arnica 200c**
Give three doses over 24 hours

To minimise the reaction in the periosteum **Ruta grav 200c, Phytolacca 30c**
Dose: *three times daily for the first five days then three times weekly long-term until the splint settles*

Where pain and swelling persist at the site of a new splint, **Asafoetida 6c**
Dose: *three times daily until the reaction subsides*

To reduce the risk of the formation of exostoses **Calc fluor 200c**
Dose: *three times weekly on a long-term basis*

For more long-standing cases where exostoses are

present **Silica 200c**
Dose: three times weekly

To prevent the formation of exostoses, **Ruta 30c** can be used with **Calc fluor** or **Silica, Heckla lava 30c**
Dose: once daily

To assist healing where there is a splint bone fracture **Symphytum 6c**
Dose: once daily

If infection is involved at the site **Silica 30c, Asafoetida 6c, Gunpowder 3x**
Dose: four times daily

External treatment

If the skin is not broken at the site of a splint, apply **Arnica** ointment initially three times daily followed by **Ruta** ointment twice daily on a more long-term basis.

Sore or bucked shins Metacarpal/(metatarsal) periostitis Dorsal metacarpal disease

This condition is a form of periostitis involving the upper or dorsal surface of the cannon bone. Most often seen in young thoroughbreds in the first weeks of training, it occurs far more frequently in the front leg in comparison to the hind. Both legs are normally involved. The most likely cause is concussion which initiates a reaction in the periosteum (periosteitis) resulting in bone reshaping together with small stress fractures and bleeding under the periosteum. In older animals direct trauma should be considered as a cause of sore shins.

The most obvious sign is swelling, pain and heat over the affected area of the bone with slight swelling of the surrounding soft tissues. Lameness will be present which will be aggravated by exercise. The outcome for this condition is good with rest and careful management. Homeopathic remedies can substantially limit the severity of the condition and provide a quicker resolution.

Suggested remedies

Preventative care for animals at risk **Arnica 6c, Ruta 6c** and **Symphytum 6c** in combination
Single dose before and after training

Where there is intermittent periosteal pain and occasional lameness in young horses with no other symptoms **Phos ac 30c** and **Phytolacca 30c**
Single dose before and after training

Where there is heat, swelling and lameness **Ruta 30c, Eupatorium perfoliatum 30c** and **Bryonia 30c** in combination
Dose: two or three times daily until the reaction subsides

If the swelling, pain and heat persist use **Asafoetida 30c** or **Kali iod 30c**
Dose: three times daily

With much swelling consider **Apis 30c**
Dose: three times daily

Once the acute symptoms resolve or where the symptoms are very minor **Ruta 30c, Heckla lava 30c, Phytolacca 30c** and **Symphytum 6c**
Dose: once daily until the condition is resolved completely

Cannon bone (third metacarpal) fractures

This type of fracture is quite common. Depending on the nature and site of the fracture, the outcome can be variable. For some animals, euthanasia is the only course of action. Some fractures can be surgically repaired and carry a favourable prognosis.

See Fractures page 170

Suspensory ligament desmitis Suspensory ligament strain

The suspensory ligament is the largest of the structures which comprise the suspensory apparatus of the fetlock. Injury is most common in racehorses and is more frequently seen in the front leg compared to the hind. The underlying cause is hyperextension of the fetlock joint although splint fractures and sesamoiditis can also be involved. The most common site for injury is where the ligament splits into two in the region of lower third of the cannon bone

Acute injuries will cause swelling and mild lameness with the horse holding his knee forward with the heel lightly on the ground at rest. In chronic cases, the suspensory ligament will become scarred and thickened. It is not unknown for the ligament to become calcified where it attaches to the sesamoid bones in very long-standing cases.

Treatment

Acute cases **Arnica 200c**, **Ruta grav 200c**, **Rhus tox 200c**, **Apis mel 200c**

Chronic cases **Ruta grav 30c**, **Calc Fluor 30c**, **Symphytum 6c**

Where there is scarring **Silica 30c**, **Thiosinaminum 6c**

For calcification **Silica 30c**, **Calc fluor 30c**

Inferior check ligament desmitis
Check (carpal) ligament sprain
Sprain of the accessory ligament to the deep digital flexor tendon

This ligament arises as a continuation of the volar (palmar) carpal ligament at the back of the knee and joins the deep flexor tendon in the middle third of the cannon bone, lying between the suspensory ligament and the deep digital flexor tendon. Injury can occur when the ligament or deep digital flexor tendon is subject to stress. This can occur due to poor shoeing or from losing a footing on a slippery surface. Lameness is often variable and is worse after exercise on hard, uneven surfaces. There is local pain on palpation of the affected area.

Treatment

Acute injuries **Arnica 200c**, **Ruta 200c**

Chronic cases **Ruta 30c**, **Sympytum 6c**, **Rhus tox 6c**

Tendon injuries
Tendonitis, tendosynovitis and bowed tendons, Tendon strains

See page 172

The Fetlock Joint
Metacarpophalangeal Joint

This is the joint formed between the cannon bone and the first (proximal) digit or phalanx and encompasses the two proximal sesamoid bones. This is a very flexible joint with a wide range of movement.

Arthritis of the fetlock joint
DJD of the fetlock joint
Osteoarthritis of the fetlock joint

This joint is one of the most commonly injured in the horse, leading to the development of arthritis or DJD. Degenerative changes can occur from repeated trauma, through wear and tear, acute injury or as a result of a chip fracture for example and can involve any of the structures that comprise the joint. Acute symptoms commonly include lameness, swelling, heat and pain. In long-standing cases, the affected joint will become enlarged due to the development of fibrous tissue and the joint will show limited degree of flexibility.

Homeopathic treatment

Acute injuries **Arnica 200c**, **Ruta 200c** (where ligaments area involved), **Apis 200c** (where there is considerable swelling/heat), **Bryonia 200c** (where there is severe pain and heat), **Rhus tox 200c** (stiffness), **Colchicum 30c** (very sensitive to touch)

Chronic cases – specific remedies **Ledum 30c**, **Actea spic 6c**, **Caulophyllum 30c**, **Rhus tox 6c**, **Ruta 6c**, **Berberis vulgaris 30c**, **Tylophora indica 1M**

Where there is fibrous enlargement **Calc fluor 30c**, **Silica 30c**

Supportive remedies **Shark cartilage 6c**, **Bamboo gum 6c**, **Argentum metallicum 6c**

Osslets, Traumatic arthritis of the fetlock joint (Periostitis of the fetlock)

The term osslet is applied specifically to a traumatic arthritis of the fetlock joint with all other degenerative changes occurring secondary to the initial trauma. Often there is an associated periostitis at the lower (distal) end of the cannon bone and the opposing surface of the first phalanx due to the stresses placed on the joint capsule (which can become thickened), disturbing the periosteum. The condition commonly affects young horse in early training around 2 years of age. The cause is concussive trauma, which may be combined with poor conformation to predispose some animals to the condition.

The most obvious sign is recurrent lameness with a gait described as choppy. In the early stages the joint will become swollen as the joint capsule becomes distended dorsally. Heat and pain will be present. This stage is often referred to as a 'green osselet'. Later, as the condition progresses and more specific degenerative arthritic changes develop, periostitis occurs and new bone may form. This can involve the joint surface or may appear in areas not involving the joint surface itself, such as the joint capsule (where it is referred to as ossification or calcification). The attachment of the lateral digital extensor may also become involved.

If treated early on, before any new bone forms, the outlook is good. Even so, where new bone does appear, if this does not encroach upon the joint surface, the outcome can be favourable.

Homeopathic treatment

Acute cases **Arnica 200c, Apis 200c, Ruta 200c, Bryonia 200c**

To prevent new bone formation **Calc fluor 30c, Heckla lava 30c, Symphytum 6c**

Chronic cases (joint capsule thickened) **Ruta 30c, Silica 30c, Phytolacca 30c**

Sesamoiditis

Inflammation of the proximal sesamoid bones is termed sesamoiditis. Strain to the fetlock joint or the effect of concussive forces may result in periostitis and osteitis of the sesamoid bones with possible demineralisation and impairment of the blood supply. The suspensory ligament and distal sesamoidean ligaments may also be involved and may develop areas of calcification as a result.

Sesamoiditis usually only causes a slight lameness although in acute cases there will be pain and swelling of the fetlock joint. In chronic cases new periosteal bone forms on the sesamoid bones which then will have a roughened outline. Treatment involves rest in conjunction with corrective shoeing to absorb the concussive forces that initiate the condition.

Homeopathic treatment

Acute cases **Arnica 30c, Ruta 30c, Asafoetida 6c** (with swelling and pain of the fetlock joint)

Chronic cases **Ruta 30c, Calc fluor 30c, Heckla lava 30c, Silica 30c**

Dose: *once or twice daily*

Sprain of distal sesamoidean ligaments Desmitis of distal sesamoidean ligaments

The two distal sesamoidean ligaments, the superficial and middle, run between the base of the sesamoid bones to the second (distal) and first (proximal) phalangeal bones respectively. Inflammation of these ligaments can occur as a result of stress to the suspensory ligament or digital flexor tendons or as a consequence of fracture of the sesamoid bones. As healing occurs scar tissue may form as well as the possibility of calcification of the damaged tissue.

Homeopathic treatment

Acute cases **Arnica 30c, Ruta 30c, Phytolacca 30c**

Chronic cases **Ruta 30c**

Where there is calcification **Calc fluor 30c**

Where there is scar tissue **Silica 30c**

Dose: *once or twice daily*

Chronic (proliferative) synovitis

This condition is caused by chronic trauma through concussion, causing inflammation in the joint capsule of the fetlock joint. The synovial pad within the joint becomes inflamed leading to the production of fibrous tissue and consequent enlargement of an area over the front of the joint. After a period of time this area can become calcified and may damage the underlying bone of the joint. Lameness is usually only very slight. Surgery is often indicated as the best course of action. The outcome is favourable if measures are taken to reduce the initiating chronic concussive trauma.

Homeopathic treatment

Prevention and treatment **Bryonia 30c**, **Ruta 30c**, **Calc fluor 30c**, **Ledum 30c**

Where fibrous tissue exists **Silica 30c**, **Thiosinaminum 6c**

For calcification **Calc fluor 30c**

Dose: once or twice daily

Constriction of palmar annular ligament

The annular ligament is a tough, fibrous sheath lined with synovial membrane that encircles the tendons at the level of the fetlock joint, preventing their displacement. Damage, infection or injury to the ligament or more importantly, to the enclosed tendons, results in inflammation, a restriction in blood supply to the tendons and subsequent formation of thickened fibrous, scar tissue and adhesions in place of the damaged area during healing. The result is a constriction that hinders movement of the structures passing through the ligament with resultant lameness and swollen tendon sheaths. Treatment is normally surgical; homeopathy should be considered in a preventative role in all cases.

Suggested remedies

Initially **Arnica 200c**, **Secale 200c** and **Ruta 200c** *three times daily for three days* then **Silica 30c**, **Calc fluor 30c** and **Thiosinaminum 30c** *twice daily* to prevent the formation of scar tissue and adhesions.

Difficult cases can benefit from **Proteus 200c** *twice weekly* over a period of several months.

Fractures

Fracture of first phalanx (long pastern bone)

This bone can fracture in a variety of ways ranging from small chip fractures to complete or incomplete breaks running down or across the bone. Depending on the exact nature of the fracture, recovery is possible either with rest and surgery where indicated. The prognosis is less favourable if the fracture involves the fetlock or pastern joints or if the fracture involves many pieces.

Fracture of second phalanx (short pastern bone)

This type of fracture is rare and most likely to occur in very athletic horses where the extreme forces generated can cause the bone to break.

Sesamoid fractures

Fractures of this type are commonly seen in racehorses and can result in severe lameness, which is worse if the limb is flexed. There will be local pain if pressure is applied to the area. The outcome depends on the exact site of the fracture.

Suggested remedies

See Fractures page 170

Luxation and subluxation of the fetlock and pastern Joints

The initiating cause of both of these conditions is acute trauma resulting in the rupture of one or both of the ligaments that hold the joints in place. The most obvious symptom is acute lameness with pain and swelling in the area of the injury. Repair is usually undertaken by applying a cast or by surgery. It very unlikely that the horse will sound enough to work properly again.

See Luxation and Subluxation page 185

The Pastern Joint

This is the hinge type joint between the first phalanx (long pastern bone) and the second phalanx (short pastern bone).

Arthritis of the pastern joint and Ringbone
DJD of the fetlock joint
Osteoarthritis of the pastern joint

Ringbone involves the formation of new bone on or

around the first, second and third phalanges, the bones that comprise the coffin and pastern joints. There are four distinct types of ringbone, which give rise to slight variations in symptoms. High ringbone occurs at the level of the pastern joint between the first and second phalanges. Low ringbone affects the coffin joint, between the second phalanx and the pedal bone. The third form is periarticular ringbone which occurs at the margins of the capsule which encompasses each joint and finally, the fourth type, articular ringbone, occurs where new bone growth is accompanied by degenerative joint disease.

Ringbone is primarily caused by trauma, often from strain placed on the collateral ligaments which hold the joints together. This condition can also be caused by stresses on the joint capsules or from tensile forces pulling on the attachment of the common extensor tendon to the first, second or third phalanx. Direct trauma to the region can also cause ringbone to develop. The cumulative effect is to damage the periosteum (the outermost covering of bone) causing an inflammatory reaction (periostitis) that eventually leads to the growth of unwanted new bone. This then impinges on surrounding tissues leading to pain and subsequent lameness. Some horses are predisposed to the condition because of poor conformation.

The exact symptoms shown by each animal will vary with the type of ringbone and are not always specific. With very minor changes the horse may remain sound. High ringbone will cause intermittent lameness with swelling which usually resolves with rest but returns when the horse is brought back into work. The pastern joint often lacks a complete range of movement especially on flexion. Low ringbone can result in heat and pain at the level of the coronary band at the front of the foot with a consequent change in the shape of the hoof wall at the toe in chronic cases. Periarticular ringbone rarely causes lameness and little pain or swelling are evident. Often the symptoms will disappear with rest in contrast to articular ringbone. This causes chronic lameness and symptoms that are most obvious when the horse turns, especially on a tight circle. Associated signs include varying degrees of heat, swelling and pain and ultimate progression to degenerative joint disease.

Homeopathic treatment

Prevention **Ruta grav 30c**, **Calc fluor 30c**, **Symphytum 6c**, **Lactic acid 30c**, **Ledum 30c**, **Phytolacca 30c**

Treatment **Ruta grav 30c**, **Calc fluor 30c**, **Heckla lava 30c**, **Silica 30c**, **Merc sol 30c** (with degenerative joint changes), **Rhus tox 6c**, **Bryonia 30c**, **Mineral 6x**

Dose: *once daily*

The Hind Limb

The hind limb is divided into several anatomically distinct regions; the pelvis and hip joint, thigh and femur, stifle joint (which includes the patella), tibia, fibula and lower leg, hock or tarsal joint, metatarsus, fetlock joint, pastern and coffin joints. The foot is detailed in a separate section.

The Pelvis

The pelvis comprises three bones, the ilium, ischium and pubis. The head of the femur or thighbone articulates with the cavity formed by the bones known as the acetabulum. This is the hip joint, a ball and socket type joint. The pelvis is joined to the spine at the sacrum by the sacroiliac joint.

Pelvic fractures

This type of fracture is quite common and inevitably the result of a bad fall. Symptoms vary depending on the exact location of the fracture and carry a poor outlook.

Hip Joint

Fractures

Fractures involving the three bones of the pelvis are rare in older animals and may occur as a result of trauma, often a fall. Fractures sometimes occur in foals following a fall and spontaneous fractures are sometimes seen in young thoroughbreds around the age of two or three. If the fracture involves the hip joint the outlook is poor. Other types of fractures will heal with box rest. Healing can be speeded by using appropriate remedies. In all cases **Arnica 200c**, **Hypericum 200c** and especially **Bellis perennis 200c** will be of special benefit at the time of trauma and in the following few days.

See Fractures page 170

Dislocation of the hip joint

Dislocation of this joint is extremely rare as considerable force is required to pull the hip out of its socket but can sometimes occur following a struggle if the horse is trapped or by falling awkwardly. Dislocation can also occur in conjunction with a fracture of the acetabulum.

See Dislocations page 185

Trochanteric bursitis
Whorlbone lameness

Inflammation of the small bursa on the greater trochanter of the femur (a bony prominence of the femur close to the hip joint), which lies under the tendon of one of the gluteal muscles, is termed trochanteric bursitis. This is a true bursitis with repetitive strain on the tendon as the initiating cause although direct injury to the area can also trigger the problem. Affected horses are lame with muscle wasting in the most severe of cases.

Suggested remedies

If traumatic injury to the area is recent **Arnica 200c**

Where there is injury from repeated low-level trauma **Ruta 30c**, **Bellis 30c**

If the area is very swollen and hot or there is marked discomfort **Bryonia 200c**

In chronic cases consider **Ruta 30c**, **Apis 30c**, **Bovista 30c**

See Bursitis page 174

Stifle Joint

The stifle joint is in fact 2 joints, that between the femur and the patella and that between the femur and tibia. It is the largest joint in the horse and also the weakest.

Stifle lameness, Gonitis

Stifle lameness, sometimes referred to by the vague term gonitis, can occur as a consequence of a number of conditions. The most common of all of these is chondromalacia of the patella (caused by partial or complete upward fixation of the patella). Other causes include meniscal cartilage damage, cruciate ligament rupture, medial or collateral ligament sprains, joint capsule injuries, joint trauma, osteochondritis dissecans and infectious arthritis.

Partial or complete upward fixation of the patella

Caused by poor conformation or poor farriery, the back leg becomes locked in extension so that the stifle and the hock are unable to flex, although the fetlock is still able to move. The leg may unlock only to lock up again after a few seconds. In other cases the leg may lock for much longer periods of time. Surgery is often used to correct the condition. In the short term appropriate symptomatic remedies include **Arnica 30c** and **Ruta grav 30c**. More long-term cases may benefit from **Gelsemium 30c**. *Dose twice daily.*

Chondromalacia of the patella

This condition occurs as a consequence of upward fixation of the patella and involves degeneration of the articular cartilage of the patella. In nearly all cases it is the pressure between the patella and the medial trochlea of the femur which erodes the cartilage surface. Other causes include ligament injuries and trauma to the stifle joint. Symptoms include lameness, local pain and swelling and grating of the patella as it moves in its groove on the femur.

Suggested remedies

This condition is best treated with a combination of **Calc fluor 30c**, **Argentum metallicum 30c**, **Ruta grav 30c**, and **Symphytum 6c**

Dose: give each remedy once every four days

Osteochondrosis of the stifle joint
Osteochrondritis (OCD) of the stifle joint
Subchondral bone cysts of the stifle

The stifle is a common site for OCD with lesions most likely to affect the lateral trochlear ridge of the femur whereas subchondral bone cysts are more likely to be seen on the medial condyle of the femur, the point of maximum weight bearing. Young horses are most likely to be affected by these problems; they are rarely seen in older animals.

Lameness may not be apparent early on until the lesions develop. Both stifles may be affected with evidence of heat and swelling of the joint capsule to varying degrees. Rest is sometimes indicated in the case of bone cysts, otherwise surgery is an option for both conditions.

Suggested remedies

Acute cases where there is lameness, heat and swelling **Bryonia 30c**, **Apis 30c**

Chronic cases, prevention & post surgery **Calc phos 6x**, **Calc carb 6x**, **Ruta 30c**, **Arg met 30c**, **Shark cartilage 30c**, **Bamboo gum 30c**

See Osteochrondrosis page 186

Patella luxation

This is a congenital condition affecting the stifle joint, usually apparent shortly after birth. The patella slips sideways out its groove, usually to the outside of the joint, so that the foal is unable to stand easily. Surgery is sometimes helpful in correcting the problem. **Gelsemium 30c** given *twice daily* may be of benefit in some cases.

Meniscal tears of the stifle

The two meniscal cartilages are situated between the femur and the tibia and are subject to injury which may result in the cartilage tearing. The condition is rare and difficult to diagnose but can occur as a consequence of severe trauma to the joint. Symptoms include chronic lameness and swelling of the joint. Treatment requires a long period of rest. Remedies such as **Symphytum 6c**, **Argentum metallicum 6c, Shark cartilage 6x** and **Ruta 30c** will help speed healing. Dose once daily for several weeks. Other remedies such as **Rhus tox 30c**, **Bryonia 30c** and **Apis 30c**, should be prescribed for the resulting lameness on a symptomatic basis.

Ligament injuries

Both the cruciate ligaments and the collateral ligaments can be injured (sprained or ruptured) as a result of trauma or as a consequence of a fracture. The stifle joint subsequently may become unstable and develop arthritic changes. Initially dose with **Arnica 200c** and **Ruta 200c** *three times daily for three days* followed by appropriate symptomatic remedies.

See Ligaments page 171

Arthritis of the stifle joint
DJD of the stifle

This is not a common occurrence but can result in chronic lameness. Suitable remedies should be prescribed on the basis of presenting symptoms.

See Joints page 179

Tibia and Fibula Region

The tibia and fibula (which is rudimentary in the horse) articulate with the femur to form the stifle joint and with metatarsus to form the hock. The tibia largely bears the full weight of the hind limb and can be fractured by a kick or awkward fall. Remedies to help can be found under fractures on page 170.

Thoroughpin

This condition is a tenosynovitis affecting the sheath that encloses the deep digital flexor tendon. The cause is not known and the condition rarely causes lameness, appearing more of an unsightly blemish than anything else. The resulting swelling can vary considerably in size and appears towards the back of the joint capsule, higher in position than the type of swelling seen with bog spavin.

Suggested remedies

In the majority of cases try **Apis mel 200c**

For stubborn cases consider **Bovista 30c**, **Thuja 30c**, **Ledum 30c**

Where there is lameness add **Bryonia 30c**

Dose: *twice daily initially, reducing to once daily to prevent recurrence*

Rupture of the peroneus tertius

Comprised of strong tendinous tissue, the peroneus tertius runs between the femur at the stifle and inserts on some of the bones of the hock joint. Its function is to mechanically flex the hock when the stifle is flexed. Rupture can occur if the hock is overextended. This can occur if the leg is trapped and the horse struggles to try to free itself. Diagnosis is straightforward. If the stifle flexes when the horse moves forward, the hock is carried without flexing so that the lower part of the leg appears to hang loosely, almost as if fractured. Recovery is possible with prolonged rest and the support of suitable remedies.

Suggested remedies

Initially **Arnica 200c**, **Hamamelis 200c**, **Apis 200c**

Follow with **Ruta 30**, **Rhus tox 1M**, **Calc fluor 30c**

See Tendon Rupture page 173

The Hock or Tarsal Joint and Metatarsal Region

The hock is a complex joint formed by three rows of bones (known as the tarsal bones) that articulate with the tibia and with the metacarpal bones. The tarsal bones are subject to considerable forces during movement and can fracture when the stresses are excessive. The outcome varies with nature of the fracture. Slab type fractures carry a poor prognosis. Chip fractures can be dealt with surgically and have a better outlook. See Fractures page 170.

Conditions Affecting the Hock

Capped hock
Bursitis of the hock

This condition refers to the appearance of a swelling under the skin over the area referred to as the point of the hock. The bone at this point, the calcaneus, is easily traumatised as it is very prominent and has very little soft tissue padding. Trauma, often from kicking a wall or horsebox ramp, leads to the development of a fluid sac over the end of the bone. This is an acquired or false bursa and is sometimes referred to as a hygroma or traumatic bursitis of the hock. Although the sac can contain a large amount of fluid and may be tender if the injury is recent, it rarely causes lameness and is more of a problem as it spoils the appearance of the horse.

Suggested remedies

Acute cases

If swelling is recent or if there is some degree of pain **Arnica 30c**

If the bone of the calcaneus has been bruised **Ruta 30c**

Damage from repeated low-level trauma **Bellis 30c**

If the area is very swollen and hot or there is some degree of discomfort **Bryonia 30c**

Use where there is swelling and fluid present **Apis 30c**, **Bovista 30c**

Dose: *once or twice daily*

Chronic cases

In some cases the condition becomes chronic and the back of the hock will remain swollen. There may be little if any fluid present and the swelling will be slight and composed mainly of fibrous scar tissue. In this situation dose with **Silica 30c** and **Calc fluor 30c**, giving *one dose of each on alternate days* over a period of several months. **Thiosinaminum 30c** or **Graphites 30c** should also be considered. *Give one dose daily*

See Bursitis page 174

Bog spavin
Tarsocrural synovitis

Bog spavin is essentially a chronic distension of the joint capsule and can arise as a consequence of one or more of a number of factors. These include poor conformation, trauma to the hock joint and surrounding structures, vitamin and mineral imbalances and osteochondrosis. Affected horses are not usually lame but will develop a number of fluctuating swellings around the joint, the largest of which will often appear over the front and towards the inside of the joint.

Smaller swellings often appear either side of the posterior (rear) area of the joint. Treatment is often undertaken for cosmetic reasons. Any underlying problems will also need attention.

Suggested remedies

If trauma is involved initially dose hourly with **Arnica 200c**

Follow with **Apis 30c**

Stubborn cases **Bovista 30c**

Where there is lameness **Bryonia 30c**, **Ledum 30c**

Dose: once or twice daily

Luxation of the hock

Trauma or injury to the hock joint, especially from sudden twisting of the joint can result in the joint luxating. Affected horses will be 10/10 lame and the joint will appear distorted. Repair can be undertaken by using a cast to immobilise the joint during healing. Useful acute remedies include **Arnica 30c**, **Ruta 30c** and **Symphytum 6c**.

See Joint luxation page 185

Bone spavin

Bone spavin is a form of osteoarthritis together with a periostitis, osteitis and ankylosing arthritis. It is a common condition, seen in all breeds of horses, particularly those with a poor conformation where abnormal stresses are placed on the joint. Trauma can also initiate the condition as well as mineral imbalances.

Affected animals will develop a bony enlargement on the inner aspect of the hock. This can vary in size and affects the third metatarsal bone and the third and central tarsal bones. As the osteoarthritis progresses, the horse will become progressively lame. In advanced cases however, the affected bones will fuse together (ankylosis) and the horse will go sound. The principal presenting symptom is lameness, often worse when the horse first moves and then easing with exercise. Pain in the joint will cause the horse to have a shortened stride with the foot landing on the toe which then becomes worn. Cases which are more advanced show aggravation of the symptoms on exercise rather than improvement.

Suggested remedies

Where trauma is involved use **Arnica 200c** and **Ruta 200c** initially, dosing *three or four times daily for a few days.*

For bony changes, bony enlargement **Calc fluor 30c**, **Heckla lava 30c**, **Ruta grav 30c**, **Silica 30c**, **Mineral 6x**

Where there is osteoarthritis **Rhus tox 6c** (symptoms ease with movement), **Bryonia 30c** (symptoms worse for movement), **Homarus 1M** (specific for the hock), **Benz ac 6c** (with cracking noises), **Lithium carb 6c** (worse for movement), **Ledum 30c**

Where the osteoarthritis is advanced **Causticum 30c**, **Aurum met 30c**, **Kali iod 30c**, **Osteoarthritic nosode 30c**, **Mineral 6x**

If mineral imbalances are involved **Calc phos 6x**, **Calc carb 6x**

Dose: once or twice daily depending on the severity of symptoms

Osteochondrosis of the hock
OCD of the hock

Seen in rapidly growing animals, OCD of the hock is second only to the stifle joint as one of the most commonly affected sites. The degree of lameness caused by OCD varies and may prove difficult to diagnose. Cases where there is no obvious lameness may respond to rest with appropriate homeopathic support. Where lameness is present, surgery can offer a viable solution.

See OCD page 186

Curb, Tarsal plantar desmitis

Curb involves injury to a small tendon known as the plantar ligament, which runs from on the underside of calcaneus (the bone which forms the point of the hock) forwards. Poor conformation predisposes horses to this condition which places undue stress on the ligament resulting in inflammation, enlargement and thickening. Affected horses are usually slightly lame with local swelling and heat over the area of the ligament.

Suggested remedies

For acute cases where there is heat and pain **Arnica 200c, Rhus tox 200c, Ruta 200c**

For established cases **Ruta grav 30c, Strontium 30c**

Relapsed cases with repetitive injury **Calc carb 30c, Causticum 30c, Ledum 30c**

Where there is scar tissue **Silica 30c, Proteus 30c**

Dose: *once or twice daily depending on the severity of symptoms*

Cunean bursitis
Cunean tendon bursitis
Cunean tendinitis

Inflammation of the cunean tendon and its bursa occurs as a consequence of poor conformation, bad shoeing or a poor training regime. Affected horses are lame, sometimes exhibiting obvious swelling over the affected region of the hock on the inside of the leg.

Suggested remedies

Acute cases **Arnica 200c, Ruta 200c, Rhus tox 200c**

Where there is swelling of the bursa **Apis 30c**

Chronic cases with lameness **Ruta 30c, Rhus tox 30c**

Dose: *twice daily*

See Bursitis page 174, Tendinitis page 172

The Back

The spinal column continues from the seven cervical vertebrae (which comprise the neck, see page 190), with a further four anatomical regions comprised of 18 thoracic vertebrae, six lumbar vertebrae, five sacral vertebrae (which are fused together) and a varying number of caudal or coccygeal vertebrae, normally numbering between 15–21. The sacral vertebrae articulate with the pelvis by the sacroiliac joint which has an imperceptible amount of movement. Back and pelvic injuries are relatively common and often require additional treatment by an osteopath or chiropractor.

Back Problems

Back pain

In the majority of cases where back pain is present, trauma is the cause with the horse twisting or falling awkwardly. Poor fitting tack can also cause back pain as can ovarian pain. The degree of pain can vary considerably and will present as any one of a number of symptoms. These include lameness, reluctance to perform or jump, uneven gait, poor tracking up, difficulty in tacking up or riding, rearing up, loss of muscling over the back and changes in behaviour.

Kissing spines
Dorsal spinal disease (DSD)

This condition can cause severe debilitating back pain rendering some horses unfit to ride and is caused by enlargement of the spines of the thoracic and or lumbar vertebrae. In the horse these spines are close together in the middle of the back and can impinge on each other causing inflammation and pain. Symptoms vary with a few cases showing no symptoms at all. Signs to look for include tense back muscles with a reluctance to dip the back. Symptoms may disappear with rest only to return when the horse is worked. It is often difficult to treat this condition, which can carry a poor prognosis.

Injury and subluxation of the sacroiliac joint

The sacroiliac joint moves very little and anatomically is designed for stability rather than movement. Severe trauma or repeated low-grade trauma can cause damage leading to inflammation and tearing of the ligaments that stabilise the joint. The surrounding muscles will go into spasm as a consequence of this, causing discomfort and lameness of the hindquarters.

Sprain of the supraspinous ligament

A fall at speed or jumping at speed can injure this long ligament which runs along the dorsal spines of the vertebrae. The main presenting symptom is restriction of movement together with muscle wasting.

Suggested remedies for back problems

Arnica Back pain arising from any injury. Symptoms worse for touch, cold and damp.

Bellis General remedy for injuries to the back especially the pelvic region. Symptoms ease with motion.

Ruta grav Pain in the lumbar area from injury or strains causing stiffness or lameness. Main remedy for sprain of the supraspinous ligament. Symptoms worse for cold and damp and on first movement.

Rhus tox Pain in the lumbar region from injury that eases with movement. Pain causes the horse to become restless and to move to ease the discomfort. Symptoms worse for cold and damp, from getting wet and at the start of the day.

Aesculus Specific for pain in the region of the sacroiliac region, hips and pelvis. Symptoms worse in the morning and for movement.

Calc phos Used for pain specifically originating at the sacroiliac junction. Symptoms are worse for cold and better for warmth.

Bryonia Suits cases where there is more severe back pain and the horse is reluctant to move preferring to stand totally still. Symptoms worse for any motion, for touch and for warmth.

Berberis Pain in the region of the lumbar spine especially over the kidney area. Pain may make urination difficult. Symptoms worse for movement.

Nux vomica Back pain where the discomfort causes the horse to become irritable. May show poor tracking with failure to bring the leg forward. Symptoms better for warmth and pressure, worse for motion.

Calc carb Back pain from the least motion. Suits horses with a 'weak back'. Important remedy for kissing spines. Symptoms worse for damp and cold, better for warmth.

Kali carb Back pain or stiffness in horses with an irritable nature. Useful where the gait is affected as well, with the horse appearing unsteady on its legs. Symptoms worse in cold weather, better in warm weather.

Lachesis Back pain linked with ovarian function. Suited to mares with a suspicious and wary nature. Symptoms worse first thing in the morning and in the period just before coming into season. Worse for the slightest touch and on the left side.

Palladium Right-sided back pain originating from the right ovary.

Sepia Lower back pain in older mares with a 'worn out, saggy' appearance. Symptoms worse before coming into season.

Chamomilla Can ease severe back pain and that seen in some cases of kissing spines. The neck may also be stiff. Affected horses may be irritable or touchy.

Belladonna Sudden onset back pain with much heat over the affected area. Symptoms worse for any motion.

Strychnine Severe stiffness or rigidity of the muscles of the neck. Stiff back causing jerky movements.

Dose with the 30c potency twice daily as needed

The Foot

The foot of the horse is a unique structure and the result of an evolutionary process that has taken place over thousands of years. The foot is flexible and lightweight, yet able to tolerate the excessive strains and mechanical stresses which movement entails. It is a complex structure consisting not only of the hoof, but also of a dermal layer, digital cushion, the bones that comprise the coffin joint, the navicular bone and navicular bursa, lateral cartilages, the laminae, sole and various ligaments, tendons nerves and blood vessels.

The hoof wall is thickest at the toe and gradually becomes thinner towards the heels. These are turned inward to form the bars and are separated from the frog by deep grooves known as sulci. The horn that makes up the hoof wall is in a constant state of growth, replacing the underside of the hoof worn away by abrasion. It takes between 8 and 12 months for new horn produced at the coronary band to grow down to reach the bottom of the foot. The quality and appearance of the horn gives some indication as to the horse's general state of health and nutrition. Regular attention needs to be paid to both hoof wall and foot as well as to nutrition and environmental conditions to ensure problems do not arise.

The Coffin Joint
The Distal Interphalangeal Joint

This joint comprises the middle phalanx, distal phalanx (coffin or pedal bone) and the navicular bone (or distal sesamoid bone) that lies at the back of the joint. As a simple hinge type joint the range of movement is almost completely limited to flexion and extension.

Fractures of pedal bone/navicular bone

The pedal bone can fracture in several places. The prognosis ultimately depends on the specific location of the fracture and whether the fracture involves the joint or not. The cause is often stress force related with a heightened risk in horses that are unbalanced. Fracture of the navicular bone results in severe sudden onset lameness and may result as a result of kicking a hard surface or object or from landing awkwardly on a stone or similar material. Injuries of this type may also fracture the pedal bone. Horses with navicular syndrome are prone to chip fractures of the navicular bone.

Suggested remedies

Aim to treat initially using **Arnica 200c** three times daily in combination with **Hypericum 200c**.
To assist healing see fractures page 170

Arthritis of the coffin joint
DJD of the coffin joint

Usually occurring through wear and tear or trauma, arthritis of the coffin joint can also occur as a consequence of navicular syndrome. Lameness is relatively non-specific.

Suggested remedies

Specific remedies **Caulophyllum 6c, Actea spic 6c, Ant crud 6c, Guaicum 6c, Sarsparilla 6c, Silica, Kali carb 6c**

General remedies **Rhus tox 6c, Colchicum 30c** (with swelling just above the coronary band), **Calc carb 30c, Causticum 30c, Rhododendron 6c, Bryonia 30c**

Where stiffness is marked **Ledum 30c, Lycopodium 30c, Rhus tox 30c, Graphites 30c**

With bony changes **Calc fluor 30c, Ruta grav 30c,**

Benz ac 6c, Graphites 6c, Ledum 30c, Lithium carb 6c, Silica 6c

Navicular syndrome
Navicular disease
Podotrochleosis

Navicular disease, more correctly referred to as navicular syndrome, is the collective name given to a number of conditions which affect the navicular bone and surrounding structures namely the navicular bursa and flexor tendons. It is a very common cause of foreleg lameness, occurring in horses aged approximately between four and twelve years of age. Male animals, predominantly geldings, are affected. Horses worked intermittently are also more likely to develop the condition. It is extremely rare for the hind limbs to be affected.

The navicular bone, sometimes referred to as the distal sesamoid, is a small, almost quarter-moon, shaped bone covered in cartilage, situated behind the middle phalanx and the pedal bone. It forms part of the functional anatomy of the coffin joint, helping to improve the bio-mechanics of the deep digital flexor tendon. A small but important cushion of fluid, known as the navicular bursa, sits between the tendon and the navicular bone and serves to help prevent damage to the tendon by reducing friction and improving lubrication. There are also a number of other structures in this area. The most important of these is a complex array of ligaments which hold the navicular bone in position and which stabilise the coffin joint.

Navicular disease was once thought to be a form of arthritis affecting the navicular bone and the impact of this problem on surrounding tissues. It is now known that there is a hereditary factor involved in the development of navicular syndrome and that the condition can be provoked by poor trimming and shoeing, working on inappropriate surfaces and by feeding a poor diet.

There are a number of theories as to why this condition occurs. One suggests that the forces exerted by the deep digital flexor tendon cause bony changes within the navicular bone. Another outlines the idea that concussion causes inflammation of the navicular bursa and consequently changes in the navicular bone. Animals with a poor conformation, low heels, small feet, which have a long toe to the hoof or which are overweight, are more likely to suffer bad effects from concussion. Another theory revolves around the blood supply to the foot and in particular to the navicular bone. Obstruction of some of the smaller blood vessels will deprive the bone of its blood supply leading to bone necrosis and remodelling of the shape of the bone. Consequences of developing navicular syndrome include the development of bony spurs on the navicular bone, the formation of adhesions to the flexor tendons and the risk of fractures developing.

The main and usually the first symptom is intermittent lameness of one or both front legs. Where both legs are usually involved, one leg will show a greater degree of lameness compared to the other. The lameness is progressive and improves with rest. Hard work, especially on hard ground, will usually make the symptoms worse.

Other signs to check for include a reduction in the length of the stride, bruising of the sole from stumbling and excessive toe wear. In long-standing cases the shape of the foot will change as the heels contract to reduce the pressure on the frog and the sole will become concave with narrowing in the quarters. These changes further complicate the situation by changing the way the horse lands on the foot.

Treating navicular syndrome involves trimming the foot with the aim of trying to return the shape to normal and to realign the foot with relation to the pastern. Ideally the toe needs to be shortened and rolled and the heels raised. Corrective shoeing is also recommended using either heart bar shoes or egg bar shoes. Padding or cushioning is also added to provide some shock-absorption to the underside of the foot. The overall aim of these procedures is to reduce the forces on the deep digital flexor tendon and to minimise the effect of concussion on the foot.

Suggested remedies

Homeopathic remedies have been used to good effect in combination with the measures outlined above.

Prevention and treatment

Arnica 30c and Ledum 30c

Using these remedies in combination will minimise the effects of the concussive forces on the feet of animals likely to develop navicular syndrome. They will help minimise further changes in animals where the problem has been previously diagnosed.
Dose: *once or twice daily on a long-term basis*

Argentum metallicum 30c

This remedy can be used to help with regeneration of the navicular cartilage. It has a more important role in maintaining the blood supply to the navicular bone and is one of the main remedies to be considered.
Dose: *once daily*

Calc fluor 30c

Calc fluor can help with the bony changes that take place in the navicular bone and will minimise the chances of adhesions developing to the deep digital flexor. It is a good remedy for long-standing cases.
Dose: *once daily on a long-term basis*

Ruta grav 30c

Ruta can help reduce the likelihood of bony changes occurring and will help reduce inflammation of the navicular bursa. It is usually more suitable for recently diagnosed cases.
Dose: *once daily on a long-term basis*

Secale 30c and Crataegus 30c

These remedies in combination will help improve the circulation to the foot and to the navicular bone.
Dose: *twice daily on a long term basis*

Heckla lava 6c

Heckla can be added where there are advanced bony (osteophytic) changes to the navicular bone.
Dose: *twice daily*

Bryonia 200c and Apis mel 30

These two remedies will help where acute navicular bursitis is a problem by reducing inflammation of the bursa.
Dose: *three times daily for five days then consider other remedies*

Aurum met 6c

Aurum can be useful in very advanced cases where the bony changes to the navicular bone are extensive and the horse is markedly lame or sore footed.
Dose: *twice daily*

Pedal osteitis

Demineralisation of the pedal bone as a result of prolonged inflammation is termed pedal osteitis, a condition more frequently seen in animals worked on hard surfaces. The main underlying cause is repeated concussion to the foot, although pedal osteitis can arise as a result of one of several other conditions including laminitis, navicular syndrome, bruising of the sole, persistent corns, puncture wounds, an abscess or low grade infection. Nutrition is also thought to be a factor in some cases.

Both feet are usually affected, leading to lameness characterised by a shortened stride. Confirmation is normally by X-ray with a proportion of horses showing bony changes as a result of periosteitis. Treatment should be instigated alongside appropriate shoeing and additional remedies for any other underlying problem.

Suggested remedies

General remedies **Calc phos 6x, Calc carb 6x, Calc fluor 30c, Symphytum 6c, Fluor ac 6c**

With infection **Silica 200c, Asafoetida 30c, Hepar sulph 200c, Calc sulph 30c**

With bony changes **Calc fluor 30c, Ruta grav 30c, Heckla lava 6c**

Where there are advanced changes **Aurum 6c**

Sidebone

Ossification of the lateral cartilages (bone formation in the cartilage) is called sidebone, a condition more commonly seen in the front feet and in horses with a poor conformation or in those that have been poorly trimmed or shod. Concussion is thought to be a contributory factor although injuries to the cartilage can also trigger the problem. To some degree ossification of the lateral cartilages takes place normally through ageing but rarely causes a problem. In cases of sidebone, ossification takes place much earlier than normal and is a rare cause of lameness. In instances where the horse appears lame there will be heat and pain over the cartilages, sometimes with bulging of the coronary band over the relevant area.

Suggested remedies

Dose: 30c daily

Calc Fluor Principal remedy to help prevent slow or ossification

Silica Should be added to work alongside Calc fluor

Ruta grav Add where concussion is a major factor

Heckla lava For more advanced cases where the bony changes to the cartilages are severe

Thiosinaminum Use alongside Heckla in more severe cases

Subchondral bone cysts

This is a condition of the pedal bone that involves the appearance of cysts within the structure of the bone. A number of causes have been suggested. One is trauma leading to avascular necrosis of the bone, another is as a consequence of osteomyelitis and finally as a consequence of osteochrondrosis. Symptoms to look out for include intermittent lameness over a period of time culminating in an episode of acute lameness. The initiating cause of lameness is concussive trauma to the affected area.

Suggested remedies

See page 186

Bear in mind **Arnica 200c** for acute cases where the horse is lame and the use of constitutional remedies particularly **Calc phos 30c** and **Calc carb 30c**. Consider **Argentum metallicum 6c** as a preventative remedy.

Buttress foot
Pyramidal disease

This is a condition affecting the pedal bone caused by excessive strain placed on the common digital extensor tendon where it inserts on the extensor process of the bone resulting in a reaction in the periosteum. The consequence of this is new bone growth, sometimes referred to as a form of low ringbone, which can also occur as result of a fracture involving the extensor process. The new bone that appears sometimes affects the hoof wall. A ridge may form, running from the coronary band down to the sole.

The resulting lameness is not specific but affected animals will show a shortened stride, with a tendency to point the affected foot and to land heavily on the heel. Acute early symptoms include pain, heat and swelling at the level of the coronary band in the centre of the wall.

Suggested remedies

Acute cases **Ruta grav 200c, Fluoric acid 30c, Apis 30c, Phosphoric acid 30c**

Long-standing chronic cases **Phytolacca 30c, Heckla lava 6c, Ruta grav 6c, Calc Fluor 6c, Silica 6c**

The Hoof and Hoof Problems

Injuries to the hoof and foot

Simple injuries such as cuts or nicks in the skin should be treated with **Arnica 200c**, **Hypericum 200c** and **Ledum 200c**.
Dose: three times daily for four–five days

Suppurating wounds can be treated with **Hepar sulph 200c** along with **Calendula 30c** to assist healing.
Dose: three times daily until healed

For slow healing wounds generally use **Silica 200c** *two or three times daily* until the area has healed. **Calendula 30c** can also be used where healing is slow.

Very small wounds that quickly become severely inflamed and infected should be treated with
Pyrogen 1M
Dose: three times daily

Overreach Injuries

This type of injury is caused by the toe of the hind limb hitting the coronary band or heels of the leg in front. This can result in severe bruising and lacerations to the affected area. The horse may or may not be lame depending on the affected area and depth of the injury.

Clean the wound with diluted **Hypercal lotion** and remove any debris and dead tissue. Dose using **Arnica 200c, Hypericum 200c** and **Ledum 200c** as detailed above. Some of the wounds arising from overreach injuries are slow to heal. Dosing with **Calendula 30c** and **Silica 200c** three times daily will speed up the process. Use **Hepar sulph 200c** if there is gross suppuration.

Nail Prick

This occurs when a nail is accidentally driven into the sensitive tissues of the foot and will cause lameness. The nail should be removed immediately and the hole flushed with diluted Hypercal lotion. *Dose:* with **Ledum 200c, Hypericum 200c** and **Hepar sulph 200c** *three times daily for three days.*

Corns and Bruising of the Sole

Corns occur predominantly on the front feet and usually arise as a consequence of improper shoeing resulting in pressure on the sole. They occur at the inner angle of the foot formed by the wall and the bar and involve the sensitive and insensitive tissues of the sole where bruising leads to the development of a haematoma. The horse may or may not be lame.

Bruising of the sole in contrast is a common cause of lameness and the result of concussion on the sole of the foot or frog often from riding on uneven ground. Poor shoeing and poor conformation are contributory factors. The horse may only show mild lameness but if the trauma is severe the horse may be extremely lame. Sometimes it is possible to see the bruise (which occurs between the sole and pedal bone) on the sole in the region of the toe or quarter area.

Both these conditions require appropriate attention from the farrier to correct any underlying problems by trimming and appropriate shoeing. Both carry a favourable prognosis. Affected horses should recover completely particularly with the help of homeopathy.

Suggested remedies

Dose: three times daily

Arnica 200c and **Ledum 200c** This combination should be used routinely in all cases

Bellis 30c Provides a good alternative to Arnica in severe cases

Hamamellis 30c Use in combination with Arnica as a preventative treatment

Hypericum 30c Indicated where the horse is lame

Sulphuric acid 30c To speed recovery from injury where this is slow

Brittle, Weak and Dry Hooves, Sandcrack and Grasscrack

Hoof problems such as these often reflect an animal's general state of health, overall condition and level of care. Bear in mind that horn quality is influenced by nutrition, type of work, environmental conditions, ability of the farrier and concurrent disease problems such as laminitis as well. As it takes between 8 and 12 months for new horn produced at the coronary band to grow down to the lower foot, problems likely to give rise to variation in horn quality may not always be immediately obvious.

Brittle, weak, flaky, poor, slow growing or dry hooves often result as a consequence of a number of factors in combination, all of which will need attention to rectify the problem fully. Poor horn will flake and is liable to crack and can predispose the horse to other conditions such as infection in unshod horses or the shoes may work loose predisposing to cracking or the horse may lose a shoe. Brittle hooves are more likely in the summer months due to loss of moisture from the hoof wall, though the reason for this is not completely understood.

Inadequate trimming or overgrown feet can lead to cracks developing in the hoof wall running from the bottom upwards. These are sometimes known as grasscracks in contrast to sandcracks, which start at the coronary band and run downward. Sandcracks originate from damage to the cells that produce horn at the level of the coronary band with length of the crack indicating the severity of the damage. Cell damage can occur as a result of trauma or from infection that has migrated upward from lower in the foot.

Depending where the crack is located, the horse may or may not be lame. Cracks are also likely to develop where there is rotation of the pedal bone (caused by laminitis) or where imbalance causing the foot to land on the ground with excessive concussive impact.

Homeopathy can help immensely with horn quality issues and is recommended alongside the use of supplements and correct management techniques including feeding and regular visits from the farrier.

Homeopathic remedies

Aim for a constitutional prescription where possible. The benefits of any treatment may not be apparent until some time has passed and new horn has grown down from the coronary band, replacing damaged or weak horn.

Use the 6c or 30c potency once daily for up to six months

Silica

Keynote: Weak horn/hooves in general, grasscrack, sandcrack, infected horn

Silica is the most widely used remedy for hoof related conditions. Indications include dry, split or cracked hooves, weak or brittle horn, grasscrack, sandcrack and hooves with corrugated ridges. It is also indicated where the hooves are grossly crippled and distorted either through neglect or disease. Silica is the remedy of choice if infection is involved and where the nutrition of the horn is, or has, been very poor. Changes as a result of laminitis should also be borne in mind particularly where the soles are tender and movement uncomfortable.

Antimonium crudum

Keynote: Thickened, distorted hoove

This is also a remedy for brittle or cracked horn where the wall of the hoof is split as in grasscrack or sandcrack. Where Antimonium crudum is needed, the horn can be slow growing or the hooves become either thickened or badly distorted as well. Other ongoing problems as well such as DJD of the coffin joint will favour this remedy over others.

Fluoric acid

Keynote: Distorted hooves with corrugations, crumbling hooves

There are some comparisons between Silica and this remedy but where Silica is a 'chilly' remedy, horses that benefit from Fluoric acid tend not feel the cold easily. Fluoric acid is indicated where the hooves are not only distorted but where there are marked corrugated ridges (as a result of laminitis for example). It is the remedy of choice where the horn/hoof is literally crumbling away. Pain in the foot due to chronic laminitis or arthritic changes in the joints is a further differentiating feature.

Graphites

Keynote: Brittle, rough hooves, grasscrack

This remedy work best on a constitutional basis. Graphites covers roughened, brittle hooves that crack from the base upwards towards the coronary band as well as hooves that are deformed or crumbling. There are several pointers for Graphites. Most cases where the remedy is needed, the foot is large and the hoof wall is naturally thick but is weak along the bottom edge. There is often a history of mud fever as well in Graphites cases.

Alumina

Keynote: Dryness, flaking or brittle horn

Dry, flaky horn where there is lack of moisture is the keynote of Alumina in contrast to other remedies. Alumina suits older horses particularly well especially where there is general weakness or where the skin is dry, chapped or sore. It is one of the remedies to consider in cases where the horn is of poor quality as a result of laminitis and where there is consequent lameness due to pedal bone rotation.

Thuja
Keynote: Brittle hooves with chronic laminitis
Thuja has a very specific indication in helping where the hooves are poor as a result of ongoing chronic laminitis.

Other useful remedies

Dose: 6c twice daily on a long-term basis

Castor equi A general remedy for brittle hooves, helping to improve horn quality

Calc carb For slow growing horn

Calc fluor Works alongside Silica to strengthen horn and improve hoof quality

Nat mur For dry and cracked hooves, best prescribed constitutionally

Sepia Used constitutionally where the hooves are distorted

Quittor

This condition, which is more common in the front leg, is cause by inflammation, infection and necrosis of the lateral cartilages of the pedal bone. The infection is often introduced by injuries (such as lacerations) to the coronary band in the area of the collateral cartilages. Quittor can also be caused by a penetrating wound to the sole or from trauma to the cartilages from wire cuts or bruising which can cause further problems by interfering with the circulation to the area.

Either cartilage can be affected initially presenting as heat, pain and swelling over the coronary band in the region of the affected cartilage. When the swelling points and bursts, a purulent discharge is released after which the area will heal only to break out again repeatedly. These sinuses, of which there may be several, are difficult to treat and may require surgery to resolve the problem. Intermittent lameness is often present and most likely during the acute stages.

Suggested remedies

Preventative measures
Injuries to the region to the coronary band should be treated using **Arnica 200c**, **Hepar sulph 200c** and **Ledum 200c**, both *three times daily for two to three days* and cleaned with diluted **Hypercal lotion** to prevent infection from gaining access.

Treating quittor

Hepar sulph 1M
This is the principal remedy to consider in the acute stage and in chronic cases where there is marked tenderness over the area of the discharging sinuses.
Dose: twice daily until resolution

Myristica sebifera 200c
This less commonly used remedy is the most effective choice for treating quittor in all but the most acute cases. It is a specific for established infections involving the tissues of the foot and especially where there are discharging sinuses.
Dose: Four times daily until resolution

Silica 1M
Silica is most useful in more chronic cases where the sinuses have been established for some time and where there is very little or no pain present.
Dose: three times daily until resolution

Pyrogen 1M
This is a remedy for the acute early stage of the condition where there is much pain and inflammation around the area. The horse is very badly lame. Pyrogen is also worth considering in the most chronic cases that appear resistant to all other remedies.
Dose: Acute cases four times daily; Chronic cases twice daily

Also consider

Anthracinum 200c Where there is gross necrosis and sloughing of the cartilages in extreme cases where the discharge is particularly foul

Asafoetida 200c As for Anthracinum but where the discharge is thin and watery

Lachesis 200c Where the problem is in part due to poor blood supply to the damaged cartilage

Kreosotum 30c Where the discharge excoriates the skin

Secale 30c To promote blood circulation to damaged cartilages

Calendula 30c After surgery to promote healing

Dose: *two or three times daily*

White Line Disease

The white line is the junction of the sole with the wall of the foot. If the horse is allowed to stand in damp, wet conditions for a long period of time, bacteria can invade the white line. Poor hoof care will be a contributory factor. Diagnosis can be confirmed by looking for the telltale dark black, foul smelling material running in a line round the junction of the sole and wall. Most horses with white line disease will not be lame unless infection spreads wider to involve the hoof wall.

Suggested remedies

Dose: twice daily

Hepar sulph 200c Initial remedy to be considered in simple cases

Kreosotum 200c For more severe or advanced cases

Myristica sebifera 200c Another alternative for severe cases

Carbo veg 30c Can be given routinely to all cases

Calc fluor 30c Add where the hoof wall is involved to strengthen the tissues

Silica 200c Use in chronic or neglected cases where the hoof wall is involved

Abscess of the Sole
Infection or Pus in the Foot
Under-run Sole

This is one of the most common causes of lameness in horses initiated by either a puncture wound to the sole or as a consequence of a crack in the white line. The majority of horses with this condition will be lame, although in the very early stages this may not be apparent. Once infection gains hold, the foot will become extremely painful, as the hoof cannot expand as the pus builds up. By this stage the horse is likely to be lame and not able to put the foot onto the ground for long. There will be heat in the foot, an increase in the digital pulse and sometimes sufficient pain to cause the horse to sweat.

The sole will be sensitive to pressure and especially at any point where it starts to track through the sole. Normally the pus will travel along the line of least resistance and will under-run the sole and travel up between the laminae to burst through at the coronary band.

Sole abscesses need to be drained to eliminate the infection and to relieve pain. Once a drainage point has been established in the sole, the area can be poulticed to draw out further infected material which normally appears as thin grey coloured fluid. Puncture wounds entering the region of the frog are much more serious as infection may gain access to the navicular bursa or pedal bone. These cases will need surgical intervention.

Suggested remedies

Initially before drainage
Dose: every three to four hours

Belladonna 1M Where the horse is extremely lames, has an increased digital pulse and heat in the hoof. Sweating may also be observed.

Pyrogen 1M Where the horse is restless and the infection takes hold quickly. Again there will be heat in the hoof and an increased digital pulse

Hepar sulph 1M To abort the abscess before any signs of lameness are present

In some cases consider
Hepar sulph 3x To promote suppuration and allow the abscess to point so that drainage can be established.

After drainage has been established
Dose: two or three times daily

Hepar sulph 1M Use where the foot is still painful although the abscess is draining

Silica 1M Indicated where drainage has been

established and pain is no longer present. Silica is also recommended for long-standing cases

Calc sulph 200c An alternative to Silica where the condition is slow to resolve. The pus will be typically thicker where this remedy is needed

Kreosotum 200c Indicated where the pus is black in colour and has a foul smell

Asafoetida 200c Where the pus is extremely watery

Anthracinum 200c Consider where the abscess keeps returning and discharging black foul pus

Myristica sebifera 200c As an alternative to Hepar sulph where this remedy fails to act. Also indicated in chronic, stubborn cases.

Thrush

Thrush is a condition that affects the lateral and central sulci of the frog characterised by the appearance of black necrotic material in the grooves. Poor hygiene (feet which are dirty and not cleaned properly) and bad environmental conditions (moist soiled bedding) are major contributory factors although it is likely that poor trimming or shoeing are also involved in a proportion of cases.

The resulting infection in the tissues of the frog leads to black, offensive, moist, purulent material accumulating in the grooves. In some instances the infection may spread to other tissues such as the horn or penetrate to more sensitive tissues. Most cases of thrush do not exhibit lameness but in such cases the horse may flinch when the area is cleaned and may be obviously lame.

Treatment involves attending to the underlying causes and removing all of the damaged, necrotic infected tissue along with the use of appropriate remedies.

Kreosotum 200c
This is the most commonly prescribed remedy used where all the characteristic symptoms are present, most notably the offensive smell of the diseased tissue.
Dose: twice daily until the condition improves

Myristica sebifera 200c
This is the second remedy of choice and is said to have excellent antiseptic powers cutting short the infection. It works well alongside other remedies.
Dose: twice daily until the condition improves

Silica 200c
Silica is most useful for cases where healing is slow or where the infection has spread to more sensitive tissues such as the laminae or to the horn. Characteristically there is little pain so the horse is not badly lame.
Dose: twice daily until the condition improves

Hepar sulph 200c
Indicated where the condition results in marked lameness and the material is especially purulent nature.
Dose: twice daily until the condition improves

Merc sol 200c
Merc sol should be used where the smell is less offensive but where the material in the sulci is particularly wet or moist in appearance.
Dose: twice daily until the condition improves

Anthracinum 200c
Useful as an alternative to Kreosotum and valuable where this remedy fails to work. It is especially good for very severe cases.
Dose: three times daily until the condition improves

Squilla maritima 30c
Add where there is obvious mild discomfort which comes and goes from day to day.
Dose: three times daily until the condition improves

Sulphur 30c
This remedy can be used on a constitutional basis to help.
Dose: three times daily until the condition improves

Canker

Canker is a chronic condition involving overproduction or hypertrophy of the horn-producing tissues of the foot. It is a rare condition and one that is most likely to affect the hind feet.

The root cause is unhygienic stabling where the horse is allowed to stand in muddy conditions or on soiled bedding coupled with poor standards of care allowing bacteria to gain access.

Lameness is unusual unless the condition has advanced to the stage where the sole or hoof wall is involved. On examination, the frog will appear ragged and the horny tissue comprising the frog will loosen easily to show a putrid smelling, cheese like, cream coloured discharge underneath. Canker is a difficult condition to treat and involves removal of all the diseased tissues, remedying underlying precipitating factors and using the following remedies.

Recommended remedies

***Dose:** 30c potency three times daily for several weeks*

Calc sulph Main remedy to consider where there is no pain or lameness

Hepar sulph Principal remedy in all cases where there is lameness

Silica For advanced cases where the condition has spread deeper

Thuja Indicated in severe or intractable cases

Ant crud Add where new tissue is slow to grow back

Secale Assists recovery in advanced cases by improving blood supply to affected tissues

Keratoma

This condition is extremely rare and is a form of cancer that involves the horn producing cells of the foot. As the condition progresses the shape of the foot becomes distorted causing the horse to become lame. Surgical treatment is possible but the condition is likely to recur. Constitutional homeopathic treatment may help combined with the use of **Thuja 30c**, **Conium 30c**, **Silica 30c** or **Antimonium crudum 30c**. Consider **Sarsaparilla 30c** when there is obvious pain present.
***Dose:** twice daily*

Laminitis, Founder

This is one of the most common of all conditions and one which all horse owners and riders should be aware of. Despite ongoing research, some aspects of the problem still remain a mystery; however, we know that correct feeding and management regimes can prevent something like 80 per cent of all cases. Laminitis, a term which specifically refers to the inflammation of the laminae and its consequences, can affect a wide range of horses, ponies and even donkeys of any age, breed or type. It can affect all four feet, although it is more commonly seen in the front feet.

The laminae are vital structures that interlock the hoof and pedal bone and provide an intricate suspension system which cushions the foot and leg from the concussion which normally occurs when the foot hits the ground. They also play an important role in the maintenance and general health of the hoof itself. If the laminae become inflamed there is effectively a lack of blood supply to the foot. The inter-linking between the pedal bone and hoof (the interlaminar bonds), start to break down and the suspension mechanism starts to fail. The attachment of the pedal bone to the hoof starts to weaken allowing the pedal bone to rotate tip downward, placing pressure on the sole of the foot and causing pain. If the rotation continues unabated, the pedal bone will eventually protrude through the sole of the foot between the front of the frog and the toe. These cases in which the hoof/pedal bone bond is totally destroyed, are known as sinkers.

Rotation of the pedal bone, also called foundering, itself causes other problems. There is tearing and shearing of the blood supply to the laminae, compromising the health of the laminae and that of the hoof wall further by preventing vital nutrients from reaching these areas. In such cases there is sometimes an additional risk of secondary bacterial infection. Other long-term effects, often seen in chronic cases, are all too obvious, as the characteristic laminitic rings on the hoof wall will testify, along with the problems of chronic pain and associated lameness, the risk of developing seedy toe, hoof abscesses and overgrown heels.

Causes of Laminitis

The causes of laminitis are well known.

Carbohydrate overload – obesity and over eating

This is by far the most common cause and most often seen in ponies which require relatively little food and which are under exercised. Obesity is a predisposing factor. Spring is the greatest period of risk, when the new lush grass contains very high levels of carbohydrate, although the autumn is also a period of risk. Soluble carbohydrate such as fructans or starch is generally regarded as the main culprit, but carbohydrates from cereal based compounded feeds will also contribute to the overall level of intake.

Excess consumption of carbohydrates caused by overgrazing lush pasture, causes a major upset in the bacteria of the horse's hindgut. In some horses only small amounts will trigger such an upset, whilst others are able to tolerate considerably more before problems arise. Very little soluble carbohydrate normally passes into the horses' hindgut. When large amounts are present, unfriendly bacteria multiply rapidly producing lactic acid, causing the bowel contents to become acid and causing the death of the normal friendly gut bacteria. Lactic acid also damages the lining of the bowel allowing toxins to enter the bloodstream. At the same time, the bacteria release toxins that activate enzymes which cause hoof detachment and consequent capillary damage as the blood vessels are disrupted. Although not clearly understood, there is also an increase in resistance to blood flow in the foot leading to the characteristic bounding digital pulse. This is likely to be due to the loss of the capillaries supplying blood to the laminae.

Carbohydrate overload – grain overload

Accidental ingestion of large quantities of grain is also a significant cause in horses that break into grain stores or bins. Overfeeding grains or high-energy grain-based feeds will have the same effect leading to the cascade of events outlined above.

Concussion or trauma to the foot, mechanical injury

Repeated concussion from working on hard surfaces or sudden acute trauma to the foot can cause damage to the laminae and trigger a bout of laminitis. Trauma is a major factor in driving horses. Improper shoeing and poor trimming can also be contributory factors. Repetitive overload, with the weight transferred to one foot due to lameness in another, can also induce laminitis. This is sometimes referred to as uneven weight bearing. Laminitis can also occur after fracture repair.

Toxaemia

Viral and bacterial infections can lead to the production of toxins that can damage the laminae. Likely triggers are septic metritis (from a retained placenta), colic, peritonitis, diarrhoea and abscesses.

Drug induced

Certain drugs, particularly steroids, can damage the laminae leading to laminitis. This action is thought to be due to constriction of the arteries to the foot restricting blood flow to the laminae. Some wormers can also induce laminitis.

Cushing's disease – pituitary dependent Cushing's disease

This is a common cause of laminitis in older horses and caused by high levels of cortisol (a natural steroid) circulating in the blood. This over-production of cortisol occurs as a result of a tumour in the pituitary gland.

Peripheral Cushing's disease or obesity dependent laminitis

This form of laminitis, which is triggered by a metabolic abnormality, can occur in animals of any age. These cases do not show the symptoms of classical Cushing's. However, affected animals are obese and have high circulating levels of cortisol.

Stress

Stress is a factor known to induce laminitis under certain circumstances. Possible triggers include travelling long distances, changing yards, exhaustion, overwork and vaccination.

Hormonally related problems

Animals suffering from hypothyroidism (an under-active thyroid), often 'easy keepers', and mares that display continual oestrus are at risk of developing laminitis.

Signs and Symptoms of Laminitis

There are three distinct phases in the development of laminitis. In the first, the **developmental phase**, separation of the laminae is triggered but no lameness or pain is evident. Other symptoms in unrelated body systems may be apparent, (such as colic) and must be attended to in addition to treating the laminitis. This phase may last anytime between about ten and 40 hours.

This is followed by the **acute phase** in which we see the consequences of the first phase that will have started some hours before any clinical symptoms are apparent. The signs of this stage are fairly characteristic when they do appear, and signify that damage to the laminae will have already occurred. Very mild cases are sometimes referred to as **sub acute**. Only minimal damage to the laminae may occur in such instances. Signs seen in the acute phase include:

- Pain, usually in the front feet but all four can be affected or just one single foot
- Reluctance to place full weight on the affected feet
- Change in posture with weight transferred to the heels or transferred to the hind feet. This produces the characteristic pose of the acutely laminitic horse rocked back onto the heels
- Changes in gait in milder cases with reluctance to move in more severe cases
- Prominent (bounding) digital pulses, sometimes the only symptom present
- Increase in temperature (heat) detectable in the hoof wall or coronary band
- Increase in body temperature, pulse and respiration in severe cases

The acute phase can be short-lived if treated promptly, but if left unattended, the pedal bone will begin to rotate (foundering) assisted by the pull of the deep digital flexor tendon. The **chronic phase** that follows is characterised by an altogether different set of symptoms and problems. Any case over 48 hours old is considered chronic.

- Recurrent bouts of laminitis interspersed with periods where there is no active inflammation of the laminae
- Chronic lameness
- Abnormal hoof growth and the appearance of rings around the hoof wall. The toes tend to grow long and there is a risk of overgrown heels
- Poor hoof quality as nutrient supply to the horn is inadequate
- Possible widening of the white line
- Weight bearing on the heels
- Dropping of the sole. The sole appears flattened and later a bruised appearance as the pedal bone rotates further
- Penetration of the sole by the tip of the pedal bone. These horses are referred to as sinkers
- Tendency to foot abscesses, seedy toe and bruising

Chronic laminitis can sometimes be difficult to diagnose and can be confused with navicular syndrome, ringbone, pedal osteitis, arthritis and fractures of the pedal bone.

Treating laminitis

Homeopathy has a good track record in treating all stages of laminitis, particularly chronic cases. However, it should not be relied on as the only therapy in acute cases. Acute laminitis is an emergency and should be treated as such. Help should be sought immediately using homeopathy in the interim until help arrives. Prevention is always better than cure. Good management is essential in preventing laminitis in those horses at risk and in assisting recovery of affected animals.

Homeopathic Treatment

Developmental and acute laminitis cases

Attend to or remove the trigger in the first instance. Where feed or grazing is a problem, lead the horse away. Where the pain is severe, try to stand the horse on a bed of deep shavings so that the soles are supported and provide complete box rest. Avoid cold water hosing or standing the horse in a stream, as there is no evidence to support that these measures are beneficial. On the contrary they may in fact be harmful. Only have the shoes removed if the soles are concave in appearance, otherwise you will be likely to increase the degree of pain. Always treat the underlying cause where this can be identified. You may be able to prevent laminitis developing.

For all acute cases

Aconite 1M

Aconite should be used routinely in all acute laminitic cases whatever the cause. This remedy is also useful where stress is a factor.
Dose: *every 20–30 minutes until the period of risk has passed*

Belladonna 1M

Add Belladonna to all cases where there is an increase in the force and rate of the digital pulse however slight. Clear indications include an increase in pulse (described an pounding) and respiratory rate, sweating, pain (with the horse leaning back with the weight on the heels), heat in the foot and coronary band and in some cases injected (intensely red) mucous membranes. Belladonna can be used alongside or alternated with Aconite.
Dose: *every 20–30 minutes until the period of risk has passed*

Secale 200c

Secale is an important remedy in that it will increase the blood flow to the laminae where this has been compromised. It should be given to all acute cases in an attempt to stop laminar separation and pedal bone rotation. The earlier this remedy can be given the better.
Dose: *every two or three hours, reducing to three times daily as symptoms ease*

Also consider:

Hypericum 1M

Hypericum should be added where there is a marked degree of pain and the horse is in a lot of discomfort, barely able to move or leaning back heavily, shifting weight onto the heels with the front legs well forward.
Dose: *every two or three hours, reducing to three times daily as symptoms ease*

Kali carb 200c

The keynote of this remedy is weakness. It is best reserved for those cases that not only have this symptom but which also show extreme pain with inability to move more than a short distance. It is also indicated where there is rapid rotation of the pedal bone. Do not use this remedy where there is toxaemia or a septic focus.
Dose: *every two or three hours, reducing to three times daily as symptoms ease*

Where trauma is involved

Arnica 200c

Use in all cases of traumatic laminitis whatever the cause.
Dose: *every two hours until the period of risk has passed*

Where there is toxaemia

Pyrogen 1M

This is the principal remedy to use where there is a toxic or septic focus. Particular indications include metritis, septic wounds and abscesses.
Dose: *every two hours until the period of risk has passed or the symptoms have abated*

Baptisia 200c

This remedy has similar indications to Pyrogen but is indicated where there is prostration and all movements are difficult, as the muscles appear sore.
Dose: *every hour until the period of risk has passed or the symptoms have abated*

Where there are dietary causes

Nux vomica 200c

Nux will drain toxins form the system and help restore balance to the digestive system. It will also act as a general tonic to the liver.

Dose: *every two hours until the period of risk has passed*

Lycopodium 1M

Lycopodium is used in a similar fashion to Nux but is ideally suited to those horses where overeating has also led to gaseous distension or flatulent colic. Lycopodium will also help restore liver function where this has been impaired by the accumulation of toxins. Acute laminitic cases where there is a history of liver disease should be given Lycopodium routinely.

Dose: *every two hours until the period of risk has passed*

Drug-induced laminitis

The use of the drug in potency will help. **Cortisone 200c** or **Prednisolone 200c** can be given *three times daily* where this has been the initiating cause.

Chronic laminitis

Chronic cases often respond well to homeopathy in conjunction with correct management. Diet or feeding and hoof care are two areas that need particular mention. The aim here is to resolve the symptoms of chronic laminitis as far as possible, to prevent recurrence in those cases that have recovered and to prevent further rotation of the pedal bone.

Avoid obesity, over eating and carbohydrate overload at all costs, ideally keeping animals at risk off grass completely. In many cases this is not practical, so ensure that they only graze when the fructan level in the grass is low in the late evening and early in the morning. Pasture management is important. Aim to maintain the pasture so that stem length is minimal, ensuring that there is more leaf as more fructans are stored in the stem than in the leaf. You can do this by cutting the pasture or by grazing sheep.

Where weight is a problem, aim to reduce this slowly by monitoring food intake carefully and by lungeing, riding or turning out to burn up excess calories. Fibre intake should be maintained. Use oat straw, last year's hay or any one of a number of approved feeds that are high in fibre and have low starch levels. Starvation is not an option as this can lead to further problems.

Regular visits from the farrier are equally important. A good farrier will help restore proper weight bearing to the foot, help prevent further tissue damage and pedal bone rotation, remove damaged or diseased horn and will help support the sole and hoof wall so that healing can occur. Special shoes or pads are often used, including egg bar shoes, heart bars and silicone pads.

Homeopathic remedies

Chronic laminitis is often best treated with remedy combinations used in low potencies (most often 6c) on a long-term basis. Experience has proved that some combinations work well together but the exact composition for each individual animal may need adjustment on the basis of a little trial and error using different combinations than those listed. Constitutional prescribing is also of great benefit.

Principal remedies

Main combinations

Dose: *once or twice daily depending on severity of symptoms*

Combination 1 (ALC) ideal for chronic laminitis cases where trauma is a factor

Arnica 6c For the effect of concussion and bruising on the foot, reduces damage to the laminae

Ledum 6c To minimise the effect of concussion and to relieve discomfort

Crataegus 6c or **30c** Improves circulation and blood flow to the feet

Caulophyllum 6c An alternative to either Arnica or Ledum to help relieve lameness

Combination 2 (CSS) for chronic laminitis where intermittent pain or lameness is a major feature

Crataegus 6c or **30c** Improves circulation and blood flow to the feet

Secale 6c Increases perfusion of blood to the laminae

Sarsaparilla 6c Helps with the pain and inflammation associated with chronic cases

Hypericum 6c An alternative to help with pain relief

Berberis 6c Excellent additional remedy where there is liver involvement or lower back pain. Helps resolve chronic laminitic pain

Combination 3 (SSA) for chronic inflammation of the laminae with poor hoof quality and associated problems

Sabadilla 6c To reduce inflammation of the laminae

Silica 6c To minimise the risk of infection and strengthen horn quality. Use where the hooves are cracked

Ant crud 6c Helps where there are pronounced laminitic rings on the hoof or where the hooves have become deformed. Helps relieve discomfort or pain

Alumina 6c Add where the soles are tender and the hooves are brittle or flaky. Useful where seedy toe is a problem

Combination 4 (SHS) for chronic laminitis with pedal bone rotation and penetration of the sole

Silica 30c Used to help prevent infections and conditions such as seedy toe occurring

Hypericum 30c Added for pain relief

Sarsaparilla 30c To ease pain and discomfort

Additional remedies

Dose: *once or twice daily depending on severity of symptoms*

General

Xanthoxylum 3x An alternative to Crataegus to help improve the circulation to the feet

Carbo veg 6c For severe cases with extensive damage to the laminae, helps improve blood perfusion of the tissues. Also useful where there is a history of repeated infections where the horn is of poor quality

Hoof care

Fluoric acid 6c Indicated where the hoof is of extremely poor quality or where there is a history of foot or sole abscesses or seedy toe

Calc fluor 6c Along with Silica this remedy will encourage good hoof growth

Graphites 30c Helpful on a constitutional basis for chronic cases where the horn quality is poor

Bony changes

Ruta grav 6c Add where degenerative bony changes are evident in the pedal bone

Heckla lava 6c Add Heckla where the bony changes are advanced

Cases with Liver dysfunction

Consider **Lycopodium 30c**, **Phosphorus 30c**, **Nux vomica 30c**, or **Berberis 6c** as appropriate

Difficult cases or where there is a specific underlying problem

Thuja 1M can be helpful generally
Dose: *once weekly for four weeks*

Hypothyroid cases

Consider **Calc carb 30c** or **Thyroid 3x**

Where continual oestrus is a factor

Specifically look at **Secale 30c**, **Sepia 30c** or **Pulsatilla 30c**

Cushing's cases

Commonly used remedies include **ACTH 30c**, **Quercus robur 30c**, **Nat mur 30c** and **Abrotanum 30c**

Seedy Toe
Separation of the Wall

This condition occurs as a consequence of chronic laminitis and involves the separation of the sensitive laminae from the hoof wall at the toe. Where the tissue breaks down, the foot is predisposed to infection and the area can fill with dry cheesy-like material. Separation of the white line can follow allowing infection to gain access leading to the condition known as gravel. Where the horse is not lame, the defect will grow out provided the foot is trimmed properly.

Suggested remedies

Dose: once daily

Silica 30c Will help strengthen the damaged horn and prevent infection

Hepar sulph 200c Indicated where there is pain, lameness or a purulent discharge

Fluoric acid 6c Indicated where the hoof is of extremely poor quality

Myristica sebifera 200c Use where the tissue is badly infected and the horn of dubious quality

Calc fluor 6c Along with Silica this remedy will encourage good hoof growth

Graphites 30c Helpful on a constitutional basis for chronic cases where the horn quality is poor

Gravel

Gravel is caused by a crack in the white line (the junction of the laminae of the wall with the sole) allowing infection to gain access and invade the sensitive structures of the foot. As there is no drainage at this point, the infection tracks along the line of least resistance, draining at the heels.

The white line can crack if the feet are too dry or crack as a consequence of laminitis or seedy toe. Affected horses will be lame, often even before drainage has occurred. Treating the condition involves establishing good drainage in conjunction with using remedies.

Suggested remedies

Dose: twice daily

Hepar sulph 200c Acute cases where there is pain and lameness before drainage has occurred

Silica 200c Use in cases where drainage has been established

Calc sulph 200c For stubborn cases where resolution is slow even with good drainage

Myristica seb 200c Consider as an alternative to Calc sulph or Silica, especially where there is gross sepsis present

The Nervous System

This section covers the nervous system and is divided into two sections. The first covers conditions which affect nerves in general, whilst the second deals with specific conditions affecting the nervous system.

The nervous system itself is divided into two main parts. The central nervous system (CNS) which comprises the brain and spinal cord (both of which are in charge of higher functions such as behaviour, sensations, coordination of movement and breathing) and the peripheral nervous system which covers the nerves which connect with all other body systems and tissues. It is these peripheral nerve fibres which allow movement by controlling the muscles and which link to the joints, ligaments and tendons. Knowledge of where the major nerves run in the lower limbs is frequently used in the diagnosis of lameness by using nerve blocks at specific sites.

Injuries or diseases which affect nerve function can interfere with the passage of nerve impulses travelling along the nerve fibres in one of several ways. They can slow the impulses down or block their passage completely. The result is either partial or complete paralysis of an area if the nerve affected supplies muscles, or complete or partial loss of sensation (feeling) if sensory nerves are affected. In some conditions the passage of nerve impulses is speeded up, resulting in convulsions or muscle spasms such as those seen in cases of tetanus.

General Conditions Affecting Nerves and the Nervous System

General Nerve Injuries

Peripheral nerves

Nerve injury can occur as the result of direct trauma to an area following an accident such as a blow, although inadvertent surgical trauma can cause similar damage. Recovery is possible providing the nerve has not been irreparably damaged. Symptoms of nerve injury depend on the exact area and nerve or nerves involved. This can range from jerky or uncoordinated muscle movements to complete or partial paralysis of an area or limb as well as loss of sensation from the area. Examples of nerve injury include facial paralysis, obdurator nerve injury and radial paralysis.

Central nervous system (CNS)

Concussion or a skull fracture can damage the nerves of the brain. Spinal injury can cause haemorrhage within the spinal canal or can crush the spinal cord. In all situations the damage may be temporary or permanent.

Basic treatment of all nerve injuries

Arnica 200c or 1M
As in all injuries give a few doses of Arnica initially.
Dose: *three or four doses over a period of one hour depending on the severity and nature of the injury.*

Hypericum 1M
This is the principal remedy for all types of nerve

injury and should be given alongside Arnica.
Dose: three or four doses in the first hour followed by dosing two or three times daily until the injury has resolved.

Bellis perennis 200c

This is a specific remedy for injuries to the pelvic region including injuries that involve pelvic nerves.
Dose: three times daily

Calendula 30c

This is another remedy with a specific action in resolving nerve injuries, particularly those that are slow to heal. Calendula can be used alongside Hypericum.
Dose: three times daily

Nerve Injuries – Concussion

Homeopathic remedies can have a remarkable effect in treating some of the seemingly more long-term problems associated with an injury to the skull, even if the original injury was some time ago. Always consider the use of Arnica and Hypericum first before using any of the remedies given below.

Aconite 1M Use immediately if there are obvious signs of fear or panic

Cicuta 200c Use where loss of balance ensues

Helleborus 200c Can help where mental dullness is a consequence

Opium 1M Where the animal appears to go into a coma like state

Natrum sulph 200c Indicated for any chronic mental changes which occur afterwards

Zincum met 200c Helpful if the after effects include restlessness or muscle twitching
Dose: Initially after the injury give several doses close together. Where the symptoms start to improve repeat with a single dose to effect as often as needed.

Nerve Injuries – Spinal Injury

Again consider the use of **Arnica** and **Hypericum** first before using any specific remedies to help with the damage to the spine itself. The consequence of spinal injury may well be muscle weakness, uncoordinated movements (ataxia), paralysis or muscle spasms. Useful remedies may be found under appropriate headings elsewhere in the book. See also the Spine.

Nerve inflammation or neuritis

Neuritis is the name given to inflammation of a peripheral nerve in contrast to involvement of the CNS. In this area we see encephalitis, which involves inflammation of the brain, myelitis inflammation of the spinal cord and meningitis, which involves inflammation of the lining of the spinal cord and brain. Meningitis and encephalitis usually have underlying infectious causes that may, on occasion, cause peripheral nerve inflammation. Neuritis can also be caused by trauma or injury. The Cauda Equina Syndrome is the only significant specific condition under the heading of neuritis.

General remedies for neuritis

Initially:
Dose: hourly until the condition improves

Aconite 1M Best given at the first sign of any trouble especially where an infection is involved

Belladonna 1M Best applied to cases where there are violent muscle spasms or movements caused by acute nerve inflammation

Hypericum 1M A good general remedy for all cases of neuritis including cases where there is loss of skin sensation and where trauma is involved

Then consider:

Allium cepa 30c This is the principal remedy for chronic traumatic neuritis

Coffea 200c Indicated where there is evidence of increased nervous activity in general such as hypersensitivity of the skin and muscle jitters

Phosphorus 30c Phosphorus can be used where neuritis leads to a degree of muscle weakness or paralysis or where there is nerve degeneration

Stannum 30c Indicated where neuritis has caused weakness of the limbs leading to stumbling

Thallium 6c Neuritis leading to hind leg weakness may respond to Thallium

Encephalitis and Encephalomyelitis

These two conditions refer to inflammation of the brain and are usually viral in origin. The most frequently encountered causes are the Eastern, Western and Venezuelan Equine Encephalomyelitis group of Viruses and the Equine Rhinopneumonitis virus (EHV-1). Both are dealt with under Infectious diseases (page 272).

Meningitis Including Neonatal Meningitis

Meningitis is the term given to inflammation of the lining of the brain and spinal cord, the meninges. Usually fatal, it is rarely seen in adult horses and is more often encountered in neonatal (newborn) foals. Bacteria are usually implicated, particularly *Streptococcus equi* (Strangles), *Escherichia coli* and *Actinobacillus equuli*.

The very first signs are of depression, weakness and inappetance although these may vary depending on the region of the brain involved and are sometimes non-specific. Newborn foals will lose the sucking reflex and show little or no interest in the mare. As the condition progresses further signs appear, with sagging of the ears, eyelids and lips, abnormal eye movements (nystagmus), tilting of the head and strabismus (abnormal rotation of the eyeballs). Blindness may also be apparent along with loss of coordination and abnormal limb movements. Further progression leads to tremors, collapse, convulsions, concave arching of the back (opisthotonus) and eventually a state of coma.

Treatment is often difficult and needs to be given as soon as possible. Homeopathy can help alongside conventional medication.

Aconite 1M

Keynote: Early stages
This remedy should be given at the earliest stage possible before more definitive signs have appeared. Restlessness or agitation would be clues to watch for.
***Dose:** every 15–20 minutes until symptoms abate or another remedy is indicated.*

Apis 30c

Keynote: Meningeal swelling
Apis should be added where there is swelling of the meninges leading to a build up of pressure in the skull. In a practical sense this would be difficult to diagnose or confirm so it would be best to give Apis routinely to any case showing signs of depression or weakness alongside Aconite if need be.
***Dose:** every 15–20 minutes.*

Helleborus 200c

Keynote: Strabismus and depression
Indicated where there is profound depression and weakness, head tilt or strabismus.
***Dose:** four times daily*

Zinc met 30c

Keynote: Drooping lips, strabismus and trembling
Tilting or rolling of the head from side to side may well respond to Zinc when accompanied by drooping of the lids. Trembling and twitching of the limbs are also part of the Zinc symptom picture.
***Dose:** four times daily*

Laburnum 30c

Keynote: Twitching of facial muscles, wobbly gait
Symptoms likely to respond include depression accompanied by an unsteady gait and twitching of the muscles around the head. There may also be unequal dilation of the pupils.
***Dose:** four times daily*

Agaricus 30c

Keynote: Nystagmus
Specifically helps where there is nystagmus along with abnormal head movements, weakness of the back legs, trembling and muscular twitching.
***Dose:** four times daily*

Stramonium 200c

Keynote: Tremors or gentle convulsions
Useful where there is trembling or twitching of the limbs or an abnormal uncoordinated gait. Convulsive symptoms will also respond where the limbs show slow, non-violent paddling movements.
***Dose:** four times daily*

Belladonna 200c

Keynote: Violent convulsions

More severe convulsive or epileptic symptoms are more likely to respond to Belladonna. Look for rapid violent trashing of the limbs, high temperature, hot, sweaty skin and dilated pupils with glaring eyes. ***Dose:*** *four times daily*

Cicuta 200c

Keynote: Opisthotonus

This remedy is a specific for treating cases that exhibit opisthotonus, concave arching of the back with the head and tail drawn together. It will also help where the head appears drawn to one side. Cicuta is one of the specific remedies cited as helping with meningitis where the symptoms match. ***Dose:*** *every two to three hours*

Myelitis

This term refers to inflammation and the consequent changes that occur in the spinal cord usually as a result of a viral infection. The symptoms include paralysis of a muscle or group of muscles, twitching or muscle spasms, paralysis of the penis (so that it hangs down) as well as paralysis of the bladder and rectum. Further symptoms may develop as the hind limbs are affected with signs of paralysis and poor coordination. Skin sensation may be lost locally, first over the skin of the hind legs and then over the back. In severe cases the front legs will be affected as the condition progresses up the spinal cord. Remedies are listed under other conditions but specific remedies include **Oxalic acid 30c** and **Thallium 30c** with many others indicated in treating the resulting symptoms. **Dose:** *three times daily*

Nerve Paralysis

This can be temporary if a nerve has been bruised, crushed or traumatised or has been damaged in some way by an infection but is still none the less intact so that recovery is possible. These cases are worth treating using homeopathy. Long-standing paralysis cases are unlikely to benefit from treatment. There are a great many remedies for dealing with the causes and symptoms of paralysis. These are the most often prescribed remedies.

Dose: *30c twice daily*

Hypericum Paralysis resulting from trauma of any kind

Causticum Paralysis following infectious diseases, bladder paralysis

Conium Progressive, slow paralysis of the hind limbs

Curare Total paralysis

Oxalic acid Paralysis from myelitis

Gelsemium Partial paralysis or weakness of affected limbs. Paralysis following illness

Phosphorus Paralysis from nerve degeneration or neuritis

Plumbum With muscle wasting

Lathyrus Spastic paralysis

Thallium Paralysis with trembling of the limbs, chronic myelitis

Oxytropis Loss of coordination and staggering as a result of nerve paralysis

Picric acid Acute symptoms of paralysis with general debility or weakness

Nux vomica Where there is dragging of the hind limbs and back pain

Zinc Paralysis with muscle tremors, trembling or involuntary limb movements

Specific Conditions Affecting the Nervous System

Wobbler syndrome
Cervical vertebral stenotic myopathy
Cervical vertebral malformation

This condition, which can be considered a developmental or growth disorder, affects the vertebrae of the cervical spine, the section of the spine running from the back of the head down to the shoulders. Wobbler syndrome may also occur as a result of direct trauma.

Occurring most often in rapidly growing thoroughbreds, the condition is seen more often in colts than fillies but can occur in older horses of all breeds. The factors underlying wobbler syndrome are complex but almost certainly include genetics, nutrition (particularly a high calorie intake and trace mineral imbalances) and traumatic injury.

As a result of these factors the cervical vertebrae do not form correctly, with the result that either the canal which carries the spinal cord is narrowed or the vertebrae are unstable. In either situation the spinal cord becomes compressed with resulting incoordination (ataxia). The hind legs are more often affected than the front. As the horse is unsure of where it is placing its legs (which may well appear weak), the gait appears unsure or 'wobbly'.

Symptoms can be slow to develop but can on occasion appear suddenly and then either progress or remain stable as time progresses. One of the initial signs is a change in gait or lameness that may jump from front to back legs and then change from day to day, sometimes even disappearing for a while. Sometimes the toes will be dragged or if the horse is turned in small circles, the back legs will be placed in odd positions often being swung out abnormally. When walking or trotting the horse may even show an unusual bounce in its gait. Although much less badly affected, the front legs can exhibit a stiffened almost spastic gait.

Treatment is aimed at reducing or limiting the damage to the spinal cord and minimizing or resolving, as far as practical, the clinical symptoms. Homeopathy has part to play here in both acute and chronic cases, although in some cases surgery is possibly the only viable option. Either way the outcome can be variable. Where the problem is considered a developmental problem, give **Calc phos 6x** twice daily in addition to the other suggested remedies.

Suggested remedies

Hypericum 1M and **Arnica 1M** should be given immediately where trauma is suspected as the initiating cause. ***Dose:*** *three times daily for five days*

Conium 30c This is the principal remedy to use where the weakness is progressive and the horse appears to unsure where it is placing its hind legs

Oxytropis 30c Acting on the nervous system in particular, this is an important remedy and can be used in all cases which show the characteristic staggering movement or gait

Gelsemium 30c Ideal for less advanced cases where the principal symptoms are those associated with weakness

Nux vom 30c Indicated where the toes drag on the ground and symptoms are worse in the morning

Lathyrus 30c Useful where there is front limb involvement with the limbs showing a spastic gait and where the muscles of the hind limb are wasted

Cauda Equina Neuritis
Cauda Equina Syndrome
Polyneuritis Equi

The term Cauda equina (which literally means mare's tail) is applied to the group of nerve fibres that emerge and run backwards from the last part of the spinal cord. Inflammation of these fibres (neuritis) is sometimes accompanied by inflammation of some of the other nerves that leave the spinal cord. Some of the nerves which emerge directly from the brain (the cranial nerves) can also be affected.

The condition is slow and progressive and involves loss of the insulating material (myelin) from around the affected nerves. The cause is unknown but may possibly involve damage from viruses or vaccines. The most common symptoms are those of weakness, lack of muscle tone and loss of sensitivity (analgesia) of the areas around the anus, tail and pelvic regions. The horse's gait may be mildly affected but more serious signs usually include incontinence of urine (with urine scald of the skin) and incontinence of dung, constipation and flaccidity of the tail. In male animals the penis may droop, as it cannot be retracted up into the prepuce.

Where the cranial nerves are involved, the horse may show signs of facial paralysis, head tilt and rapid movement of the eyes from side to side (nystagmus).

The long-term outlook is poor but the following remedies may be of value.

Phosphorus 200c

Phosphorus is best used in the early stages when the

symptoms are only just apparent.
Dose: twice daily

Hypericum 200c

This is another remedy indicated in treating symptoms of neuritis and may well be worth consideration alongside Phosphorus. Lack of sensation (analgesia) of some of the areas of skin around the tail and perineum are an indication for the use of this remedy.
Dose: twice daily

Thuja 1M

Indicated where the symptoms arise after vaccination.
Dose: once daily for ten days then consider a more specific remedy

The following remedies are more concerned with the symptoms of paralysis which are a feature of this condition

Picric acid 30c Cases most likely to respond will show signs of paralysis accompanied by general weakness and in particular, dribbling of urine

Causticum 30c Useful where the bladder is paralysed and there is lack of skin sensation

Plumbum 30c Where there is muscle wasting and paralysis of both the bladder and rectum

Oxytropis 30c Best used where the gait is affected and there is incontinence of dung

Nux vomica 30c Indicated where there is bladder weakness gait abnormalities as the hind limbs are weak. The toes may be dragged on the ground

Alumina 30c Suitable for older animals where the hind limbs are weak and the dung is passed only after some effort. The feet may be flaky cracked and the dung dry where Alumina is needed

Gelsemium 30c For generalised weakness where the hind limbs tremble and show weakness, the bladder is paralysed and fills with urine to the extent that it dribbles out. The rectum shows partial paralysis

Conium 30c For progressive weakness of the hind limbs where urine is passed intermittently with difficulty and the gait is badly affected

Agaricus 30c Use alongside other remedies where there is nystagmus and head tilt

Cocculus 30 Add where there is facial paralysis

Dose: three times daily

Facial Paralysis

The facial nerve supplies some of the structures of the side of the face, specifically the muscles of the lips, cheeks, nostrils, ears and eyelids. Where the nerve passes behind the back of the lower jaw it is vulnerable to injury, which can result in paralysis of the affected side of the face. The typical symptoms of facial paralysis include drooping of the upper and lower lips, a sagging eyelid and ear and collapse of the nostril. The area around the mouth often looks distorted as the muscles on the good side of the face pull the lips from the affected area over to one side. Recovery usually takes some time and there may be some difficulty in feeding.

Initially treat with **Arnica 1M** and **Hypericum 1M**, giving five or six doses of each spaced out over the first day. Subsequently dose with **Hypericum 1M** twice daily for the following ten days along with the most appropriate remedy:

Causticum 30c

This is the most frequently prescribed and single most effective remedy with a predilection for being more effective where the problem is right sided. A specific pointer is where the condition arises after exposure to cold or wet weather.
Dose: twice daily for as long as needed

Cocculus 30c

Should be considered an alternative where there appears to be some discomfort when the horse opens its mouth.
Dose: twice daily for as long as needed

Other remedies which may possibly help include:

Nux vom 30c Where the problem is left sided and the horse has an irritable nature

Ammon phos 30c May help where there is a concurrent respiratory infection or where there are problems with bony changes in the joints

Gelsemium 30c Indicated where the patient appears dull, quiet or lacks interest

Senega 30c Helps where the symptoms are left sided and accompanied by a chronic, rattling cough

Other remedies worthy of consideration include: **Plumbum 30c** (where there is muscle wasting) and **Cadmium sulph 30c** (where the left side is affected) and **Curare 30c** in refractory cases.
Dose: twice daily

Sweeny, Suprascapular Nerve Paralysis, Shoulder Slip

Sweeny refers to wasting or atrophy of the two muscles that cover the shoulder blade, the supraspinatus and the infraspinatus. This arises as a result of trauma to the suprascapular nerve that supplies these muscles. Passing over the front of the shoulder blade, the nerve is subject to damage if the horse collides with a hard object, falls onto the shoulder or moves the limb backwards suddenly with considerable force.

Signs of lameness may follow the initial injury which then resolves after a few days followed by a gradual muscle wasting which appears slowly over the following few weeks. Depending on the nature and severity of the injury, the paralysis may be permanent. Where the injury is of a more minor extent, recovery will be slow and is likely to take several months. Prompt homeopathic treatment will increase the likelihood of recovery. Along with rest, other therapies such as acupuncture, ultrasonic stimulation, physiotherapy and massage are all likely to help.

Start the treatment with both **Arnica 1M** and **Hypericum 1M** *dosing alternately every 30–60 minutes for the first day and then both twice daily for the subsequent ten days.* Continue with **Hypericum 30c** on alternate days *dosing for several months if needed,* adding the following remedies where indicated:
Dose: twice daily

Curare 30c Indicated where there is complete paralysis

Causticum 30c As an alternative to Curare, especially in older horses

Gelsemium 30c Where there is partial paralysis

Plumbum 30c To slow down muscle wasting

Silica 6c To slow the development of any scar tissue around the recovering nerve

Radial Paralysis

The radial nerve supplies the muscles of the front leg which extend the elbow, knee and foot. Originating from a complex group of nerves known as the brachial plexus, the radial nerve spirals down over the humerus before branching to supply the various muscle groups. It is at this point that the nerve is most susceptible to damage either from trauma (from a kick, knock or fall for example) or from pressure (from lying down during surgery or illness).

The exact nature of the symptoms associated with radial paralysis varies and will depend on the area of the nerve that has been damaged and the nature of the injury involved. Where there is total paralysis, the elbow drops with the knee and fetlock both flexed and the toe dragging behind. The horse is unable to extend the leg forward but may compensate during movement by swinging the leg outwards. Where there is severe damage the chance of recovery is slim and the muscles of the affected limb will slowly waste.

Recovery is often very slow and may take several months. As well as using homeopathy, other therapies such as acupuncture and massage are extremely useful.

Arnica 1M and **Hypericum 1M** should be used initially *dosing alternately every 30–60 minutes* for the first day and then *twice daily for the subsequent ten days.* **Ruta 200c** can be added if the bone underlying the nerve has been traumatised and **Secale 200c** where there has been damage from pressure. *Both should be given twice daily.* Treatment should be continued with the most appropriate of the following nerve remedies which need to be given *twice daily*:

Curare 30c Indicated in complete paralysis where there is no extensor action at all

Causticum 30c Indicated in near complete paralysis

Hippomanes 30c For partial paralysis resulting in joint weakness below the elbow

Gelsemium 30c Use where there is partial paralysis and the leg is weakened or the horse's gait is affected, causing stumbling

Plumbum 30c Muscle wasting is the chief indication for this remedy

Lathyrus 30c Indicated where the toe is dragged along the ground but there are slow signs of recovery

Obdurator Paralysis

The obdurator nerve supplies some of the muscles of the hind limb and can be come damaged during foaling. Pressure on the nerve as the foal is born causes the nerve to become pinched, leading to partial paralysis of the affected back leg.

Immediate treatment with **Arnica 1M** and **Hypericum 1M** as above will help. **Bellis 200c** (every two hours) is a good alternative to Arnica if there has been considerable trauma to the pelvic region during foaling. During recovery dosing with **Gelsemium 200c** twice daily will speed up the healing process.

Crural Paralysis
Paralysis of the Femoral Nerve

The femoral nerve supplies the quadriceps group of muscles that cover the front and sides of the femur. Injury to the femoral nerve can occur as a result of trauma (over stretching of the leg), from being tied up in a recumbent position or from azoturia. Paralysis results in the horse being unable to put weight on the leg. Standing with the affected limb flexed there is difficulty moving the limb forward with the horse compensating in its gait.

Suggested remedies:

Initially **Arnica 1M, Hypericum 1M**

Follow with **Conium 30c, Curare 30c or Plumbum 30c**

Stringhalt

Stringhalt is an unusual condition that affects the back legs, the precise cause of which is unknown. One theory is that plant toxins are implicated, causing nerve damage or impairment. Plants suspected of causing problems include Catsear or False Dandelion (*Hypochaeris radicata*) in Australia and possibly Dandelion (*Taraxacum officinale*). Potentised preparations of these plants may possibly help in treatment but have not been tried. Another theory suggests that stringhalt is a manifestation of sciatica resulting from local nerve irritation or inflammation of the hip. One fact that is known for certain is that either the lateral digital extensor muscle or tendon is involved as surgical removal eases the signs associated with stringhalt.

The symptoms are normally characteristic (but may be confused with upward patella fixation) and involve an over exaggerated flexion of the hind leg or legs resulting in an odd goose-stepping gait. The degree to which this occurs can vary. It is often slight at first and appears nothing more than a mild flexion. However, in more advanced cases, the flexion can be extreme with the foot slamming down to the ground with some considerable force as the horse moves forward or the fetlock may even hit the stomach. Often as the horse warms up or when working at a faster pace, the symptoms will disappear and the horse will appear normal. If both back legs are affected the horse may exhibit a bunny hopping like gait. Severe or advanced cases may also show other neurological signs that can include muscle wasting or paralysis of the left-hand side of the larynx causing the horse to 'roar'.

Stringhalt is not easy to treat by any means although recovery is possible. The following remedies are useful in managing the condition:

Mag phos 30c

Keynote: Mild cases

Mag phos has a reputation as an antispasmodic remedy and is one of the chief remedies to be considered in treating this condition when the symptoms are not extreme. Its symptom picture covers the involuntary muscle spasms seen in stringhalt as well as nerve pain that might be associated with sciatica.

Dose: once or twice daily depending on the severity of the condition

Strychnine 1M

Keynote: Key remedy for severe cases
More severe cases are more likely to respond to Strychnine, where the flexion is violent and the foot slams down onto the ground with considerable force.
Dose: once daily

Cuprum 200c

Keynote: Where there is spasmodic flexion
Cuprum is an alternative to Mag phos and is more suited to cases where the spasmodic flexion of the leg is held for some time before the limb is relaxed. Jerking or twitching of the leg muscles is a further pointer.
Dose: once or twice daily depending on the severity of the condition

Other useful remedies

Lathyrus 30c

The nerves of the spinal cord come under the influence of this lesser known remedy whose symptoms include spastic paralysis of the hind limbs. Lathyrus should be considered where there is associated muscle wasting or where both back legs are affected.
Dose: twice daily

Cina 30c

Cina is suited to horses that have an irritable temperament and could be considered where this is accompanied by the characteristic sudden violent jerking seen with this condition and where only the left side is affected.
Dose: twice daily

Colocynthis 30c

This is another remedy linked with anger and irritability that has cramping and spasms within its symptom picture. Colocynthis should be considered for the more severe cases where the symptoms are marked and the affected leg is drawn up high.
Dose: twice daily

Causticum 30c

Causticum can be added where laryngeal paralysis is evident.
Dose: twice daily

Shivering, Shivers

Horses with this condition are sometimes described as being 'stringy'. Often confused with stringhalt, this condition affects the back legs, which are periodically bent or flexed upwards for several seconds at a time. Although this may happen when the horse is standing still, it is most likely to occur when walking, backing or turning. The affected leg may also shake and the tail may show tremors or be held up in an elevated position. In rare cases, the thigh muscles may waste a little.

Some of the remedies used for stringhalt are appropriate and should be considered namely **Mag phos**, **Strychnine**, **Cuprum**, **Colcocynthis**, **Zinc** and **Lathyrus**. The following remedies might also prove useful:

Lycopodium 30c In animals with the typical Lycopodium constitution.

Secale 30c Where there is poor circulation to the affected limb.

Strontia 30c Where there is also swelling of the hock.
Dose: twice daily

Tetanus, Lockjaw

Tetanus is one of the oldest recorded conditions in the world and one to which horses are especially susceptible in comparison to other domestic animals. Today the disease is relatively rare due to widespread conventional vaccination. Nonetheless, it is a serious condition which can include worrying complications such as pneumonia and laminitis. Tetanus is nearly always fatal; few cases survive.

The symptoms of tetanus are caused by toxins (more correctly neurotoxins which affect the nerves) released from a species of bacteria known as *Clostridium tetani*. In spore form, this bacterium can survive in the soil for a great many years. The spores do not present any problem until they gain entry to the body, which is usually through a wound. Deep penetrating wounds are the most worrying, as the spores may be deposited deep into the tissues in an anaerobic environment (one with a very low oxygen level) which favours their growth. However, Clostridial spores can gain entry to the body by a whole variety of other routes including during routine surgery such as wound stitching or castration, during foaling, from seemingly minor lacerations or small wounds and even through the umbilicus in foals.

Following entry to the body, there is an incubation period that is usually between 7 and 21 days, after which the organism multiplies and produces the toxins responsible for the symptoms characteristic of tetanus. The principal toxin causes abnormal muscle contractions or spasms triggered by even slight degree of stimulation, a condition sometimes referred to as hyperaesthesia.

The clinical signs that we associate with tetanus vary between individual animals and will depend on age, vaccination history, size of the animal and the amount of the toxin produced by the bacteria. The first symptom to be seen is usually progressive stiffness with reluctance to move which may present as an abnormality in the gait. Other symptoms of tetanus include a restriction in the range of normal jaw movement, an anxious alert expression, flaring or dilation of the nostrils, prolapse of the third eyelid, sweating and raising of the tail which is held out rigidly.

As the disease progresses the classical lockjaw symptoms appear with all four legs in spasm, held in rigid extension (the saw horse posture) together with spasm of the neck and jaw muscles. In the early stages the animal will continue to eat and drink, but as the spasms become more intense, feeding and swallowing become difficult. Saliva may run from the mouth and food may also be regurgitated.

Additional distress ensues as the animal falls over and is unable to get up. Death eventually follows a few days after the onset of symptoms from a combination of exhaustion, respiratory failure, aspiration pneumonia or cardiac arrest.

Treating tetanus

Treatment of tetanus cases is difficult and often unrewarding, despite intensive management aimed at neutralising the toxin, eliminating the bacteria responsible and alleviating the spasms. Homeopathy should be considered an adjunct to conventional treatment and as first aid therapy while waiting for conventional help. Ideally the indicated remedies should be administered in liquid potency dripped onto the mucous membranes to minimise stimulation of the patient.

Remedies for tetanus

Aconite 1M

This remedy needs to be given in the very early stages to have any effect on the course of the disease, ideally after any injury that gives rise to concern as a potential tetanus risk. Due to varying incubation time, Aconite should also be given as soon as symptoms appear.

***Dose:** hourly for six hours, longer if needed; discontinue if another remedy is indicated*

Belladonna 1M

Indications for Belladonna include rapid bounding pulse, pronounced sweating, hot feel to the skin and particularly the symptom of hyperaesthesia, which is especially marked where Belladonna is needed.

***Dose:** hourly as needed*

Cicuta 200c

This is one of the main remedies for muscle spasm and one that acts particularly on the nervous system. The keynote to its use is the intense muscle spasm associated with tetanus leading to bending of the neck, head and spine backwards. Cicuta is also indicated where spasms of the throat make feeding or swallowing difficult.

***Dose:** hourly as needed*

Strychnine 200c

The later spasmodic stages of tetanus are likely to respond well to this remedy whose symptoms include the stiffness in the muscles of the face and neck and the spasmodic arching back of the neck and spasm of the muscles of the back and those of the tail. The muscle spasms ease between paroxysms but are stimulated by the slightest touch to the body or even sounds.

Dose: every 20–30 minutes

Nux vomica 1M

Muscle spasms, particularly of the limbs and back characterise this remedy, which also has marked hypersensitivity linked with its symptom picture. The spasms are not as intense as those associated with Strychnine.
Dose: hourly as needed

Hypericum 1M

Hypericum will slow the progression of the disease along the nerve endings and is a specific remedy indicated in the treatment and prevention of tetanus.
Dose: hourly as needed

Ledum 200c

Along with Hypericum, Ledum is also indicated in the prevention and treatment of tetanus. A specific indication for Ledum is spasmodic twitching of the muscles near the site of entry of the Clostridial bacteria associated with tetanus.
Dose: hourly as needed

Opium 30c

Indicated in the early stages when there are signs of facial twitching and twitching of the limbs prior to the intense spasms of the later stages. Opium is also useful where the third eyelid is prolapsed.
Dose: every 15 minutes

Passiflora 1x

Passiflora is a general calming remedy and indicated as an antispasmodic remedy in the treatment of tetanus.
Dose: every 15 minutes

Upas 30c

This lesser known remedy is another specific for treating the symptoms of tetanus and used to help relieve the spasms seen in the later stages of the condition. Upas is also a remedy for asphyxia and can be utilised in the last stages of tetanus when muscles involved with respiration start to become affected.
Dose: every 10–15 minutes

Oenanthe crocata 30

A specific remedy for the facial area and in particular lockjaw, Oenanthe may be of help in relieving the spasms of the jaw muscle allowing the mouth to be opened a little to allow feeding support.
Dose: every 20–30 minutes

Tetanus nosode 30c

Also known as **Tetanotoxinum**, this nosode can be given alongside any of the other remedies.
Dose: once daily

Prevention of tetanus

Any suspect wound should be cleaned well and bathed well with **Hypercal mother tincture** (**Hypercal Ø**). Dilute 1 teaspoon with 1 pint of cold boiled water and bathe the wound twice daily or as needed. Where tissue trauma is involved give **Arnica 200c** routinely twice daily for five days as well.

Both **Ledum 30c** and **Hypericum 30c** should be given routinely as a preventative. *Give one dose of each twice daily for three weeks.* If the risk of tetanus is high give the **Tetanus nosode 30c** (**Tetanotoxinum 30c**) as well.

Other remedies which have a preventative role and which could be considered include: **Physostigma 30c** and **Thuja 30**.

Equine Rhinopneumonitis Virus (EHV-1) Equine Herpes Virus Type 1, Subtype 1

Infection with this virus can cause neurological symptoms. See Infectious diseases, page 272, for more details.

Epilepsy Seizures, Convulsions, Fits

Epilepsy in horses is not very common and is a condition that has not been widely investigated or researched, so that knowledge about the condition is relatively scant. Fits occur where there is abnormal electrical activity in the brain. There are a number of known triggers and conditions that can give rise to epilepsy, which is classified into two types –

idiopathic, arising from within the brain itself, and secondary, where fits occur as a result of other disease conditions.

Horses that have been poisoned or which have ingested toxins may develop epileptic fits, as can animals with liver or kidney disease, heart and circulatory problems and those with inflammatory conditions involving the brain, some of which may be viral in origin. Some nutritional and metabolic problems, brain tumours and trauma to the skull can also lead to horses developing seizures. Recorded triggers include bright lights, sudden noises, hormonal fluctuations (as in the oestrus cycle), tacking up and stress.

The symptoms can take several different forms and patterns. In some horses the seizures are very intermittent and may last only a minute or two with long gaps in between episodes of up to several months or years. Some animals will show a period of abnormal activity before a fit (the prodromal phase) that may include a period of depression or wandering around aimlessly, staring into space or pawing the ground for no reason. Others will show a depressive or sleepy phase after the fit is over, in the postictal phase. Some will show no warning symptoms before a fit occurs and will proceed to recover quickly.

During a fit, a number of symptoms can occur rapidly, which vary in severity or intensity between patients. A few horses will collapse suddenly with no warning. The limbs will jerk violently for a minute or so along with some vocalisation and then this will stop and the horse will remain recumbent for a while before getting up. With this type of fit, recovery in the postictal phase is slow.

In other horses, the fits can take a different form. The muscles go rigid, forcing the body into unusual contortions with the head and neck pulled backwards towards the chest. Remaining conscious throughout, the horse will recover quickly but will lean against the stable wall or a fence for stability.

The epileptic horse provides a challenge for both rider (in terms of safety) and for the veterinary surgeon on the grounds of safety for the rider and the horse. Riding a horse which has seizures is particularly dangerous and hazardous. Veterinary treatment using anti-convulsants will now be considered by a few veterinary surgeons.

Homeopathy can be used in some cases under the guidance of a homeopathic vet and should be considered as complementary or supportive to any other measures taken.

Suggested remedies

Dose: this depends on the frequency and severity of the fits and may range from once weekly to daily. Professional help is advised

Belladonna 1M

Keynote: Violent fits with thrashing limbs
Violent fits with dilated pupils, bounding throbbing pulse, much heat, sweating and thrashing legs.

Stramonium 1M

Keynote: Triggered by bright lights, staring into space
Fits with whinnying, pupils dilated, slower paddling of limbs, often triggered by bright lights or objects. May stare into space in the prodromal phase.

Hyoscyamus 1M

Keynote: Violence, aggression, suspicious nature
Fits in horses with an aggressive nature and which may kick out if approached, usually very vocal. Muscles may twitch along with pupil dilation. Symptoms worse during oestrus.

Cicuta 200c

Keynote: Body contorted or rigid
Body and neck contorted as muscles in total spasm. Head bent back over towards the chest along with jerky muscle movements. Pupils dilated.

Oenanthe crocata 30c

Keynote: Worse during oestrus
Fits that occur during the oestrus period usually starting with twitching of the facial muscles progressing to trashing of the limbs. Jaws are clenched tight and the pupils dilated. Back can be arched with the concave side facing upwards and legs outwards (opisthotonus).

Silica 200c

Keynote: Worse at full moon, after vaccination
Epileptic fits arising as a sequel to vaccination or

which occurs specifically at full moon.

Cuprum met 200c

Keynote: Spasms or twitching in the legs
Convulsions originating in the lower limbs suggest cuprum especially where the facial muscles are in spasm and pulled back tightly. Legs tend to go into jerky spasms or twitch in short episodes.

Strychnine 200c

Keynote: Tetanic spasms, triggered by least stimulation
Violent tetanic spasms with opisthotonus with the muscles relaxing between spasms. These are triggered by the slightest stimulation be that touch, movement or noise. Muscles of the neck and back are tight and very hard when touched.

Plumbum 30c

Keynote: Debility
Convulsions in debilitated horses with weak muscles or in those horses with kidney disease.

Ignatia 1M

Keynote: Emotional trigger, hysteria
Epilepsy in flighty, sensitive horses that tend to be jumpy or nervy. Epilepsy arising from grief or emotional shock. Muscles tend to twitch.

Other useful remedies:

Lachesis 200c Keynote: Suspicious nature, worse before oestrus

Passiflora 3x Keynote: From anxiety

Phosphorus 30c Keynote: Where there is concurrent liver disease

Bufo 30c Keynote: Fits occurring during sleep

Agaracus 30c Keynote: With persistent ataxia

The Skin

The skin is by far the largest visible organ in the body and performs a variety of vital functions. It acts as a barrier, protecting the body from trauma and injury, from infection by micro-organisms, from the harmful effects of sunlight and prevents the entry of toxic or poisonous substances. It prevents dehydration and yet helps regulate body temperature through sweating, shivering and control of the position of the hair shafts. It allows the body to be aware of its environment through the sensations of touch, pain, pressure and the appreciation of temperature. The many glands that the skin contains secrete some of the body's waste products whilst others produce important hormones called pheromones that are involved in stimulating sexual behaviour. The skin also manufactures vitamin D and is an integral part of the body's immune system.

There are two very distinct layers to the skin. The epidermis is the outermost protective layer and has no blood supply and it composed of soft keratin. This layer is further sub-divided into several other layers the outermost of which is the hardened, dryer, horny layer of the epidermis. The epidermis varies in thickness depending on the area of the body being thickest over the back and thinner on the face, lower abdomen and neck. Where the climate is temperate or cold, hair is produced in the winter months to provide extra insulation. Other than the hair of the mane and tail, new hair grows annually, stimulated by the increasing daylight length of the spring, gradually replacing the old hairs, which are shed.

Underlying the epidermis is the layer known as the dermis. This layer is composed of collagen and other interwoven fibres connecting the epidermis to the subcutaneous tissues underneath. The dermis contains blood and lymphatic vessels, nerves, hair follicles, sweat and sebaceous glands and provides nutrition, support and strength to the epidermis. It also contains the small arrector pili muscles which attach to the hair shafts and control the position of the hairs. These play an important part in temperature regulation of the body. The subcutaneous layer under the dermis is composed of loose fatty connective tissue allowing mobility of the skin over deeper layers. This layer also contains the panniculus muscle, a large sheet of muscle which contracts to generate body heat by shivering.

As the skin is such a vital part of the body, its condition reflects the general state of health of the animal and the environment in which it is living. Poor conditions and poor nutrition will be reflected in the condition of the skin. Concurrent conditions such as liver disease, cancer, diarrhoea, dehydration, parasitic infections (including heavy worm burdens), bowel damage and ingestion of certain poisonous plants can all have an impact on the way the skin appears or how it reacts. The result may be hair loss, itching, inflammation, scaling, scabbing, alteration in elasticity, thickening and a variety of other changes.

Basic Skin Conditions

This section deals with the fundamental and basic skin conditions that are seen in horses as opposed to specific skin conditions which are dealt with in a later section. Detailed are the most commonly used remedies to help with each condition.

Alopecia

Alopecia is the term applied to loss of hair which can be complete or partial and either temporary or permanent. The latter occurs where the hair follicles have been destroyed and replaced with fibrous tissue. This can occur following third degree burns, severe infections, chemical damage or severe skin injury. There is no definitive treatment for this type of alopecia unless appropriate remedies are used to minimise any scarring during healing in the hope of saving some follicles. Indicated remedies include: **Graphites**, **Silica**, **Calc fluor** and **Thiosinaminum**. *Dose: using the 30c potency three times daily whilst healing takes place*

Temporary alopecia is far more common and results from self-inflicted trauma which is secondary to a primary cause which need to be established. In general the following remedies will help with the re-growth of hair if correctly matched to the underlying accompanying symptoms.
Dose: twice daily with the indicated potency

Arsenicum album 30c
Hair loss associated with itching and scaling (dandruff).

Fluoric acid 6c
General hair loss associated with ageing, ulcers or scars which appear to cause irritation.

Natrum muriaticum 30c
Indicated where the condition is linked with pining or grief and where the horse appears depressed and lacks energy. Hair loss resulting from some types of eczema will also respond.

Carbo veg 30c
Indicated for aged animals where there is general loss of vitality and condition.

Abrotanum 30c
This is an excellent remedy for aged horses where there are signs of alopecia accompanied by weight loss yet despite a good appetite. The hair loss is often patchy and the remaining hair dry and without lustre.

Pix liquida 6c
Alopecia accompanied by intense irritation with cracked and sore skin often responds to this remedy.

Phosphoric acid 30c
Indicated for hair loss accompanied by generalised debility from another underlying condition.

Selenium 30c
Will help with hair loss over head area and over the lower limbs where there is scaling and slight itching.

Sepia 6c
Helpful where there is hair loss associated with greasy skin or where the skin is thickened. Alopecia linked with some types of eczema will also respond.

Lycopodium 6c
Will help with hair loss resulting from liver disease.

Thallium 6c
Thallium is a general remedy that will help stimulate the growth of hair irrespective of cause.

Thyroidinum 6x
Another remedy to generally stimulate the growth of hair. It will also help where hair loss is associated with malnutrition or where the skin looks very dry or in poor condition.

Abrasions or grazes

An abrasion is superficial patchy loss of the epidermis often resulting in a little capillary bleeding but with some degree of pain. This sort of skin injury is likely to be seen in horses that slip when being loaded into horse boxes or which slip on rough surfaces like concrete. The area should be cleaned with diluted **Hypercal lotion** to remove debris and dirt, dried and then **Calendula** cream applied to stimulate healing. This should be carried out twice daily. *Dose with:*

Arnica 30c *three times daily* until the area is healed. Helps to stimulate healing and to reduce bruising and risk of infection.

Hypericum 30c *three times daily* if there is evidence of pain. This remedy will also reduce the chance of tetanus developing.

Abscesses

The definition of an abscess is a collection of pus or infected material within an enclosed area or cavity. Abscesses form under the skin for a variety of reasons, often initiated by entry of an infection through a minor wound. Penetration of the skin by a

foreign body can also result in the formation of an abscess, which develops as the body tries to expel the foreign or infected material. Encouraging the abscess to burst by poulticing is often beneficial to bring it to a head and then to draw out the material inside. Remedies to help include:
Dose: three or four times daily

Hepar sulph 6x
Keynote: Abscess promotion/maturation
This low potency will encourage developing abscesses to increase in size, with the aim of bringing the problem to a head so that the abscess will burst and discharge its contents. After this stage has been achieved, switch to one of the other indicated remedies.

Hepar sulph 200c
Keynote: Suppuration with pain
In higher potency this remedy will help abort acute abscesses which are painful to the least touch. It will also help with discharging abscesses either acute or chronic in nature, where pain is a marked feature and the discharge is of a foul suppurative nature.

Silica 30c
Keynote: Chronic suppuration without pain
Silica is the primary remedy to consider where a foreign body is involved as it will help the push the material to the surface for discharging to the exterior. Silica is also indicated in chronic conditions where the abscess is draining and discharging pus but has not yet resolved. The affected area shows little or no pain in contrast to Hepar sulph. This remedy will also help break down and shrink chronic hardened abscessed areas and will abort small cold abscesses before they have a chance to develop further.

Calc sulph 30c
Keynote: Stubborn discharging abscesses
This remedy is useful where an abscess is open and discharging, particularly if the pus is yellowish in colour and thick in texture. Long-standing discharging abscesses will often respond where other remedies have failed to help.

Arnica 200c
Keynote: After local injury
Helpful where an abscess develops locally after an injury where there is tissue degeneration. Arnica will also help abscesses that fail to mature.

Lachesis 200c
Keynote: With skin discoloration
For abscesses where the skin is markedly discoloured with a blue or purplish tinge and where there may be a surrounding area of cellulitis. The affected area feels hot. Lachesis will also help if any of the skin areas involved have become gangrenous.

Pyrogen 1M
Keynote: With fever and sepsis
For abscesses accompanied by sepsis and fever and where the pus is very foul in character. Pyrogen is also useful where the most minor of wounds becomes grossly septic.

Merc sol 200c
Keynote: Green coloured pus
Useful where the pus is green in colour and which may contain traces of blood.

Asafoetida 30c
Keynote: Watery pus and local swelling
Most useful where the pus is of a more watery appearance and where the surrounding tissues are swollen and puffy.

Tarentula cubenisis 30c
Keynote: With acute pain and skin discoloration
Indicated in abscesses where pain is a very prominent feature and where the surface of the skin is discoloured.

Myristica sebifera 30c
Keynote: Difficult cases
This little known remedy has great antiseptic powers and will often help with acute and chronic abscesses where other indicated remedies have failed to have any effect. Helps especially where trauma is involved.

Calc carb 30c
Keynote: Deep abscesses
This remedy will help with the resorption of pus in

abscesses that are deep within the tissues of the body.

Bites and stings

Hypercal lotion should be the first line of treatment to clean the area, which should then be inspected to ascertain the damage. Always give **Ledum 30c** *every 15 minutes for four doses as soon as possible*. This remedy is indicated in all puncture type wounds whatever the cause and should be used alongside the most appropriate other remedies. Dosing with Ledum will also significantly reduce the risk of tetanus occurring.

Bites from other animals

Arnica 200c ***Dose:*** *three times daily* until the wound has healed.

Hepar sulph 200c ***Dose:*** *three times daily* to reduce the risk of infection.

Calendula 30c ***Dose:*** *twice daily* where healing is slow.

Clean the area with diluted **Hypercal lotion** *twice daily* until the area has healed completely.

From insects

Apis 200c ***Dose:*** *three times daily* if puffy, swollen, large patches appear over the skin like hives.

Vespa 30c ***Dose:*** *three times daily* if the puffy areas are small and very itchy.

Urtica 30c ***Dose:*** *three times daily* if there is much skin irritation.

Antipyrine 6c where there is intense itching all over with the sudden appearance of small swollen plaques of skin. ***Dose:*** *four times daily*

Bovista 30c use where large areas of skin puff up after a bite or where affected areas go weepy and then crust to form scabs. ***Dose:*** *three times daily*

Rhus tox 30c use if cellulitis develops. ***Dose:*** *four times daily*

From snakes

Snakebites need urgent veterinary help. Clean the area with diluted **Hypercal lotion** as needed.

Whilst waiting use:

Lachesis 200c indicated if the skin around the bite is discoloured with a bluish or purple hue. The affected area will be swollen, and oozing dark fluid. Cellulitis may be present. ***Dose:*** *hourly*

Crotalus horridus 30c works best where there is considerable swelling and pain. This remedy will also help where lymphangitis has developed as a result of a bite or where the area has become grossly septic. ***Dose:*** *hourly*

Echinacea 6x can be added where there is sepsis, lymphangitis or risk of gangrene.

Burns and scalds

Pour cold water over the affected area as soon as possible to take away the heat. For smaller areas a cold compress can be used instead. Dose immediately with:

Arnica 200c *every ten minutes for three doses* to limit tissue damage then:

Cantharis 30c *every 10–15 minutes for up to ten doses* then *three times daily* until the area is healed. Cantharis will help reduce the pain and blistering of serious burns.

Urtica 30c can be used if the area is very uncomfortable. ***Dose:*** *three times daily*

Apis 30c for more minor burns with pain, swelling and inflammation. ***Dose:*** *three times daily*. Apis is often the remedy of choice for chemical burns.

Carbolic acid 6c can be used if the burnt area ulcerates with an offensive discharge. ***Dose:*** *four times daily*

Causticum 30c is indicated where healing is slow or where there is scarring of the area with residual pain. Causticum is also useful for older burns that remain painful or uncomfortable. ***Dose:*** *three times daily*

Burns should be cleaned twice daily with **Calendula**

lotion to soothe the area and to stimulate healing. Alternatively use a combination of **Cantharis Ø** and **Urtica Ø** (mother tinctures), diluting 1 teaspoon (5ml) with 500ml of water. Applying **Urtica** ointment after cleaning will also help soothe affected areas.

Bruising and contusions

A contusion occurs when there is trauma to the skin and underlying tissues without the skin being broken. The underlying tissues will be bruised, painful and swollen to a varying degree depending on the extent of the injury. In many horses, the purple, black discoloration of the skin due to the bruising and subcutaneous bleeding is not always easy to see.

The main remedy to consider here is Arnica. For slight to moderate bruising use **Arnica 30c** and *dose three times daily* until the area has healed. For more severe bruising use **Arnica 200c**, dosing *three times daily for five days* and then twice daily until the bruising has resolved. There are also several other remedies to consider.

Dose: two or three times daily according to the severity of the symptoms.

Bellis perennis 30c is a specific remedy for deep bruising and is also useful after surgery to the abdomen. It works especially well for bruising to the pelvic area.

Ledum 30c can be used for bruising around the site of a puncture wound. Ledum is helpful for contused bruises or where the area remains swollen long after the injury despite the use of other remedies.

Hamamelis 30c will help reduce congestion around the bruised area, especially where there is swelling.

Sulphuric acid 30c can help where severe bruising leads to damage of the underlying tissues and the overlying skin is livid purple or blue in colour. This remedy will also help where damaged areas of skin are likely to become gangrenous or are slow to heal.

Haematoma

A haematoma is a sizeable accumulation of blood under the skin, which forms a clot following local trauma. Initially the area will be painful with surrounding areas of skin often showing evidence of contusion. Typical causes include falls, kicks or blows from blunt objects. The brisket area is a common site for a haematoma to appear after a fall. Treatment should involve dosing with **Arnica 30c** or **Arnica 200c** (depending of the severity of the problem) *twice daily*, along with **Hamamelis 30c** *twice daily* until the haematoma has resolved. Where progress is slow consider changing remedies and using both **Silica 30c** and **Calc fluor 30c** *once daily* over a period of several weeks. **Lachesis 30c** *given twice daily* is useful where the skin takes on a purple hue and the blood is slow to clot. **Phosphorus 30c**, **Secale 30c** or **Crot horr 30c** can also be effective in resolving haematomas that fail to clot easily or which do not reabsorb effectively. *Dose three times daily.*

Cellulitis

Cellulitis is a term applied to an infection, normally bacterial, which spreads along the tissues underlying the surface of the skin. Affected areas are swollen or puffy and painful to touch. Ideal remedies to help are:

Arnica 200c *give two or three doses over 15–20 minutes* followed by:

Rhus tox 30c Is the most useful remedy in resolving this condition.

Apis 30c Can be used where there is much swelling, pain and heat.

Hepar sulph 200c Where there is pus like discharge or where the area is painful to the slighted touch.

Manganum acetate 30c Is indicated for cellulitis around the areas of joints.

Lachesis 200c Useful where the skin is grossly discoloured (blue, black or with a purple colour) and hot to touch.

Myristica sebifera 6c A good general antiseptic remedy to consider where the skin is inflamed as well.
These remedies should be used two or three times daily depending on the severity of the problem.

Cysts

A cyst is a fluid filled cavity where no inflammation is present. Remedies useful in the treatment of cysts in the skin are:

Graphites 30c Where the cyst weeps a clear, sticky fluid.

Baryta carb 30c A general remedy for cysts in older horses.

Calc carb 30c For cysts in the heavy breeds.

Sabina 30c Is useful where there are also warts present.

Silica 30c For cysts which are harder in texture or which have become fibrosed or scarred internally.

Dose: once daily for a period of six or seven weeks.

Gangrene

Gangrene is tissue death or necrosis through lack of blood supply. This can arise through swelling and inflammation of the affected area of skin or from a wound or cut which interrupts or cuts off the blood supply. Indicated remedies are:

Secale 30c For dry gangrene and where the skin appears shrivelled up.

Carbo veg 30c Where there is general loss of condition and deep ulcers with gangrenous skin on the outer edges or where dead skin overlies an offensive and purulent infection.

Lachesis 30c Gangrene from wounds which result in a septic infection and where the edges are blue-black in colour.

Arsenicum album 30c For gangrene with inflammation and from wounds where the affected part of the body feels cold.

Causticum 30c Is recommended for gangrene arising from old burns or deep ulcers which are not healing well.

Anthracinum 30c Gangrene from burns and from gross sepsis where there is swelling

China 30c Indicated in cases of gangrene where the affected tissues are moist rather than dry.

Use the most appropriate remedy and dose four times daily

Excoriation or intertrigo

This occurs when the superficial layer of skin, the epidermis, is rubbed or chaffed away from an area of the body leaving the underlying tissues sore and inflamed. Affected areas should be bathed twice daily in **Hypercal lotion** to soothe and clean up the area. Initially give a single dose of **Arnica 200** as soon as the problem is noticed followed by:

Hypericum 30c If the area is especially sensitive and painful. *Dose: twice daily until healed.*

Calendula 30c To initiate healing. *Dose: twice daily until healed.*

Graphites 30c Indicated if the area is raw and weeping a clear coloured fluid. *Dose: twice daily until healed.*

Causticum 30c Indicated if the lesions are in folds of skin and where there is much rawness and soreness. *Dose: twice daily until healed.*

Sulphur 6c Can be used for older infected areas that are healing poorly. *Dose: three times daily until healed.*

Fissures and Cracked Skin

A fissure is a crack or a split in the skin, usually due to dryness or loss of elasticity. Secondary infection can lead to further problems. Remedies to help include:

Graphites 30c The best remedy to use if the skin is exuding a sticky, honey-coloured secretion. Graphites is useful if the cracked or fissured areas of skin are painful.

Petroleum 30c Will help where the skin has become very dry, thick and leathery. The cracks in the skin bleed easily and the affected area is sensitive to touch.

Pix liquida 6c A remedy to consider where there is excessive irritation associated with the cracks. Bleeding from the skin may also be noted.

Kali ars 30c Indicated for fissures which are present

in the bends of the joints. Itching is a feature and is worse in warm weather.

Sarsaparilla 6c Will help in older horses where there has been loss of condition resulting in some degree of emaciation. Check for areas of skin that are cracked and hard, especially in the folds.

Dose: once or twice daily over a period of several weeks depending on the severity of the problem.

Hyperkeratosis or thickening
Flakey feathers

This is basically an increase in the thickness of the horny layer of the epidermis. The overall effect is to make the skin leathery, hard and less pliable. Callouses fall into this category. In some areas the thickened skin will become fissured and may become infected, sore and weepy. Where the condition occurs behind the carpal joints (knees) or pasterns in horses with feathers, the condition is referred to as flakey feathers and can be associated with chorioptic mange (see page 258).

The remedies listed need to be given *twice daily*.

Antimonium crudum 6c Will help where there are thick scabs present as well. Other skin lesions may also be evident including pustules, warts and dry areas of skin.

Hydrocotyle 6c Will help where there is excessive skin thickening and lots of scaling (dandruff) present.

Graphites 30c Indicated where the affected areas are weepy, exuding a sticky, honey coloured secretion.

Petroleum 30c Will help where the skin has become very dry, thick, leathery and cracked. The cracks in the skin bleed easily and affected areas are sensitive to touch.

Rhus tox 6c Helpful where the thickened areas are sore, inflamed and very itchy.

Sepia 30c Is useful where the skin is thickened, itchy and has a bad odour. Sepia works best if the affected areas are near the bends of the limbs.

Sulphur 30c Will help where the skin looks generally unhealthy.

Eczema and dermatitis

These are general non-specific terms used to describe skin problems that cannot be identified easily as specific conditions. The triggers for these problems are varied and may involve factors such as stress, feeding, and environment. The underlying cause may be bacterial, viral, fungal or even allergic in nature. Visible lesions and symptoms may include hair loss, scabbing, weeping, crusting, dandruff, inflammation and reddening of the skin, swelling, pustules, vesicles, nodules, itching, rubbing, changes in skin texture and pigmentation, seborrhoea and ulceration.

Try to identify the problem and refer to the relevant skin section. Where this is not possible check the list at the end of this section to find the remedies that most accurately match the symptoms.

Dandruff or pityriasis
Scaling

Dandruff or scaling is not a condition in its own right, but rather a symptom of another underlying problem. Where there is mild scaling, this may simply be associated with poor diet, a heavy parasitic burden, bad stabling and care or lack of proper grooming. More severe cases may be linked with other underlying conditions as liver disease, skin parasites (such as lice and mange) or with other skin conditions.

Typically the scales appear of a bran-like nature or as white flakes, either on the surface of the skin or intermingled with the hair. Remedies to help on a symptomatic basis include:

Arsenicum album 200c

Arsenicum suits fine-skinned animals that show signs or either being anxious or restless. The scales are small and fine in nature and most commonly found in the hair of the mane, withers region and tail base area.
Dose: three times weekly

Arsenicum iodatum 200c

This remedy will help where the skin is dry and scaly and where the scales are larger. The skin underlying the scaly lesions is sore and weepy. Some areas of skin in chronic cases will show thickening.
Dose: three times weekly

Kali sulph 30c
The scaling which responds to this remedy is more yellow in colour and may be associated with ringworm, non-specific eczema, greasy seborrrhoeic skin or a rash.
Dose: *once daily*

Sepia 200c
This remedy will help where there is thickening of the skin, ringworm or greasy, oily skin. Mares are more likely to respond, especially those of a more sullen, slow character.
Dose: *three times weekly*

Lycopodium 1M
Lycopodium suits horses of a lean build with an apprehensive nature. Scaly areas of skin most likely to respond include areas where the skin is thickened with dry patchy hair loss, wrinkling or where there is seborrhoea.
Dose: *three times weekly*

Sulphur 30c
Sulphur will help where the skin is generally unhealthy and looks poorly cared for. Some animals will also have a musty skin odour and show signs of mild irritation and other skin lesions such as scabs, pustules or sores.
Dose: *once daily*

Nat mur 30c
Nat mur will help where the skin and coat are especially dry or show greasy areas. Scaling is particularly evident around the bends of the joints and along the mane and region of the withers as well as the tail base. Horses which respond well to this remedy are thirsty, sometimes sullen in character and do not always socialise well with other animals.
Dose: *once daily*

Badiaga 30c
This remedy will help where there is scaling confined to the head area only.
Dose: *once daily*

Seborrhoea, Greasy skin

This term refers to an excess of sebum production by the skin, so that it appears greasy or oily and sometimes has a musty odour as well. Seborrhoea in horses does not often occur as a primary condition as it does in humans but is normally associated with some other type of skin condition such as eczema, dermatitis or skin allergies. In horses, seborrhoea sometimes occurs as an exudative dermatitis, more commonly known as greasy heel or mud fever, and is restricted to the lower limbs (see page 225). Remedies listed under this heading will help.

More generalised seborrhoea is less common, nevertheless some horses do show seborrhoeic dermatitis over large areas of the body. Useful remedies which should be used constitutionally where possible include: **Lycopodium** (which has a special regulatory effect on sebaceous secretions from the skin), **Sepia**, **Sulphur**, **Kali sulph**, **Nat mur**, **Psorinum**, **Selenium**, **Arsenicum album**, **Iodum** and **Vinca**.
Dose: *use the 30c potency twice daily until an improvement is seen*

Scarring

A scar forms where a wound or lesion has healed leaving fibrous (scar) tissue behind. This is often visible as a blemish on the skin. Due to the nature of fibrous tissue and depending on the area of the scar, there will be some loss of elasticity. The following remedies will help reduce scarring.

Silica
This is a key remedy in helping to prevent scarring and in the reduction of old scars. It will help where old scar tissue becomes sensitive or painful or where there is along standing infection present. Silica has a good reputation in the dissolution of old scar tissue and of hardened fibrous nodules.
Dose: *30c once daily until the problem has resolved.*

Graphites
The keynote for Graphites is acute suppuration or infection. Where there are infected wounds, this remedy will assist healing and help prevent the formation of scar tissue at the site at the site of the injury. Graphites will also help with scars that have a very hard texture and scarring arising from burns.

Dose: 30c once daily until healing is complete.

Calc fluor
Will help with scar tissue in general but works especially well where the scar tissue feels very hard and knotty.
Dose: 30c once daily

Fluoric acid
Fluoric acid will help where there is scarring accompanied by irritation.
Dose: 6c once daily for many weeks

Thiosinaminum
This remedy has a reputation for dissolving scar tissue and adhesions and can be used to help reduce or dissolve away old scars.
Dose: 6c potency once daily for many weeks

Acetic acid
Over a period of months, this remedy can dissolve away some of the fibrous nodules that can arise in scarred tissue.
Dose: 6c potency once daily for many weeks

Calendula
Calendula will help where a wound is not healing properly and where there is a risk of scar tissue forming. The main action of this remedy is to ensure that wounds heal cleanly with the minimum of scarring.
Dose: 6c potency three times daily until the area has healed

Sinus or fistula

This is a channel that opens to the outside through the skin and which allows drainage of infected material (usually pus) to the exterior of the body from underlying tissues. The origin of the infection should be determined and surgically dealt with where practical. Remedies that will help include:

Silica
This is the most important remedy to try to help resolve sinus problems especially in long-standing cases where there is a discharge of pus-like material. A pointer to its use is the absence of pain in the region of the sinus. Where foreign material is the root cause, this remedy will help the body to expel the offending material. Care needs to be exercised where surgical implants are involved (such as screws) as the remedy may cause unwarranted problems unless the implants are removed first. Silica is also the primary remedy of choice where lymphatic glands are involved.
Dose: 30c potency once or twice daily increasing to 200c daily as the problem resolves

Fluoric acid
The special sphere of action of this remedy is the face and teeth where it will help with dental fistulae and sinuses that involve the region of the upper jaw.
Dose: 30c twice daily until the problem resolves.

Calc carb
Useful for deep-seated sinuses in heavy breeds where it can be used alongside Silica to help resolve a problem
Dose: 200c three times weekly

Calc sulph
This remedy is indicated in stubborn cases where the discharge is thick, lumpy or yellow in colour.
Dose: 30c twice daily

Other less important remedies to be considered are:

Hepar sulph 30c Indicated where there is much pain around the area of the sinus.

Phosphorus 30c An alternative to consider where lymphatic glands are involved.
Dose: twice daily

Proud flesh or exuberant granulation

Proud flesh occurs at the site of a wound when the body overreacts and produces an excessive amount of healing granulation tissue. This type of tissue normally forms during the healing process and encourages the wound to contract whilst protecting it at the same time. When produced in excess, the tissue will stand proud of the wound and will need attention if the area is to heal properly. This problem is common and often occurs on the limbs as the result of a cut or similar wound. Suitable remedies to help are listed below. In most cases you should seek professional help as well.

Nitric acid 200c
This is the principal remedy to consider using to help treat this condition.
Dose: twice daily until the area has healed

Thuja 30c
Thuja should be considered for stubborn cases or where Nitric acid fails to act.
Dose: twice daily

Calendula 30c
This remedy is also recommended in the treatment of proud flesh and will help speed up the healing process.
Dose: twice daily

Arsenicum album 30c
Useful where the condition is linked with poor general vitality and ongoing sepsis in the affected area.
Dose: twice daily

Other useful remedies to consider include **Flouric acid**, **Graphites** and **Silica**.
Use the 30c potency and dose twice daily.

Decubitus or pressure sores

Saddle sores or saddle galls also come under this heading. Persistent pressure on a particular area of skin (such as might occur in a recumbent animal) will result in the death of the skin at the point of most pressure followed by an ulcer. Similarly poor fitting tack (which includes the saddle and bridle in particular) which rubs and chaffs underlying skin can cause hair loss, inflammation, skin thickening and eventually ulceration. Needless to say, all tack should be checked regularly and the necessary adjustments made. Recumbent animals should be turned regularly to avoid pressure sores occurring and adequate bedding should be provided.

Ulcerated areas of skin should be cleaned regularly with **Hypercal lotion** and then **Calendula cream** applied. Useful remedies include **Secale 6c**, **Muriaticum acidum 6c** and **Calendula 30c**.
***Dose** twice daily. Some of the ulcer remedies listed below may also help.*

Ulcers

An ulcer occurs when there is complete loss of the epidermis revealing the underlying dermis. The most common cause of ulcers is wearing away of the skin over pressure points. Remedies that will help include:

Nitric acid 30c Will help with ulcers that bleed freely or those associated with cancerous skin lesions.

Mezerium 30c Will help with ulcers that have an overlying crust or where there is a yellow discharge. Ulcers of this type usually itch.

Kali bich 30 Will help with very deep ulcers.

Merc sol 30 Suits dirty or mucky looking ulcers with a rough margin.

Silica 30 Will help ulcers which are associated with a sinus or fistula. It will also help with stubborn or slow healing ulcers.

Muriaticum acidum 6c Suits ulcers which appear on the lower parts of the legs and which have a foul discharge.

Arsenicum album 30c Helps where there is an offensive discharge or with suppurating cancerous ulcers. This remedy will also help with ulcers associated with gangrene.

Dose: twice daily until the area has healed.

Vitiligo or hypopigmentation

This is the loss of skin pigmentation and is not at all common. It is most likely to be seen in Shires or Arabians where the areas affected include the sides of the face and the eyelids. Affected areas appear pink with some hair loss as well.The cause is unknown but it can occur following surgery or cryosurgery as this destroys the pigment producing cells in the skin. **Thuja 30c** and **Sepia 30c** are the two remedies most likely to help.
Dose: twice daily.

Wounds

In general

Initial treatment depends on the cause and nature of the wound. Regardless of the type of wound, start treatment with *three or four doses* of **Arnica 200c** given over the first day. Continue over the following days, *dosing twice daily* until the wound has healed. All wounds should be cleaned with diluted **Hypercal lotion** *twice daily*.

Where a fever develops following a wound, use **Pyrogen 1M,** dosing every hour until an improvement is seen. For suppurating, infected wounds use **Hepar sulph 200c**, *three times daily* and for slow healing, chronic wounds use **Silica 200c** or **Graphites 200c**.

The other remedies which will help with slow healing wounds are **Calendula 30c** and **Carcinosin 30c**. Wounds which bleed should be treated with **Lachesis 30c** where there is dark oozing blood, **Phosphorus 30c** where there is continued bleeding from even the smallest wound and **Millefolium 30c** for wounds that bleed freely.

Dose every hour until the bleeding stops.

Puncture wounds

This type of wound is caused by the penetration of the skin by a sharp object such as a stake or from a bite. Injection sites can also be considered to be puncture wounds.

Use **Ledum 30c** (*dose three times daily*) to reduce the risk of tetanus and to prevent infection. **Hepar sulph 200c** should be used where the risk of infection is great or where the wound is very sensitive to touch. This remedy should be used where infection or suppuration is already apparent. *Dose three times daily.* Where much pain is evident add **Hypericum 30c** *three times daily.*

Cuts, lacerations and tears

Injuries of this nature are often the result of becoming entwined with barbed wire. Use **Hypericum 30c** *three times daily* to help with the pain and to reduce the risk of tetanus. Where there is continued bleeding try **Phosphorus 30c** dosing *every 30 minutes* until the bleeding stops. **Calendula 30c** will help specifically with healing wounds of this nature. *Dose three times daily.*

Incised wounds

This type of wound can be caused maliciously with a knife or blade and has clean clear, cut edges. Surgical wounds also fall into this category. Giving either **Hypericum 30c** or **Staphysagria 30c** (especially where the horse appears irritable) *three times daily* can help with the pain aspect. Where there is seepage of blood following wound suturing consider *dosing every 30 minutes* with **Millefolium 30c** or with **Strontia 30c** where there is also evidence of shock.

Specific Skin Conditions

Photosensitisation and Sunburn

This is an uncommon condition in which the skin becomes reactive to ultraviolet light in those areas that lack pigmentation. This means that the condition is normally limited to the white areas of the skin which naturally lack pigmentation and is essentially a form of sunburn. Exposed, hairless areas are particularly likely to be affected including the ear tips, nose and muzzle.

There are two underlying types. In primary or direct photosensitisation the skin becomes susceptible to UV radiation due to ingestion of plants containing photosensitising agents. These compounds can be found in plants such as St John's Wort (*Hypericum perforatum*) and dried Buckwheat plants and seeds (*Polygonum fagopyrum*). Initially there is an increase in skin irritation seen as rubbing and ear flicking. As the condition progresses the skin becomes inflamed, red and swollen and will eventually start to peel and will ooze serum from the exposed red raw areas. As the inflammation subsides, scabs will form and healing will slowly take place. In some horses, such as skewbald and piebald animals, large areas of skin can become involved.

Underlying liver disease or damage can trigger secondary or indirect hepatogenous photo-sensitisation. In this case, liver damage (caused by ingestion of poisonous plants in most cases), results in poor excretion of a compound called phylloerythrin. This is a normal breakdown product of chlorophyll, the pigment found in green plants. As this substance builds up, the skin is sensitised to UV light and reacts as detailed above.

Moving the horse out of direct sunlight is the first and most obvious immediate course of action. You should also prevent ingestion of any further poisonous material. The choice of remedies to use will depend partly on the initiating cause and partly on the stage of the condition.

Early stages – rubbing and itching

Dose: four times daily

Urtica 30c useful in the very early stages where the only symptoms are those of itching or rubbing.

Fagopyrum 6c can be used where Buckwheat ingestion is involved. It is also indicated where there is much itching and there are a few sore red blotches appearing.

Sol 6c can be used as a general remedy in the early stages.

Hypericum 30c is indicated where St John's Wort is the initiating cause and where itching is the only symptom to be seen.

Proteus 30c. This remedy can be used for severe burn cases. It is also an excellent remedy for recurrent cases of photosensitisation. The dose in this instance should be **Proteus 200c** given *once every four weeks.*

Intermediate stage–inflammation, reddening and swelling

Dose: three times daily

Apis 200c is useful where the skin is swollen and has a red or purple appearance. Apis will also help where there are a few weepy sores present. Affected animals will be restless.

Belladonna 1M can be used where the inflammation is extremely severe and the area is red, hot, painful and very swollen.

Later stages – blistering and weeping

Dose: four times daily

Rhus venenata 30c Useful where itching and irritation are prominent symptoms with evidence of blisters and accompanying dermatitis.

Rhus tox 30c Again this remedy is useful where irritation is much in evidence. Affected areas of skin are swollen, weepy and moist. Underlying tissues may show evidence of cellulitis.

Cantharis 30c Cantharis will help where the skin is intensely inflamed and where there are vesicles and blistering. The skin appears very raw and sore.

Later stages – scabbing and healing

Dose: three times daily

Ant crud 6c This remedy is best used in later stages where scabs have formed over the affected areas and healing has started. This remedy helps especially where the nose is involved.

Calendula 6c This useful remedy helps speeds healing in the final stages.

Where the liver is involved

Dose: once daily

Chelidonium 30c This can be used as a good general remedy to stimulate the liver and aid repair.

Nux vomica 30c Ideally best used where there are symptoms of poisoning accompanying other liver symptoms.

Skin Conditions with an Allergic Basis

Urticaria
Hives
Allergic reactions
Nettle rash
Anaphylaxis

The sudden appearance of variable sized plaques or wheals on the skin is usually the result of an allergic reaction and is a relatively common problem. There are various different causes. Most often insects are involved (such as the stable fly) but the list of allergens also includes foods (such as concentrate proteins or the proteins in fresh grass), drugs, vaccines, plants and trees (such as willow), as well as a number of specific, often unidentifiable, allergens. Reactions resembling urticaria can also occur in a condition known as purpura haemorrhagica (see page 103). This can occur following certain infections including strangles and some viral infections.

The size of the plaques can vary considerably from small round elevated lesions to raised swellings which can involve large areas of the body. The extent of the reaction depends on the nature of the allergen and the individual sensitivity of the animal. Whatever the type of allergen, the horse must have had previous exposure at which time sensitisation must have taken place.

The smaller swellings often tend to disappear quickly and cause little concern with the minimum of irritation. Where larger areas are involved, the horse may show other symptoms as well, such as marked itching, poor appetite and malaise. Severe reactions can result in a condition termed anaphylaxis where there are widespread swellings over the skin including around the eyelids, as well as the release of fluids into the respiratory tract causing breathing difficulties. Such cases constitute an emergency situation where veterinary help should be summoned quickly.

Remedies for treating urticaria

Dose: 200c every two to three hours until symptoms resolve

Apis mel This is the principal remedy to consider, especially where there is extensive swelling or very oedematous plaques.

Urtica Urtica is suited smaller swellings (1–2cm in diameter) with or without irritation.

Bovista Helps in more severe cases where the plaques are large (4–5cm in diameter) and show pitting on pressure and a degree of itching. Bovista is one of the remedies to consider in chronic cases.

Rhus tox Ideally suited to urticaria which appears in wet weather and particularly where there are also symptoms of stiffness. Consider Rhus tox in cases where there is also concurrent fever.

Histamine This is a good general remedy to use alongside other remedies.

Astacus Another useful general remedy effective where the symptoms resemble nettle rash and where there is itching. Swollen glands are a guiding symptom to the use of this remedy.

Arsenicum album, Calc carb, Hepar sulph, Graphites, Sulphur, Psorinum and **Nat mur** can be considered in chronic cases and used on a constitutional basis.

Anaphylaxis

Camphor

Indicated in acute cases of anaphylaxis where there are symptoms of collapse and the horse feels cold to the touch. Depending on the skin symptoms, dose alongside either **Apis 200c** or **Urtica 200c**.
Dose: Alternate dosing with 200c potency along with other appropriate remedies every five minutes

Prevention

Aim to determine the underlying allergen if possible and avoid exposure where practical.

From insect bites

Ledum 6c, Apis 6 and **Urtica 6c**
Where insect bites cause recurrent problems consider dosing with a combination of these remedies on a daily basis.

Dose: once or twice daily depending on the severity of the symptoms

From other causes

Consider **Urtica 6c, Apis 6c, Histamine 6c** or **Bovista 6c** depending on the symptoms.

Dose: once or twice daily depending on the severity of the symptoms

Sweet Itch

Culicoides hypersensitivity
Summer eczema, Summer dermatitis
Summer seasonal recurrent dermatitis
Queensland itch, Dermite estivale

This is a common condition that occurs worldwide including the UK, Japan, France, North America and

Australia and is known by a number of different names depending on the geographical location.

Underlying this condition is an allergic reaction to the bite of the female Culicoides midge, *Culicoides pulcaris* (in the UK). These midges, sometimes known as sandflies, are avid blood-suckers and will direct their bites at specific regions of the body, especially the mane and tail areas. With each bite, they inject a small amount of saliva into the horse's skin which causes an allergic or hypersensitivity reaction resulting in itching, rubbing and irritation; the familiar symptoms of sweet itch.

There is some considerable variation in the way in which each individual horse reacts to the midge bite. Ponies in particular seem to react badly, but the condition occurs in all breeds. Some animals show relatively few symptoms with little itching and few skin lesions. Others will show intense irritation, rubbing themselves against stable walls and fencing, often causing considerable damage to themselves and their surroundings. The signs, however, are usually easy to spot but occasionally can bear some resemblance to other skin problems such as rainscald, lice infestation and pinworms. If you are unsure of the diagnosis, then it is best to get a vet to confirm the diagnosis.

Typical sweet itch symptoms include rubbing with associated hair loss along the back, rump, tail base and sometimes withers, poll and ear region. The most severely affected horses will have lesions on the sides of their body, neck, legs, face and tail as well. After a time the skin can appear thickened, fissured, flaky or crusty as a result of continual rubbing. Much of the skin damage seen is self-inflicted.

There are a number of factors which influence the chances of sweet itch developing. One of the most important is the environment close to where the horses are grazed and stabled. Culicoides midges thrive in areas close to water, in damp regions and where there is decaying vegetation. Areas near to ponds, lakes, rivers, marshland, forests and woods are the most likely to favour the midges. The weather also has a part to play. The midges are most active on days which are humid and when the air is calm and are most likely to appear in the early morning and in the evening, towards dusk. Sweet itch is a seasonal condition and appears only when the midges are present. Normally this is between April and October, but with changes in the climate, this period often extends a month either side.

The successful control and treatment of sweet itch depends on two factors. The first is management to minimise exposure to the midges. Affected horses should be grazed and stabled as far away as possible from watery, marshy or wooded areas. Since the midges are most active before 10am and after 4pm it is best to stable horses during the periods of risk where practical. If this is not possible, provide a field shelter or even use a light rug to prevent midges gaining access to the skin. Use a hood if the face area is targeted or reacts badly. Special rugs are now available for horses which react very badly to midge bites. Think about using fly strips or deterrent aromatherapy oils (such as lavender) in stables to deter midges from entering.

Treating sweet itch

Management guidelines need to be combined with the second factor; that is treating the condition successfully. Homeopathy can be particularly effective in dealing with sweet itch. Suitable remedies are listed below.

Dose: *unless otherwise indicated use the 30c potency two or three times daily depending on severity of the problem; once symptoms improve reduce to once or twice daily as appropriate*

Sulphur

Keynote: Dirty coat and skin

Sulphur suits untidy looking, sometimes overweight, animals, where the general coat condition is poor and may appear dirty. Some horses which respond to Sulphur may, however, be thinner and lean in stature. Symptoms are worse for heat and in general sulphur type horses will prefer shade. Check for sores and scaly areas on the skin as well as areas of hair loss.

Psorinum

Keynote: Unhealthy coat and skin

In general where this remedy is needed the coat and skin appears unhealthy and greasy with a seborrhoeic odour. Horses, which respond to Psorinum feel the cold easily and are often rugged up on relatively mild days. Psorinum should only be used for up to five days before changing to another remedy.

Tuberculinum

Keynote: Difficult cases, stubborn nature
Where the response to indicated remedies is poor, consider giving a few doses of Tuberculinum before continuing with an appropriate remedy. This remedy can also be used constitutionally. Typically dose using the 200c or 1M potency, once daily for five days.

Arsenicum album

Keynote: Dandruff, thin-skinned animals
This can be one of the most effective remedies in treating sweet itch. Horses that suit Arsenicum are neat, tidy and clean in their appearance and generally have skin of a thin or fine texture. Affected areas of the skin will feel burning hot. Scaling with dandruff-like flakes is a classic feature, especially over the mane and tail. Symptoms can be worse at night and affected animals tend to be restless or agitated by the skin problem. Moving around often seems to ease the symptoms.

Arsenicum iodatum

Keynote: Scaling with large flakes
This remedy is most useful where the dandruff flakes are particularly large and where the skin appears thickened or raw in patches.

Petroleum

Keynote: Cracked and thickened skin
Cracked, dry and thickened skin is an indication for this remedy, especially where the skin appears leathery with hair loss. Crusting and scaling are also a feature where Petroleum is useful, especially where the tail, mane and withers are affected.

Graphites

Keynote: Weepy, sticky skin lesions
Graphites suits lazy animals with a stout build and where the skin lesions are raw, weepy and sticky as opposed to dry and flaky. Weepy lesions tend to exude a clear honey-coloured fluid. This remedy will also help where there are areas of the skin that appear hard and rough.

Calc carb

Keynote: Larger, heavily built animals
Heavily built and slower stocky horses such as Shires are most suited to this remedy, helping where the skin appears sore and is slow to heal.

Kali arsenicum

Keynote: Severe itching worse with heat
Kali ars will help where the itching is extreme and where the skin is very dry and scaly. Covering the skin or the least rise in temperature will make the symptoms much worse. Numerous small nodules may be apparent in various areas of the skin.

Sulphur iodatum

Keynote: Stubborn cases
This remedy is worth consideration where other remedies have failed to act.

Caladium

Keynote: Marked attraction to insects
This remedy is good where the irritation is intense and the skin feels rough. Excessive sweating and increased attraction to insects is a clue to its use.

Rhus tox

Keynote: Small scabs, symptoms worse in autumn
This is another remedy which is useful where the irritation is intense and where there are sores, small scabs and scaling. Rhus tox is particularly good for cases that continue late into the year, well into the autumn.

Formica rufa

Keynote: Burning, red, itchy skin
This remedy is a good choice where the skin appears red, itchy and feels hot to the touch with little flaking.

Culicoides nosode

Keynote: General additional remedy
This remedy is made from the midge itself and can be used alongside other remedies.

Histamine

Keynote: Additional remedy
This remedy is worth considering in stubborn cases.

Topical (external) and preventative treatment for sweet itch

From a conventional perspective, the application of

topical fly treatments is normally the first line of treatment, aimed at trying to prevent the midges biting. Benzylbenzoate is commonly used, although many veterinary surgeons will use a combination of both benzylbenzoate and liquid paraffin. More modern preparations are based upon permethrin or related compounds and produced as pour-on products, although some are used as concentrates or creams.

Calendula cream can be used to help soothe and heal lesions with the additional benefit of added remedies. To each 100g of cream add 5ml each of the mother tinctures of **Urtica** and **Ledum** and 5ml (100 drops) of **Arsenicum 6c**. This preparation should be mixed well and applied twice daily to flaky sore areas.

Ledum 30c

This remedy can often be used on a preventative basis to minimise the reaction from the midge bites.
Dose: once daily throughout the season.

Petroleum 30c and Berberis vulgaris 30c

Both of these remedies can be used together acting as remedies to 'drain' the skin of toxins. This principle will often help in refractory cases and will improve the chance or increase the effectiveness of other remedies working.
Dose: once daily with alternate day dosing of both remedies; ideally dose for about one month prior to using other remedies or throughout the season in difficult cases

Thuja 1M

Can be used in a situations where other remedies fail to work. Thuja is the remedy of choice where vaccination is thought to be involved in the development of the condition or as acting as an obstacle to other remedies working effectively.
Dose: once daily for five days

Other allergic skin based problems

A fair number of horses show skin symptoms which have an allergic basis but which do not have either sweet itch, hives or urticarial plaques. Many of these animals only rub on a seasonal bias, which suggests they are reacting to specific allergens present only at particular times of year. This list might include tree or plant pollens, grasses, moulds or even chemical sprays. Other horses rub more or less all year round, suggesting that they are exposed to the allergen or a combination of allergens all the time. It is often worth looking at the feed in these cases. Often, removing any molasses will help ease the symptoms slightly.

If the allergen can be identified it can be used in homeopathic potency along with other remedies.
Dose: 30c potency once or twice daily depending on the severity of the symptoms.

In general most of these animals will also have some form of non-specific eczema or dermatitis accompanying the itchy symptoms. The actual choice of remedy to use to treat the problem will depend on matching the skin symptoms to those of the remedy. Where possible a constitutional remedy should be used. Many of the remedies already mentioned are applicable but it is also worth looking at the guide at the end of this skin section to outline other possible choices.

Skin conditions associated with fungal, bacterial and viral infections

Ringworm, Dermatophytosis

This is a common contagious skin condition of horses caused by fungal infection of the superficial layers of the skin. Spread is normally due to direct contact between infected animals or indirectly by using contaminated tack, grooming equipment (such as brushes), or by sharing blankets and rugs. Ringworm is of some concern as it is transmissible to humans.

Infection is very slow to appear and it may take up to four weeks after infection, before any signs are apparent. Even then it is possible to confuse ringworm with other skin conditions such as rainscald. Skin scrapings will often be needed to confirm the diagnosis, along with possible culture. Checking samples for fluorescence under an ultra violet lamp is also a valuable aid to diagnosis. Of the two types of fungi involved only Microsporum will show this phenomenon. Trichophyton, the other species involved, does not react to UV light but is the more common of the two infections. The actual lesions that develop vary with the species of fungi involved.

Trichophyton equinun causes small round patches which slowly grow larger. Vesicles can also form in areas that lack hair. These can rupture and form scabs with some minor irritation.

Trichophyton mentagrophytes tends to form lesions on the head, neck and tail base, appearing as round or irregular areas with grey looking crusts.

Trichophyton verrucosum is often seen in horses that have been in contact with infected cattle and produces symptoms similar to *Trichophyton mentagrophytes.*

Microsporum species produce much smaller round lesions with some scaling. Some species produce larger inflamed lesions with red, sticky ulcers underneath crusting.

Ringworm often responds well to homeopathic treatment but it is important to also clean any contaminated tack to avoid any re infection. Suitable remedies include:

Bacillinum 200c

A good general remedy and one which is specifically indicated for treating ringworm.
***Dose:** one dose daily for three days, then one dose weekly until the condition is resolved.*

Tellurium 30c

Indicated where the lesions are classically circular. This remedy also works well where the head and ears are particularly affected.
***Dose:** one dose daily until the problem has cleared*

Sepia 30c

Helpful where ringworm is associated with some slight skin irritation or where the condition appears in the springtime. Sepia suits mares in particular.
***Dose:** one dose daily until the problem has cleared*

Chrysarobinum 6c

Helpful where there are thick scabs and considerable itching. Evidence of vesicles will confirm the use of this remedy.
***Dose:** twice daily until all the lesions have cleared*

Bacterial folliculitus Furunculosis, Acne

Folliculitis is a condition that involves inflammation of the hair follicles either by bacteria (commonly staphylococci) or by fungi, and which occurs more often in mild wet conditions. Where the infection spreads to the surrounding tissues it is referred to as furunculosis or acne. Check for small raised pimples or boils which are painful and clumped together. Pustules are rarely seen. In severe instances there can be swelling or an abscess starts to form as the infection spreads. The most likely site for this problem to occur is under the saddle or areas that are in contact with tack. Dirty tack, poor grooming and poor management are underlying factors that need to be attended to in the course of treating the problem.

Remedies listed should be given three times daily for ten days

Hepar sulph 30c The most useful remedy where pimples or boils are present and affected areas are painful or sensitive to the touch.

Calc sulph 30c Ideal for pimples and pustules where there is absence of pain.

Sepia 30c Useful in mares with lesions on the head.

Silica 200c For chronic situations or where there is abscessation.

Sulphur 30c Useful where the skin condition is poor in general.

Nat mur 6c For folliculitis where there is loss of hair or where there is general emaciation.

Viola tricolour 30c Indicated for lesions occurring on the face and where pus is a feature.

Kali brom 6c Indicated where pustules are present on any area of the body with itching.

Staph nosode 30c Can be used alongside other remedies.

Rain scald
Dermatophilosis
Rain rot

Rain scald is one of the more common skin conditions and usually seen in horses over the winter period when there are prolonged periods of damp and wet weather. In some instances signs may persist into the warmer weather if the condition happens to become chronic. The other, less common name for this condition is dermatophilosis, which is derived from the name of the type of bacteria involved, *Dermatophilus congolensis*. Occasionally other bacteria are involved, such as *Staphylococci*, but these are normally considered secondary invaders.

The characteristic skin symptoms of rain scald give the impression that large droplets of water have scalded the skin. Check for affected areas of skin over the rump, loins, saddle area, lower limbs and along the lines of natural water drainage over the skin. Problems start with the skin exuding a sticky secretion which mats the hair together, forming tufts which give a 'paintbrush' type of appearance to the hair in affected areas. Eventually scabs will form which, when removed, will reveal areas of pink, moist skin that may bleed a little. These sore areas are painful when touched but surprisingly, are not usually itchy. In short-haired horses the scabs tend to be small with the hairs embedded within the scab, but where the hair is longer, the scabs can reach a diameter of around 2cm or so. On the lower limbs you will see much the same sequence of events with the additional swelling of the skin, cracking of the skin, further weeping, swelling and pain which can result in lameness. These are essentially the lesions associated with mud fever (see page 255)

Rain scald is usually easy to diagnose but as always you should have your horse checked if you are uncertain. It is possible to confuse the symptoms of rain scald with ringworm (especially in the early stages) and with seborrhoea (excess grease production). Samples taken from the skin can be examined microscopically for the bacteria to confirm the diagnosis.

Affected horses should be kept dry and exposure to wet weather and muddy conditions cut to a minimum. Try, as far as is practical, to stop mud splashing up onto the skin of the body and lower limbs as this is a definite contributory factor. Animals under treatment should be stabled in a dry box and any damp bedding removed. Good grooming is just as important. Pay particular attention to cleaning any grooming kit to avoid spreading the infection by contamination with infected scabs and tufts of hair.

Treatment of rain scald often involves cleaning the affected areas of skin with an antiseptic type scrub (such as surgical scrub) and applying a solution of one per cent potash alum. More severe cases may need antibiotics. As an alternative, clean the areas with diluted **Hypercal lotion** and use the most appropriate homeopathic remedies to deal with the infection.

Dose: *two or three times daily (depending on the severity of the condition), until the symptoms have cleared*

Dulcamara 30c

Keynote: Scabs and crusts overlying sores
Dulcamara is one of the most effective remedies for this condition and will help heal the skin quickly especially at the stage where scabs have formed.

Graphites 30c

Keynote: Skin oozing a sticky clear secretion
This remedy is best used in the initial stages when the areas are sticky (oozing a clear honey coloured fluid) and essentially before the scabs have formed. Graphites works best in the heavier breeds and in lazy show ponies.

Antimonium crudum 30c

Keynote: Aggravated by touch, skin thickened and hard
The type of skin lesions which respond to this remedy are a little like Graphites but the weepy areas will have dried and formed crusts which are extremely hard. There is a marked dislike of the affected areas being touched.

Hepar sulph 30c

Keynote: Irritability and suppuration
Used on a more constitutional basis where the horse is irritable, angry and extremely sensitive to touch or noise, Hepar will help if the lesions are badly infected.

Rhus tox 30c

Keynote: Small scabby or moist sores
Rhus tox will help where there are either small scabby lesions or sticky sores. It works best where the affected areas are particularly sore to touch or where there is some slight irritation.

Mancinella 30c

Keynote: Large sticky and crusty sores
This is an unusual and less well-known remedy and is effective where there are sticky, oozing areas of skin accompanied by crusts that are particularly large and thick.

Mezerium 30c

Keynote: Thick scabs overlying pus and deep ulcers
Mezerium is most useful where there are very thick scabs on the skin complicated by secondary bacterial infection underneath. Affected areas will show pus-like fluid under the scabs and skin, which is more deeply ulcerated, compared to other remedies.

Vinca minor 6c

Keynote: Affected areas very sensitive
This remedy will prove useful where the material underlying the scabs is foul in nature and irritates the skin sufficiently to make the affected areas very sensitive to touch.

Thuja 30c

Keynote: Very acute cases
Thuja should be considered if the symptoms of rain scald appear very suddenly and in a very acute form. This is also the remedy to consider using in cases that appear shortly after vaccination.

Arsenicum album 30c

Keynote: Dry rough scaly areas
Consider Arsenicum in cases where the lesions are dry in nature and where there are flaky dandruff-like scales intermingled with the hair. This remedy follows Thuja well in treating acute cases that keep relapsing.

Dermatophilus nosode 200c

This remedy can be used alongside other remedies in treatment or in a preventative role in advance of a potential problem arising.
Treatment: *dose once daily for five days at the start of treatment*
Prevention: *dose once weekly throughout the period of risk*

Mud fever
Greasy heel
Cracked heels
Scratches
Pastern dermatitis
Gale de boue

Mud fever is a common skin condition of horses and is known by a variety of different names depending on the geographical location. It occurs predominantly during the damp and wet winter months and is seen in all breeds but often affects those animals with long hair around the fetlock area and those kept in poor or unhygienic conditions. Areas that are usually affected include the bulbs of the heels as well as the fetlock and pastern regions of the legs. The back legs are more often affected than the front.

The condition is usually started by damage to the skin from local contamination by dirt or grit. This adheres to the skin in the damp and wet conditions causing irritation and inflammation particularly to the skin and underlying tissues at the back of the pastern and heel region. One of the organisms most frequently implicated is *Dermatophilus congolensis.* This is the same organism that is responsible for rain scald, but other bacteria such as Staphylococci, Streptococci or Corynebacteria, can be involved as well.

Once infection is established, the affected area gradually swells and the skin stretches and starts to weep. After a while, cracks appear in the skin and the hair in the surrounding area falls out. Crusts form as the weepy secretion dries and glues the strands of hair together, forming hard, scabby lumps. Removing the scabs will reveal areas of moist, pink skin underneath which are often raised and round in shape. If the infection continues, it will progress from the bulbs of the heel and gradually creep around to the front of the fetlock and pastern areas.

As the horse moves, the cracks in the skin may open up further, leading to pain and discomfort. In the most severe cases the horse may go lame and the legs can swell. Further bacterial complications ensue to the extent that there can be severe skin irritation. Badly affected areas may even have a foul, putrid odour.

Treating this condition not only involves the use of homeopathic remedies, but also necessitates the correction of any bad management practices. As far as practical, avoid contact with wet and muddy areas and keep susceptible horses out of the rain as much as possible. For stabled animals, always ensure that the bedding is clean and dry. When wet, try to dry your horse's legs before stabling. Brushing out any mud and grit that is clogging the hair, and removing excessive feathering by clipping will make this easier and much less of a problem. Avoid clipping the legs out completely if you can. Scabby material should be gently eased off the skin by gentle washing with tea tree shampoo. Very weepy or sore areas can dabbed with witch hazel.
Ideal remedies, which can be used in the *30c potency and given two or three times daily,* depending on the severity of the problem, include:

Graphites
Keynote: Clear sticky, weepy secretions
This is an important remedy and one that often gives good results. It is ideally suited to cases where the skin is cracked, raw and sore with a honey-coloured, weepy, sticky secretion. Graphites works at its best before there is extensive scabbing.

Malandrinum
Keynote: Scabs and cracks
This remedy is of most use in more severe cases and can be combined with Graphites. It is one of the remedies to be considered in cases that arise after vaccination.

Petroleum
Keynote: Cracks and fissures
This remedy is most suited to cases where there are severe cracks in the skin and where there are sores covered in thick scabs.

Thuja
Keynote: Stubborn cases
This is most useful for stubborn cases and notably where the condition seems to start within a few weeks of the horse having been given a vaccination.

Rhus tox
Keynote: Inflammation, swelling and irritation, cellulitis
Use this remedy where the surrounding and underlying tissues are inflamed and there is a degree of skin irritation. Rhus tox is helpful where there is evidence of cellulitis, where the infection has advanced to involve the deeper tissues of the skin.

Hepar sulph
Keynote: Severe or foul infections, area sensitive to touch
Animals with severe mud fever which show lameness often respond to Hepar sulph. Affected areas of skin are extremely sensitive to touch and exude a foul smelling discharge. Cracks and fissures will be fairly deep and extensive.

Mezereum
Keynote: Thick scabs with itching
Lesions which respond well to Mezereum characteristically itch but may also normally have very thick scabs overlying infected, purulent material.

Sanicula
Keynote: Greasy, dirty skin with fissures
Sanicula is a less well known and used remedy which will help treat mud fever where the skin is dirty, greasy and show evidence of fissures.

Other remedies worth consideration are:

Selenium 30c
Suited to greasy areas on the lower limbs.

Vinca minor 6c
Where the skin is very sensitive to the touch and appears raw.
Dose: once or twice daily.

For very difficult cases consider the use of a constitutional remedy given at the very beginning of the treatment. This can then be followed with a more local remedy. Constitutional types to identify include:

Sulphur, **Nat mur**, **Lycopodium**, **Sepia**, **Arsenicum album**, **Phosphorus** and **Calc carb**.
Dose: using 1M potency once daily for three days at the start of the treatment.

Skin Conditions Associated with Parasites

Lice
Pediculosis

Two different species of lice affect the horse, the biting louse *Haematopinus asini* and the sucking louse (which sucks blood), *Damalinia equi*. Lice infestations are most likely to occur over the winter period and affect younger animals and those whose general condition is poor. Lice are visible to the eye and are slow moving, spending their entire life on the animal. Their eggs (known as nits) can be seen attached to hair shafts and are extremely difficult to brush off.

The most common place to find lice is on the neck and shoulder region as well as under the tail base. Symptoms include a dull and scaly coat with signs of itching and rubbing. Self inflicted damage leads to breaking of the hairs and areas of hair loss so that the skin ends up with a moth-eaten appearance. Very severe cases of lice infestation may lead to anaemia and loss of general condition. Long-standing cases may also develop thickening of the skin with chronic irritation and debility.

Treatment can be helped by:

Psorinum 1M
Indicated where the skin has a moth-eaten appearance and is associated with itching. In general the condition of the skin is poor and the hair looks dry and lacks shine. Horses that respond well to this remedy feel the cold easily.
Dose: once daily for five days

Sulphur 1M
Sulphur will help in situations similar to those of Psorinum. Sulphur is indicated in individuals where the skin appears untidy, scaly and in general unhealthy. Itching when present will be worse in the evening and on warmer days. Animals that respond better to Sulphur tend to tolerate cold weather better.
Dose: once daily for five days

Arsenicum album 200c
Indicated where there is excessive scale formation and the horse is constantly rubbing, so much so that the skin becomes excoriated and may bleed. Arsenicum is best suited to finer skinned animals.
Dose: once daily until the symptoms resolve

Oleander 30c
Can be used where there has been a lot of self-inflicted damage to the skin resulting in oozing or bleeding lesions which are sensitive to touch as well as itchy.
Dose: three times daily until the symptoms resolve

Ichthyolum 6c
This remedy will help in difficult cases where the lice prove resistant to treatment and where the skin remains scaly and itchy.
Dose: three times daily until the symptoms resolve

Petroleum 30c
Petroleum is useful in chronic cases where the skin has become thickened and cracked.
Dose: twice daily until the symptoms resolve

Harvest mites
Neotrombiculosis
Trombiculosis
Berry bug
Heel bug

It is only the larval stages of this mite, *Neotrombicula autumnalis,* which are parasitic, as it spends most of its life cycle in the soil. In the warmer weather around May to October, the larvae climb up blades of grass, having emerged from the soil, and attach themselves to the horse's legs or muzzle. The mites are visible to the naked eye as small orange specks that cause local irritation (itchy feet or pedal irritation) and occasionally papules. Where the irritation is pronounced consider:

Sulphur 6c As a general remedy to cleanse the body of toxins and to reduce irritation.

Psorinum 30c If the animal is in poor condition

Rhus tox 6c Where there are papules

Calc carb 6c Suited to larger, heavier breeds to help reduce irritation

Dose: twice daily for ten days

Mange
Acariasis
Scab
Itch

Mange is caused by small mites which infest the skin and is more likely to be seen in horses kept in poor, unhygienic conditions. Eliminating the mites means cleaning the tack effectively and treating the animal with an appropriate external preparation to eradicate the infestation.

There are several different types of mange. The most common form in the UK was once Sarcoptic mange, also known as scabies, but this form has been eliminated and is no longer seen. In other countries where still prevalent, the symptoms include very intense irritation around the region of the head, shoulders and neck with then appearance of small hairless patches of skin. In bad cases the whole body can be involved. The lesions tend to become sticky as serum exudes which dries completely to form scabs. The following remedies will help to resolve the problem:

Psorinum 1M Best given in the very early stages.
Dose: once daily for five days followed by:

Sulphur 30c Where the itching is still intense but there are no sticky areas or scabs.

Graphites 30c If the skin lesions are sticky or weepy and before the scabs have formed.

Staphysagria 30c If there are many dry scabs and the itching is still intense.

Dose: three times daily until the symptoms change or resolve

Chorioptic mange is the most common type of mange now seen in horses in the UK and is caused by the mite *Chorioptes equi*. This parasite, which is just about visible to the naked eye, lives on the surface of the skin where it burrows into the skin and causes intense irritation leading to self-inflicted damage. Hair loss leads to small areas of alopecia with excoriated areas, some exudation (weeping) and formation of crusts. The skin can appear thickened in some areas, a condition referred to as hyperkeratosis. Usually the lower limbs are affected, with the irritation causing the horse to stamp its legs restlessly. In more severe cases, the condition can spread to the inside of both the front and back legs as well as along the underside of the chest and abdomen. An exact diagnosis can be made from examination of the scales or crusts from affected areas.

Initially use either:

Sulphur 1M can be used as a general remedy to help cleanse the system and to reduce irritation.
Dose: once daily for three days

or

Psorinum 1M where the general condition of the animal is poor.
Dose: once daily for three days

Followed by

Selenium 30c Where only the skin around the feet is affected and the lesions are sticky.

Graphites 30c Indicated where the larger areas of the body are affected and the skin is sore and weepy.

Lycopodium 30c Will help animals with a lean stature and apprehensive nature where the irritation is intense and the skin is excoriated. If the condition has continued for some time then the skin will show signs of thickening.

Dulcamara 30c Will reduce the intense irritation at the stage where the lesions have become crusty and dry.

Arsenicum album 30c Can be prescribed where the irritation continues to lead to self-inflicted skin damage and the affected areas start to look dry and rough.

Dose: three times daily

The third form of mange to affect horses is **Psoroptic mange** caused by the mite *Psoroptes equi*. The initial areas to be affected are normally the base of the mane and the base of the tail although the condition can appear in any areas where the hair is thick. This mite can also affect the ears and will live in the ear canals where it causes excess wax production. The irritation can cause the horse to shake its head so that it may present as a head shaker.

Check the skin for alopecia, papules and crusty, scabby lesions that remain moist rather than dry. Remedies to help:

Initially use **Psorinum** or **Sulphur** as described above, followed by

Elaps 30c Is useful where only the ears are affected and there is excess production of wax. Itching leading to headshaking is a notable feature.

Graphites 30c Will help where there are scabby lesions that are sticky to the touch and where the horse is either lazy in nature or of stout build.

Rhus tox 30c Will help where there are moist sticky scabs and where there is marked irritation.

Merc sol 30c Is useful where the lesions are very moist and the crusts are yellowish brown in colour and intermingled with the hair. Horses which respond well have a tendency to sweat easily.

Staphysagria 30c Can be used where the animal has an irritable nature and there are a great many small moist scabs intermingled with the hair down the mane and tail base.

Dose: three times daily

Ticks

Ticks do not often affect horses but occasionally the sheep tick, *Ixodes ricinus*, can be found attached to the thinner areas of skin on the underside of the abdomen. They can be removed by applying a wad of cotton wool soaked in spirit for a few minutes before pulling the tick off gently. Sometimes the site where the tick was attached can become septic. If this occurs treat with both **Ledum 30c** and **Silica 30c** *three times daily* until the reaction subsides.

Conditions Caused by Flies

Fly strike

Wounds and open areas where the skin is damaged can attract flies, which will then lay eggs. When the larvae develop they will penetrate through the tissues leading to damage and the possibility of secondary bacterial infection. The area will need extensive clipping, removal of the larvae and cleaning with diluted **Hypercal lotion**.

Infected or suppurating areas of tissue can be treated with:

Hepar sulph 200c
Where the affected areas are oozing pus and are very sensitive to touch
Dose: three times daily

Anthracinum 6c
Where the affected areas are decomposing badly and swollen. There is a discharge from the skin that is thick and tar-like in nature. Sloughing areas of dead skin are an additional pointer to its use.
Dose: four times daily

Tarentula cubensis 30c
Will help where the skin takes on a purple colour and is very inflamed due to the underlying problem of sepsis caused by fly strike.
Dose: three times daily

Gunpowder 6x
Is indicated where the skin is affected in small patches and is pitted where the larvae have burrowed down into the deeper tissues underlying the skin.
Dose: four times daily

Fly worry
Musca infection

This is a form of ulcerative dermatitis, which affects the inner corners of the eyes (leading to increased tear production and irritation), is caused by flies. Occasionally other areas of the body may be affected, including the eyelids, lips, nose and vulval regions. Remedies to help include:

Argentum nitricum 30c
Is indicated where the inner corner of the eye is very inflamed and red looking and the discharge from the eye is thick, discoloured and irritates the skin. The eyelids may also be affected.

Arsenicum album 30c
Will help where the discharge from the eye is more watery and excoriates and inflames the skin over which it flows. Affected horses will appear markedly restless due to the fly irritation. The more severe cases are sometimes better served by using **Ars iod 30c** instead.

Euphrasia 30c
Can help where the eyes water excessively and the discharge is thicker and irritates the skin. The eyelids may appear swollen.

Rhus tox 30c
Will help where the skin around the eyes is very inflamed, swollen, puffy and ulcerated.

Nat mur 30c
Can help where there is excessive tear production to the extent that the tears run right down the face. This remedy will also help where the lips are affected as well.

Nitric acid 30c
Will help where the corners of the eyes, eyelids, lips and vulva are showing signs of ulceration and irritation.

***Dose:** three times daily to treat the condition, once daily as a preventive*

Stable flies

The stable fly, *Stomoxys calcitrans*, can cause painful bites that may need treatment. Ideal remedies to help alleviate the discomfort are **Ledum 30c** which should be given routinely (*four doses over a two hour period*) adding **Hypericum 30c** if pain is evident and **Apis 200** if there is much swelling. (See bites section above.)

Non-Infectious Skin Conditions

Equine nodular skin disease
Necrobiosis
Sweat bumps
Allergic collagen necrosis
Eosinophilic granulomata/granuloma

This condition goes under the guise of several names, the simplest of which is sweat bumps, but it is more often referred to as equine nodular skin disease or necrobiosis and, rarely, as allergic collagen necrosis. The exact cause is not known but various ideas include allergic-based reactions or a response to microfilariae in the skin. Fibrous lumps of varying size appear under the skin and in particular, seem to appear mainly under the saddle, but can also occur over the shoulder region, flanks, neck and prepuce. The nodules are non-painful and can be up to about 2cm in diameter.

The fibrous nodules are diagnostic of the condition but can occasionally become confused with pressure sores caused by an ill-fitting saddle. If there is any doubt a biopsy can be taken to confirm the diagnosis. In a few cases, the nodules will regress spontaneously, but this is rare, and in the majority of affected animals, the nodules will remain. Usually they will not cause problems, other than appearing unsightly. However, in some instances the nodules will be in a particular area such as under the saddle and may be uncomfortable and lead to rubbing.

This condition, which is difficult to treat with conventional medicine, often responds well to homeopathy which can act both in a preventative role and in reducing the nodules in size by dissipating the fibrous tissue.

Treatment
Best results can be achieved by using a trio of remedies:

Silica 30c

Graphites 30c

Thiosinaminum 30c
All three of these remedies help to dissolve scar tissue and should be given over a period of several

weeks until the nodules have reduced as far as possible. An ideal regime is to use Silica the first day, Graphites the second and Thiosinaminum the third before repeating the trio.

Kali ars 30c or **Kali iod 30c** (where there is a general tendency to react to insect bites with skin swellings) are worth consideration if these remedies fail to act. **Acetic acid 6c** can also help in dissolution of the nodules where they are slow to clear.
Dose: *once daily*

Cenchris contortrix 200c should also be considered in cases where the nodules seem to lie in a chain as if following a blood or lymphatic vessel. This remedy is specific in this instance. Its use can be confirmed if other symptoms such as restlessness, anxiety or tendency to show signs of jealousy are present.
Dose: *once daily for ten days*

Prevention

In horses prone to develop this condition, the following remedies can be used on a long-term basis:

Ledum 30c should be given in all cases ***Dose:*** *once daily*

Urtica 6c can be used where the reactions in the skin are small ***Dose:*** *once daily*

Apis 6c can be used where the skin reactions are larger ***Dose:*** *once daily*

Histamine 6c for difficult cases ***Dose:*** *once daily*

Kali iod 30c as above ***Dose:*** *once daily*

Pemphigus

This type of skin condition is rare and occurs as a consequence of the body's own immune system attacking the skin and mucous membranes so that these areas then become diseased. The underlying trigger for this autoimmune disease is not completely understood, but concurrent respiratory infections or cancer can sometimes be involved. The end result is that the body is no longer able to recognise either the skin or mucous membranes as 'self' and as a result the body's defences start to attack these areas as they are considered foreign tissue.

Pemphigus is difficult to treat both conventionally and with homeopathy. There are two basic types of equine pemphigus which are similar, but which have slightly different symptoms:

Pemphigus foliaceus occurs if the immune system attacks the area between the upper and lower layers of skin and is the most common form seen in horses. Initial symptoms appear as tiny blisters following which, the skin starts to peel off in either circular or large irregular areas. You will also notice flaky grey areas of skin and in severe cases, extensive hair loss, where the hair simply just falls out on the slightest touch. Some weeping from the damaged skin areas will follow, with crusts developing as a consequence.

Commonly affected areas include the head, neck and body. The legs can also be involved but this occurs less frequently, however it is not unusual for the coronary band to show severe signs of the disease. The borders of the ergots and chestnuts may also show signs at the same time. In such cases, the growth of the horn is affected, so that the hoof wall flakes and is of poor quality. It is not unusual to see other signs. The horse may appear depressed and may show signs of poor appetite and weight loss. Itching of the skin may or may not be present depending which areas of the body are affected.

The much rarer form, **Pemphigus vulgaris**, occurs if the mucous membranes of the mouth, anus, vulva, nasal cavity or eyelids are involved leading to extensive tissue destruction. Considerable pain is involved so that the animal will have trouble eating or drinking.

Remedies which may help:

Cantharis 200c

Most valuable where the skin is severely blistered and weepy. The animal will also appear agitated.

Rhus tox 30c

An important remedy which will ease the symptoms where the skin is severely inflamed, red and notably swollen with patches of oozing skin intermingled with scabs.
Dose: *three times daily initially reducing to twice daily as symptoms improve*

Bufo 30c

A remedy for the blister stage where the skin starts to

peel off leaving irregular slightly raw areas underneath.
Dose: three times daily

Mancinella 30c
Will help with cases of pemphigus foliaceus where there are large areas of skin involved and where the skin appears blistered with either crusts or scabs present.
Dose: three times daily initially reducing to twice daily as symptoms improve

Caltha palustris 3c
Indicated where there is itching present or where the eyes specifically are involved.
Dose: three times daily initially reducing to twice daily as symptoms improve

Ranunculus sceleratus 3c
Guiding symptoms include itching which is a marked feature or where large areas are involved which weep a sticky discharge that irritates the skin locally.
Dose: three times daily initially reducing to twice daily as symptoms improve

Arsenicum album 30c
Suited to finer skinned, anxious animals where patchy scaling is more of a feature than ulceration and where hair loss is evident.
Dose: twice daily

Nitric acid 200c
This is the principal remedy for cases of pemphigus vulgaris, where the mucous membranes of the mouth, eyelids, anus, vulva and nose may be affected. These areas show severe inflammation and ulceration of the membranes such that these areas are painful.
Dose: twice daily until improvement is seen, then once every two days

Also worth considering dosing using *30c potency two or three times daily* as appropriate: **Lachesis**, **Merc sol**, **Merc corr**, **Phosphorus**, **Sepia** and **Thuja**. Where poor horn has occurred as a result think about using **Thuja**, **Ant crud** and **Graphites**.

However, the most useful remedy of all and most likely to improve horn quality is **Silica**. *Dose: 30c once daily over several months*

Warts, sarcoids and melanomas

All three of these conditions can be treated to some extent using homeopathic remedies. As well as using remedies given orally, external treatment is also of great help:

Thuja mother tincture, Thuja Ø
This can be applied externally once daily using moistened cotton wool to help reduce any of these skin masses. With an alcohol base Thuja mother tincture is sometimes apt to sting a little in which case dilute 50:50 with water.

Thuja cream
This can be used as an alternative, especially on sensitive or larger lesions as it is less likely to irritate. The cream should be applied once daily.

Thuja and witch hazel cream
This is a better alternative and is especially effective on ulcerated, bleeding, infected, sticky or sore lesions where the astringency of the **Witch hazel** is an advantage in drying up and shrinking skin growths. This cream can be made up easily from base ingredients. To 100g **Calendula** base cream add 5ml **Thuja** tincture and 5ml distilled witch hazel mixing well before applying once daily. Where bleeding is a particular problem you can also add 5ml of **Nitric acid 6c** liquid potency.

Warts
Viral papillomatosis
Verrues

Warts are one of the most easily identified of all skin conditions in the horse and typically appear in animals under three to four years of age. The underlying cause is a virus which will spread easily between animals by direct contact so that a whole group may be affected at one time.

The incubation time after exposure to the virus is between one and two months. Initially the warts will appear as smooth raised bumps in the skin, gradually increasing in size up to about 2cm in diameter. The most common location for warts to appear is around the muzzle and nasal area, sides of the face and eyelids. From time to time they may also be seen on the neck and forelegs. After several months, the warts will regress spontaneously. However, treatment with an appropriate remedy will often hasten this process dramatically.

Success hinges on the choice of remedy which depends on the characteristic of the warts and a few other guiding factors.

Selecting a wart remedy

Thuja 200c Large, bleeding or moist types, may appear after vaccination, commonly used remedy

Antimonium crudum 30c Rough, hard or horny warts

Calc carb 200c Fleshy warts, works best in larger breeds of horse

Dulcamara 30c Large, flat, smooth warts, especially on the face

Lycopodium 30c Smaller warts with a more nodular, smooth appearance

Sabina 30c Useful where the warts bleed and are itchy

Causticum 200c Pedunculated, bleeding, jagged, sore or inflamed warts

Nitric acid 200c Pedunculated, bleed very easily, sticky or moist

Natrum sulph 30c Warts appearing near the anal region or on the flaps of the nostrils

Staphysagria 200c Warts very sensitive to touch, dry in texture, irritable animal

***Dose:** 200c twice weekly or 30c alternate days*

Sarcoids
Angleberries

Sarcoids are common and can affect all horses regardless of breed, age, sex or colour. Regarded as a type of non-malignant skin tumour, the exact cause is unknown, but thought to be viral in origin.

There are several types of sarcoids. The first type tends to appear quite suddenly, and grow quickly and somewhat aggressively often resembling red raw chronic granulation tissue. This type bleeds easily. These **fibroblastic sarcoids** will initially appear as hard fibrous nodules which erode through the skin and consequently become damaged, taking on the appearance of proud flesh. This type is more often seen on the legs, underside of the abdomen and on the head. The **warty** or **verrucous** type of sarcoid grows more slowly, is usually less than 6 cm in diameter and will consist of areas of thickened skin and have a scabby grey appearance. This type can also appear on stalks and is typically dry and horny or cauliflower-like in appearance.

A third type of sarcoid is the **benign nodular** form consisting of small nodules surrounded by an area of hair loss and slight skin scaling. This type (sometimes seen on the ears and eyelids) can remain inactive for many years and may ultimately regress and disappear altogether. They may appear in many hundreds and can often be removed surgically. Unfortunately, in some cases if disturbed (by surgery or trauma for example), this type may start to grow significantly.

Another type of similar appearance are sometimes referred to as **occult sarcoids** which are characterised by a circular shape, hair loss and a scaly grey appearance.

Mixed sarcoids are not unknown, consisting of the verrucose (warty), nodular and fibroblastic types which can be aggressive in nature. However, the most worrying type is the malevolent form which, although rare, is very aggressive. They are most likely to be seen on the face or elbows.

Sarcoids often respond favourably to homeopathic remedies, providing that the remedy is selected with care.

Thuja 200c

Thuja is the principal remedy to consider and will help in most cases, especially those that look like granulation tissue or proud flesh. Success is also likely where the sarcoids are either cauliflower-like or are fairly large in size. Sarcoids, which appear suddenly or become active following vaccination, should also be treated with this remedy.
***Dose:** twice weekly*

Nitric acid 200c

This remedy can be used in those sited near body orifices (mouth, eyes, rectum, vulva etc.) and for

those which tend to ulcerate and bleed. Its main sphere of action, however, is to help with those sarcoids which appear to be of the granulation tissue type of appearance and which grow aggressively.
Dose: *twice weekly*

Antimonium crudum 200c
The cauliflower types, which are hard and horny in nature, will respond best to this remedy.
Dose: *twice weekly*

Silica 30c
This remedy is worth consideration for those fibroblastic type sarcoids which are at the early nodular stage before any skin erosion has occurred. Silica is most likely to help those animals that appear to have a weaker general constitution or those where the problem appears to arise following vaccination.
Dose: *once daily*

Ranunculus bulbosus 30c
Ranunculus will help where the sarcoids are very hard and dry in texture.
Dose: *once daily*

Conium 1M
The small inactive nodular type of sarcoid will respond best to this remedy. Conium can also be considered in the early nodular stages of the fibroblastic type of sarcoid.
Dose: *twice weekly*

Sabina 200c
Sabina can help those sarcoids which appear to resemble exuberant granulation tissue. The keynote to this remedy is that the sarcoids appear to cause irritation, causing the animal to rub affected areas.
Dose: *twice weekly*

Medorrhinum 1M
Giving a few doses of Medorrhinum and then repeating a more specific remedy can help difficult and non-responsive cases.
Dose: *once daily for five days*

Carcinosin 1M
This remedy can help when given on a constitutional basis.
Dose: *once daily for five days*

Beryllium 200c
This remedy can be used where there are other skin masses such as cysts or nodules present.
Dose: *twice weekly*

Sarcoid nosode 30c
A basic nosode is available and can be used alongside other remedies. It is, however, better to produce a specific nosode from sarcoid material from the animal under treatment. This form of treatment, referred to as isopathy, is likely to give better results than the standard nosode.
Dose: *once daily*

Melanoma

A melanoma is a type of tumour which commonly occurs in the skin, but which can also occur at other sites. It is composed of the same type of cells that produce the skin pigment called melanin which is responsible for the darkened area of skin (such as around the muzzle) which we see in many horses. Uncontrollable multiplication of these cells, gives rise to the type of tumours recognised as melanomas.

Most, but not all, melanomas in the horse are benign and do not spread around the body. They appear either as single, firm, darkly pigmented nodules or in clusters composed of several nodules close together. Although they can appear at any location on the body, melanomas tend to occur at specific sites. Melanomas occurring on the skin are often found near the anus, the vulva, the penis, the tail and the ears. They can also occur on the eyelids and actually inside the eye where they can seriously interfere with vision. Rarely, they can be found in the abdomen where they can interfere with the digestion.

Grey horses, especially those over six years old, are most at risk of developing melanomas, although they can occur in any animal. Coloured horses tend to have single tumours on the legs or body wall, whereas multiple tumours are likely to be malignant in horses of this type compared to isolated single masses. Wherever the location, melanomas can grow at different rates. Some will remain as slow growing nodules and cause few problems. Others will grow much quicker, ulcerate, bleed or discharge a foul black liquid.

There are a few lumps and bumps which can resemble melanomas including sarcoids, cysts and other types of nodule. Samples taken from a suspect mass or excision of the whole tumour can aid diagnosis when subject to a detailed microscopical examination. With a confirmed diagnosis, isolated skin melanomas, and small tumours on the eyelid, can often be left alone. Other options are to remove the growth surgically, freezing the masses using cryosurgery or using one of human drugs used to treat stomach ulcers. Homeopathy provides another viable alternative.

Suggested remedies

Thuja 200c

This remedy can be used routinely in most cases but it is also one of the main remedies to consider where the condition appears following vaccination or where pre-existing masses appear to increase in size after vaccination. Thuja should certainly be used in those melanomas which discharge dark coloured fluid and those which appear on or near the eyelids or on the penis.
Dose: *twice weekly*

Lycopodium 30c

The type of melanomas which respond well to Lycopodium appear as smooth single or clustered pigmented masses in the skin. Animals which are likely to respond well are those which display typical Lycopodium traits such as apprehension, lean stature and tendency to digestive problems.
Dose: *three times weekly*

Sabina 30c

Sabina works well alongside Thuja so both remedies can be used in tandem. This remedy is more suited to mares but can be used in any situation to help treat melanomas which are darkly pigmented but small in size. Sabina will also help where there is a likelihood of the melanomas bleeding.
Dose: *three times weekly*

Fluoric acid 30c

Horses which respond well to Fluoric acid are most likely to be elderly and may show slight signs of weight loss or loss of condition. The type of melanoma most likely to respond are those which show signs of inflammation around the base of the mass or those which appear to itch or bleed slightly.
Dose: *three times weekly*

Nitric acid 200c

Nitric acid is best reserved for those melanomas which appear ulcerated and which bleed bright red fresh blood profusely from time to time. This remedy is also useful for any melanomas appearing near the orifices of the body such as the anus, tip of the penis (especially if they bleed) and vulva as well as on the eyelids.
Dose: *three times weekly*

In cases where there is acute and profuse bleeding from a melanoma *dose using Nitric acid 200c every 30 minutes until the bleeding ceases.*

Carcinosin 30c

Carcinosin is of most value in cases where the melanomas are most likely to be malignant or where multiple nodules appear rapidly.
Dose: *once daily*

Condurango 30c

Ulcerated melanomas which bleed and which are located near the body orifices (the anus and vulva particularly), are most likely to respond to this remedy.
Dose: *once daily*

Melanoma nosode 30c

The standard melanoma nosode can be used alongside any other remedies. However, a specific nosode made from a sample taken from the animal under treatment will be of greater benefit.
Dose: *three times weekly*

Simple Pointers to Common Skin Remedies

Brief details are included of the most important skin remedies to aid selection of the most appropriate remedy.

To help identify some of the problems, some of the most common skin terms are explained in more detail first.

Crusting A scab or dried secretion from the skin that lies on top of a lesion

Fissure A crack or split in the skin

Lesion An abnormality that differs from normal

Nodule Raised area of skin, usually firm to touch and larger than 1cm across and extending into the deeper skin layers

Papule Small hard raised solid area of skin less than 1cm across

Plaque A solid raised area of skin more than 1cm in diameter but flat on top

Pustule A small, very slightly raised area of skin that contained pus

Scaling The same as dandruff or scurfy pieces on the skin on in the hair

Vesicle Raised area of skin filled with fluid like a blister

Skin remedies

Ars alb Fine skinned animals, itching with small dandruff-like flakes in the hair, often seem anxious

Ars iod Itching with larger dandruff-like flakes

Anacardium Itchy swollen areas of skin, marked mental irritability, suspicious nature

Ant crud Urticaria, dry areas of skin, scales and pustules, vesicles with thick honey-coloured scabs

Apis mel Red inflamed skin with swelling, puffy skin areas, sensitive to touch, restless nature, difficult to examine, burns

Bacillinum Ringworm

Bovista Itching with moist eczema and thick crusts

Calc carb Stout, heavy build, unhealthy skin, itching, skin feels damp

Calc sulph Itching with many small crusty scabs in the skin

Cantharis Itching with burning red hot, raw areas of skin, possibility of vesicles, burns

Dolichos Intense itching with no visible lesions, worse across the withers and around elbows and stifles

Dulcamara Itching with red spots or small scabs or thick crusts that bleed when removed, crusts tend to matt the hair together

Fagopyrum Itching with small red skin blotches, worse in sunlight

Formica rufa Red, burning, itching skin

Graphites Itchy moist areas of skin, weeping a clear honey-coloured fluid, lazy nature, often overweight

Hepar sulph Papules, bacterial infections, suppurating lesions, unhealthy skin, infected easily, itching, irritable nature

Hippozaenium Eczema or dermatitis with pustules

Kali arsenicum Itching with dry scaly skin, chronic problem, worse in warm weather

Kali sulph Itching with seborrhoeic greasy skin, papules

Lycopodium Itching with thickened skin, dry areas which may bleed, cracks and fissures, bad skin odour, lean build, apprehensive nature

Malandrinum Skin problems arising from persistent contact with water, fissured or cracked, swollen, sore areas of skin

Mancinella Thick brown crusts, red inflamed areas with itching, oozing of sticky fluid that dries to form crusts

Manganum acetate Itching around the joints, cracked and fissured skin, cellulitis

Merc sol Moist sticky eczema with purulent discharge, possibly vesicles and pustules, suppurating areas

Mezerium Manic itching, vesicles, ulcerated areas of skin covered by thick scabs

Nat mur Greasy itchy skin, crusty lesions in folds of skin especially around the limbs, red raw areas of skin, hair loss, withdrawn, sullen nature

Nux vomica Skin feels very hot, red blotchy areas, itching, and irritable, impatient nature

Petroleum Rough and cracked skin, suppurates, thick crusts, raw thickened skin, bleeding cracked or fissured skin

Psorinum Dirty skin with a bad odour, poor skin in general, rough coat, lacks shine and lustre, seborrhoea, crusty eruptions, always feels the cold, and always needs covering with rugs

Pulsatilla Gentle nature, often mares, itching particularly underside of body

Radium Generalised eczema or dermatitis with itching, skin inflamed

Rhus tox Intense itching, urticaria, scaling, many small scabs or sores, symptoms worse in wet weather, cellulitis

Rhus venata Itching, skin very inflamed with dark colour, vesicles

Rumex crispus Itching around the legs, worse in cold weather

Selenium Vesicles and greasy skin with itching around the legs

Sepia Itching especially around elbows and stifles, thickening and increase in skin pigmentation, greasy skin, ringworm

Silica Unhealthy skin, urticaria and itching, poor general conformation, timid nature

Staphysagria Itching with dry thick scabs, irritable or aggressive nature

Sulphur Unhealthy skin, poor coat and skin, dry and scaly, rough, bad odour, pustules, soreness, especially in folds of skin, itching worse in warm weather and in damp conditions

Tellurium Eczema in circular patches, ringworm

Thuja Warts, melanoma, proud flesh, sarcoids, thickened skin, chronic eczema or dermatitis

Urtica Urticaria, itchy skin blotches, burns

Vespa Hives with intense itching, redness of skin

Vinca minor Red and sore areas of skin from rubbing, possibly pustules, hair mats together

Viola tricolour Eczema affecting the head, thick scabs with cracks and yellow pus

The Endocrine System

The endocrine or hormonal system controls some of the major functions of the body through a number of chemical intermediaries or chemical messengers referred to as hormones. These are produced and secreted by a number of glands and circulate in the blood to their target organs. Hormones, for example, control the oestrus cycle, influence hair growth, maintain blood sugar levels and regulate metabolism. Endocrine problems are relatively rare in the horse. The most common condition is Cushing's disease but on occasion diabetes mellitus, diabetes insipidus and hypothyroidism may be seen.

Cushing's Disease Hyperadrenocorticism

Cushing's disease is named after an American surgeon, Harvey Cushing, who first described the condition in people in 1932 whilst researching the brain and function of the pituitary gland. Mainly seen in older horses, it has been diagnosed in horses as young as seven.

Symptoms arise due to high levels of the hormone cortisol circulating in the blood secreted by the adrenal glands which are located near the kidneys. Cortisol secretion is governed by a hormone known as adrenocorticotrophic hormone (ACTH), which is produced by the tiny pituitary gland, located near the base of the brain. Cushing's disease develops when the gland develops cancerous changes. Classified as a pituitary adenoma (sometimes referred to as pituitary hyperplasia or adenomatous hypertrophy of the pars intermedia of the pituitary gland), this slow growing, benign tumour secretes excess quantities of ACTH which in turn causes excess production of cortisol by the adrenal glands. The stable balance between the pituitary gland and the adrenal gland (together with a closely linked area of the brain known as the hypothalamus) normally maintained and regulated by a negative feedback mechanism, is no longer stable. The effects on the body of the excess cortisol are varied and include an anti-insulin action, an increase in blood glucose level (caused by stimulating the liver to break down stored protein) and constriction of blood vessels (vasoconstriction).

One of the earliest symptoms is an increase in thirst (polydipsia) and consequently an increase in urination (polyuria), signs often difficult to spot in animals kept outside. Other signs are more obvious. One of the most common is retention of the long, shaggy winter coat, which is not shed in the spring or summer as normal and an increase in the rate of growth of the coat (hirsuitism) which often appears unusually curly. These can often be the first symptoms to be noticed and may be accompanied by a tendency to sweat more (hyperhydrosis).

Other symptoms include an increase in appetite without weight gain and often with some slight loss of condition especially over the topline and the development of laminitis which can become a recurrent problem. Affected horses will also have a weakened immune system, which can lead to a variety of problems such as abscesses, skin and respiratory infections, ulcers within the mouth and slow wound healing. Less commonly seen symptoms include abnormal oestrus cycles and milk production in mares, general lethargy, depression, heavy parasite burdens, the appearance of supra orbital fat deposits – bulges over the eyes and of fat pads elsewhere over the body.

The course of the disease is slow but as the tumour enlarges it can put pressure on other parts of the brain affecting temperature regulation and the optic nerve (leading to blindness). In very advanced cases, symptoms can include dementia and head tilting.

Treating Cushing's Disease

Problems such as laminitis, diabetes and abscesses can be dealt with as they arise. The remedies listed below are specific for helping with Cushing's.

ACTH and Quercus robur

This combination of two remedies has been the most successful homeopathic approach to treating Cushing's disease.
Dose: 30c twice daily

Carduus marianus

Use this remedy in low potency to routinely provide liver support in all Cushing's cases. In addition to this it will help regulate the metabolism of sugar and improve the blood flow to the periphery of the body, counteracting the vasoconstrictive effects of the cortisol.
Dose: 6x twice daily

Abrotanum

Abrotanum has been useful in cases where there is muscle wasting.
Dose: 30c twice daily

Thuja

Thuja can be added as general remedy to help slow the growth of the pituitary adenoma.
Dose: 30c twice daily

Nat mur

This is another remedy to consider where there is weight loss, depression or withdrawal, together with a marked increase in thirst.
Dose: 30c twice daily

Echinacea 30x

Echinacea can be used to support the immune system alongside other remedies for Cushing's disease.
Dose: 30x two or three times daily

Hypothyroidism

Underactivity of the thyroid gland is termed hypothyroidism; however, there is some question as to whether this condition really exists in horses. Animals diagnosed with this condition are overweight, sluggish and sometimes referred to as 'easy keepers'. There are two other clinical signs that may be apparent. One is chronic laminitis and the other is abnormal deposits of fat in the neck and at the base of the tail. Occasionally, poor performance syndrome and tying up have also been associated with hypothroidism. Treatment with conventional synthetic thyroid medication often produces good results.

Tests aimed at diagnosing the condition, which measure the levels of thyroid hormone in the blood, give inconsistent results and do not always accurately measure thyroid function, casting doubt onto the existence of the condition. However, from a homeopathic viewpoint, suspect cases can be treated in accordance with the presenting symptoms irrespective of having a totally accurate diagnosis.

Treating hypothyroidism

Thyroid 3x

Thyroid in low decimal potency can be used in all cases and can be given alongside other remedies.
Dose: twice daily

Calc carb 30c

This remedy is suited to animals that are overweight, slow and sluggish and which appear depressed. Other features which point towards this remedy include stiff joints, a general aversion to work and unhealthy looking coat and skin.
Dose: twice daily

Graphites 30c

Graphites has features which are very similar to Calc carb. Horses that will benefit from this remedy also tend to be overweight, slow and tire easily. The main differentiating feature is the skin, which in this case, will be thickened in places and will show cracked areas suggested a tendency to mud fever. The hair will tend to be untidy and in poor condition possibly with tangles.
Dose: twice daily

Kali carb 30c
Horses needing Kali carb have an irritable nature and are stubborn, show a general lack of energy and tire easily. Often they have a history of back pain but do not show the skin symptoms seen in either Calc carb or Graphites.

Sepia 30c
The nature of Sepia which stands this remedy apart is indifference, along with a dull nature and general appearance of being worn out. More often suited to mares, horses benefiting from this remedy will have a greasy skin, which will show areas of thickening and hair loss.
Dose: twice daily

Alumina 30c
Alumina is indicated where the coat is dry and flaky and where the hooves are similarly dry and may be cracked. Mentally horses that require this remedy will be slow both physically and mentally.
Dose: twice daily

Diabetes Mellitus

Diabetes is rare in horses and caused by a failure of the pancreas to produce enough of the hormone insulin. The consequence of this is that the cells of the body are unable to take up glucose which then raises the level of glucose in the blood to abnormally high levels, a condition referred to as hyperglycaemia. Glucose will appear in the urine, causing the animal to pass more urine than normal (polyuria) and changing its odour so that it smells sweet. Affected horses will be thirsty and may show weight loss due to breakdown of body tissues to supply energy in place of the glucose, which cannot be absorbed into the cells to be metabolised.

Hyperglycaemia is a feature of Cushing's disease as is glycosuria, the presence of glucose in the urine and ketonuria, the presence of ketones (formed from the excessive breakdown of fat) in the urine. Urine tests performed to detect both glucose and ketones and blood tests to detect hyperglycaemia are often used in the initial diagnosis of Cushing's disease before performing more specific tests.

Remedies to help with diabetes
Dose: two or three times daily

General remedies **Syzgium 6x**, **Insulin 6x**

As general pancreatic remedy **Iris vers 30c**

With marked thirst and nervous temperament **Phosphorus 30c**

Affectionate, friendly animals **Carcinosin 30c**

With liver involvement **Lycopodium 30c**. **Phosphorus 30c**

With irritable nature, needs to be kept busy **Helonias 6c**

With debility **Phos ac 6c**

With emaciation **Uranium nitrate 30c**

With very high levels of glucose in the urine **Uranium nitrate 30c**

Diabetes Insipidus

This form of diabetes, which is extremely rare, involves the hormonal mechanism that controls water regulation within the body and is caused by a tumour within part of the pituitary gland. Symptoms include excessive thirst, an increase in frequency and volume of urine passed, weight loss, exercise intolerance and general weakness. The urine is very dilute, pale in colour and does not contain glucose. Principle remedies that may help include **Uranium nitrate 30c**, **ADH 6c** (antidiuretic hormone) and **Apoc cann 30c**. *Dose: twice daily.*

Equine Metabolic Syndrome (EMS)

This condition is seen in older adult horses which are genetically predisposed. The main symptom is obesity due to the deposition of fatty tissue in the body together with the development of insulin resistance and the subsequent risk of laminitis. Affected horses acquire fat stores during periods when there is an abundant food supply, more often than not due to simple over-feeding, inappropriate diet and or lack of exercise. Aim to reduce the risk of developing EMS by restricting the intake of soluble carbohydrate whilst maintaining the bulk of the ration, increasing the level of exercise and avoiding obesity in horses when they are younger. The following remedies may be of help in treating the problem, bearing in mind that the remedies used to treat diabetes mellitus and laminitis should be considered alongside any others used:

***Dose:** twice daily*

As a general remedy **Capsicum 30c**

Used constitutionally **Calc carb 30c, Graphites 30c, Phosphorus 30c, Arsenicum album 30c**

Where there is depression **Aurum 30c**

Infectious Diseases

This section covers conditions caused by bacterial, viral, protozoal and fungal infections as well as a number of other organisms. Some of the diseases are covered in other sections of the book. Not all the diseases are present in the UK.

By law, in the UK, some of the conditions listed are notifiable[11].

Infections Caused by Viruses

Viral infections Characterised by Respiratory Symptoms

Equine Rhinopneumonitis Virus (EHV-1)
Equine Herpes Virus Type 1, Subtype 1
Equine Herpes Virus Type 1, Subtype 2, EHV-4
Stable Cough
Snotty Nose
Rhinopneumonitis
Viral Abortion

There are two different subtypes or serotypes of EHV-1. The first, known as subtype 1, causes neurological signs, respiratory symptoms (principally rhinopneumonitis – inflammation of the upper airways and lungs) and carries the risk of abortion. Subtype 2, also known as EHV-4 also causes respiratory symptoms that are indistinguishable from the symptoms caused by subtype 1. Infections are common within horses up to a year old and in horses starting training. In fact the majority of horses will encounter this highly contagious virus during their lifetime with infection occurring by inhalation of infected particles spread around by nasal droplets in the air. In a proportion of horses the virus can lie dormant and become reactivated if the immune system is stressed.

EHV-1 subtype 1 is the more serious of the two, starting as a respiratory infection and then travelling to the unborn foal or to the spinal cord or brain. The virus can enter the white blood cells and stay lodged there for some time, affecting the horse's performance and ability to fight off other infections.

Symptoms appear between two and 12 days of infection and initially include fever (with a rise in temperature up to 41°C, 105.8°F) and with a cough or slight whitish nasal discharge with possible enlargement of the lymph nodes in the throat. Conjunctivitis is also common as is a cough. In rare cases the virus can progress beyond the respiratory phase and involve the nervous system of adult horses with symptoms apparent six to ten days after infection.

Neurological signs (myeloencephalopathy) may present as a vague lameness or stiffness progressing to obvious hind limb weakness, ataxia or incoordination, progressing forwards to affect the front legs as well. Other symptoms follow and can include urinary incontinence, flaccidity of the vulval lips, prolapse of the penis, retention of faeces, swelling of the legs, colic and eventual recumbency with the horse sitting in a dog-like position.

Pregnant mares are at risk of abortion, which is most likely to occur at around seven months gestation (and anytime up to full term) without any clinical signs being present beforehand in those affected. A large number of mares may abort together (termed an abortion storm) or it is possible that just one or two may be affected. Foals infected by EHV-1 in the womb may be stillborn or die shortly after birth. Some foals that appear apparently normal after birth may have a weak immune system and quickly succumb to either viral or bacterial infections.

Homeopathic Treatment of EHV-1[10]

Respiratory symptoms – Rhinopneumonitis (EHV-1, EHV-4)

Once symptoms are apparent, if left untreated the signs of fever may last up to five days. The nasal discharge and cough can last from anywhere between one and three weeks. The following remedies are for the initial stages. Where a cough persists see the respiratory section, page 87, for the most appropriate remedies.

Aconite 1M

Aconite needs to be given at the very earliest stages of the disease as soon as the symptoms of fever or respiratory symptoms are detected.
Dose: once every 15 minutes until symptoms abate or another remedy is indicated

Ferrum phos 200c

Use Ferrum phos when it is too late to use Aconite effectively and where the lymph nodes in the throat are enlarged or where there is a fever and a slight nasal discharge or slight cough present.
Dose: once every 30 minutes until symptoms abate or another remedy is indicated

Arsenicum album 200c

This remedy is useful where respiratory symptoms continue to predominate and where neurological signs are evident. Indications include a watery nasal discharge or a cough with a slight wheeze. The hind legs will show heaviness or weakness. Developing paralysis will be apparent. Restlessness and anxiety will be additional features where this remedy is indicated.
Dose: four times daily

Rhus tox 200c

Another remedy to use in the earlier stages where the only symptoms appear to be vague stiffness with some slight signs of weakness along with a dry cough and a watery, fluid nasal discharge.
Dose: four times daily

Kali iod 200c

Kali iod is indicated where conjunctivitis is a prominent feature or where the respiratory symptoms are more severe and include a more violent type of cough.
Dose: four times daily

Neurological symptoms (EHV-1)

The symptoms of myeloencephalopathy often progress for 48 hours, and then plateau out before improving slowly. Full recovery can take many months but this may be shortened by a correct homeopathic prescription. A few horses may show progression of the symptoms and may fail to recover.

Agaricus 30c

This is the principal remedy to help with the symptoms of ataxia in the earlier stages, where the gait seems uneven and is obviously progressing to the stage where signs of paralysis or weakness can be seen.
Dose: four times daily

Gelsemium 200c

Gelsemium encompasses many of the symptoms seen with this disease; the general ataxia, lack of co-ordination, hind limb weakness, urinary incontinence and faecal retention. As such it is one of the most important remedies to be considered in treating symptoms associated with the EHV-1 virus. As a fever remedy it can be considered as an alternative to Aconite in the early stages where the symptoms are slow to appear and including trembling or shivering. Horses that are likely to respond best will show additional signs of apathy, general listlessness or dullness.
Dose: every one to two hours

Conium 30c

The key feature of Conium is progressive hind limb weakness where symptoms include heaviness, weariness and unsteadiness. It is best used before the stage of paralysis is reached where the horse is unable to get up.
Dose: four times daily

Causticum 30c

One of the keynotes of Causticum is paralysis and

hence its application in treating the symptoms which predominate in the later stages. These include hind limb weakness and paralysis. Causticum should always be used where urinary incontinence is present.
Dose: four times daily

Nux vomica 30c
Indicated where the hind legs are affected and where the horse drags one or both legs, wearing away the tip of the toe. These cases show slow progressive weakness. Inflammation of the nasal membranes causes the nose to appear stuffed so that the horse 'snuffles'.
Dose: three times daily

Plumbum 30c
Plumbum is best reserved for the stage where paralysis and ataxia are both evident and accompanied by faecal retention.
Dose: four times daily

Phosphorus 30c
Phosphorus covers many of the neurological symptoms of this condition and can be put to use to slow down the progressive symptoms of weakness and paralysis which eventually lead to horse sitting in the classic dog sitting position. Animals likely to respond well will show symptoms of increased thirst and restlessness.

Additional remedies used in the homeopathic treatment of EHV-1

Echinacea 30x
This remedy is indicated where the virus has entered the white blood cells and is suppressing the immune system, reducing ability to fight off other infections.
Dose: three times daily

Selenium 30c
Add where the immune system is suppressed as indicated by a low white cell count (leucopaenia)
Dose: two times daily

Vanadium 6c
Vanadium can be used alongside Echinacea to support the immune system, acting to increase the activity of the white cells in fighting off infection.
Dose: three times daily

Caulophyllum 200c
Exposed pregnant mares should be dosed with Caulophyllum in an attempt to prevent abortion.
Dose: once weekly for the first seven months of pregnancy then three times weekly

Equine Influenza Virus – Equine Flu Infectious Equine Bronchitis Infectious Equine Cough Newmarket Cough

Infection with this virus (which occurs through contact with infected horses) is common. It results in flu-like symptoms as a result of the virus attacking the cells that line the respiratory tract from the nose down through to the lungs. Foreign material such as debris, dust or bacteria cannot be cleared from the respiratory tract with the possible risk of bronchitis or pneumonia. Oedema or swelling of the legs can also occur in such cases.

Symptoms arise within three days of infection with affected animals running a fever (up to 41°C, 105.8°F) accompanied by a drop in appetite.This is followed by a deep, hacking cough (dry at first and moist later on) and a watery nasal discharge (which may be absent altogether or minimal in amount) that can rapidly change colour if secondary bacterial infection occurs. The lymph nodes under the jaw are often enlarged.

Homeopathic treatment of equine flu

Untreated, uncomplicated cases should recover in about ten days, although a cough may remain for some weeks afterwards. Affected horses should be kept away from all other horses and rested and then only returned to work gradually. Recovery time is hastened by using appropriate homeopathic remedies.

More complicated cases, where secondary bacterial infection occurs, carry the risk of death as a result of pneumonia (See respiratory system, page 84), pleurisy (see respiratory system, page 86), or purpura haemorrhagica. (See blood and blood vessels, page 103.)

Further complications include the risk of developing allergy-based problems (such as COPD), guttural pouch infections and sinusitis. (See pages 78, 80 and 90.)

The remedies listed are for the initial stages. Where a cough persists see respiratory system page 87.

Aconite 1M
Use Aconite at the very onset of the condition where fever is present with the absence of other symptoms.
Dose: *every 15 minutes until the symptoms abate or another remedy is indicated*

Gelsemium 200c
Indicated where the horse appears extremely dull and every movement appears a great effort. There is a general appearance of apathy.
Dose: *every 15 minutes until the symptoms abate or another remedy is indicated*

Baptisia 1M
Horses that require Bapitisa are extremely ill with symptoms appearing suddenly and progressing rapidly with a high fever, risk of pneumonia and very marked lethargy.
Dose: *every 15 minutes until the symptoms abate or another remedy is indicated*

Pyrogen 1M
Specifically to be used where the horse has a high temperature but low pulse rate. A keynote is that the horse is restless and has to keep moving around to ease the symptoms.
Dose: *every 15 minutes until the symptoms abate or another remedy is indicated*

Bryonia 200c
Use Bryonia early in those animals where there appears to be the likelihood of pleurisy developing. Affected horses may appear thirsty, irritable and will have a dry cough.
Dose: *every 15 minutes until the symptoms abate or another remedy is indicated*

Nat mur 200c
The key pointer to Nat mur is the production of a profuse clear nasal discharge which can appear like the consistency and colour of egg white. Affected horses avoid fuss, appear dull, withdrawn and depressed and develop a slight cough that progresses to a much deeper cough.
Dose: *every 15 minutes until the symptoms abate or another remedy is indicated*

Equine Viral Arteritis (EVA)
Pinkeye
Infective Equine Cellulitis
Equine Typhoid

Caution – notifiable disease

The virus responsible for EVA causes an acute, severe, upper respiratory tract infection (more severe than both EHV-1 or Equine Flu) as well as carrying the risk of causing abortion in pregnant mares. EVA also has a specific effect on small arteries causing inflammation termed medically as arteritis.

The virus can be found in fluid from the nose of infected animals as well as the urine, faeces and vaginal secretions and is transmitted by inhalation of aerosol droplets. Infected stallions, however, can appear totally healthy but yet transmit the virus to mares during breeding. After contacting the virus, there is an incubation period of up to six days before clinical symptoms appear. One of the first symptoms is a fever that can vary from between 39–41°C (102.2–105.8°F) as well as a watery nasal discharge, cough and a decrease in appetite. The eyes become puffy as the eyelids swell and the eye becomes cloudy as the cornea is affected (a condition referred to as keratitis) along with excess production of tears that run down the side of the face. A variety of other symptoms are also seen. These can include diarrhoea and abdominal pain, jaundice, swelling of the limbs, udder, prepuce or scrotum, congestion of the mucous membranes with small haemorrhages (petechiation), dehydration and muscle weakness. Abortion is also a feature of the illness and occurs much earlier on in pregnancy than with infections with EHV-1. Foals that are not aborted and born with the infection usually die after a few days.

The illness will run a course of between three and

eight days. Where secondary bacterial infection occurs, the nasal discharge will become coloured and thickened with the risk of a bad cough developing along with difficulty breathing and congestion of the lungs (pulmonary oedema).

Homeopathic Treatment of EVA

Initial stages

Aconite 1M
Use Aconite in the early stages before there is a high fever, where there is a slight drop in appetite and a slight clear nasal discharge.
Dose: *every 20 minutes until improvement or another remedy is indicated*

Belladonna 1M
Indicated in the next stage where there is a high fever accompanied by a more profuse nasal discharge and slight cough.
Dose: *every 30 minutes until improvement or another remedy is indicated*

Nat mur 200c
Worth considering in the early stages where the animal appears depressed and withdrawn and where there is profuse tear flow from both eyes, puffy eyelids with a profuse clear nasal discharge as well.
Dose: *every 30 minutes until improvement or another remedy is indicated*

Principal remedies

Ars alb 1M
Ars alb is the main remedy for treating EVA covering all the main symptoms of the condition including fever, swelling around the eyes, watery discharge from the eyes and nose, petechial haemorrhages and diarrhoea.
Dose: *one dose every hour*

Apis mel 200c
Apis should be considered in those horses that show symptoms not only of severe conjunctivitis with very swollen eyelids, acutely inflamed conjunctival membranes, profuse discharge and keratitis, but also of pulmonary oedema, swollen limbs and swelling of the scrotum or mammary glands.
Dose: *one dose every hour*

Rhus tox 200c
The eye symptoms are also covered by this remedy, which encompasses cellulitis involving the region around the eyes, severe swelling of the eyelids, a profuse yellow coloured discharge from the eyes and corneal inflammation. Swelling of the scrotum is also covered as well as the petechial haemorrhages seen in the skin.
Dose: *one dose every hour*

Kali iod 200c
Kali iod covers the symptoms of severe keratitis, red inflamed conjunctival membranes, swelling of the lids and watery nasal discharge and is a key remedy in treating pulmonary oedema where present. Kali iod should be used where there is a violent cough and where there is a risk of pneumonia developing.
Dose: *one dose every hour*

Other useful remedies

Dose: *four times daily*

Argentum nit 30c
Add where the eye symptoms prove unresponsive to other remedies, especially where there is a marked keratitis.

Phosphorus 30c
Indicated where petechiation is marked and where jaundice is present.

Crot horr 30c
Can be used to limit effects of arteritis and subsequent petachiation of the skin.

Millefolium 30c
Can be used in a similar situation to Crot horr but specifically in cases where the fever is slow to resolve.

Ant tart 30c
Can be added where there is an imminent risk of pneumonia, and a noisy moist cough.

Equine 'Cold' Viruses
Equine Rhinovirus

The Rhinovirus is similar to the cold virus that infects humans and causes the appearance of acute onset, but usually mild, respiratory symptoms. Young horses are at most risk.

Spread and infection of this virus is by aerosols originating from infected nasal discharge, faeces or urine, following an incubation period of up to eight days. The first symptom is normally fever in conjunction with inflammation of the back of the mouth (pharyngitis) and lymph node enlargement. This is followed by a nasal discharge and a cough, which may be present for up to as long as three weeks. Most horses recover, but treatment can be useful in limiting the illness and in reducing or treating the effects of secondary bacterial infection.

Equine Adenovirus

Infection with the Equine Adenovirus is very common, especially in younger horses after weaning, leading to symptoms of an upper respiratory tract infection that ranges from moderate (in adult animals) to severe (in foals). In some foals, the infection can lead to severe pneumonia, which can prove fatal. Most horses will recover with good nursing care and support.

Following infection through a virus secreted by another animal (by means of nasal discharge, urine or faeces), a fever develops, along with a nasal discharge, conjunctivitis and a cough. This is a less prominent symptom than with infection with Rhinovirus. Diarrhoea is also a common symptom with transient softening of the dung.

Homeopathic Treatment of Equine Rhinovirus and Equine Adenovirus Infections

Aconite 1M

Aconite is best used early on before symptoms become too advanced. Affected animals will show a high fever accompanied by restlessness and anxiety. Where pharyngitis is a symptom, swallowing may be uncomfortable.

***Dose:** every 20 minutes until the symptoms abate or another remedy is indicated*

Belladonna 1M

With Belladonna, the symptoms are more intense. There is a high fever and the horse feels hot to the touch. There is a marked resentment of the throat region being examined. The pulse rate will be elevated and of a bounding nature.

***Dose:** every 15 minutes until the symptoms abate or another remedy is indicated*

Ferrum phos 200c

The symptoms related to Ferrum phos fall midway between those of Aconite and Belladonna and focus on the back area of the throat especially. This remedy is useful in early cases of Rhinovirus infection before the symptoms become too intense and before any real quantity of nasal discharge is apparent.

***Dose:** every 15 minutes until the symptoms abate or another remedy is indicated*

Eucalyptus 30c

Eucalyptus acts best after the initial stage is passed and where there is a watery clear, nasal discharge present, gradually turning coloured due to secondary bacterial infection. The nose will sound congested and an irritating cough may have just started to develop.

***Dose:** four times daily*

Phytolacca 30c

Add this remedy specifically in cases of Rhinovirus infection where the lymph nodes in the throat region remain enlarged along with an obvious watery nasal discharge.

***Dose:** four times daily*

Nat mur 30c

This remedy is indicated there is a watery nasal discharge with bouts of coughing and where the horse appears depressed and withdrawn. Conjunctivitis may be an additional feature where the eyes appear watery or have a very 'wet' appearance.

***Dose:** four times daily*

Ars alb 30c
An ideal remedy for cases where diarrhoea is present as well as early stages where the respiratory symptoms include a watery discharge from the eyes, a watery nasal discharge and a dry cough with a high temperature.
***Dose:** four times daily*

Viral Infections Characterised by Neurological Symptoms

This group of conditions have very similar symptoms and can often only be differentiated by laboratory tests. Treatment is given on a symptomatic basis.

Rabies is excluded from this list as it is invariably fatal and poses a significant and serious health risk to persons handling infected (rabid) horses.

Venezuelan encephalitis virus (ve)
Eastern equine encephalitis (ee)
Western encephalitis virus (we)
Equine arbovirus encephalomyelitis

Caution – notifiable disease

The most common causes of equine encephalomyelitis in the USA, are the Eastern, Western and Venezuelan equine encephalomyelitis viruses. All three are strains of arbovirus. Rarely seen in the UK, these viral infections are notifiable under the Animal Health Act 1981. This means that they must be reported to DEFRA if an animal is suspected of developing any of these viral forms of encephalomyelitis.

All three viruses are individual, distinct strains and vary in degree of virulence, yet produce very similar clinical signs and are spread by insects, usually mosquitoes. Initial signs can include depression although some horses may show aggressive behaviour or hyperexcitability followed by the depression stage later. Most affected animals will stop eating or drinking as the illness progresses. Food may be seen hanging from the mouth as swallowing becomes difficult. A fever will be present which will wane before a second fever phase begins accompanied by the main symptoms which affect the CNS. These include drowsiness, excitability, head pressing, blindness, circling, epileptic fits, prostration, coma and eventually death. The final outcome depends on the strain of the virus and the degree of nursing support available. As such, there is no specific treatment but homeopathic remedies can offer support with some hope of recovery.

West Nile Virus or West Nile Fever

Caution – notifiable disease

West Nile Virus was originally only seen in Africa, Asia and Southern Europe but emerged in North America in 1999 in birds. This virus is mosquito borne and is spread between birds when they are bitten by infected mosquitoes. In this way the virus multiplies. Horses can become infected when bitten by a mosquito carrying the virus but are unable to spread the virus any other animals.

Following infection, symptoms occur after an incubation period of between five and 22 days, leading to signs associated with meningitis and encephalitis. Initially there is fever with lethargy and sweating together with a drop in appetite. Weakness or paralysis of the hind limbs follows, along with muscle twitching or twitching of the muzzle. Movement is impaired and uncoordinated with aimless wandering, circling or head pressing. Swallowing can become difficult and teeth grinding may be observed in a number of horses. Convulsions, excitability, collapse, coma and death follow. About 30 per cent of all infected horses die or are put down.

Borna disease

This form of encephalitis was first seen in Germany and is caused by a virus that is relatively resistant to environmental factors compared to some of the other encephalitis viruses. It is thought to be spread by inhalation or ingestion. Symptoms appear after an incubation period of four weeks with the appearance of a fever, paralysis of the throat, muscle tremors and hyperaesthesia (excessive sensitivity to external stimuli such as being touched or to noise). In the later stages affected horses appear lethargic and lose muscle tone so that a flaccid type of paralysis results. Many of these cases will unfortunately die.

Japanese encephalitis

This condition is primarily one which affects humans and which is then spread to horses. Symptoms vary widely in severity, with some showing fever, a drop in appetite, jaundice and slow, sluggish movements for a few days followed by recovery. In severe cases there is extreme lethargy, fever and sleepiness. Jaundice is also a feature along with difficulty in swallowing, incoordination and ataxia (staggering). Other short lasting symptoms may also be seen, including rigidity of the muscles of the neck, paralysis of the radial nerve and of the lips and finally blindness. The very worst of all the cases exhibit a high fever along with hyperexcitability, sweating, muscle tremors and violent uncontrollable movements. Recovery is likely in all but the worst cases.

Homeopathic Treatment of Viral Infections Characterised by Neurological Symptoms

Early stages

Aconite 1M
Of most use on initial diagnosis where there is fever with few other signs.
Dose: *every 20 minutes until an improvement is seen or another remedy indicated*

Belladonna 1M
This is an important remedy to consider. Use where fever is present (especially with sweating) or where there are signs of aggression or violent epileptic fits or seizures characterised by thrashing of the limbs.
Dose: *half hourly until symptoms abate or another remedy is indicated*

Baptisia 200c
Baptisia is recommended where there is a fever that has proved unresponsive to Belladonna. Pain in the throat region makes swallowing very difficult and the horse has a confused, besotted, subdued look.
Dose: *half hourly until symptoms abate or another remedy is indicated*

Gelsemium 1M
Use in the early stages where dullness or lethargy are prominent signs and before any CNS involvement is apparent. Gelsemium is also an important remedy to use in later stages where there are signs of weakness or paralysis of the legs, especially the hind limbs but also where swallowing is difficult due to the muscles of the throat being affected.
Dose: *every 15 minutes until an improvement is seen or another remedy indicated*

Later stages

Agaricus 200c
Agaricus covers the symptoms of hyperexcitability, muscle twitching and weakness resulting in uncoordinated (ataxic) movements. Difficulty in swallowing is another observed symptom as the throat becomes very dry. It is also a remedy for the later stages of these viral conditions where there is mental depression, drowsiness or indifference, after the stage of muscle twitching is past.
Dose: *every 15 minutes*

Helleborus 200c
This is a specific remedy to use where head pressing is a symptom. Helleborus can also be used in later stages where there is sensorial depression preceding the coma stage. ***Dose:*** *every 15 minutes*

Zincum metallicum 200c
Another remedy for head pressing but should only be considered with the accompanying symptoms of muscular twitching, rolling of the head from side to side or restless movements of the legs.
Dose: *every 15 minutes*

Hyoscyamus 1M
A remedy to be considered at the epileptic stage where there are also signs of violence or aggression. Symptoms of delirium and vocal activity distinguish this remedy from Belladonna.
Dose: *every 15 minutes*

Conium 200c
Principally used in cases where the hind limbs are weak and getting progressively worse, tending

towards paralysis.
Dose: twice daily

Strychnine 200c
Used where there is marked violent muscular twitching, involuntary limb movements and hyperaesthesia. Strychnine also covers the symptoms of stiffness of the neck and contraction/rigidity of the neck muscles as seen particularly in cases of Japanese encephalitis.
Dose: twice daily

Plumbum 200c
Plumbum is more specific for cases such as Borna disease where symptoms include flaccid paralysis and hyperaesthesia.
Dose: twice daily

Final stages

Camphor 30c
This remedy is worth considering in the later stages of the disease, following the epileptic stage, where the animal is collapsed and verging on coma or near death. There is a clear indication for Camphor if the horse is cold to the touch.
Dose: every ten minutes

Opium 200c
This remedy is an alternative to Camphor. Indications are very similar but more likely to help if the animal does not feel chilly.
Dose: every ten minutes

During recovery

Causticum 30c
Useful in those horses that are undergoing recovery where there are signs of residual weakness or paralysis.
Dose: twice daily

Phos ac 30c
Similarly used during recovery where the animal has become debilitated or weak.
Dose: twice daily

Viral conditions characterised by skin lesions

Equine herpes virus 3 (EHV-3)
Coital exanthema
Spots

See Reproductive System, page 151

Equine papilloma virus

See Skin (warts), page 262

Horse pox virus

This is a rare condition that occurs in Europe from time to time. There is a small risk of younger horses not surviving if the disease is severe. Other badly affected horses may become debilitated. The cause is a pox virus that is related to the virus of cowpox and spread by handling, grooming and contaminated tack.

Pox lesions develop in the mouth (the buccal form of the disease), first on the inside of the lips, then over the whole of the inside of the mouth occasionally spreading to the pharynx, larynx and nostrils. Stomatitis (inflammation of the inside of the mouth) develops and is painful, leading to salivation and fall in appetite. In severe cases, pox lesions can develop on the vulva and on the rest of the body. Symptoms, which can be confused with mud fever, can also develop at the back of the pastern (the leg form), and involve the typical pox lesions that start as a small papule, progressing through to the vesicular stage followed by the formation of pustules and scabs.

Homeopathic treatment of horse pox virus

Ars alb 30c
Can be used in the early stages where the mouth is affected and vesicles are present especially on the upper lips. Affected horses appear restless. Arsenicum is also indicated where there are lesions on the legs.
Dose: four times daily

Nat mur 30c
Helps where there are initially vesicles on the lips and before any other lesions develop. Horses that respond well to Nat mur appear thirsty, depressed and withdrawn.
Dose: four times daily

Cantharis 200c
Indicated in cases where the symptoms of stomatitis are evident and where there are a great many vesicles. The whole of the mouth may be affected, including the larynx and pharynx. Pain leads to the production of sticky, thick mucus which drools from the mouth.
Dose: three times daily

Borax 30c
An alternative to Cantharis but where the symptoms are less pronounced. Salivation is evident but is less profuse and not so thick on comparison.
Dose: four times daily

Kali chlor 30c
Another alternative remedy to use where there are signs of severe and extensive stomatitis where the whole of the inside of the mouth appears red, swollen and inflamed.
Dose: four times daily

Ant crud 30c
Indicated where there are extensive lesions that cover the whole body or where there are vesicles, pustules or honey-coloured scabs.
Dose: four times daily

Kali iod 30c
Matches the symptoms of both forms of the disease and can be used where both are both present at the same time.
Dose: four times daily

Vesicular stomatitis virus

Caution – notifiable disease

Vesicular stomatitis occurs not only in horses, but also in cattle and pigs. It is spread by insects and by contact between individual horses leading to sporadic outbreaks in both North and South America. After an incubation period, which takes on average nine days, a fever develops, following which the virus causes vesicular lesions to appear on the tongue (often badly affected) and lips. Rarely vesicles can also appear on the udder and prepuce. When the vesicles (which can be as large as 2cm) burst, they leave raw ulcerated areas that heal quickly (in three or four days) but cause the production of thick, ropy saliva. Some horses will show difficulty eating until the ulcers heal.

Homeopathic treatment

Aconite 1M
Dose during the incubation period before any vesicles are present.
Dose: hourly

Baptisia 200c
Indicated where there is a fever along with early lesions on the tongue that are obviously painful as the horse has some trouble eating.
Dose: hourly

Arsenicum album 30c
Should be used where there is fever and vesicles present on both the lips and tongue.
Dose: four times daily

Natrum mur 30c
Used in a similar situation to Arsenicum, but where affect horses appear sullen and depressed. The tongue appears sore and is uncomfortable.
Dose: four times daily

Nitric acid 200c
Use at a more advanced stage where the tongue shows painful vesicles, especially along its edges and where the lips also show uncomfortable vesicles.
Dose: three times daily

Capsicum 30c
Indicated where the vesicles have ulcerated leaving raw painful areas and where secondary bacterial infection causes a bad odour from the mouth.
Dose: four times daily

Merc sol 30c
Merc sol is best saved for those horses where ulceration of the lesions has caused production of ropy, thick saliva.
Dose: four times daily

Equine viral papular dermatitis

This condition is caused by pox viruses and spread by insects. Infection causes the appearance of rounded pimples or papules only, covered with crusts, which form after about a week. Areas of hair loss are left (alopecia) as the scabs fall off. The condition is self-limiting but can be helped by using the following remedies: **Calc sulph** 30c (initial lesions), **Kali iod 30c** (if itchy), **Tellurium 30c** (alopecia), **Thallium 6c** (marked alopecia).
Dose: twice daily

Equine molluscum contagiosum

This skin problem is also caused by pox viruses and leads to the appearance of greyish white pimples with a waxy appearance under the front legs, thighs, on the mammary glands, penis and prepuce. The principal remedies to help clear the condition are **Ars alb 30c** (lean horses), **Calc carb 30c** (heavier horses) and **Molluscum contagiosum nosode 9c**.
Dose: twice daily

Other viral infections

Equine infectious anaemia (EIA) Swamp fever

Caution – notifiable disease

This is a contagious viral disease of horses that is transmitted by biting insects and which occurs worldwide in low-lying swampy regions. Spread can also occur through blood-contaminated needles, surgical instruments and tack. Following an acute initial illness, some horses may subsequently go on to develop recurrent symptoms so that the disease becomes a chronic, long-term problem. A few horses may develop an illness that is sub-clinical in which no obvious symptoms are to be seen. These animals are classed as carriers and can spread the disease to other horses.

Following infection there is an incubation period of up to four weeks on average, although this period can last as long as several months. At first the horse may appear depressed, uncoordinated and weak with some loss of condition. A variable fever (up to 104–108°F, 40–42.2°C) develops with temperature variations that appear to fluctuate rapidly. Other signs that develop include severe anaemia, jaundice, petechial haemorrhages (on the mucous membranes at the base of the tongue and eye), oedema (swelling) of the legs, prepuce and underside to the abdomen and an increase in the heart rate. Myocarditis (inflammation of the heart muscle) is a common finding, as is enlargement of the spleen.

It is not uncommon for horses to recover from this acute stage, while a few become weaker and weaker over a period of time and will subsequently die. Recovery in many cases is only temporary, with symptoms returning after a few weeks, albeit in a less severe (subacute) form. Even at this stage, some animals may not survive the illness. This pattern of recovery and relapse can become a chronic situation with stress a contributory factor and with many months between episodes. Relapses are characterised by bouts of fever, weight loss, weakness, heart problems, pale mucous membranes and anaemia.

Homeopathic treatment of EIA

Recovering animals present a risk as carriers and may be destroyed as part of a control programme in some areas. There is no specific conventional treatment.

Acute cases

Aconite 1M
Best used very early on as soon as symptoms appear
Dose: every 20–30 minutes

Belladonna 1M
Indicated at the stage of high fever where the pulse is rapid
Dose: every 20–30 minutes

TNT 30c
TNT can be used in acute cases to limit the anaemia and to help treat the subsequent jaundice.
Dose: four times daily

Phosphorus 30c
Can be used to treat symptoms of anaemia, jaundice incoordination, weakness and especially where there are petechial haemorrhages present.
Dose: four times daily

Chronic cases

China 30c
China is best used where the disease has become chronic and where a relapse has occurred with symptoms of fever, weakness, anaemia and debility. A good supportive remedy during recovery that can be given daily over a long period of time.
Dose: relapses four times daily
Recovery and support once daily

Ferrum metallicum 30c
Ferrum can be used to assist recovery where the anaemia is profound and where pallor of the mucous membranes is very marked, a symptom that will often only appear in later stages of the disease. This remedy can also be used where there are mild relapses and where there is a fever that is not high.
Dose: three times daily

Chininum arsenicosum 30c
Protracted weakness with heart problems indicate this remedy which can be used to encourage recovery between bouts.
Dose: twice daily

Abrotanum 30c
Another remedy offering support where the animal is debilitated, despite eating well.
Dose: twice daily

Additional remedies

Apis 30c Where there is oedema

Ceanothus 30c For splenic enlargement

Crataegus 6c, Adonis 6c, Digitalis 6c, Strophanthus 6c To support the heart where there is myocarditis

Chelidonium 30c General liver support where jaundice is present

Dose: two or three times daily

African Horse Sickness
Caution – notifiable disease

This serious viral condition, which is spread by insects, occurs in horses in some areas of Africa, with incidents in the Middle East and Southern Europe recorded. There are three distinct forms of the illness, an acute pulmonary form, a subacute cardiac form and horse sickness fever. Rarely, mixed forms are seen as well. Following infection, there is an incubation period of between five and seven days with a fever of 40–41°C (105–106°F) in all forms of the illness.

Acute pulmonary (respiratory) form
This form of the illness is the most common. Laboured breathing and bouts of coughing along with a frothy, yellow, fluid discharge from the nose follow the fever stage. Severe sweating ensues, along with weakness, incoordination, collapse and eventual death four to five days after the initial appearance of the symptoms. In the small proportion of horses that survive, laboured breathing is observed for some weeks afterwards.

Subacute cardiac form
Following a longer period of incubation of up to three weeks, fever develops slowly accompanied by oedema (swelling) of the head (including the temple area, the eyelids and lips) with spread to the neck, brisket and chest. The mucous membranes in the mouth take on a blue tinge (cyanosis) with small petechial haemorrhages on the tongue. Fluid collects around the heart (hydropericardium) with endocarditis and accumulation of fluid in the lungs (pulmonary oedema). Affected horses often appear restless and may show signs of mild colic. Paralysis of the oesophagus with regurgitation of food and water and difficulty swallowing, can also be a feature. Fewer horses die with this form of the disease, but there is a prolonged recovery period.

Horse sickness fever

The symptoms of this form may go unrecognised, as there may be no clear diagnostic signs. A fever develops of up to 40.5°C (105°F) within three days and then returns to normal after a further three days. A drop in appetite is common along with a mild conjunctivitis and some difficulty in breathing.

Homeopathic treatment of African Horse Sickness

Fever stage

Aconite 1M

Useful only in the very early stages of the disease before other symptoms have developed.
Dose: hourly

Acute pulmonary (respiratory) form

Arsenicum album 200c

Principal remedy to use in this form of the illness where the symptoms include laboured breathing, coughing and frothy nasal discharge.
Dose: every two to three hours

Antimonium tart 200c

Useful where breathing is laboured and where rattling noises can be heard from the chest along with repeated coughing.
Dose: every two to three hours

Stannum 30c

Stannum is best reserved for those cases where the paroxysmal bouts of coughing are the most prominent symptom along with difficulty breathing. Limbs appear weak and movements are uncoordinated. It is a good remedy to use during the recovery phase for those horses that survive the most severe stages.
Dose: four times daily

Alumina 200c

Use where there is very laboured breathing with very marked ataxia.
Dose: three times daily

Conium 200c

Indicated where there is marked weakness of the hind limbs with incoordination and laboured breathing.

Opium 200c

Use in the later stages where there is laboured breathing, weakness and the animal is approaching a state of collapse.
Dose: every 30 minutes

Subacute cardiac form

Arsenicum alb 200c

One of the most important remedies to consider at the stage where petechial haemorrhages on the tongue are evident along with the problems of both endocarditis, hydropericardium or where paralysis of the oesophagus is apparent. Breathing is laboured almost as if the horse appears to be suffocating. Mucous membranes appear to have a blue (cyanotic) colour due to lack of oxygen and poor circulation.
Dose: every two hours

Apis 200c

Add where there are signs of swelling (oedema) of the head, neck, eyelids, lips or pulmonary oedema. Breathing is laboured and difficult. Any increase in ambient heat causes the symptoms to intensify.
Dose: every two hours

Antimonium tart 200c

Laboured breathing with rapid short breaths, due to pulmonary oedema, along with rattling noises in the chest suggests Ant crud. Again it appears almost as if the horse was suffocating.
Dose: every two hours

Phosphorus 200c

Phosphorus can be added where the petechial haemorrhages on the tongue are very marked.
Dose: three times daily

Gelsemium 200c

Consider where there are signs of paralysis of the oesophagus and difficulty swallowing. Cases that fail to respond to Arsenicum may respond to this remedy.
Dose: three times daily

Cactus 6x
Can be used to support the heart generally and can be prescribed alongside other remedies. Cactus is especially useful where endocarditis and oedema is present.
Dose: three times daily

Other indicated remedies include **Lachesis 30c** (pulmonary oedema), **Cuprum 30c** (cyanosis), **Opium** 200c (cyanosis and oesophageal paralysis), **Kalmia 6c** (endocarditis).
Dose: three times daily

Horse sickness fever

Belladonna 30c
Belladonna can be used in this form of the illness where symptoms are apparent.
Dose: four times daily

Equine rotavirus

Rotavirus, which can be naturally present in healthy animals, can cause acute diarrhoea in young foals that is profuse, watery and foul smelling. Infection occurs when foals come into contact with contaminated feed or surfaces. As the infection is self limiting most animals will recover within seven days, unless complications ensue. The virus attacks the cells lining the bowel, not only causing diarrhoea, but also leading to dehydration, depression, abdominal pain, teeth grinding, lethargy and weakness as the foal fails to suck from the mare, which will then have a full udder.

Treatment of Rotavirus infection

Podophyllum 30c
Podophyllum is the remedy to select where there is abdominal pain accompanied by teeth grinding. Watery diarrhoea is passed painlessly and can appear greenish in colour.
Dose: four times daily

Elaterium 30c
Diarrhoea which is green and frothy and which squirts out with some force suits Elaterium. Signs of mild abdominal discomfort may be present.
Dose: four times daily

Gratiola 30c
Gratiola can help where the diarrhoea is watery, green, frothy and passed without effort or pain.
Dose: four times daily

Crot tig 30c
Signs of straining and discomfort are present where Crot tig is useful. Watery diarrhoea (which is copious in quantity) is shot out with some force and followed by urging. Gurgling sounds may be audible from the bowel. Symptoms are worse for suckling or feeding.
Dose: four times daily

Gambogia 30c
Gambogia suits diarrhoea which is profuse and watery and which is accompanied by straining, abdominal distension, rumbling sounds and pain. Symptoms are worse in the evening and at night.
Dose: four times daily

Jatropha 30c
This remedy is indicated where the diarrhoea is not only watery but appears like rice water and is expelled with some considerable force.
Dose: four times daily

More serious cases may well warrant the addition of the following remedies, which should be given *four times daily*

Forceful watery diarrhoea with prostration or collapse, animal cold to the touch **Veratrum album 200c**

Total collapse, icy feel to body **Carbo veg 200c**

Collapse with weak pulse, body cold, breathing laboured **Camphor 200c**

Where there is dehydration **China 200c**

Infections Caused by Bacteria

Strangles

Strangles is an acute condition, seen worldwide, caused by infection with *Steptococcus equi*. The main symptoms involve the upper respiratory tract and the adjacent lymph nodes, affecting mainly younger horses up to about five years of age and especially those in large groups.

Horses contract the infection by direct contact with the nasal discharge of infected animals, through contaminated pasture, water and feed troughs, clothing and equipment. Infection can be spread for up to a period of four weeks after the appearance of clinical signs. The bacteria are relatively resistant to environmental factors and may remain a risk for up to four weeks after the source of the infection has been removed.

Following infection there is an incubation period of between four and eight days after which the symptoms appear suddenly. A drop in appetite is accompanied by a fever (39.5–40.5°C, 103–105°F), a watery nasal discharge that becomes coloured and purulent, inflammation of the pharynx (pharyngitis) and larynx (laryngitis), a moist cough, which causes discomfort and occasionally conjunctivitis. The throat area may become painful so that the head is extended out in an attempt to relieve the discomfort and swallowing may become so difficult that food or water is regurgitated through the nose. After two or three days the fever abates but returns as the characteristic abscesses develop in the lymph nodes of the throat region. Affected lymph nodes swell, become both hot and painful and, if left untreated, discharge serum followed by thick, creamy yellow pus.

In severe cases, other lymph nodes are affected and abscesses may occur superficially at any point on the body, but especially on the face and limbs. Obstruction of local lymphatic vessels can lead to accumulation of fluid (oedema). Infection can also spread to the sinuses and guttural pouches (see respiratory system, pages 78). It is rare for horses to die from this condition unless infection spreads to internal organs. The illness can last for up to three weeks in duration. One of the consequences of infection with *Steptococcus equi* is sensitivity to streptococcal proteins, leading to a condition known as purpura haemorrhagica (see blood and blood vessels, page 103).

Homeopathic treatment of strangles

Initial stages

Aconite 1M
Dose with Aconite in the very early stages before any other symptoms develop
***Dose:** every 15–20 minutes until an improvement is seen or another remedy indicated*

Belladonna 1M
Indicated where there is a high fever and swallowing is already a little difficult as lymph nodes local to the throat are enlarged. There will also be a drop in appetite. Other signs to look for include a bounding full pulse and irritability.
***Dose:** half hourly until symptoms abate*

Ferrum phos 30c
Use Ferrum phos where the symptoms are past the Aconite stage but are not yet as intense as for Belladonna. Throat symptoms including laryngitis are present but there will also be a cough, which is hard and dry.
***Dose:** half hourly until symptoms abate*

Lachesis 200c
Symptoms centred on the throat are the key to using Lachesis. There is great sensitivity to handling around this area with the horse kicking out at the least touch. Symptoms are worse on the left-hand side. The throat area is painful so that swallowing is difficult with the neck extended. These signs are accompanied by a dry cough.
***Dose:** hourly until symptoms abate*

Where a nasal discharge is present

Merc sol 30c
Use where the nasal discharge is predominantly green or yellow green, thick and purulent and may make the nostrils sore.
***Dose:** three times daily*

Kali bich 30c
In this instance the nasal discharge is extremely thick, stringy and greenish-yellow in colour. The lymph nodes around the throat are swollen.
***Dose:** three times daily*

Hydrastis 30c
Hydrastis fits the picture where the nasal discharge is thick, yellow and ropy but is initially watery and accompanied by much sneezing.
***Dose:** three times daily*

Pulsatilla 30c
Here the nasal discharge is creamy, bland and slightly greenish as opposed to thick and yellowish. Catarrh in the throat causes the horse to cough up bland looking mucus.
***Dose:** three times daily*

Stage of abscessation

Hepar sulph 6x
This remedy in low potency will promote suppuration and hasten ripening of any abscesses that need to mature so that they can discharge their contents.
***Dose:** four times daily*

Hepar sulph 200c
In higher potency Hepar sulph can be used to resolve discharging abscesses where the affected lymph nodes are quite painful to touch.
***Dose:** three times daily*

Silica 200c
Use in a similar situation to high potency Hepar but where the discharging lymph nodes are relatively painless to touch.
***Dose:** three times daily*

Calc sulph 200c
Calc sulph covers many of the symptoms seen in strangles and suits horses of a heavier build. It acts best where there is a yellowish, purulent nasal discharge accompanied by discharging lymph nodes where the pus is yellow, thick and possibly lumpy.
***Dose:** three times daily*

Phytolacca 30c
Phytolacca is an ideal remedy
affected lymph nodes arounc
the touch as well as hot and
which occur during the sec
swelling of the lymph nodes can narro
and make swallowing difficult. Additional symptoms include pharyngitis and a dry hacking cough.
***Dose:** four times daily*

Where there is oedema

Apis mel 200c
This is the main remedy to consider where obstruction of the lymphatic vessels has led to local oedema.
***Dose:** three times daily*

To assist recovery

Sulphur iodatum 6c
Indicated once the main infection has cleared but where there is residual throat pain.
***Dose:** three times daily*

Prevention

Strangles nosode 30c
Routine use of the nosode may help prevent an outbreak. This remedy can also be used in treatment of cases alongside other remedies.
***Prevention:** dose twice daily for five days in anticipation of a period of risk*
***Treatment:** dose twice daily*

Contagious Equine Metritis (CEM)

Caution – notifiable disease

This is a bacterial disease of horses which is spread venereally and which involves infection with a number of contagious bacteria. *Taylorella equigenitalis* (the contagious equine metritis organism – CEMO), *Klebsiella pneumoniae* and *Pseudomonas aeruginosa*. Spread is either by direct transmission between horses at the time of mating or teasing, but can also be through semen from infected stallions (used for artificial insemination) or through water, instruments or accidental human transfer.

The disease in mares can vary in severity and

ıe appearance of a vaginal discharge (due ımation of the uterus) between one to six ıter infection in the acute situation. The ease can also exist in a chronic form with less obvious symptoms due to a deep-seated infection that may not result in the appearance of a vaginal discharge until some 80 days after infection. The chronic state can be difficult to clear.

A carrier state can also exist where there are no signs of infection but where the mare remains infectious. Stallions and teasers are normally just carriers and rarely show clinical symptoms but nevertheless, are able to transfer the infection to mares during mating.

Homeopathic treatment of mares with CEM[12]

Homeopathic remedies can clear the infection from the reproductive tract of the mare. The choice of remedy depends principally on the nature of the discharge amongst other symptoms. As a guide consider:

Milky discharge **Pulsatilla**, **Calc carb**

Makes perineal skin sore **Nitric acid, Sepia**, **Silica**

Bland, creamy **Pulsatilla**

Dark coloured **Kreosotum**

Very profuse **Graphites**, **Sepia**, **Lycopodium**, **Thuja**

With lumps **Sepia**

With bad odour **Kreosotum**, **Sepia**

Stringy, thick **Sabina**, **Nitric acid**, **Kali bich**, **Hydrastis**

Watery, thin **Graphites**, **Nitric acid**, **Pulsatilla**

Clear, transparent **Nat mur**, **Sepia**

White **Borax**, **Graphites**, **Nat mur**, **Sepia**

Yellow **Arsenicum**, **Calc carb**, **Hydrastis**, **Kreosotum**, **Sepia**

Dose: *30c two or three times daily until symptoms resolve*

For difficult cases, particularly chronic cases, consider either **Medorrinum 200c** *once daily for five days* or **Syphilinum 200c** *once daily for five days.*

Salmonella
Salmonellosis

Salmonella can cause serious illness in horses with a number of different species involved. Approximately 75 per cent of infections involve *Salmonella typhimurium*. Other species implicated can includes *S. newport*, *S. enteritidis* and *S. dublin*. In the majority of cases, affected animals are often debilitated or unduly stressed, with a smaller proportion infected through contaminated feed or water. A number of horses can act as carriers of the bacteria and, although they have no symptoms, they pass the organism continuously or intermittently in their dung. The illness takes four different forms: peracute (septicaemic form), acute, chronic and atypical. Homeopathic treatment can be used to augment conventional medicine.

Peracute salmonella infection

This form of the illness affects mainly foals and appears suddenly with a fever of 40–41°C (104–106°F) along with evidence of septicaemia, depression, appetite loss, diarrhoea containing blood and material from the lining of the bowel, abdominal pain, dehydration, an increase in respiratory and heart rates (with a weak pulse), blue tinged mucous membranes with small haemorrhages on the surface and finally circulatory collapse. Many of the affected animals die – but along with conventional treatment the following remedies could prove useful:

Dose: *200c every 20 minutes*

Baptisia Septicaemia with moderate fever plus thin, watery, foul smelling diarrhoea with dark blood.

Pyrogen Septicaemia with rapid rise to high temperature with brown or blackish foul smelling diarrhoea passed painlessly. Horse very restless.

Cantharis Evidence of bowel lining with bloody diarrhoea, mucus and straining along with shivering. Feels cold to touch.

Capsicum Bloody diarrhoea with mucus with much straining, shivering and a marked increase in thirst

Colchicum Painful diarrhoea with straining, mucus, blood and shredded particles, evidence of weakness tending towards collapse.

Merc corr Abdominal pain with slimy diarrhoea with blood and frequent ineffectual straining. Sweating can be a feature.

Veratrum album Forcefully evacuated, watery diarrhoea with ensuing weakness and debility. Animal very thirsty and extremely cold to the touch along with blue coloured mucous membranes and eventually collapse.

Arsenicum album Diarrhoea with dark-coloured blood and foul smell, with straining together with abdominal pain. Restless and thirsty for small amounts of water each time. Feels icy cold to touch.

Carbo veg Final stages where the animal is collapsed, dehydrated and extremely cold.

China Can be added to help with dehydration.

Phos ac Helpful during recovery in debilitated horses.

Acute salmonellosis

This form occurs mostly in adult horses. Symptoms appear suddenly, the first sign of which is a fever, ranging from 40–41°C (104–106°F) with an increase in heart rate and respiratory rate. Depression, with a drop in appetite follows, along with weakness. Diarrhoea follows with mild abdominal discomfort but may not appear for several days. Septicaemia develops in many cases, together with dehydration and collapse of the circulation. These symptoms in fact resemble the peracute illness, but the illness runs a longer course with many surviving as long as three weeks. Some animals may survive with care and appropriate use of homeopathic remedies. Some of these will become salmonella carriers.

The remedies listed above are all useful in treating this condition.

Chronic salmonellosis

This can follow on from the acute condition or can arise in its own right and is believed to be a consequence of damage to or changes occurring in the bowel lining. The prognosis can be poor. Affected horses may die or subsequently be destroyed. Symptoms involve weight loss, soft dung with episodes of more acute diarrhoea with accompanying fever and loss of appetite. Affected horses constitute a health risk.

Use the **Salmonella nosode** (in **30c** potency given *once daily for ten days*) along with an appropriate remedy from those given in the list of general remedies for chronic diarrhoea (Digestive system, page 121) such as **Gaertner-Bach**, **Silica**, **Nat mur**, **Acetic acid**, **Abrotanum**, **Iodum**, **Podophyllum**, **Phosphorus** and **Sulphur** adding **Aconite**, **Belladonna** or **Baptisia** where bouts of fever recur.

Atypical (asymptomatic) salmonellosis

This form is triggered by stress, which can include competitions and events, transportation and veterinary procedures including surgery. Signs of depression, a drop in appetite with a fever, slight abdominal pain and soft dung are the main signs to look for. Recovery normally occurs within a week. Homeopathy can be used to minimise stress and reduce the chance of the condition being triggered.

Useful remedies are given below.

Dose: *one dose 30 minutes before stressful situation and repeated to effect.*

Where there is

Fear **Aconite 1M**

Restlessness or agitation **Arsenicum album 200c**

Excitement **Argentum nit 200c**

Pre-event nerves **Lycopodium 200c**, **Argentum nit 200c** or **Dys co 200c**

A change in feeding routine **Nux vomica 200c**

Risk of becoming over heated **Ant crud 200c**

Clostridial diseases

Clostridium perfringens type A enterotoxaemia
Colitis X
Oedematous bowel syndrome
Equine intestinal clostridiosis

In adult horses *Clostridium perfringens* can cause an acute form of colitis (inflammation of the colon) sometimes referred to as colitis X. This particular species of bacteria normally inhabits the bowel in small numbers and under certain circumstances can produce a type of toxin, known as an enterotoxin. Symptoms of the illness develop extremely rapidly with signs of acute toxaemia including fever, rapid weak pulse and injected (muddy, red coloured) mucous membranes. The majority of affected horses exhibit signs of acute pain and may die before any signs of profuse diarrhoea (enteritis) are apparent, although some animals may show signs of distension of the bowel with gas build-up. Body temperature rapidly falls and becomes subnormal although the skin will feel cold and clammy quite early on during the disease. Most horses will survive no longer than 24 hours, many considerably less. Emergency intensive conventional care is needed if the horse is to survive.

Homeopathic treatment

Dose: *200c or 1M every five to ten minutes*

Initial stages of acute enterotoxaemia **Pyrogen**

Where there is pain **Belladonna**, **Merc corr**

With signs of enteritis/diarrhoea **Veratrum album** (diarrhoea evacuated with great force), **Carbo veg** (diarrhoea dribbles out), **Merc corr** (with straining)

Gaseous distension of the bowel **Colchicum** (with pain)

With cold clammy skin **Carbo veg**

Final stages – collapse **Arsenicum album**, **Carbo veg**

Tetanus

See Nervous System, page 232

Botulism

See The Foal, page 159

Sleepy Foal Disease
Shigellosis

See under The Foal, page 158

Tyzzer's Disease

See The Foal, page 160

Ulcerative Lymphangitis

See the Lymphatic System, page 106

Glanders
Farcy

Caution – notifiable disease

Glanders or Farcy is an old disease of horses, which is contagious, often fatal and still prevalent in particular areas of the world. It is caused by an organism known as *Pseudomonas* (*Actinobacillus*) *mallei*. The illness occurs in both acute and chronic forms and is typified initially by a high temperature, dry cough, a foul-smelling nasal discharge and acute pneumonia and in the later stages by ulcers or nodules in the respiratory tract or on the skin. Animals that apparently recover can become carriers and are an important source of infection. Clinically infected cases are best destroyed and should not be treated as the illness is transmissible to humans and can prove potentially fatal.

The best homeopathic approach is to dose animals at risk in order to try and prevent infection with **Hippozaenium 30c** (also called **Ozeana 30c**) once daily. Ironically, Glanders is one of the diseases mentioned in many of the older veterinary homeopathic texts where successful cures were reported using **Arsenicum album**, **Crot horr**, **Kali bich**, **Lachesis**, **Merc sol**, **Belladonna**, **Hepar sulph** and **Hippozaenium**.

Lyme Disease

Lyme disease occurs worldwide, including in the UK, and is caused by a corkscrew shaped, spirochete bacterium called *Borrelia burgdorferi* that is transmitted to the horse (and other animals as well as man) by ticks of a species known as Ixodes. Sometimes called blacklegged or deer ticks, the immature tick larvae become infected when they ingest blood from infected rodents. The infection rate among the ticks varies with geographical location and specific species of tick. For example, in the USA, Lyme disease is especially prevalent in New York State, Connecticut, Massachusetts, Rhode Island and New Jersey as well as Minnesota, Wisconsin and Northern California. In these regions a greater percentage of the ticks will be infected.

Infected ticks transmit the organism to new hosts when they attach themselves, feed and take a blood meal. Ticks have to undergo three distinct stages to become an adult starting with the larval stage, progressing to the nymph and finally to the adult stage. They have to feed on blood at each stage before progressing to the next phase and before they can transmit the bacteria to the new host. Ticks at the middle stage of the life cycle (nymphs) can feed on a variety of wild and domesticated animals including horses, cattle, goats, dogs and cats. Deer are the main host for adult ticks but horses may also act as host for this stage. Ticks are most likely to be picked up in forested areas as well as woodland and parkland, preferring in general, areas where moisture is present.

In many animals, including horses, infection can be subclinical without any apparent symptoms. This situation is quite common in horses, with as few as ten per cent showing clinical signs, making diagnosis quite difficult. Clear evidence of having seen ticks (particularly adult ticks) is a useful pointer. Present over the winter and during the spring, ticks may be found during routine grooming, especially around the head area, throat, belly and near the tail.

Infected horses can show a variety of symptoms involving several body systems including the joints, musculoskeletal system and nervous system. A shifting lameness is often present and involves the larger joints caused by a progressive, chronic arthritis with animals appearing generally stiff or sore. Laminitis can also be another consequence of infection. Fever is noted in some cases with loss of appetite and swelling of the glands. Behavioural abnormalities such as irritability or changes in attitude are also seen.

Homeopathic treatment of Lyme disease

Ledum 1M

Ledum is the principal remedy for treating Lyme disease and the ensuing symptoms in horses as well as other species. It covers the shifting joint symptoms seen in many cases as well some of the symptoms seen in horses where laminitis is a feature. Other laminitis remedies are listed on page 217.

Dose: one dose daily for five days

Rhododendron 200c

This remedy is a good second choice where Ledum fails to act. Pointers include joint swelling (worse on the right hand side of the body) and joint pain which is worse at rest and in wet, stormy weather. Symptoms are eased by warmth.

Dose: one dose daily for five days

Kalmia 200c

Kalmia is another remedy that acts on joints and can be used to treat cases of Lyme disease. Again there is swelling of joints with pain and consequent lameness which appears periodically and then abates quickly to return later. Symptoms are worse for movement.

Dose: one dose daily for five days

Bryonia 200c

Use Bryonia where the symptoms include fever, hot swollen and painful joints and where the horse shows irritability and an increase in thirst. Affected horses are very reluctant to move. Symptoms are worse in hot weather and eased when it cools down.

Dose: one dose daily for five days

Borrelia burgdorferi nosode 30c

The nosode can be used alongside any of the other remedies listed.

Dose: twice daily for five days

Other useful remedies

The following have been reported as being useful in treating cases of Lyme disease: **Lac caninum, Carcinosin, Thuja, Syphilinum, Arsenicum album**.

Prevention of Lyme disease

In areas of risk there are number of measures that can be used to avoid infection. Routine daily grooming is essential along with looking for and removing ticks. This method works effectively as the ticks need to feed for 12–24 hours before transmitting the organism. Tick repellents can also be used and are best applied in the early part of the spring and in the autumn, periods where the adult ticks are active. Mowing pasture and keeping it short also helps as this provides an inhospitable habitat for ticks. Dealing with rodent infestations will also help.

Homeopathically, dose horses at risk using **Ledum 1M**, *one dose weekly* and **Borrelia burgdorferi nosode 30c**, *one dose weekly.*

Leptospirosis

Leptospirosis is caused by infection with motile, spiral shaped bacteria classified as spirochetes, the same class of organisms responsible for Lyme disease. These organisms are further classified into a number of different groups called serovars and serogroups. Leptospirosis is common in both wild and domestic animals but clinical infection in horses is thought not to be common. Leptospirosis can occur in humans and therefore poses a health risk.

Infection is often due to excretion of the organism by an infected animal, however, some wild animals (such as rodents) can act as reservoirs. When the organisms are shed into the environment they can invade damaged mucous membranes or skin and then migrate around the body. In horses a variety of symptoms can occur depending on the site of infection. In pregnant mares, abortion can occur due to localisation of the organism in the uterus, placenta or the foetus. Infection in the mare can also result in stillbirth and in the birth of a weak, sick foal. If the kidneys are involved (which is extremely rare), kidney disease can ensue. By far the most common problem in the horse involves the eye, leading to moon blindness (periodic ophthalmia or recurrent uveitis). In this case, however, the cause is not due to a direct infection of the eye by leptospiral organisms, but rather by an immune-mediated reaction as a consequence of a previous leptospiral infection.

Treatment of Leptospirosis

The choice of remedy depends on where the infection localises. In all instances, treatment can be combined with use of the nosode, **Leptospira 30c**, which can be given *once daily.*

Where there is risk of abortion or stillbirth the following remedies may be of some help in prevention: **Viburnum opulus 6c** or **Caulophyllum 6c** once daily for the duration of the pregnancy.

For acute renal problems think of: **Apis mel 200c, Cantharis 200c** or **Terebinthina 200c** (see page 132)

Where periodic ophthalmia is a problem, initially consider the following remedies **Aconite 1M, Merc corr 30c** or **Rhus tox 30c**. See page 71 for more details.

Infections Caused by Rickettsia

Potomac Horse Fever (PHF) Equine Monocytic Ehrlichiosis

This condition is seen in the mainly in the North-Eastern United States and Canada and is spread by an insect vector via blood transmission, rather than by direct infection. The organism responsible, *Ehrlichia risticii*, can infect any age of animal, with infections occurring sporadically and usually involving only small groups of horses at any one time. Once an area or farm has affected animals, there is a high chance of recurrence of the disease.

Symptoms of infection appear in about 10–15 days and can vary considerably in intensity. Common signs include fever, depression, a drop in appetite, diarrhoea, reduced or increased bowel motility, colic, small haemorrhages on the mucous membranes (petechiation) and laminitis. In some horses the symptoms can be so severe as to send the animal into a state of shock. Prompt conventional treatment is needed if the horse is to survive. Homeopathy can provide additional support.

Homeopathic treatment of Potomac Horse Fever

Belladonna 1M
Belladonna is the principal remedy for the early fever stage where other symptoms include poor appetite, colic, depression, thin watery diarrhoea and a likelihood of laminitis.
Dose: *every 20–30 minutes*

Baptisia 200c
Another remedy for the fever stage but where the fever is less intense than with Belladonna and where the diarrhoea is characteristically dark-coloured, foul-smelling and watery. Increased sounds are heard from the bowel, which may show signs of distension.
Dose: *every 20–30 minutes*

Colocynthis 200c
Indicated where there are signs of colic and the horse is agitated, irritable, keeps looking round at its flank or wants to be left alone. The diarrhoea has a slimy appearance.
Dose: *every 20–30 minutes*

Arsenicum album 200c
Restlessness is the key feature of this remedy with added symptoms of watery, foul smelling diarrhoea that dribbles down the back legs making the skin sore. Petechial haemorrhages are visible on the mucous membranes as an additional pointer.
Dose: *every 20–30 minutes*

Merc sol 200c
Here the dung is loose, slimy and passed with some discomfort and straining which continues even when there is nothing further to pass. Colic is a feature.
Dose: *every 20–30 minutes*

China 30c
Principally used as an additional remedy in any case where there is dehydration and where fluid therapy has been instigated. Can be used to help in cases where there is watery diarrhoea that is passed with no effort but which debilitates the horse.
Dose: *every 20 minutes*

Camphora 30c
Camphora is reserved for the most acute cases where signs of shock are quickly evident and the horse is cold to the touch and weak to the point of collapse. The diarrhoea is dark and watery in nature and accompanied by signs of colic.
Dose: *every 20 minutes*

Potomac Horse Fever Nosode 30c
This nosode can be used in treatment (alongside other remedies) and in possible prevention of horses at risk.
Treatment: *twice daily*
Prevention*: one twice daily for five days during each period of risk*

Infections Caused by Protozoa

Babesiasis or Babesiosis
Biliary fever
Piroplasmosis

This disease, which is transmitted by blood-sucking ticks, occurs throughout the world. Various species of *Babesia* are involved depending on the exact geographical location. Once infected, there is an incubation period of up to ten days. The protozoa multiply in the blood vessels leading to breakdown of blood cells (haemolysis) along with the related symptoms of anaemia, jaundice and the presence of blood in the urine although this last symptom is not commonly seen in horses. Some horses will appear unable to move or will be found lying on their side with no attempt to get up if prompted. Fever is often present although may only last for a short period. Swelling of the hocks, head and underside of the abdomen can occur as well as colic. Affected horses can die within 24 hours of the first symptoms. Some horses can become carriers.

The disease causes a much more serious illness in younger animals which can become badly jaundiced and weakened with small haemorrhages present on the mucous membranes.

Homeopathic treatment of Babesiasis

Belladonna 200c
Use in the initial stages where a fever is present and before any other symptoms are evident.
***Dose:** hourly until improvement*

TNT 30c
TNT is one of the best remedies to use prior to the stage where haemolysis takes place (as a preventative) and to use where it has already occurred and signs of jaundice and anaemia are just apparent.
***Dose:** every 30 minutes*

Manganum acetate 30c
Can be used in a very similar way to TNT also but specifically suits cases where the horse appears unable to move or is recumbent.
***Dose:** every 30 minutes*

Phosphorus 30c
Use alongside TNT to help limit haemolysis and to help treat jaundice. Also indicated in more severe cases where petechial haemorrhages are present on the mucous membrane and in treating the subsequent anaemia.
***Dose:** every 30 minutes in acute situations; twice daily in treating anaemia*

Millefolium 30c
Add where blood is present in the urine (haematuria).
***Dose:** every hour*

Apis mel 200c
Added where symptoms of oedema are present.
***Dose:** three times daily*

During recovery

Phosphorus 30c
As above.

Ferrum met 6c
As a general remedy to help resolve anaemia.
***Dose:** twice daily*

China 30c
Helps with recovery in cases where the animal is weak, anaemic and debilitated.
***Dose:** twice daily for several weeks*

Dourine
Caution – notifiable disease

A protozoan called *Trypanosoma equiperdum* is the cause of the contagious venereal disease known as dourine. It is transmitted through mating and affects the external genital organs, the skin and may also cause paralysis. It occurs in Africa, Asia, South America, South East Europe and Eastern Europe. Following infection, the incubation period is between two and four weeks but may be as long as 12 weeks in some animals, following which there are initial signs of fever and a drop in appetite.

Clinical signs in the stallion include oedema of the prepuce, penis and scrotum, which may run forward as far as the chest. An infected, mucus-like urethral discharge is also a common finding and local lymph nodes may be swollen. Some stallions may also exhibit paraphimosis (see page 155). In mares there is a profuse fluid vaginal discharge along with vulval oedema that spreads to the udder region and floor of the abdomen.

Involvement of the nervous system follows on from the symptoms centred around the genital system and presents as stiffness, progressive weakness and incoordination of the legs. The muscles of the back legs waste away slowly, along with a general loss in condition progressing to state of emaciation, which may necessitate destruction. Where skin symptoms are evident, these comprise swellings (urticarial plaques) up to 5cm in diameter on the body and the neck. These may disappear in a few days but others may successively appear over the following weeks.

The course of the disease is more severe in Europe with many horses not surviving. Conventional treatment gives variable results with cases taking as long as 12 months to recover. Some horses act as carriers but remain free of symptoms following infection and subsequent treatment. Homeopathy can act help with the recovery of those animals that have not reached an advanced stage of deterioration.

Homeopathic symptomatic treatment of Dourine

Aconite 1M

Aconite can be used in the very early stages where signs of fever and a drop in appetite are the only observed symptoms.
Dose: every 15 minutes until an improvement is seen or another remedy indicated

Sulphur 30c

Following on from Aconite, Sulphur is the main remedy of choice in treating this condition, encompassing the majority of the symptoms of disease, including muscle wasting, emaciation, neurological symptoms, the urethral or vaginal discharge and skin symptoms.
Dose: three times daily

Apis 30c

Apis is the main remedy to consider in helping to reduce oedema where the prepuce, penis or scrotum is swollen in the stallion and the vulva in the mare. Apis will also alleviate the characteristic urticarial plaques where present on the skin.
Dose: four times daily

Urtica 200c

This remedy can also be used to help alleviate the skin symptoms where urticarial plaques are present. In addition it will reduce scrotal and vulval swelling.
Dose: four times daily

Plumbum 30c

This is the key remedy to slow the wasting of the muscles of the back limbs and the accompanying emaciation together with the incoordination and weakness seen where the nervous system is involved.
Dose: three times daily

Conium 30c

Add where hind limb incoordination is very marked and the muscles weak
Dose: three times daily

Abrotanum 30c

Can be added as an additional remedy where there is marked emaciation of the back legs in more long-standing cases.
Dose: three times daily

Equine Protozoal Myeloencephalitis (EPM)

This debilitating disease is often difficult to diagnose as it often mimics other diseases. It is widespread in the USA with over 50 per cent of horses having been exposed to the organism, a protozoal parasite called *Sarcocystis neurona*. Transmission between horses is not directly from horse to horse, but by another host, the opossum. Sporocysts, the infective stage of the organism, are passed in the opossum's faeces and are ingested by the horse during feeding or drinking. Once in the gut, the sporocysts migrate into the bloodstream and travel to brain. Here they attack the horse's central nervous system leading to a range of symptoms that can appear suddenly or over a longer period of time. Some animals are infected with the organism for many, many months before symptoms start to appear. In undiagnosed and untreated cases, permanent damage can occur to the nervous system.

Numerous symptoms are recorded principally centred around he nervous system. These include incoordination (ataxia), odd gait or lameness, stiff, stilted movements, spasticity, weakness, muscle wasting (especially of the muscles of the hind limb), difficulty swallowing, epilepsy, paralysis of the muscles of the face, mouth, eyes (seen often as drooping eyelids), excessive sweating, loss of skin sensation, loss of balance (with some horses leaning against the stable wall for support) and tilting of the head.

Treatment is on a symptomatic basis. The exact symptoms will depend on the site of the infection within the central nervous system but nearly always occur symmetrically, i.e. on both sides of the body.

Homeopathic symptomatic treatment of EPM

Dose: Acute cases: 200c three times daily
Chronic cases: 30c twice daily

Incoordination **Agaricus**, **Oxytropis**, **Conium**,

Alumina, Zinc, Phosphorus, Onosmodium (with weakness)

Stilted movement **Lathyrus**

Spasticity **Strychnine, Nux vomica**

Weakness of the limbs **Gelsemium, Picric acid** (acute cases only), **Onosmodium, Cocculus**

Muscle wasting **Plumbum**

Difficulty swallowing **Hyocyamus, Lachesis, Nux vomica, Plumbum, Stramonium, Strychnine**

Epilepsy **Belladonna, Stramonium, Hyoscyamus, Cuprum, Zinc**

Paralysis:

Face **Causticum, Cocculus**

Mouth **Gelsemium, Plumbum**

Eyes **Causticum, Gelsemium**

Excessive sweating **Eupion, Belladonna, Nux vomica, Phosphorus, Zinc**

Loss of skin sensation **Causticum, Hyoscyamus, Nux vomica, Phosphorus, Plumbum, Stramonium**

Loss of balance **Agaricus, Belladonna, Gelsemium, Phosphorus**

Head tilt **Agaricus**

Infections Caused by Coccidia

Coccidiosis

This condition is very rare and affects younger horses, normally those less than one year of age. The organism responsible is *Eimeria leuckarti*, which is often naturally present in the small intestine. Characteristic symptoms include diarrhoea with haemorrhage from the bowel which may be either of dark or bright red blood. Although the illness is self-limiting the following remedies will assist recovery.

Merc sol 30c
This is the main remedy to consider and indicated where the diarrhoea is bloody and slimy, accompanied by great straining even when there is no material to pass.
Dose four times daily

Capsicum 30c
Best used where there is bloody mucus in the dung and straining is a feature.
Dose four times daily

Crot horr 30c
Indicated where the blood is dark and the dung watery and foul smelling.
Dose four times daily

Ipecac 30c
Ipecac is indicated where the dung is dark green in colour and contains frothy, slimy material with shreds of mucus with bright red blood.
Dose four times daily

Infections Caused by Fungi

Ringworm

See Skin, page 252

Epizootic Lymphangitis
Pseudofarcy
Pseudoglanders
Equine Blastomycosis
Equine Histoplasmosis

Caution – notifiable disease

Usually affecting horses under six years of age, this condition is caused by a fungus, *Histoplasma farciminosum*. It is prevalent in parts of Africa, Asia and in countries bordering the Mediterranean. Spread occurs quickly between horses by direct contact by means of spores and has a long incubation period of up to three months.

Invading the tissues under the skin, the fungus sets up granulomatous reactions or ulcers and spreads along the lymphatic vessels. Nodules and abscesses appear, especially on the neck, head, shoulders and limbs (especially around the hock areas), which can be come swollen. In rare cases, the vulva and the scrotum can be affected as can the eye (causing keratitis and conjunctivitis) and the sinuses. The abscesses burst and discharge oily, creamy, thick pus. There is also local enlargement of lymph nodes. All the skin lesions are painless.

Recovery is very slow as the course of the disease can last up to 12 months with many animals becoming debilitated and unable to work. Homeopathic remedies can shorten the recovery period.

Homeopathic remedies for Epizootic Lymphangitis

Calc sulph 30c
The remedy most likely to help reduce the recovery time where the pus is characteristically yellow, thick and may contain lumps. Calc sulph is best used early on in the course of the disease.
Dose: twice daily on a long-term basis

Calc sil 30c
Indicated in cases where the pus is thick, yellow and creamy but also where the animal has become emaciated as in the later stages of the illness. Affected animals appear weak.
Dose: twice daily on a long-term basis

Silica 30c
Best reserved for chronic cases where other indicated remedies have failed to act or have not worked sufficiently well.
Dose: twice daily on a long-term basis

Kali iod 6x
Recommended in treating any illness where a fungal infection is involved and can be prescribed alongside other remedies. Helpful where a large number of nodules are present along the course of the lymphatic vessels.
Dose: twice daily on a long-term basis

Pulsatilla 1M
Bland creamy pus can indicate Pulsatilla, which should be used on those horses that have this type of constitution alongside other indicated remedies.
Dose: one dose weekly

Calendula 6c
Calendula can be used in the later stages of the illness to help the affected areas to heal.
Dose: twice daily as long as needed

Tuberculinum 200c
Also useful in the later stages to assist recovery in horses that have become weak and debilitated.
Dose: twice weekly

Behavioural Problems

This section covers behavioural problems relating to the horse and is divided into two sections. The first deals with more specific conditions whilst the second acts as a quick reference for more common everyday problems. Remember that some changes in behaviour have their roots in physical problems, especially pain, which can alter normal behaviour significantly.

Specific Problems

Stereotypic Behaviour or Stable Vices

Crib-Biting
Wind-Sucking/Aerophagia
Weaving
Box-Walking, Pacing
Circling
Head Twisting
Self-Mutilation
Rug Tearing
Teeth Grinding
Tongue Flicking or Curling

Stereotypic behaviour occurs in all ages and breeds of horses and in those working in a wide variety of different disciplines. Occurring in foals as young as two months of age, this type of behaviour is more prevalent in older animals. By far the most common types of stereotypic behaviour are crib-biting in conjunction with wind-sucking and weaving with box-walking whilst the remainder of the problems occur much less frequently but, are nonetheless, characteristic of stereotypy.

Some other forms of unusual behaviour may appear stereotypic, but in fact occur as a result of other problems. Coprophagia (eating dung) and wood chewing, for example, arise from dietary deficiencies and door banging and hay dipping are both types of learned behaviour. Medical conditions that involve the brain, nerves and skin can both cause symptoms resembling stereotypy and will need investigation and treatment in their own right. Typically, horses displaying stereotypic behaviour tend to show variations in the behaviour pattern (such as changing the direction of circling) between episodes and continue to respond to routine handling and to environmental stimuli in contrast with behavioural changes resulting from other causes or medical conditions.

Behaviour that is classified as stereotypic has no obvious aim or function and is, by nature, repetitive (showing no change in sequence, number and length of episodes) in comparison to learned behaviour traits which show variation and which have a definite aim. The repetitive aspect of stereotypy in fact causes release of stress hormones and neurotransmitters that have a calming effect upon the horse, the ultimate aim or goal of the behaviour. Stressful situations consequently will usually serve only to increase the intensity of the behaviour in contrast to learned behavioural problems that will halt or at least stop temporarily in such situations. Punishment will also halt learned behavioural traits, in contrast to stereotypic behaviour which will continue regardless of any threat or pain induced in an attempt to stop the horse behaving in such a way.

Stressful situations (many of which may occur close together in a short time period) that are likely to induce or trigger stereotypy include:

- Changes in normal daily routine
- Change of owner, handler or rider
- Change of stable/yard

- Turning out into a new paddock
- Differences in feeding (increased palatability or an increase in protein level)
- Movement away from close companion animals
- Isolation or lack of social contact
- Travelling
- Increased work load
- A reduction in the level of fitness
- Frustration, especially at feeding time
- Weaning

Other situations include feeding or anticipation of feeding and excitement which can stimulate stereotypic behaviour (such as box-walking and crib-biting) and a number of clinical conditions. Pain for example can lead to crib-biting or pacing around, tooth abscesses can induce wind-sucking and crib-biting and some tumours can cause the animal to self-mutilate. Stereotypy is not caused by boredom or learned from watching other horses. In any group of horses subject to repetitive (chronic) stress only a few will develop stereotypic behaviour; the susceptibility is determined genetically.

Managing stereotypy or stable vices

Careful management and attention to husbandry combined with homeopathic treatment can prove successful in resolving many of these problems. Aim initially to make sure that there are no physical causes (such as an abscess) underlying the problem. Basic approaches include:

- Improve social contact and reduce isolation (recommended for horses that weave)
- Avoid strict routines
- Increase the level of fitness
- Changes in feeding (especially useful for crib-biters)
- Increase the length of time spent feeding
- Mix concentrate feed with forage to reduce level of excitement
- Feed protein sources such as grass nuts in preference to oats, maize or soya
- Reduce the protein content of the diet

Homeopathic help

One of the most powerful ways of dealing with behavioural problems of this type is to treat using constitutional remedies often in increasing potencies over several weeks to several months. In many cases, improvement will only be noted with higher potencies as problems of this type are deep seated. Professional help is often needed at this stage. ***Dose:*** Start with *30c potency* and *dose twice daily for ten days* observing any effect. If the remedy fails to act or an improvement is seen which then fades, repeat using *200c given daily for five days.* Consider going higher based on the response with the *1M potency giving three doses over 24 hours.* This can be repeated if needed if the response wains.

Pointers to useful remedies

Causes

Upset by changes in routine **Arsenicum album, Lycopodium**

Change of owner, handler, rider **Ignatia, Nat mur, Pulsatilla**

Change of yard or stable **Bryonia, Ignatia, Capsicum, Phos ac, Merc sol, Carbo animalis**

Loss of companion **Ignatia, Nat mur, Carcinosin, Staphysagria, Graphites, Pulsatilla, Causticum, Aurum**

Weaning (for mare) **Ignatia, Nat mur**

Isolation **Aurum, Psorinum, Pulsatilla, Argentum nitricum, Arsenicum album, Lycopodium, Phosphorus, Lac caninum, Hyoscyamus**

Travelling **Petroleum, Sepia, Cocculus, Gelsemium, Tabacum, Iris, Nux vomica**

Increased work load **Nux vomica, Bryonia**

Consequences

Crib-biting **Stramonium, Anacardium, Hyoscyamus,**

Cuprum, Nux vomica, Staphysagria, Tatentula hisp, Veratrum alb, Cina, Nat mur, Arsenicum, Arum triphyllum, Medorrhinum, Sulphur

Wind-sucking/Aerophagia **Platina** (specifically), **Lycopodium, Phosphorus, Pulsatilla**

Weaving **Hyoscyamus, Agaricus, Tarentula hisp, Arsenicum album, Argentum nitricum, Lycopodium, Kali carb, Phosphorus, Pulsatilla**

Teeth grinding **Belladonna, Apis, Cina, Hyoscyamus, Tuberculinum**

Circling **Stramonium, Thuja**

Pacing/Box-walking **Argentum nitricum, Sepia, Arsenicum album, Chamomillla, Stramonium, Tuberculinum, Lyssin**

Self-mutilation **Anacardium, Staphysagria, Lilium tigrinum, Arsenicum album, Tuberculinum, Natrum sulph, Lyssin, Tarentula hisp**

Rug tearing **Tarentula hisp, Stramonium, Sulphur Veratrum, Hyoscyamus**

Head twisting **Hyoscyamus, Nat mur, Lycopodium, Belladonna, Tuberculinum, Medorrhinum**

Tongue flicking **Lachesis, Helleborus, Lycopodium**

Anticipatory Anxiety

This is the type of anxiety experienced before a testing event such as an exam or driving test. Many horses experience the same type of feeling before racing, jumping or performing in the dressage ring. Homeopathic remedies can help enormously without fear of breaking the FEI rules on prohibited substances or causing sedation.
Dose: *unless otherwise stated, 200c, one dose 30 minutes before event and repeated shortly before performing and then as needed*

Lycopodium

Keynote: Anxious beforehand but always performs impeccably
The horse that needs Lycopodium is always very anxious before performing, appears restless, passes wind or dung frequently and normally lacks confidence. However, inevitably once work starts, everything calms down and the animal performs extremely well. In humans the equivalent problem is similar to the fear of appearing in public.

Argentum nitricum

Keynote: Diarrhoea caused by anxiety, wants to escape
The nervous horse that requires this remedy often passes loose dung (diarrhoea) prior to an event or may even attempt to escape from any situation of stress. Argentum nitricum type horses are hardly ever at ease and often appear hurried.

Dysentry co

Keynote: Anticipatory anxiety with insecurity and apprehension, easily flustered
This bowel nosode is suited to animals that show evidence of nervous tension before an event. Typically they are likely to be both insecure and apprehensive, taking little to disturb their concentration so that they do not perform well. They may be reluctant to load into the horsebox before an event or to enter the show arena when they arrive. Sometimes described as 'highly strung', they also lack confidence and may exhibit phobias and irrational fears.

Gelsemium 1M

Keynote: Anxiety roots the horse to the spot
The key to using this remedy is anticipatory anxiety which almost roots the horse to the spot so it is unwilling to move. If the fear is extreme then the animal may tremble. Frequent (nervous) urination is another pointer to this remedy.

Aconite 1M

Keynote: Acute anxiety with fear
Aconite is useful in the short term if no other remedy is available or matches the symptoms. It is useful if the animal also appears fearful. The dose often needs repeating frequently to maintain an effect.

Arsenicum album

Keynote: Anxiety with restlessness and pacing
The anxiety displayed by the horse needing Arsenicum results in pacing and restlessness such that the horse cannot settle at all. Profuse sweating is another clue to using this remedy.

Nat mur

Keynote: Anxiety with irritability
Horses needing Nat mur are not keen on fuss and are easily upset by the commotion involved in preparing for an event. This results in an irritable animal that resents any fuss and may become withdrawn or uncooperative on arrival at the show ground.

Silica

Keynote: Lacks confidence and willpower
Horses needing Silica lack confidence. They may also lack stamina and are prone to frequent illness as a result of stress.

Phosphorus

Keynote: Anxiety leading to excitement or jumpiness
The anxiety of Phosphorus is expressed as excitement or over-sensitivity to any external stimuli, especially noise. Horses that are likely to respond are jumpy and react to the least noise or any unusual movement around them. If excited, they are unable to concentrate until they calm down.

Grief and Pining

By nature horses are extremely sensitive emotionally. They often become closely attached to another horse or to one person in particular, sometimes far more bonded than would at first seem apparent. It is only with the loss of a companion through death, change of yard or ownership that this may become obvious by a change in behaviour or mood. This may manifest as becoming withdrawn, isolated, moody, dull or indifferent and possibly in more extreme cases show loss of condition or body weight However, some horses will grieve or pine silently and show no symptoms initially of the mental stresses at play inwardly. Continued unresolved grief can be a trigger for physical illness and is an important part of looking at any illness arising close to the loss of a companion or change of circumstances. Homeopathy has a good track record of helping resolve grief and pining issues.
***Dose**: initially with 200c daily for seven days repeating with the 1M potency if warranted to resolve the problem. Repeat using the 1M potency if the symptoms return.*

Ignatia

This is the principal remedy to consider in treating grief, both silent grief and pining, and for the deeper effects of these emotional problems. Ignatia is still appropriate even if the trigger was some time in the past. It is a key remedy for emotional shock.

Nat mur

Prolonged unresolved grief, especially where the horse appears to be depressed, withdrawn or unusually irritable suggests Nat mur as the prime remedy. Consider Nat mur also in cases where Ignatia has only partially resolved the problem. A keynote to the remedy is that fuss or attention is not tolerated well.

Phos ac

Consider Phos ac where grief and pining have caused weakness through mental exhaustion.

Carcinosin

This is also another remedy suited to treating the long-term weakening effects of grief. Along with Ignatia, Nat mur and Causticum, it ranks as one of the most important remedies in treating grief associated with the loss of a very close companion.

Pulsatilla

The motherly, submissive and gentle Pulsatilla type can hide feelings of grief well and may appear totally unaffected by the loss of a companion animal or human. Termed silent grief, the suppressed feeling may cause subsequent physical illness.

Causticum

Causticum type horses are sensitive emotionally and are concerned about the welfare of others. Consequently this remedy is used to treat cases where long-lasting grief and its effects are a problem.

Staphysagria

Grief along with feelings of resentment or indignation are clues to the use of Staphysagria. The main clue to look out for is a change in behaviour with normally balanced animals becoming irritable, angry or aggressive for no obvious physical reason.

Physical illness/conditions arising as a result of grief

The following remedies have proved useful in treating a variety of physical problems where the trigger has proved to be a change of circumstances or the loss of a companion. Included alongside each remedy is the most likely target area that will be affected (although, of course, the underlying problem can express itself through any part of the body) along with some of the chief guiding mental symptoms as pointers. In each individual case, aim constitutionally where possible.
Dose*: initially with 200c daily for seven days repeating with the 1M potency if warranted to resolve the problem. Repeat using the 1M potency if the symptoms return*

REMEDY	TARGET AREA	EMOTIONAL STATE/MENTAL SYMPTOMS
Aurum	Bone	Depressed, sensitive
Carcinosin	Skin growths, cancers	Sad, emotionally sensitive, caring, concerned
Causticum	Joints, muscles	Affectionate
Cocculus	Nervous system	Slow, dull
Crataegus	Heart	Apprehensive
Gelsemium	Nerves, muscles	Weakness, apathy
Ignatia	The senses	Nervous, excitable, moody uncontrollable
Lachesis	Immune system	Touchy, irritable, noisy (talkative)
Nat mur	Endocrine system	Withdrawn, sad
Nux vomica	Digestion	Overly sensitive, irritable
Phos ac	Physical weakness	Listless, apathetic
Phosphorus	Respiratory system	Excitable, sensitive, jumpy
Pulsatilla	Reproductive system	Shy, gentle
Staphysagria	Skin	Resentful, irritated, anger

Transportation problems

This covers difficulty loading and problems experienced during travel
Dose: *200c repeated as needed*

Loading

Fear in general of loading **Aconite**

Fears the inside of the horsebox specifically **Succinum**

Becomes very excitable on trying to load **Stramonium**

Will only load if accompanied by another horse **Lycopodium**

Apprehensive of loading **Dysentry co**

During travel

Appears agitated **Arsenicum album**, **Chamomilla**

Becomes angry or irritable **Bryonia**, **Nux vomica** (irritated by noise of vehicle), **Chamomilla**

Acts violently **Hyoscyamus**, **Lachesis**

Uncontrollable **Lyssin**

Profuse diarrhoea **Argentum nitricum**

Flatulent colic **Lycopodium**

Spasmodic colic **Colocynthis**

Becomes withdrawn or sad **Nat mur**

Sweats profusely **Arsenicum album**

Dehydrated **China**

By road
Upset by motion of vehicle **Bryonia** (becomes irritable) **Cocculus, Petroleum, Tabacum, Sepia, Pulsatilla**

By sea
Upset by rolling of ship **Borax** (with anxiety, dislikes up and down motion); **Sanicula** (agitated by up and down motion)

By air
Upset by movement of plane **Cocculus**

'Jet lag' in general **Melatonin**

Resultant weakness **Gelsemium**

With stiff muscles **Arnica**

Slow recovery **Cocculus**

Other behavioural problems and traits

The following list details those remedies which are the most likely to help with the behavioural problems outlined or which serve as clues to finding suitable remedies for treating other conditions. Mental symptoms often act as excellent pointers to suitable remedies.
The principal (main) remedies are shown in **bold**. Remedies with a weaker association with the behavioural trait or problem are shown in *italics*.

Affectionate	**Pulsatilla**, *Carcinosin, Ignatia, Phosphorus, Causticum*
Aggression	*Belladonna, Nux vomica, Lyssin, Stramonium*
Anger	**Aconite** (from fright), **Anacardium** (easily upset – short tempered), **Bryonia** (with irritability), **Chamomilla** (with pain), **Cina** (younger horses), **Hepar sulph, Ignatia** (with anxiety), **Kali carb, Lycopodium, Natrum mur** (also withdrawn), **Nux vomica** (easily roused), **Sepia** (with indifference), **Staphysagria** (with sudden kicking out), **Sulphur, Tarentula hisp** (if touched)
Anxiety	**Aconite** (in general also in crowded areas or at night), **Arsenicum** (if left alone or with pain), **Phosphorus** (if left alone or with excitement, during thunderstorm), **Lycopodium** (with unfamiliar animals or people, if unable to see companion animal), **Theridion** (unable to calm down), **Argentum nitricum** (appears hurried and impulsive, with irrational behaviour), **Carcinosin, Causticum, Kali phos, Nitric acid, Pulsatilla, Rhus tox, Secale, Sulphur,** *Gelsemium*
Apprehension	See Anxiety
Boredom	**Lycopodium** (also lacks confidence), **Medorrhinum, Merc sol, Sulphur** (looks untidy), **Tuberculinum**, *Alumina, Nux vom* (with an irritable nature)
Confidence (lack of)	**Lycopodium, Dysentry co, Silica, Baryta carb** (younger animals), **Kali phos, Carcinosin, Graphites**
Coprophagia	**Veratrum alb, Merc sol, Viscum alb, Sulphur, Silica, Calc carb, Calc phos**
Destructive nature	**Stramonium**, *Anacardium, Belladonna, Cantharis, Cuprum met, Nux vom, Staphysagria, Tarentula hisp*
Excitability	**Belladonna, Carcinosin, Chamomile, Coffea, Hyoscyamus, Lachesis, Nux vom, Phosphorus, Staphysagria**

Fear (general)	**Aconite** (acute sudden onset), **Argentum nitricum** (hurried), **Phosphorus** (over-sensitive), **Arsenicum album** (nervous), **Calc carb** (sluggish) **Carcinosin** (sensitive), **Graphites** (lazy), **Ignatia** (mood varies), **Lycopodium** (apprehensive), **Lyssin** (hypersensive), **Platina** (haughty), **Sepia** (indifferent), **Stramonium** (vocal)
Fears (specific)	*Strangers:* **Lycopodium**, **Baryta carb** (especially younger animals), **Causticum** (older horses), **Cuprum met, Thuja,** *Natrum carb* (to specific people)
	Crowds: **Lyssin, Aconite, Ambra grisea** (over-sensitive, lean, nervous horses), *Argentum nitricum, Natrum mur, Pulsatilla, Nux vom, Kali arsenicum*
	Water: **Lyssin**, **Belladonna**, **Hyoscyamus**, **Stramonium**, *Phosphorus*
	Heights: **Argentum nitricum**
	Vehicles approaching: **Phosphorus, Lyssin**
	Clipping: **Chamomila, Antimonium crudum,** *Aconite, Hepar sulph, Lachesis, Arnica, Tarentula hisp*
	Unfamiliar objects: **Lycopodium**, **Arsenicum**
	Enclosed spaces: **Argentum nitricum, Aconite, Stramonium, Pulsatilla, Natrum mur, Lycopodium**
Fright	*Bad effects from:* **Aconite** (with anxiety), **Argentum nitricum**, **Carcinosin** *(severe cases),* **Gelsemium** (with resultant weakness), **Ignatia**, **Lycopodium**, **Natrum mur** (withdrawn), **Opium** (fear remains long after the event), **Pulsatilla, Silica**
Frightened easily	**Argentum nitricum**, **Arsenicum album** (in anxious horses), **Borax** (at sudden sharp sounds), **Graphites**, **Natrum carb** (sensitive to noises), **Nux vomica** (with an irritable nature), **Phosphorus** (in oversensitive animals), **Sepia**, **Stramonium** (terrified), **Kali carb** (by the least thing)
Gentle nature	**Arsenicum**, **Pulsatilla**, **Phosphorus**, **Silica**, *Lycopodium*
Greedy	**Lycopodium, Iodum, Cina**, *Ferrum met, Sepia*
Haughty	**Platina** (mares especially), **Lycopodium**, **Veratrum alb**, **Stramonium**
Homesickness, pining	**Bryonia**, **Capsicum**, **Carbo animalis**, **Ignatia**, **Mag mur**, **Merc sol**, **Phos ac**
Indifference, apathy	**Alumina**, **Anacardium**, **Calc carb**, **Gelsemium**, **Helleborus**, **Natrum mur**, **Nux vomica**, **Opium**, **Pulsatilla**, **Sepia**, **Sulphur**, *Silica, Arsenicum*
Insecurity	**Arsenicum**, *Lycopodium, Bryonia*
Irritability	*In general:* **Apis, Bryonia, Chamomilla, Hepar sulph, Kali carb, Lycopodium, Lil tig, Lycopodium, Natrum mur, Nux vom, Sepia, Silica, Staphysagria** (resentment), **Sulphur**
	When shown affection: **Ignatia, Natrum mur, Silica, Sepia**
	When touched: **Ant crud**, *Lachesis, Tatrentula*
Jealousy	**Lachesis** (dislikes touch and suspicious), **Nux vom** (with irritability), **Hyoscyamus** (also suspicious), *Apis* (restless), *Lycopodium, Cenchris, Platina, Staphysagria, Stramonium*
Kicks out	**Hyoscyamus**, **Hepar sulph**, *Nux vomica, Lachesis, Phosphorus, Platina* (at own offspring), *Staphysagria*
Laziness	**Graphites**, **Lachesis**, **Lycopodium**, **Natrum mur**, **Nux vom**, **Sepia**, **Sulphur**, **Tuberculinum**, *Calc carb*
Mareish behaviour	See page 150

Mischievous	**Anacardium**, **Cannabis indica**, **Nux vomica**, **Stannum**, **Tarentula hisp**, *Stramonium, Lachesis, Hyoscyamus, Merc sol*
Moody	**Carcinocin**, **Ignatia**, **Iodum**, **Zinc**, **Nux moschata**, **Pulsatilla**, **Graphites** (better in the morning), **Sarsaparilla**, *Platina* (with a haughty nature)
Nymphomania	See page 151
Obstinacy, stubborn	**Anacardium, Argentum nitricum, Cal carb, Chamomila, Cina, Nux vomica, Tarentula hisp, Tuberculinum**
Panic	**Aconite** (acute), **Argentum nit**, **Kali arsenicum**, **Phosphorus** (excitable nature), *Cannabis indica, Chamomilla* (angry), *Cocculus* (during travel), *Hyoscyamus* (hysterical), **Lycopodium** (lacks confidence)
Quarrelsome nature	**Bryonia**
Resentment	*Staphysagria, Lachesis*
Restlessness	**Arsenicum album**, **Aconite**, **Carcinosin**, **Kali arsenicum**, **Lycopodium**, **Natrum carb**, **Natrum ars**, **Tarentula hisp**
Sensitive nature	**Carcinocin, Gelsemium, Phosphorus, Pulsatilla, Stramonium, Staphysagria** (with anger or resentment)
Sensitive to noise	**Phosphorus**, **Borax**, **Theridion**, **Asarum**, **Coffea**, **Nux vom**, **Opium**, **Silica**
Sensitive to bright lights	**Belladonna**, **Nux vom**, **Stramonium**, **Lyssin**, **Phosphorus**
Sensitive to reprimand	**Staphysagria**, **Natrum mur**, *Ignatia, Medorrhinum, Carcinosin*
Shyness, timidity (bashful)	**Pulsatilla**, **Coca**, **Arsenicum**, **Dysentry co**, *Baryta carb, Ignatia, Calc carb, Graphites*
Spooking	**Phosphorus**, **Borax**, **Theridion**, **Arsenicum album**, **Lycopodium** (at anything new), **Ignatia** (if frequently), **Hyoscyamus**, **Natrum mur**, **Natrum carb**, **Natrum phos**, **Silica**
Startled easily	**Borax**, **Kali carb**, **Kali phos**, **Natrum carb**, **Natrum phos**, **Natrum mur**, **Phosphorus**, *Nux vom, Stramonium, Theridion*
Suspicious or wary	**Anacardium**, **Arsenicum album**, **Causticum**, **Cenchris**, **Lachesis**, **Lycopodium**, **Pulsatilla**, **Stramonium**
Trauma/injury	*Effects from past trauma:* **Opium**, **Stramonium**, **Carcinosin**, **Natrum sulph** (mental consequences), *Helleborus* (mental consequences)
Wood chewing	**Alumina, Calc carb, Calc phos, Silica, Nitric acid, Lachesis**

Miscellaneous Conditions

The Immune System

At its most basic level, the function of the immune system is to protect the body from potential invaders such as bacteria, viruses and parasites. To enable it to do this effectively it has three essential functions. The first is the ability to recognise foreign material and substances. The second is the ability to react specifically to each invading pathogen and the third is the ability to remember the encounter and to react quickly the next time the body encounters the same pathogen again. To enable all this to happen the immune system has two inbuilt defensive responses.

The first is the production of antibodies or immunoglobulins and termed the humoral response. This is targeted against organisms such as viruses and bacteria. The second type of response is cellular based, termed cell mediated immunity, and involves mobilisation of an array of cells (lymphocytes or white cells) to engulf and destroy foreign material, damaged or cancerous cells and the like.

The efficient and correct functioning of the immune system is vital to good health and to effectively deter invaders. A weakened immune system opens up the body to infection, disease and a whole host of other problems. Homeopathy can do much to help maintain the immune system and to support it where it is working ineffectively and where the immune response has become changed or altered in some way. The latter is evidenced by inappropriate or over-exaggerated responses. Such responses can be to a variety of allergens, such as pollens or dust, resulting in COPD, for example, or to mosquito saliva as in the case of sweet itch. In addition, there can be problems where the immune system attacks the bodies' own tissues resulting in conditions that have an autoimmune basis such haemolytic anaemia of the newborn foal.

Post-Viral Syndrome (PVS)
Post- Viral Fatigue
Equine ME

Lack of stamina, lethargy and an air of depression characterise this condition, which is sometimes likened to the human illness referred to as myalgicencephalomyelitis or ME. Symptoms appear following a viral infection, although other causes are cited such as change in ownership, change of stable or following vaccination.

The clinical signs of the disease (such as a cough) will appear to abate but the animal fails to recover completely. Some horses will show a persistent nasal discharge with enlarged lymph nodes in the region of the neck. Additionally, the majority will tire easily even on the least exercise. Others will have a dull coat, reduced appetite and may show signs of weight loss. Blood samples often reveal a low white cell count.

Treatment

Aim to treat constitutionally where possible, otherwise approach the case on the basis of key presenting symptoms. The following remedies (which are briefly outlined) fit the main key and common symptoms seen in nearly all cases, namely weakness, lethargy, lack of stamina, dullness and weariness.

***Dose:** 30c three times daily unless otherwise indicated*

Carcinosin

Carcinosin is a key remedy for treating PVS and suited to animals that have had a history of recurrent illness such as bouts of fever, fatigue, poor appetite and loss of condition. Typically Carcinosin patients are likeable animals which are affectionate, sensitive by nature and hard workers.

Gelsemium
Gelsemium can be used for generalised weakness following a viral illness where signs include dullness, listlessness, lack of energy and a desire to be left alone.

Graphites
This remedy is suited to overweight horses which have a timid nature and which appear extremely sluggish.

Lachesis
Guiding symptoms for Lachesis include a suspicious nature and dislike of being touched or examined.

Phos ac
This is a major remedy for horses that have PVS and can be used alongside other remedies. A keynote of Phos ac is debility, both mental and physical, with exhaustion, listlessness and apathy. It is best suited to younger animals.

Silica
Indicated where the horse's constitution is intrinsically weak and resistance to disease is low. Silica animals appear chilly and feel the cold easily. A key symptom to check for is chronic enlargement of the lymph nodes in the neck.

Calc carb
Calc carb is suited to horses which have a heavy build and which are slow and sluggish by nature. These traits are pronounced in cases that have post-viral syndrome.

Calc phos
Younger animals with a lean, athletic appearance are suited to Calc phos.

Ferrum met
Ferrum phos is indicated where there is a clear history of a viral respiratory infection preceding the onset of symptoms. This remedy can be used where there is evidence of further problems, such as recurrent infections with a slight rise in temperature.

Nat mur
Marked depression is the keynote of Nat mur. Horses requiring this remedy appear very withdrawn along with signs of weight loss, weariness and weakness. They also tend to feel the cold and need rugging up.

Phosphorus
This is another remedy suited to lean-looking horses that are normally athletic and extremely friendly and affectionate. They are sensitive to noises and start easily. Some of the cases requiring Phosphorus will show evidence of liver impairment.

Sepia
Sepia type horses, often mares, are slow and sluggish by nature and appear worn out. These signs are more prominent in horses with PVS. Their general nature is one of indifference.

Zinc
Zinc acts best in animals where the symptoms of illness have appeared slowly with a gradual loss of vitality. There may also be evidence of anaemia, stumbling gait, restlessness and back pain.

Sulphur
Sulphur is worth consideration where there is no clear indication for any other remedy as it may help stimulate the recuperative powers of the patient. Used constitutionally, it suits lazy, untidy looking animals.

Psorinum
With similar indications to Sulphur, Psorinum can reinforce the immune system. It works best in horse with PVS which feel the cold easily as their immune system is not functioning well.

The following have also proved useful:

Tuberculinum
Consider using Tuberculinum where all other remedies have failed. Included within its symptom picture are low resistance to disease, susceptibility to illness in general, fatigue, weight loss and depression.
***Dose:** 200c potency twice daily for three days then consider other remedies*

Arsenicum iod
Indicated for animals that have never been quite right since a viral respiratory infection. Clues to its use include evidence of a chronic, thin watery nasal discharge and swollen lymph nodes around the neck.
Dose: *6c potency three times daily*

Vanadium
A general remedy that can be used to raise the white cell count and to stimulate the activity of the white cells to fight infection. It works best in cases where weight loss is coupled with a drop in appetite.
Dose: *6c potency three times daily*

Echinacea
This is another general remedy which supports the immune system and which can be used alongside any other remedy.
Dose: *30x potency three times daily*

The Body's Response to Infection

Fever

Fever is a common symptom of illness and defined as a rise in body temperature in response to infection. However, a rise in body temperature can also occur where there is pain such as in colic and in a number of other situations such as cases of heatstroke for example. Homeopathy can be regarded as an adjunct to help the body fight the infection and to abort the illness if the symptoms are noted quickly or to at least shorten the course of the illness and hasten recovery. The choice of remedy lies closely on the observation of the symptoms.

Principal remedies and indications

Aconite
Fever of sudden onset especially after exposure to cold weather or a cold wind. The patient appears restless and anxious.
Dose: *1M every 20–30 minutes*

Arsenicum album
Fever with anxiety and extreme restlessness. The patient seeks warmth and is thirsty for small amounts.
Dose: *200c every 20–30 minutes*

Baptisia
Fever with dullness and confusion, muscles appear sore. An abnormal odour from the body may be present.
Dose: *200c every 20–30 minutes*

Belladonna
Sudden high fever with inflammation. The horse is hot to touch, sweaty, the pulse and respiratory rates are elevated, the pulse quality is full and throbbing and the pupils may be wide open and dilated. In severe cases there may be slight delirium and the horse may seem unaware of its surroundings. Any discharge noted (as from the nose for example) will be clear and non-purulent where this remedy is needed.
Dose: *1M every 20–30 minutes*

Bryonia
Fever of slower onset and usually accompanied by inflammation where pain is a feature. The horse is unwilling to move, thirsty and irritable.
Dose: *200c every 20–30 minutes*

Ferrum phos
Fever which lacks the acute onset of Aconite, the intensity of Belladonna and the sluggishness of Gelsemium characterises Ferrum phos. This is a remedy that needs to be used early on where the symptoms match and in cases where there are throat symptoms.
Dose: *30c every 20–30 minutes*

Gelsemium
Slow onset fever with weakness. The horse appears cold, shivery and sluggish, almost half asleep. There may be some trembling of the limbs. There is an absence of thirst.
Dose: *200c every 20–30 minutes*

Nux vomica
High fever peaking at 6pm but where the horse appears irritable, cold and the muscles stiff.
Dose: *200c every 20–30 minutes*

Pyrogen
High fever as a result of sepsis. Where this remedy is indicated, the pulse rate is characteristically slow even where the fever is very high. The opposite may also occur with a rapid pulse rate accompanied by a low fever. Aching muscles will sometimes cause the horse to become restless.
Dose: 1M every 20–30 minutes

Septicaemia 'Blood poisoning'

This is a serious condition where invading bacteria and the toxins they produce enter the bloodstream and circulate around the body and throughout the tissues. Causes include infection gaining access after foaling, from wounds, nail penetrations to the sole, from burns, ruptured intestines, from specific bacterial infections and rarely from surgery.

Symptoms can include a high temperature, sweating, an increase in the pulse and respiratory rates, small petechial haemorrhages on the mucous membranes, inappetance, weakness and depression. Severe cases can result in death.

Toxaemia

This is the term given to the presence of toxins in the blood either as the result of septicaemia or from absorption from the gut as in some cases of laminitis.

Remedies for septicaemia and toxaemia

Dose 200c every 30 minutes unless otherwise stated

Arsenicum album, Aconite (1M) and Pyrogen (1M) See above

Echinacea (30x) A good general remedy. Can be used alongside other remedies

Carbo veg Feels cold to touch or collapsed, lifeless, weak

Crotalus horridus With jaundice or haemorrhage of dark blood

Lachesis From septic wounds where the skin is deeply discoloured

Anthracinum Where sepsis (infection) is involved (especially involving the skin) or where there is an abscess.

Tarentula cubensis More centred on toxaemia where sepsis is involved. Painful abscesses where the skin is discoloured can respond.

Headshaking Headshaking Syndrome

Headshaking is a relatively common and at times distressing condition that presents both a challenge in terms of accurately diagnosing the cause and in treating the symptoms successfully. Although poorly understood, continuing research may ultimately reveal some further insight into a condition that can ultimately prove frustrating to treat. The condition occurs world-wide and in all types of horses, young and old. It is said to be more of a problem in dressage horses and possibly thoroughbreds.

The symptoms are well known to most horse owners and vary in type and in severity. The most obvious is shaking of the head up and down, ranging from nothing more than a few signs of simple annoyance or discomfort, to extreme up and down movements which render the horse unsafe to ride. Admittedly most horses will headshake from time to time. This is normal behaviour and often due to irritation from flies or due to anxiety or impatience before a ride. This is not to be confused with horses that genuinely headshake involuntarily or uncontrollably. Added to this headshakers may show a range of other definitive signs. These may include nasal irritation causing the horse to rub its nose on a foreleg or stable wall, sneezing and snorting, coughing, sudden jerky movements, forward kicking of the forelegs and a symptom referred to as photophobia – squinting in bright light. Some animals may show more extreme and distressing signs. The headshaking symptoms may be so severe that the horse may become terrified and will panic and rear up. Others may show signs of deep and intense pain, striking their head against the wall of the stable, against trees or even fencing. Symptoms often are very mild at the start of a ride and intensify as the horse warms up.

There are a number of possible causes. One of the most common is allergic rhinitis caused by a reaction to pollens from trees, rapeseed and a variety of other plants found in the hedgerows. Such cases tend to be seasonal, with symptoms appearing in early spring and continuing until September or October. Often the horse will only headshake when ridden and will be free of symptoms when stabled or if ridden in an indoor school. Signs are worse on hot, bright sunny days where there is little wind and when riding near trees or between hedgerows.

The fact that some horses will headshake at other times and over the winter, points to the fact that not all cases are allergy related. Other possible causes include ear mite infestation, guttural pouch infections, trigeminal neuritis, photic headshaking (due to bright light stimulating the trigeminal nerve), head injuries, mechanical problems with the articulation of the head and upper spine, poorly fitting tack, behavioural issues possibly linked with stress and problems with the teeth.

Treatment

Conventional treatment is often cited as unsuccessful. In about 90 per cent of cases the cause cannot be determined accurately. Where ear mites are involved, these can be dealt with successfully. Problems with the teeth, guttural pouches and with the spine and head can likewise be corrected. For the remaining cases, it is worth trying to treat these on a symptomatic basis, using homeopathy.

Main non-specific remedies

Lycopodium

This is one of the principal remedies to consider and one of the more effective and worth trying in the absence of any other clearly indicated remedy. It can be prescribed on the basis of shaking of the head without an apparent cause although additional signs that can include twisting of the face and lips, snuffling noises from the nose and flapping movements of the nostrils. A ticking cough may also be present.
Dose: *30c three times daily*

Agaricus

As another frequently effective remedy, Agaricus can be combined with Lycopodium if needed. Horses that will benefit will show constant headshaking which will be worse in bright sunlight and which will increase with exercise. Agaricus covers a host of other headshaking-related symptoms including jerky movements of the head, neuralgic pain in the head, itching of the nose, twitching muscles and coughing.
Dose: *30c three times daily*

Allergy based cases

Mixed pollen and rapeseed pollen

Where the cause is seasonal, a combination of pollens in potency has frequently proved effective along side other remedies.
Dose: *30c two or three times daily*

Arundo

Arundo is a specific remedy for cases where itching or rubbing of the nose is a prominent symptom. Suitable cases may also exhibit itching of the ears and discomfort in the mouth.
Dose: *30c two or three times daily*

Arum triphyllum

Horses that require this remedy have extreme symptoms associated with the head and nose. The discomfort associated with the condition is such that the horse will bury its head and nose hard against a wall or tree. An additional clue is the presence of a nasal discharge that makes the nostrils sore.
Dose: *30c two or three times daily*

Wyethia

This lesser known remedy suits animals where there is mild itching of the nose accompanied by a hacking, dry cough.
Dose: *30c two or three times daily*

Cina

This is another remedy where nasal itching is prominent and the horse may bury its nose into the horse in front or into the hedgerow. The key pointer to the use of Cina is an irritable, cross, short-tempered nature.
Dose: *200c twice daily*

Arsenicum album
Symptoms of headshaking accompanied by obvious anxiety and restlessness suggest Arsenicum album. Affected horses will squint in bright light and will have a thin watery nasal discharge.
Dose: *30c two or three times daily*

Arsenicum iodatum
The symptoms associated with this remedy are similar to those of Arsenicum album except that there are two additional prominent symptoms to distinguish the two. Sneezing is an obvious sign together with a very dry irritating cough.
Dose: *6c two or three times daily*

Natrum muriaticum
Very violent sneezing with symptoms of depression and withdrawal suggest this remedy. Affected horses are touchy which may suggest that there is pain around the head area as well.
Dose: *30c two or three times daily*

Nux vomica
Suited to animals with violent headshaking that sneeze repeatedly and heavily. There will be a scant but clear nasal discharge along with puffy eyes that may swell at times to obscure vision. The ears may also be itchy.
Dose: *30c two or three times daily*

Gelsemium
This is another remedy where the eyes are swollen along with sneezing but the main guiding symptom for Gelsemium is general weakness so that affected horses appear lethargic and lack stamina.
Dose: *30c two or three times daily*

Sabadilla
Sabadilla is characterised by bouts of violent sneezing, with a watery, runny nasal discharge. The eyes also water considerably and appear very inflamed and red.
Dose: *30c two or three times daily*

Solidago
Again there are paroxysms of sneezing with this remedy together with the likelihood of watery eyes. Standing apart from Sabadilla is the fact that the nose is irritated with the production of large amounts of mucus causing the horse to headshake violently. Evidence of bronchitis is usually apparent with an accompanying cough and wheezy breathing.
Dose: *30c two or three times daily*

Sulphur
Sulphur is indicated where the horse has a general untidy appearance and where there are skin symptoms accompanying signs associated with headshaking. A guiding symptom for Sulphur is that the top of the head feels unusually hot.
Dose: *30c two or three times daily*

Histamine
This remedy is also worth considering in cases which have failed to respond to other allergy-based remedies.
Dose: *6c two or three times daily*

Cases with suspected trigeminal neuritis

Spigelia
Included within the symptom picture of this remedy is pain in the head extending to the eyes and pain around the head like a tight band. Assuming that some affected horses may have this sensation it is worth trying this remedy. Symptoms are worse on motion.
Dose: *30c three times daily*

Belladonna
Belladonna is one of the remedies for very violent headshaking where the symptoms are so extreme that the horse cannot be ridden. Horses that need this remedy may show associated aggression by kicking out and may prove difficult to handle.
Dose: *200c twice daily*

Bryonia
Horses needing Bryonia will have also a dry hacking cough as well as headshaking symptoms linked with pain in the region of the sinuses and an irritable, short-tempered nature. The symptoms are worse on movement and intensify when the weather is hot.
Dose: *30c three times daily*

Tuberculinum
This remedy is worth trying in cases where intense pain around the head is suspected and the horse appears depressed. Suited to horses which are lean and which have low resistance to illness. Tuberculinum is worth trying when no other remedy seems to work.
Dose: 200c twice daily for three days then consider other remedies

Photic headshakers

Sol
Sol is potentised sunlight and can be used in any horse where bright sunlight seems to be a factor.
Dose: 30c two or three times daily

Allium cepa
Allium is needed where the horse is sensitive to bright sunlight along with a watery discharge from the eyes. Sneezing is also a prominent symptom, worse on warm days and with a watery nasal discharge.
Dose: 30c two or three times daily

Stramonium
This remedy is indicated where bright sunlight causes severe headshaking so much so that it is difficult to ride the horse. The animal may become agitated, distressed, difficult to handle and may try to escape.
Dose: 30c two or three times daily

Nux vomica
Nux vom suits horses with an irritable nature, which are sensitive to noise and which dislike being handled by strangers. Headshaking symptoms are caused by pains in the head induced by bright light. There will be evidence of photophobia, the eyelids may be swollen or puffy and the skin region around the ears will be itchy.
Dose: 30c two or three times daily

Behavioural based cases

See behavioural section, page 303

Cases with pain originating from the teeth

Consider **Belladonna, Chamomilla, Hepar sulph, Merc sol, Hypericum** and **Staphysagria**.
Dose: 30c two or three times daily

Poor Performance Syndrome

This syndrome encompasses a range of conditions, any one of which, singly or in combination, can cause a number of symptoms which collectively can lead to poor performance. The type and severity of the symptoms can vary considerably and in part depend on the type of work the animal undertakes.

One of the most common signs is simply poor stamina, lack of energy or loss of form. Horses that would normally finish an event easily lag behind, appear sluggish, fail to finish or do not recover afterwards as they would do normally. Their respiratory rate, temperature or pulse rate may remain elevated far longer than is considered normal. Other horses might appear irritable, show difficulty in moving easily, stumble or fall, show a drop in appetite or develop vague, ill-defined symptoms.

Once investigated, many cases of poor performance can be linked to common identifiable conditions which are detailed within this book. These include:

- Arthritis or degenerative joint disease (DJD), page 179
- Azoturia and related conditions, page 177
- Navicular disease and other conditions relating to the foot, page 209
- Heart and circulatory problems, page 95
- COPD, page 90
- Exercise induced pulmonary haemorrhage, page 93
- Laryngeal paralysis, page 83
- Gastric ulceration, page 112
- Cervical vertebral myelopathy or wobbler syndrome, page 227

To this list of common conditions we can add two additional causes

- Post-viral syndrome or post-viral fatigue, page 306
- Reactions to vaccination, page 322

Anhydrosis
Non-sweaters
Puffers
Dry-Coated Horses
Shy Sweaters

Anhydrosis is the inability to sweat or to produce sweat in normal quantities. Horses regulate their body temperature in a number of different ways. Thermoregulation not only involves the movement of blood from deeper tissues in the body to the skin and panting, but also sweating which is by far the most important way of losing the excess heat generated during exercise.

Sweat evaporates from the surface of the skin and reduces body temperature. This cooling effect is critical, as even short periods of exercise can result in an increase in body temperature to near 104°F. If the body temperature is allowed to rise to around 105/106°F, then temperature related injuries become inevitable. The brain is particularly likely to be affected, resulting in heat stroke.

Symptoms of anhydrosis, which are most often encountered in athletic horses, can appear slowly over a period of time or may develop suddenly. Signs include exercise intolerance, an increase in heart rate and respiratory rate, panting, a rise in body temperature, hair loss (especially around the face), a dull, rough coat and flaky, itchy skin and the most obvious sign, either dry skin or unexpectedly light sweating.

Some of the horses affected by this condition show evidence of electrolyte imbalance. Low levels of sodium, potassium and chloride in the diet may result in low sodium and chloride levels in the blood. Where this is the case, the diet needs supplementation in addition to careful management.

Treatment of anhydrosis

Use the 30c potency two or three times daily unless otherwise indicated

- Main remedy, but especially where there is dry flaky skin **Alumina**
- With anger **Chamomilla**
- Where there is muscle stiffness **Rhus tox, Dulcamara**
- With scaly skin and lacklustre hair **Sulphur**
- Where heat stroke has been evident or a risk **Belladonna, Stramonium**
- Where touch is resented **Lachesis**
- With poor conformation **Silica**
- For fat overweight horses **Graphites**
- Irritable nature with hair loss **Kali carb**
- With anger and resentment **Staphysagria**
- Where there is electrolyte imbalance **Nat mur 6x, China**
- Worth consideration **Thyroid 6x, Thallium**

Excessive Panting
Thick in the Wind
Fat Inside

This problem is seen in endurance and racing horses that continue to pant for about 20 minutes or so after stopping work. These animals are normally very fit and would not be expected to pant for so long.

Panting is a way of losing excess heat along with sweating. If the horse has a thick coat, is unable to sweat properly or is dehydrated, it will be unable to lose heat sufficiently to cool down. Resolving the problem entails attending to the coat, treating any sweating problems and ensuring proper hydration.

To minimise the problem before riding give a single dose of **Arnica 30c** along with **China 30c** and **Belladonna 200c**. if the horse is exceedingly overheated on return from a ride, dose with **Belladonna 200c** and **Glonoine 30c** every ten minutes.

The condition may also arise where a horse sweats heavily, with the loss of potassium and chloride salts. This results in a build up of alkaline salts in the blood which initiates an increase in frequency and depth of respiration.

To reduce the problem before a ride dose with **China 30c,** and the tissue salts **Nat mur 6x** and **Kali mur 6x**.

Heat stroke
Equine heat stress

This is a potentially life-threatening condition if not spotted early on and dealt with effectively. The period of most risk is during the summer but heat stroke can occur in other situations especially during transportation. It is important to spot the signs as early as possible and take action before the situation becomes critical.

Exercise causes an increase in the heat production of the body. Up to 50 per cent more is produced during periods of intense exercise. To lose heat, the horse sweats, breathes faster and diverts blood flow to the capillaries in the skin to allow release of the heat. Where heat production exceeds loss, the symptoms of heat stroke/stress will appear. Horses that suffer from anhydrosis are much more at risk of developing symptoms compared to normal animals.

The most common signs initially are profuse sweating, rapid pulse rate and rapid breathing – signs of heat stress. As the condition develops the risk of heat stroke increases. The skin becomes dry and hot, both pulse and respiratory rates exceed what is considered normal and the rectal temperature will rise from normal (101 °F) to near 104 °F. If the body temperature hovers for any length of time around this level then the condition becomes critical and life-threatening.

Once the condition becomes apparent, stop work and place the horse in a shaded area if possible. The uses of fans to improve airflow will help increase the evaporation of sweat from the skin as will the wind or any breeze. If neither are available, walk the horse slowly in the shade to allow evaporation of some of the sweat. In all cases spray cool water onto the legs or if practical, place ice-packs over areas where large blood vessels run. Cold wet towels can also be used, but will need changing frequently as the water in the towels will heat quickly. Ensure that your horse is not dehydrated as sweating involves the loss of large amounts of fluid. Check by pinching the skin. If the animal is dehydrated the skin recoil will be slow compared to returning immediately in normal, hydrated animals. Where heat stress or stroke is apparent, allow small amounts of water to be taken frequently, avoiding consumption of large quantities at any one time to reduce the risk of colic.

Treatment

Glonoine 200c

This is the main remedy to consider. The pulse is rapid and pulsating and the horse is unable to move, showing signs of weakness and confusion.
Dose: every 15 minutes

Belladonna 1M

Keynotes are sudden appearance and development of symptoms, rapid pulse and respiration, dilated pupils, staring eyes, dry hot skin, thirst for large amounts of water and signs of physical and mental distress. Belladonna is the remedy of choice as a preventative (and treatment) for animals at risk travelling by air.
Prevention: dose hourly
Treatment: every 15 minutes

China 30c

This is the main remedy to use where dehydration is evident
Dose: every 15 minutes

Phos ac 30c

Add where there is dehydration, weakness and apathy.
Dose: every 15 minutes

Gelsemium 30c

Use where acute symptoms have abated and the period of risk is over and where the body temperature and pulse and respiratory rates are normal yet the horse remains confused and weak.
Dose: every 30–60 minutes

Poisoning

Poisoning in horses is thankfully rare, however, if you believe that your horse has been poisoned, then you should summon veterinary help immediately. Diagnosis is often difficult because the symptoms displayed are very similar between different poisons, often making exact identification of the poison very difficult. However, careful examination of the environment, feed and water supply can reveal some clues as to the cause. Making a careful note of the exact symptoms will provide the information needed to establish an appropriate homeopathic prescription, although many of the remedies will crop up repeatedly regardless of the cause of the poisoning. You can use homeopathy to provide interim treatment whilst waiting for veterinary help and continue to use this form of treatment in tandem with any treatment your vet may give. Always remember to isolate and remove the cause of the poisoning as quickly as possible.

Poisons can be ingested, inhaled or absorbed through the skin. In horses, however, by far the most common route of absorption is by ingestion. Broadly speaking poisons can be divided into the following categories: plant-based, heavy metals and other elements, chemical poisons, anticoagulants and mycotoxicosis (poisoning by fungi). To this list we can add snakebites and stings by bees or wasps as well.

In all cases use the 30c or 200c potency if available. Any potency will suffice in an emergency and is better than not dosing the patient at all. Doses should be gauged to the severity of the symptoms. In acute cases doses should be given every ten minutes or so. Less acute symptoms can be treated by dosing every one to two hours.

Plant-based Poisons

Ragwort (*Senecio jacobaea*)

Horses will not ingest fresh ragwort as they find it unpalatable but they will eat the dry plant if it included in hay, silage or haylage. The plant usually needs to be consumed over several weeks or months before any clinical symptoms are apparent, unless a large amount is consumed in one go. Toxicity is due to a group of compounds known as pyrrolizidine alkaloids, which cause liver damage.

Symptoms include muscle weakness and tremors, jaundice, photosensitisation, difficulty in swallowing, yawning, regurgitation of food and water, blindness, compulsive walking, head pressing, weight loss, diarrhoea and subcutaneous oedema (fluid under the skin).

Suggested remedies

On a symptomatic basis

Liver support **Chelidonium**, **Phosphorus**, **Nux vomica**

Muscle tremors **Zinc**

Head pressing **Helleborus**

Difficulty swallowing and regurgitation **Baryta carb**

Photosensitisation **Hypericum**, **Apis mel**, **Cantharis**

Oedema **Apis mel**, **Arsenicum**

Diarrhoea **Arsenicum album**

Yawning **Chelidonium**

Bracken *(Pteridium aquilinum)* and Horsetails (*Equisetum spp*)

Poisoning is due to compounds known as thiaminases which are present in both these species of plant. Normally horses will not eat bracken but may do so if the pasture is poor. A large amount needs to be consumed over several weeks before symptoms appear. These include incoordination and staggering (Bracken staggers), severe muscle tremors, weight loss (emaciation) and muscle spasms (opisthotonus) and finally death.

Suggested remedies

On a symptomatic basis

Incoordination and staggering **Agaricus**, **Nux vomica**

Muscle tremors **Agaricus**, **Strychnine**, **Zinc**

Muscle spasms **Mag phos**, **Strychnine**, **Cicuta**

Emaciation **Phos ac**

St John's Wort (*Hypericum perforatum*)

This plant contains compounds which cause photosensitisation to ultraviolet light in the areas of skin that lack pigment. As a consequence, the white areas of skin blister, become puffy and develop an exudative (moist), itchy, dermatitis. Areas most affected are the muzzle region and around the eyes. This type of photosensitisation needs to be differentiated from the type caused by liver dysfunction.

Suggested remedies

On a symptomatic basis

Where the skin is blistered or swollen **Cantharis**, **Apis mel**, **Urtica**, **Bovista**

Yew (*Taxus baccata)*

Yew is extremely toxic and can cause death within a few minutes of ingestion. Usually there is little opportunity to start any treatment. Symptoms include difficulty breathing, staggering, hypothermia (subnormal temperature), weakness followed by collapse and death.

Suggested remedies

On a symptomatic basis

In an emergency use **Nux vomica**, **Carbo veg**
Dose every five minutes

Acorn Poisoning

Horses will some times accidentally ingest acorns or oak leaves, both of which contain tannins, compounds that damage the gut, liver and kidneys. Unripe acorns are usually considered more of a problem, as they are more toxic. Commonly observed symptoms, which develop gradually, include listlessness, a drop in appetite and diarrhoea. Treatment with liquid paraffin is usually successful.

Suggested remedies

On a symptomatic basis

Dose with **Nux vomica**

Hemlock (*Conium maculatum*)

Poisoning with hemlock produces symptoms of abdominal pain, diarrhoea and neurological signs. The toxic alkaloid present in this plant has an action like nicotine, initially stimulating and then depressing parts of the autonomic nervous system. Look for dilation of the pupils, a slow, then rapid but weak pulse and slow, laboured breathing. Hemlock also paralyses the nerves that supply the muscles causing muscle weakness and paralysis.

Suggested remedies

On a symptomatic basis

Principal remedy **Aethusa cynapium**

Add for muscle paralysis **Conium**, **Curare**

Heavy Metal and Other Elements

Lead

Lead poisoning in horses causes a neuritis (inflammation of nerves) leading to general weakness, pneumonia and paralysis of the muscles of the pharynx (throat) accompanied by anaemia, apparent blindness with a tendency to head press.

Suggested remedies

On a symptomatic basis

Principal remedies **Arsenicum album**, **Alumen**, **Opium**, **Sulphuric acid**

Muscle weakness **Plumbum**

Pharyngeal paralysis **Causticum**

Head pressing **Helleborus**

Anaemia **Plumbum**, **Ferrum met**, **Arsenicum album**

Arsenic

Horses may accidentally consume products that contain arsenic. Inorganic arsenic compounds are found in industrial waste and some older types of wood preservative and weedkiller. Organic arsenic is included in some pig rations. The effect of arsenic is to irritate the lining of the bowel and to produce symptoms of salivation, abdominal pain, increased thirst, staggering gait, weakness, trembling and paralysis.

Suggested remedies

On a symptomatic basis

Principal remedies **Hepar sulph**, **Nux vomica**, **Phosphorus**, **Arsenicum album**

Where there is salivation **Ipecac**, **Merc sol**

Where there is paralysis **Nux vomica**, **China**

Cadmium

Cadmium is a heavy metal that can contaminate pasture near old mine workings and waste dumps through airborne contamination or by water seepage. Absorbed by plants, especially the daisy, cadmium accumulates in the body through grazing. Symptoms of poisoning include diarrhoea, jaundice, fatty changes to the liver, poor appetite and incoordination.

Suggested remedies

On a symptomatic basis

Principal remedies **Phosphorus**, **Conium**, **Agaricus**

Jaundice **Phosphorus**, **Chelidonium**, **Chionanthus**

Fatty changes in the liver **Phosphorus**

Incoordination **Alumina**, **Phosphorus**, **Plumbum**, **Conium**, **Gelsemium**

Mercury

Poisoning with mercury is rare in horses. Toxicity can occur when it is absorbed into the body in the form of inorganic compounds used in seed dressing. The most obvious symptom is a severe gastroenteritis along with inflammation of the mucous membranes in the mouth, incoordination, a drop in appetite, kidney damage (nephritis) and anxiety. Treatment by washing out the stomach needs to be done quickly in order to save the horse.

Suggested remedies

On a symptomatic basis

Principal remedies **Aurum**, **Merc sol**

Gastroenteritis **Veratrum album**, **Carbo veg**

Incoordination **Alumina**, **Phosphorus**, **Plumbum**, **Conium**, **Gelsemium**, **Hepar sulph**

Nephritis **Kali iod**

Selenium (Alkali Poisoning)

Selenium is absorbed by plants growing in areas where there is a high concentration in the soil such as some parts of America. Chronic cases of selenium poisoning, often referred to as alkali poisoning, show signs of hair loss from the mane and tail regions, develop rings on the hoof below the coronary band and exhibit lameness due to lesions developing on the surface of the joints in the limbs. Acute cases of poisoning, referred to as blind staggers, develop a staring coat, salivate, show signs of paralysis and wander aimlessly as their vision is impaired.

Suggested remedies

On a symptomatic basis

Principal remedies chronic cases **Fluor ac**, **Arsenicum album**

Principal remedy acute cases **Agaricus**, **Arg nit**, **Zinc met**, **Nux vomica**

Hair loss **Thallium**

Chemical Poisons

Organophosphates

Farm chemicals are the main source of this class of poisons though toxicity is less likely than it used to be. The main symptom is excess salivation, increased tear production, muscle twitching, colic, sweating and in the final stages convulsions.

Suggested remedies

On a symptomatic basis

Principal remedies **Belladonna, Zinc**

Also consider **Chelidonium**, **Agaricus**, **Alumina**, **Calc carb**

Ionophores (antibiotics added to feed)

Horses are susceptible to poisoning by certain antibacterial drugs added to compound feeds for cattle, sheep and poultry feeds, if ingested. Signs to check for include poor appetite, incoordination and intermittent bouts of sweating.

Suggested remedies

On a symptomatic basis

Principal remedies **Alumina**, **Gelsemium**, **Nux vomica**, **Phosphorus**

Nitrates and Nitrites

High rainfall after the application of nitrogen fertilisers to pasture can lead to concentrations of nitrates in grass and in water ditches or ponds through soil leeching. These are converted to nitrites that are potentially more toxic. Nitrites also accumulate in plant material after herbicide treatment and in sugar beet tops. Poisoning results in liver damage as well as signs that include abdominal pain, difficulty breathing, dark coloured mucous membranes and weak pulse.

Suggested remedies

On a symptomatic basis

In all cases **Nux vomica**, **Carbo veg**, **Colocynthis**

Also consider **Kali nit**, **Arsenicum album**

Anticoagulants

Warfarin

Warfarin is the most commonly used anticoagulant (drugs which prevent blood from clotting). It is one of the main poisons used against rodents so accidental ingestion is possible. Symptoms include prolonged bleeding from wounds, internal bleeding which can cause colic, areas of swelling under the skin, especially near joints and pale mucous membranes. Veterinary help should be sought immediately.

Suggested remedies

On a symptomatic basis

In all cases **Millefolium**

Also consider **Erigeron**, **Ficus religiosa**
Dose*: every five minutes*

Mycotoxicosis

This term applies to the symptoms caused by poisoning from mycotoxins, compounds formed by the growth of fungi or moulds on feeds, especially those with a high moisture content. Symptoms vary and include depression, drop in appetite, anaemia, bleeding from the nose, blood in the dung, abnormal gait (ataxia) and convulsions. Cases that are less acute may show evidence of jaundice.

Suggested remedies

On a symptomatic basis

Main remedies **Phosphorus**, **Conium**

Where there is nasal bleeding **Millefolium**

Ataxia **Conium**

Convulsions **Aconite**, **Belladonna**

Jaundice **Chelidonium**

Snake Bites

Horses are prone to snake bites but fortunately a bite that would kill a small dog will have much less serious consequences in the horse. Bites can be identified by the fang marks usually on the leg with an area of swollen tissue around the wound that may ooze darkened blood. Antiserum should be given where appropriate and the animal kept quiet to reduce the spread of the poison.

Treatment

Initially **Ledum**, **Arnica** *Dose every five to ten minutes for five doses*

Follow with **Lachesis** *Dose hourly until symptoms abate*

Also consider **Vipera** (for adder bites), **Crot horr** (rattlesnake bites)

Insect Bites

Insect bites are much less serious than snake bites but may cause considerable local irritation with a varying degree of swelling.

Treatment

Initially **Hypericum**, **Ledum**

Follow with **Apis** (where there is local swelling)

Pre- and Post-Operative Homeopathy

This section covers remedies that can be useful pre- and post-operatively to the animal's advantage to speed recovery and minimise some of the complications that can arise.

Pre-operative remedies

Normally used to calm animals prior to surgery
Use the 30c potency unless indicated otherwise indicated

Anxiety Generally **Aconite 1M**
With restlessness **Arsenicum album**
With desire to escape **Argentum nitricum**
Rooted to the spot **Gelsemium 200c**

Fear Generally **Aconite 1M**
Approach of strangers **Arnica**, **Lycopodium** (apprehensive)
Of being touched **Arnica**, **Lachesis** (will kick out)
Enclosed places **Argentum nitricum**, **Lycopodium**, **Succinum**
Specific fear of surgery **Phosphorus**

Panic Generally **Phosphorus**
Consider **Aconite 1M, Argentum nitricum**

Excitability Generally **Stramonium 200c**
With violence **Hyoscyamus 200c**
With sweating **Belladonna 200c**
Consider **Phosphorus 200c** (reacts badly to noise)

Anger/Irritability Generally **Staphysagria 1M**
Consider **Chamomilla**
With irritable nature **Nux vomica**

Separation anxiety Generally **Ignatia 1M**
With depression/sadness **Nat mur 200c**

Post-Operative Remedies

Used to help the recovery phase
***Dose:** two or three times daily for ten days starting on the day of surgery*
In general for all surgical procedures **Arnica 30c**

Add additional remedies as follows:

Where the pelvic area is involved or deep tissues

Also for trauma to soft organs – spleen, liver, uterus etc. **Bellis 30c**

To speed wound healing **Calendula 30c**

Wounds that won't heal consider **Causticum 30c**, **Carcinosin 30c**, **Hepar sulph 30c**, **Silica 30c**

Septic wounds **Pyrogen 1M**, **Calendula 200c**, **Anthracinum 30c**, **Ledum 30c** (with soft swelling)

Wound suppuration **Calc sulph 30c**, **Silica 30c**, **Hepar sulph 30c** (painful to touch), **Calendula 30c**

If proud flesh develops **Calendula 30c**, **Graphites 30c**, **Fluor ac 6c, Nitric acid 30c**

For deep bruising, slow to resolve **Sulphuric acid 30c**

Severe bruising, skin purple **Lachesis 30c**

Where the swelling at the site persists **Kali mur 6c**

To reduce pain
For incised wounds **Hypericum 30c**
Where there is anger/violence **Chamomilla 200c**
Wound cannot be touched **Chamomilla 200c**
With resentment **Staphysagria 200c**
Abdominal pain **Colocynthis 30c** (back arched), **Dioscorea 30c** (better for stretching and moving around)

General pain
Unable to move **Bryonia 30c**
Bone pain **Eupat perf 30c, Stillingia 30c**
Periosteal pain **Ruta grav 30c, Phos ac 30c, Asafoetida 30c, Mezerium 30c**
Eye pain **Symphytum 6c**
Kidney pain **Berberis 30c**
Sacro-iliac pain **Aesculus 30c**
Sore wounds **Rhus tox 6c, Staphsagria 30c**
Distraught with pain **Aconite 1M, Coffea 200c** (very agitated),**Chamomilla 200c**
Where the eye is involved generally **Ledum 30c, Senega 30c**
Where joints are involved **Ruta 30c, Symphytum 30c**
After fracture repair **Ruta 30c, Sympytum 30c, Calc phos 6c**

For spinal surgery and where nerves are involved **Hypericum 30c, Nat sulph 6c, Bryonia 30c, Conium 6c**

Surgery where blood vessels are involved **Millefolium 30c**

For surgery on the bowel with gas build-up **Raphanus 30c**
Bowel stasis **Nux vomica 30c** (patient also very irritable)
Also consider **Opium 1M**

Where tooth extraction is involved **Hypericum 30c**

Surgery involving sphincters or the bladder **Staphysagria 30c**

Where there is bladder paralysis **Causticum 30c, Nux vomica 30c**

Where there is bleeding
Generally in addition to **Arnica** add **Millefolium 30c**
For active haemorrhage, bright red blood **Nitric acid 30c**
For active haemorrhage, watery blood **Phosphorus 30c**
Slow bleeding, dark blood **Hamamelis 30c, Elaps 6c**
Haematoma **Hamamelis 30c, Lachesis 30c, Crot horr 30c**
Blood seepage from wounds postoperative **Strontia 30c**
Passive seepage **China 30c**
Bleeding from tooth socket **Phosphorus 30c**
Bleeding from the bladder **Erigeron 30c**

Post-operative fluid build up (oedema) **Apis 30c**

Bad effects from the anaesthetic
Generally **Nux vomica 30c**,
Also **Acetic acid 30c, Phosphorus 30c**
Consider **Potentised anaesthetic 30c**

Adhesion prevention **Calc fluor 30c, Thiosinaminum 6c, Graphites 30c, Carcinosin 30c**

Irritant itchy scars **Fluoric acid 6c**

Slow recovery generally **Kali sil 30c, Kali phos 30c** (with weakness), **Opium 200c** (very drowsy)

Restless after surgery, cannot settle **Arsenicum album 30c, Rhus tox 30c**

Irritable after surgery and upset **Nux vomica 30c, Chamomila 30c, China 30c**

Post-Operative Sepsis

Septicaemia **Pyrogen 1M**, Echinacea **30x**, **Arsenicum album, Crot horr 30c**

Acute infections with pain **Hepar sulph 1M, Myristica seb 30c**

Chronic infections **Silica 200c**

Post-Operative Emergencies

Surgical shock
Generally **Aconite 1M, Arnica 200c**

Cold and collapsed **Carbo veg 200c, Veratrum album 30c**

Weak pulse, cold and collapsed **Camphora 30c**
With fluid loss **Strontia 30c**
With depressed respiration **Carb ac 30c**

Dehydration
Generally for fluid loss **China 30c, Phos ac 30c**
With hind limb weakness **Phosphorus 30c**
With general weakness **Phos ac 30c, Secale 30c** (with cold limbs)
Subsequent anaemia **Arsenicum album 6c, Ferrum phos 6c, Phosphorus 6c**

Vaccines, Vaccine Reactions, Vaccinosis and Nosodes

Conventional Vaccines

In the UK, horses are routinely vaccinated against Equine influenza using an inactivated vaccine and against tetanus using a vaccine containing tetanus toxoid, enhanced by the use of an adjuvant such as aluminium phosphate.[13] Only healthy, immune competent horses should be vaccinated in order to ensure that there is a good immune response to the vaccine. However, it is generally accepted that a small number of horses will fail to respond to vaccination successfully (for a variety of reasons) and will therefore have no (or very weak) protection. No one would dispute the advantages of vaccination in protecting horses against disease but a small proportion of horses will exhibit a reaction of some types of vaccine.

Vaccination Reactions

Reactions fall basically into three categories:

1. Physical reactions

This is a rare occurrence and manifests as swelling and pain at the site of the injection. Palpation of the affected area is often resented and the horse may back away if an extensive area is involved. Inflammation of local muscles results in difficulty in moving the head and neck. The reaction usually subsides in a few days.

Treatment

Initially **Arnica 200c** and **Ledum 200c** *every two to three hours* until the condition improves. If the symptoms persist continue treatment with:

Where there is heat, swelling and considerable pain **Belladonna 1M**

Difficulty moving the neck **Bryonia 200c**

Persistent stiffness in the neck **Rhus tox 30c**, **Ruta 30c**

Threatening abscessation **Hepar sulph 200c**

Chronic abscessation **Silica 200c**

Dose: two or three times daily

2. Allergic reactions

In mild cases there will be little more than slight swelling at the injection site; however, more serious allergic or anaphylactic reactions can also occur, requiring immediate veterinary treatment. In the most severe cases, anaphylaxis will result in the horse collapsing through a sudden drop in blood pressure, narrowing of the airways and oedematous swellings on the surface of the skin.

Treatment

Mild cases – skin symptoms only

Where there is oedematous swelling at the injection site **Apis 200c**

With more generalised skin swellings (hives) **Apis 200c**, **Urtica urens 30c**, **Histamine 30c**

With puffing up of large areas of the body **Medusa 30c**

Dose: every five to ten minutes

Severe cases – anaphylaxis/collapse

In general **Apis 1M**, **Urtica urens 200c**

With collapse and weak pulse **Carbolicum acidum 200c**

Where difficulty breathing **Arsenicum album 200c**

Dose: every five minutes

3. Reactions which have an Impact on General Health

The most minor reactions will involve a transient period of being 'off colour' which will pass in a day or two and may result in mild respiratory symptoms where flu vaccination has been given. Treatment with the **potentised vaccine** in **30c** potency or the relevant **nosode** in **30c** potency *twice daily for five days* will help cut short this period.

The nosode can also be given *twice daily for five days*, commencing the day before the injection is given as a preventative measure.

More serious vaccination reactions can have a more profound effect on the health of the animal possibly triggering symptoms of chronic illness. Conditions observed to arise following vaccination include symptoms of chronic malaise and poor performance syndrome, sweet itch, chronic obstructive pulmonary disease (COPD), behavioural changes and mud fever. It is quite likely that other conditions can also be triggered by vaccination.

Vaccinosis

Illness arising or triggered by vaccination is termed vaccinosis by homeopaths and may involve components of the vaccine (including not only the antigenic material but also chemical additives such as aluminium or mercurial compounds) influencing the immune system adversely. Vaccinosis is a contentious issue amongst the medical and veterinary community but has been highlighted many times by homeopaths as a factor that can influence health adversely.

Prevention of vaccinosis

In general dose with **Thuja 200c** *twice daily for five days* starting the day before vaccination. This treatment can be combined with using **Hypericum 30c** and **Ledum 30c** *twice daily* if need be as an extra preventative measure.

Treatment of vaccinosis

Where vaccinosis has been identified in the medical history, consideration needs to be given to treating this problem first (in effect to clear the path ahead) before embarking on treatment with other remedies.

The most widely used remedy is **Thuja** but the list of suitable remedies includes **Carcinosin**, **Maladrinum**, **Mezerium**, **Sarsaparilla**, **Silica**, **Sulphur** and **Tuberculinum**.

Dose *using the 200c potency twice daily for five days with the most appropriate remedy*

For specific conditions arising after vaccination consider:

COPD or other respiratory symptoms **Ant tart**, **Silica**, **Thuja**

Back pain **Silica**

Epilepsy **Silica**

Skin symptoms **Mezerium**, **Thuja**, **Sulphur**

Mud fever **Malandrinum**

Dose initially with the 200c potency *twice daily for five days* considering higher potencies if warranted to resolve the symptoms. Alternatively consider other remedies if any vaccinosis issues have been cleared.

Nosodes

A nosode is a homeopathic remedy produced from diseased material; the term nosode itself is derived from the Greek *nosos* meaning disease. The original material may be bacterial, viral, diseased tissue, pus, mucus or any other type of discharge associated with a particular disease. Nosodes are often used in the prevention of disease and are sometimes loosely termed 'homeopathic vaccines' as they are used by homeopaths as an alternative to conventional vaccines. However, nosodes are also remedies in their own right and can be used in the treatment of a patient.

Using Nosodes in a Preventative Role

As energetic homeopathic medicines, nosodes are thought to provide protection against the diseases they are prepared from, although the mechanism of this protection is unknown at this time. Unlike conventional vaccines, there is no antibody production (and for pregnant mares there will be no antibodies to pass onto the foal) and therefore nothing measurable to substantiate the claim of protection. However, anecdotal evidence suggests that nosodes do have an action on the body and do offer some form of protection against illness. They also have the advantage of freedom from side effects. The ultimate choice as to use nosodes in place of conventional vaccines, however, must lie with the reader who must weigh up the pros and cons of each method for themselves.

Guidelines on the Use of Nosodes in Place of Vaccination

Where nosodes are to be used prophylactically in place of vaccination, a dosing regime has been devised through the experience of homeopathic veterinary surgeons and homeopathic pharmacists originating from the use and application of nosodes in practice. Like all homeopathic remedies, nosodes should be stored carefully and not administered at the same time as either garlic or peppermint. The suggested recommended dosing regime is given below. There is some variation between individual practitioners in dosing frequency so alternative suggestions are given in brackets.

One dose twice daily for three (five) days, then

one dose weekly for four weeks, then

one dose monthly for four (six) months.

Following this, a booster course of one dose twice daily for three (five) days should be given every six months, starting six months after the completion of the primary course.

The Use of Nosodes in the Treatment of Disease

As individual remedies, nosodes can be used in the treatment of illness in their own right. However, where necessary, they can be used alongside other remedies. For example, the Lyme nosode (*Borrelia burgdorferi* 30c) can be used in treating the illness alongside other remedies.

There are, however, other ways of utilising nosodes in treating horses. Their use involves using remedies at an advanced level and details are only included here in brief outline.

Constitutionally

This is where the patient's symptoms match the mental, physical and particular symptoms characteristic of the nosode. As an example, Tuberculinum, (a nosode prepared from tubercular abscess) suits horses that are lean, impatient, show initial enthusiasm for a ride that wanes quickly and which are prone to respiratory problems and which have slow recuperative powers.

Where other remedies fail to act

In this case a suitably (and accurately) chosen remedy fails to produce a reaction. The use of a nosode can open the way for the remedy to act. The nosode selected may be relevant to a past infection or may be selected on current symptoms of the patient. There are also links here with miasmic illness (see page 16), which can cloud, mask or alter the patient's symptoms.

Where there are no real symptoms

Here the patient presents with no real clear symptoms and the use of a nosode may bring forward new symptoms on which to prescribe. Tuberculinum or Psorinum are often good remedies to use in horses in such cases. Again there are miasmic links.

Where the symptom picture is confused and suggests more than one constitutional remedy

Use of a carefully chosen nosode can clarify the symptom picture, often revealing the true constitutional remedy.

Where an animal has never been well since a specific infection

Using the relevant nosode can improve the health of an animal or help reveal the constitution by uncovering a layer of disease that may mask the patient's true symptoms.

First Aid and Emergency Care

This section is a quick-reference guide to the most common remedies used in emergency situations. It also includes some of the remedies to help deal with the consequences of such problems. In some cases you will need to use the list in conjunction with a materia medica (or the relevant sections of this book) in order to establish the most ideal remedy to use. Those remedies in **bold** type are the most important. Those in *italics* are a little less significant but nevertheless worth consideration.

Potency Selection

Ideally in most cases, aim to give **30c** or **200c** *every 60 minutes* until the symptoms abate. Where the case is very acute the dose intervals should be shorter. Likewise in less acute cases the interval between the doses can be several hours. If the suggested potencies are not readily at hand, it is best to give any available potency rather than give no remedy at all. Remedies used to help with the consequences of an injury should be used in the **30c** potency and given *once or twice daily* until the condition resolves.

Where the skin or wounds are involved, affected areas can be cleaned or bathed with diluted **Hypercal lotion**. To encourage healing and to soothe sore areas, **Calendula cream** can also be used.

Abscesses
Hepar sulph, **Silica**, **Merc sol**, **Calc sulph**, *Anthracinum, Tarentula cubensis*

Acute anxiety – panic
Aconite, **Argentum nitricum**, **Phosphorus**

Allergic reactions – acute
Apis, **Urtica**, **Histamine**

Azoturia
Very acute **Aconite**, **Belladonna**
Acute **Aesculus**, **Berberis**, **Bryonia**, **Actea rac**, **Rhus tox**

Bites
Animal **Hypericum**, **Ledum**, *Lachesis, Apis, Belladonna, Arsenicum*
Insect **Hypericum**, **Ledum**, *Cedron, Apis, Arsenicum album*
Snake **Belladonna**, **Lachesis**, *Ledum, Cedron, Hypericum. Crot horr, Vipera*

Bleeding – poor clotting
Crot horr, **Ferrum phos**, **Ipecac**, **Lachesis**, **Nitric acid**, **Phosphorus**, *Millefolium*

Bruising (contusions)
Arnica, **Bellis**, **Hamamelis**, **Ledum**, **Phosphorus**, **Ruta**, **Sulphuric acid**

Burns
Cantharis, **Urtica**, **Arsenicum**, **Sol**, *Apis*

Choking – acute
Lycopodium, **Pulsatilla**, **Hyoscyamus**, **Aconite**

Colic
Spasmodic **Colcocythis**, **Nux vomica**
Flatulent **Dioscorea, Mag phos, Lycopodium, Chamomilla, Carbo veg**
Impacted **Nux vom, Plumbum, Alumina, Opium, Bryonia**
Thrombo-embolic **Bothrops**

Collapse

In general **Carbo veg**, **China**, **Arsenicum album**, **Camphora**
From diarrhoea **Arsenicum**, **Camphora**, **Carbo veg**, **Veratrum album**

Concussion

Arnica, **Cicuta**, **Hypericum**, **Helleborus**, *Nat sulph*

Cyanosis (lack of oxygen)

Carbo veg, **Camphora**, **Cuprum met**, **Digitalis**, **Lachesis**, **Laurocerasus**, **Opium**, **Veratrum album**, *Ant tart*, *Ammon carb*

Dehydration

China, **Chin sulph**, **Phos ac**, **Calc carb**

Dislocations

Rhus tox, **Ruta**, **Lycopodium**, **Calc carb**, **Natrum carb**, *Bryonia*

Electric shock

Phosphorus, *Helleborus*

Exhaustion see Collapse

Falls

Arnica, **Calendula**, **Hypericum**, **Nat suph**, **Ruta**

Fever from trauma

Arnica, *Aconite*, *Arsenicum album Lachesis*, *Pyrogen*

Fever (pyrexia) from infection

Aconite, **Belladonna**, **Baptisia**, **Pyrogen**, **Echinacea**, **Arsenicum album**, **Gelsemium**, **Eupat perf**

Foaling

Arnica, **Caulophyllum**, **Causticum**, *Bellis*, *Calc phos*, *Secale*, *Pulsatilla*, *Kali carb*, *China*

Fractures (to heal)

Symphytum, **Calc phos**, *Ruta*, *Silica*, *Calendula*, **Bovista** (to reduce swelling where the fracture involves a joint)

Fright

Aconite, **Gelsemium**, **Ignatia**, **Opium**

Gangrene

Secale, **Anthracinum**, **Arsenicum album**, **Cantharis**, **Causticum**, **Lachesis**

Haematoma

Arnica, **Hamamelis**, *Phosphorus*, *Secale*, *Calc fluor*, *Silica*, *Crot Horr (if recurrent)*

Haemorrhage

Bright red in general **Aconite**, **Ipecac**, **Millefolium**
Bright and watery **Phosphorus**, *Ferrum*,
Dark, black and watery **Crocus**
Dark and decomposing **Crot horr**, **Lachesis**, **Vipera**
Dark and slow **Hamamelis**
Thin **Ferrum**, **Secale**
With clots **Sabina**, **Rhus tox**, **Platina**, **Chamomilla**
With dark clots **Crocus**, **Elaps**
Post-operative **Strontium carb**, **Calendula**
Post-foaling, intermittent gushes, bright red **Ipecac**, **Trillium**
Bright red, persistent **Sabina**, **Nitric acid**,**Millefolium**
Bright red, watery **Phosphorus**
Dark-coloured, persistent **Secale**
From torn blood vessels **Erigeron**
After trauma **Arnica**, **Millefolium**
With fear or anxiety **Aconite**

Heat stroke/exhaustion

Belladonna, **Glonoine**, *Gelsemium*, *China*, *Phos ac*

Hives (urticaria)

Apis, **Arsenicum album**, **Histamine**, **Ledum**, **Nat mur**, **Rhus tox**, **Sulphur**, **Urtica**

Infection, sepsis, septicaemia

Hepar sulph, **Pyrogen**, **Baptisia**, **Anthracinum**, **Arnica**, **Arsenicum**, **Echinacea**, **Lachesis**, **Crot horr**, **Crot horr**, **Tarentula cubensis**

Injuries, in general

Arnica, **Calendula**, **Hypericum**, **Ruta**, **Nat sulph**, **Bryonia**, **Hamamelis**, **Ledum**, **Rhus tox**, **Silica**, **Staphysagria**, **Symphytum**
Bone – fractures **Arnica**, **Bryonia**, **Calc phos**, **Carbolic acid**, **Ruta**, *Symphytum*, *Calendula*, *Calc carb*, *Eupat perf*, *Silica*, *Hypericum*
Bone – crushed or splintered **Carbolic acid**

Back **Arnica**, **Bellis**, **Hypericum**, **Rhus tox**, **Ruta**, *Kali carb*
Blood vessels **Millefolium**
Brain (concussion) **Arnica**, **Cicuta**, **Helleborus**, **Hypericum**, **Nat sulph**, **Opium**, *Cocculus*, *Ledum*, *Kali phos*
Eye **Aconite**, **Arnica**, **Calendula**, **Hypericum**, **Ledum**, **Silica**, **Symphytum**
Muscles **Arnica**, **Conium**, *Calendula*, *Pulsatilla*, *Rhus tox*, *Sulphuric acid*, *Symphytum*, *Bellis*
Neck **Bryonia**, **Hypericum**, **Rhus tox**, *Ruta*, *Calc carb*, *Symphytum*
Nerves **Arnica**, **Hypericum**, **Bellis**, **Calendula**, *Phosphorus*, *Curare*, *Mag phos*
Joints **Bryonia**, **Ruta**, **Rhus tox**, *Arnica*, *Bellis*
Pelvis **Bellis**, **Arnica**, *Aesculus*, *Hypericum*, *Carbolic acid*, *Silica*, *Mezerium*
Periosteum **Fluoric acid**, **Ruta**, **Mezerium**, **Phos ac**, *Asafoetida*, *Symphytum*, *Aurum*, *Phosphorus*
Sphincters **Staphysagria**
Spine **Hypericum**, *Helleborus*
Spleen **Ceanothus**
Tendons **Arnica**, **Ruta**, **Rhus tox**, *Ledum*, *Hamamelis*, *Calendula*, *Arg met*
Udder **Conium**, **Arnica**

Laminitis
Very early stages **Aconite**, **Belladonna**, **Secale**
With more obvious symptoms add **Hypericum**, **Pyrogen**, as appropriate **Kali carb**, **Arnica**, **Nux vom**, **Lycopodium**

Lightning strike
Phosphorus

Lymphangitis
Very early stages **Aconite**, **Belladonna**
With more obvious symptoms **Bothrops**, **Apis**, **Mang acetate**, **Rhus tox**, **Bufo**, **Bovista**
Severe **Crot horr**

Oedema
Apis mel

Over-exertion
Arnica, **Rhus tox**, *Hamamelis*, *Millefolium*, *Arsenicum album*

Pain
In general **Hypericum**, **Chamomilla**, **Coffea**, **Staphysagria**, **Bryonia**, **Arnica**, **Mag phos**, **Colocynthis**, **Spigelia**
Abdominal – see Colic
With anxiety or restlessness **Aconite**, **Arsenicum album**, **Phosphorus**
With anger or violent behaviour **Chamomilla**, **Hepar sulph**, **Aurum**, **Staphysagria**
Severe **Chamomilla**, **Coffea**, **Aconite**, **Hepar sulph**

Post-operative – See Pre- and Post-Operative Remedies, page 320.

Paralysis, in general
Hypericum, **Causticum**, **Conium**, **Curare**, **Gelsemium**, **Zinc**

Poisoning – see page 315

Proud flesh
Nitric acid, **Thuja**, *Calendula*, *Arsenicum album*, *Silica*

Shock
Traumatic **Aconite**, **Carbo veg**, **Arnica**, **Camphor**, **Lachesis**, **Opium**, **Veratrum album**
Mental **Opium**, **Aconite**, **Arnica**, *Gelsemium*, *Ignatia*

Skin
Abrasions **Arnica**, **Hypericum**, **Calendula**
Blunt trauma **Arnica**, **Bellis**, **Bryonia**, **Ledum**
Cuts **Arnica**, **Calendula**, **Staphysagria**
Cellulitis **Mang acetate**, **Rhus tox**, **Apis mel**
Grazes **Arnica**, **Hypericum**
Lacerations **Calendula**, **Hypericum**

Strain – See Over-exertion

Sprains
Arnica, **Bryonia**, **Rhus tox**, **Ruta**, *Causticum*, *Calc carb*, *Strontium*

Sunburn (photosensitisation)
Apis mel, **Rhus tox**, **Rhus venata**, **Cantharis**, **Sol**, **Proteus**

Tetanus (prevention)
Ledum, Hypericum, Tetanus nosode

Vaccination reactions – localised
Belladonna, Apis, Rhus tox, Ruta, Hepar sulph

Vaccination consequences from (vaccinosis)
Thuja, Sulphur, Silica, Carcinosin, Malandrinum, Mezerium, Tuberculinum

Wounds
In general **Arnica, Calendula, Hypericum, Ledum, Pyrogen, Staphysagria**
Bleeding (freely) **Millefolium, Phosphorus, Lachesis, Nitric acid**
Puncture **Ledum, Hepar sulph, Hypericum**
Gunshot **Arnica, Hypericum, Ledum, Apis mel**
Stab **Hypericum, Staphysagria, Apis mel**
Surgical **Arnica, Hypericum, Staphysagria**
Infection threatened **Ledum, Hepar sulph**
Infection present **Hepar sulph, Anthracinum, Pyrogen, Gunpowder, Apis mel, Lachesis, Crot horr, Calc sulph, Silica, Myristica seb**
Painful **Staphysagria, Hypericum**

Remedies for the First Aid Kit

These are remedies that you should consider having in your first aid box. Start with a few and learn how to use them correctly before adding to your collection. The remedies are graded. The **Vital** remedies are those that you should always have without doubt. The remedies in the **Essential** list are those that would complete a practical, basic, homeopathic first aid kit for horses. The remedies included in the next list, the **Extras**, are for the more experienced user with specific additions for the **yard** and **stud** as well as for **endurance horses**. The most practical potencies are given for each remedy and are best obtained as tablets packaged in amber glass vials for long-term storage. The final list covers **External** (topical) remedies.

Vital

Aconite 1M
Apis 30c
Arnica 30c
Belladonna 1M
Bryonia 30c
Colocynthis 30c
Echinacea 30x
Hepar sulph 200c
Ledum 30c
Nux vom 30c
Rhus tox 30c
Ruta grav 30c
Silica 30c

Bach Recovery or Rescue Remedy – for routine use for panic, anxiety, fear and fright. Ideal for both rider and horse before any event. A combination of Bach Flower Essences: Clematis, Cherry Plum, Impatiens, Rock Rose and Star of Bethlehem.

Essential

Agaricus 30c
Argentum nitricum 30c
Arnica 200c
Arsenicum album 30c
Bellis perennis 30c
Calc fluor 30c
Calendula 30c
Cantharis 30c
Euphrasia 30c
Ferrum phos 30c
Gelsemium 30c
Graphites 30c
Hypericum 30c
Lycopodium 30c
Phosphorus 30c
Pulsatilla 30c
Secale 200c
Staphysagria 200c
Symphytum 6c
Urtica 30c

Recovery Plus Emergency Spray – for extreme fear and panic; for major crisis situations. A combination of Bach Flower Essences; Aspen, Cherry Plum, Clematis, Impatiens, Mimulus, Rock Rose, Star of Bethlehem and White Chestnut in a non-alcoholic base.

Extras

Antimonium tartrate 30c
Arsenicum album 200c
Calc carb 30c
Chamomilla 30c
Chelidonium 30c
Heckla lava 6c
Hamamelis 30c
Kreosotum 30c
Kali bich 30c
Lachesis 30c
Merc sol 30c
Millefolium 30c
Nat mur 30c
Petroleum 30c
Senega 30c
Sepia 30c
Silica 200c
Sulphur 30c
Thuja 30c
Tuberculinum 30c

Extra remedies for the yard

Bacillinum 200c
Colocynthis 200c
Dioscorea 200c
Ferrum phos 30c
Gelsemium 200c
Hepar sulph 1M
Rhus tox 200c
Ruta 200c
Sarsaparilla 30c

Extra remedies for the stud

Calc phos 30c
Carbo veg 30c
Caulophyllum 30c
Causticum 30c
China 30c
Cimicifugia 30c
Ignatia 1M
Kali phos 30c
Mag phos 30c
Opium 200c
Pyrogen 1M
Sabina 200c
Strontia 30c

Extra remedies for the endurance horse

Aesculus hippocastanum 30c
Arnica 1M
Berberis vulgaris 30c
China 30c
Cuprum met 1M
Phos ac 30c

External or topical treatments for the first aid kit

Arnica cream – Applied to bruised or traumatised tissues provided the skin is not broken

Calendula (Marigold) cream – Applied to soothe and heal sore skin or wounds

Calendula (Marigold) lotion or Cicatrin* lotion – Used to bathe and clean wounds of any type

Hypercal tincture (Hypericum and Calendula tinctures mixed) – Used to bathe, soothe and heal sores, wounds, cuts and ulcers. Dilute 1:25 with water before use

Euphrasia Ø, Euphrasia mother tincture – Used to treat eye problems. Dilute 2–3 drops in an egg-cupful of cold boiled water or cold Chamomile tea

Ruta ointment – Applied topically to strained tendons or ligaments

Witch-hazel (distilled) an astringent – Applied using cotton wool to arrest local bleeding

Bach Recovery Plus Emergency Cream – Can be applied topically to any wound or sore area of skin to assist healing

* From Dr Reckeweg – see Suppliers' List in Useful Addresses

Equine Materia Medica

This section of the book covers the individual homeopathic remedies in more detail and is divided up into four sections:

- The main Materia Medica covering the majority of remedies in significant detail
- Information on minor and less frequently used remedies covered in less detail
- Information on the bowel nosodes, a special group of remedies
- Information on the tissue salts, another special group of low-potency remedies

Information covered in the Materia Medica

Remedy Keynotes and Main Indications

The main Materia Medica, and to a lesser extent the other sections, covers the important symptoms and key pointers characteristic of the remedies listed in this book, together with useful details that include the following:

- The **homeopathic name** or names of the remedy, together with its abbreviated homeopathic name where this exists in common usage
- The **common name** of the remedy. This is the everyday, colloquial name of the remedy
- **Remedy classification**. This is a classification of the base material as animal, vegetable or mineral origin with further classification where appropriate
- **Method and material** from which the remedy is produced. This is the way in which the remedy is produced homeopathically together with details of the starting (base) material used
- **Keynotes**. This lists the key pointers and features of the remedy in a general. This has an overall veterinary bias but is not exclusively focused on horses
- **Modalities**. This is a list of the factors that influence the patent as a whole or the patient's symptoms, either aggravating (making them worse) or ameliorating (improving or easing) the symptoms
- **Remedy interactions**. This lists which remedies are incompatible (where their actions will nullify each other), remedies which work well together, either before, with or after the remedy and those remedies which could be considered as close alternatives in treating certain conditions[14]
- Main **therapeutic (clinical) indications** as regards horses. This section lists the most appropriate uses of the remedy in treating conditions seen in horses

Abrotanum

COMMON NAME: Southernwood, Lady's love, *Artemesia abrotanum*
CLASSIFICATION: Plant: Asteraceae (Compositae) family
PREPARATION: Mother tincture prepared from the plant stems and leaves

Keynotes
- Gradual wasting or loss of muscle mass (especially of the hind limbs) accompanied by a good appetite
- Conditions arising from poor nutrition or weak digestion
- Oozing of blood or moisture from the navel
- Residual weakness after respiratory infections
- Loss of hair with a loss of general condition
- Flabby looking tissue and loose skin
- Hard lumps in the abdomen

Modalities
WORSE/AGGRAVATED BY: Cold air, getting wet
BETTER/AMELIORATED BY: Moving around

Remedy Interactions:
WORKS WELL WITH: Aconite, Bryonia, Hepar sulph, Lycopodium, Kali bich

Principal Equine Indications
- Cushing's disease
- Alopecia linked with debility
- Slow recovery after viral respiratory infections
- Debility
- Chronic diarrhoea with wasting or weight loss
- Malabsorption syndrome
- Generalised muscle wasting
- Equine infectious anaemia
- Dourine
- Navel ill in foals

Acetic acid, Aceticum acidum

COMMON NAME: Glacial acetic acid, vinegar
CLASSIFICATION: Mineral: Acetates
PREPARATION: From solution in rectified spirit for higher potencies

Keynotes
- Wasting and debility
- Tendency to bleed/haemorrhage
- Anaemia
- Fluid retention
- Thirsty
- Frequent passing of pale-coloured urine
- Ability to dissolve scar tissue
- Reduces the chances of scar tissue forming
- After-effects of anaesthesia

Modalities
WORSE/AGGRAVATED BY: Cold weather, at night
BETTER/AMELIORATED BY: Rest

Remedy Interactions
CONSIDER ALSO: Apis, Arsenicum album, Uranium nitrate, China, Digitalis

Principal Equine Indications
- Emaciation with anaemia
- Chronic diarrhoea with emaciation
- Malabsorption syndrome
- Ascites
- Filled legs
- Lymphangitis
- Diabetes associated with Cushing's disease where urination is frequent
- Symptoms arising after anaesthesia including slow recovery
- Equine nodular skin disease
- Dissolution of fibrous nodules
- Dissolution of scar tissue especially problems arising after trauma or surgery
- Pericarditis; to stop adhesions forming
- Dissipation of blood clots

Aconite, Acon

COMMON NAME: Monkshood, Wolfsbane, *Aconitum napellus*
CLASSIFICATION: Plant: Ranunculaceae family: Polycrest
PREPARATION: Mother tincture made from the whole plant and root made at the time of flowering. The active part is an alkaloid, aconitine.

Keynotes
- Symptoms appearing acutely or suddenly
- Shock
- Haemorrhage of bright red blood
- Fever
- Injury
- Anxiety
- Restlessness
- Great fear
- Conditions arising after exposure to dry cold air or drafts
- Sensitivity to touch and noise
- General affinity with serous membranes and muscles
- Acutely inflamed, red eyes
- Red, hot swollen joints

Modalities
WORSE/AGGRAVATED BY: Dry cold winds, evening and at night, in warm areas
BETTER/AMELIORATED BY: In the open air

Remedy Interactions
WORKS WELL WITH: Arnica, Belladonna, Bryonia, Phosphorus, Sulphur (considered the chronic of Aconite), Coffea
INCOMPATIBLE WITH: Acetic acid
CONSIDER ALSO: Ferrum phos, Rhus tox, Sulphur

Principal Equine Indications
- Anxiety and restlessness
- Nervous tension, anticipatory anxiety
- Difficulty loading into horseboxes
- Shock
- Fears especially of being touched and of crowds
- Starting or jumpy behaviour
- Oversensitivity to noises
- Fright and its consequences, diarrhoea from fright
- Early on in cases of fever especially where the horse is restless and thirsty
- The early stages of many infectious diseases
- Acute infections, septicaemia, toxaemia
- Peritonitis
- Equine influenza, rhinitis
- Tyzzer's disease
- Strangles (early stages)
- Uveitis
- Periodic ophthalmia
- Acute conjunctivitis with photophobia, redness, swollen lids and excess tear production
- Dry, hacking cough with difficult breathing, bronchitis, pneumonia (early stages)
- Tympanic colic with extreme restlessness and anxiety
- Acute synovitis with great heat, acute joint inflammation
- Acute laminitis
- Septic arthritis
- Meningitis, neuritis
- Tetanus (early stages)
- Haemorrhage of bright red
- Exercise induced pulmonary haemorrhage (EIPH)
- Epistaxis, nosebleed

Actaea racemosa

See Cimicifuga racemosa

Actea spicata, Actea spic

COMMON NAME: Baneberry, Bugbane, Toadroot, Herb Christopher
CLASSIFICATION: Plant: Ranunculaceae family
PREPARATION: Mother tincture prepared from the root

Keynotes
- Action is focused on muscles and the smaller joints of the body
- Special focus of action on the knee (carpal) joint
- Swelling of the smaller joints with heat
- Symptoms worse on the right-hand side

Modalities
WORSE/AGGRAVATED BY: Movement, slightest motion, touch, cold weather
BETTER/AMELIORATED BY: None listed

Remedy Interactions
CONSIDER ALSO: Caulophyllum, Cimicifugia, Causticum, Ledum, Guaiacum

Principal Equine Indications
- Arthritis (DJD) affecting the knee (carpus), hock (tarsus), fetlock, pastern or coffin joints
- Joint swelling appearing after exercise

Adonis vernalis

COMMON NAME: Pheasant's eye
CLASSIFICATION: Plant: Ranunculaceae family
PREPARATION: From tincture of the fresh plant

Keynotes

- Acts on the heart and circulation
- Kidney disease
- Oedema, ascites
- Distorted damaged heat valves, endocarditis
- Myocarditis
- Rapid, irregular pulse
- Hydrothorax, fluid in the chest cavity

Modalities

WORSE/AGGRAVATED BY: Cold weather
BETTER/AMELIORATED BY: In the open air

Remedy Interactions

CONSIDER ALSO: Digitalis, Crataegus, Convallaria, Strophanthus

Principal Equine Indications

- Equine infectious anaemia (EIA)
- As a cardiac tonic
- Swelling of the limbs from poor circulation, ascites
- Weak circulation
- Myocarditis
- Endocarditis
- Hydrothorax
- Pneumothorax

ACTH, Adrenocorticotrophin hormone

COMMON NAME: Corticotrophin
CLASSIFICATION: Animal: Sarcode
PREPARATION: From the pituitary gland

Keynotes

- Deposits of fat under the skin
- Glucose in the urine (glycosuria)
- Excessive growth of hair
- Excessive sweating
- Greasy skin
- Depressed nature
- Desire to stand away from other animals
- Constriction of peripheral blood vessels

Modalities

WORSE/AGGRAVATED BY: From riding
BETTER/AMELIORATED BY: In the afternoon

Remedy Interactions

CONSIDER ALSO: Quercus robur

Principal Equine Indications

- Cushing's disease
- Diabetes insipidus

Aesculus hippocastanum, Aesculus

COMMON NAME: Horse chestnut
CLASSIFICATION: Plant: Hippocastanaceae family
PREPARATION: Mother tincture prepared from the whole fruit and its capsule

Keynotes

- Main action centred on the lower bowel and organs of the pelvis
- Sluggish digestion, liver, heart and circulation
- Venous congestion
- Swelling of the mucous membranes of the rectum
- Weakness of the sacral area and lower back
- Swelling and synovitis of the hock joint

Modalities

WORSE/AGGRAVATED BY: Morning, from riding, after feeding
BETTER/AMELIORATED BY: Cool air, in the open air

Remedy Interactions

WORKS WELL WITH: Carbo veg, Lachesis
CONSIDER ALSO: Aloe, Hamamelis, Nux vomica, Paeonia, Sulphur

Principal Equine Indications

- Lower back pain
- Pain around the sacral, sacroiliac and hip area
- Weakness of the back legs with occasional stumbling
- Tying up, azoturia
- Bog spavin
- Sluggish haemorrhage of dark venous blood
- Rectal prolapse
- Variocele

Aethusa cynapium

COMMON NAME: Fool's parsley
CLASSIFICATION: Plant: Apiaceae (Umbelliferae) family
PREPARATION: Mother tincture made from the whole flowering plant

Keynotes

- Action focussed on the brain and nervous system
- Gastro-intestinal upsets
- Digests milk poorly
- Swollen udder

Modalities

WORSE/AGGRAVATED BY: In the evening, from milk, 3–4am
BETTER/AMELIORATED BY: In the open air

Remedy Interactions

WORKS WELL WITH: Calc carb
INCOMPATIBLE WITH: Antimonium crudum, Cicuta, Opium
CONSIDER ALSO: Antimonium crudum, Arsenicum album, Calc carb, Mag carb, Natrum carb, Natrum mur, Opium

Principal Equine Indications

- Diarrhoea from mare's milk
- Engorged mammary glands, swollen with milk
- Hemlock poisoning

Agaricus muscarius, Agaricus

COMMON NAME: Toadstool, Bug agaric, *Amanita muscaria*
CLASSIFICATION: Plant: Fungi: Amanitaceae family
PREPARATION: The mother tincture is prepared from the fresh fungus

Keynotes

- Jerking, trembling, twitching and other involuntary movements
- Spasms and cramping of muscles
- Stumbling, drunken-like gait
- State of delirium with whinnying
- Transient paralysis of the hind legs
- Small intensely itchy skin lesions

Modalities

WORSE/AGGRAVATED BY: Open air, cold air, before a thunderstorm, after feeding
BETTER/AMELIORATED BY: Gentle exercise

Remedy Interactions

CONSIDER ALSO: Cuprum met, Rhus tox, Zinc, Nitric acid, Argentum Nitricum

Principal Equine Indications

- Headshaking
- Poisoning-symptomatic treatment
- Blepharospasm
- Epilepsy/convulsions
- Meningitis
- Loss of balance
- Tying up
- Stringhalt
- Cauda equina neuritis
- EHV-1-neurological symptoms
- Viral infections with neurological signs, encephalitis
- Equine protozoal myeloencephalitis
- Eclampsia, hypocalcaemia
- Dermatitis with excessive irritation and multiple small scabs
- Temporary limb paralysis following overexertion

Agnus castus

COMMON NAME: Chaste tree, Monk's pepper, *Vitex agnus castus*
CLASSIFICATION: Plant: Verbenaceae family
PREPARATION: The mother tincture is prepared from the ripe berries

Keynotes

- Action focused on the reproductive system
- Impotency
- Agalactia

Modalities – None listed

Remedy Interactions

WORKS WELL WITH: Arsenicum album, Bryonia, Caladium, Ignatia, Lycopodium, Pulsatilla, Selenium, Sulphur
CONSIDER ALSO: Selenium, Lycopodium

Principal Equine Indications
- Poor libido in the stallion
- Lack of interest in the mare
- Total lack of milk or poor lactation
- Retained placenta
- Urethral discharge in geldings and stallions

Alfalfa

COMMON NAME: Lucerne, California clover, *Medicago sativa*
CLASSIFICATION: Plant: Fabiaceae (Leguminosae) family
PREPARATION: Mother tincture is prepared from the leaves and stem

Keynotes
- Main action is to influence nutrition
- Improves appetite and digestion
- Flatulence
- Improves mental and physical ability
- Increased thirst
- Poor kidney function
- Assists elimination of urea
- Improves the production and quality of milk

Principal Equine Indications
- Malnutrition and debility
- To tone the digestive system
- Poor appetite
- Weak digestion
- Chronic flatulence associated with impaired nutrition or digestion
- Kidney disease
- Lack of milk, agalactea
- To improve milk quality

Allium cepa

COMMON NAME: Common red onion
CLASSIFICATION: Plant: Alliaceae family
PREPARATION: From tincture of the whole fresh plant gathered in July and August

Keynotes
- Profuse watery irritating nasal discharge with sneezing
- Sore nostrils
- Watery eye discharge
- Sclera red
- Photophobia
- Dry hacking cough

Remedy Interactions
WORKS WELL WITH: Phosphorus, Thuja, Pulsatilla
CONSIDER ALSO: Arundo, Euphrasia, Sabadilla, Wyethia

Modalities
WORSE/AGGRAVATED BY: In the evening, when stabled, springtime
BETTER/AMELIORATED BY: In the open air

Principal Equine Indications
- Conjunctivitis with redness, watery discharge and photophobia
- Dry hacking cough worse in cold air
- Upper respiratory tract viral infections
- Rhinitis with a profuse watery discharge
- COPD, RAO
- Photic headshaking
- Chronic traumatic neuritis

Aloe

COMMON NAME: Socotrine aloes, *Aloe socotrina*
CLASSIFICATION: Plant: Alocaeae
PREPARATION: Trituration or from solution in spirit of the gum

Keynotes
- Helps to re-establish physiological equilibrium where the symptom picture has been confused by the use of drugs
- Congestion of the portal system
- Conditions arising from lack of use or under use
- Conditions arising in the later stages of life
- Tendency to laziness
- Problems arising from failure to pass dung
- Abdominal distension caused by gas accumulation
- Watery dung with mucus and gas
- Uncontrolled passage of dung containing mucus
- Abdominal pain after passing dung

Modalities
WORSE/AGGRAVATED BY: Early morning, summertime,

heat, hot damp weather from eating
BETTER/AMELIORATED BY: Cold weather, open air, passing gas

Remedy Interactions

WORKS WELL WITH: Sulphur, Kali bich, Sepia
CONSIDER ALSO: Aesculus, Nat sulph, Sulphur, Podophyllum

Principal Equine Indications

- Confused symptom pictures
- Tympanic colic
- Colitis X
- Diarrhoea containing a mixture of solid and loose material
- Acute 'spluttery' diarrhoea with gas and mucus
- Drug induced diarrhoea
- Weakness of the anal sphincter

Alumen, Alumn

COMMON NAME: Potash alum
CLASSIFICATION: Mineral: Aluminiums
PREPARATION: From trituration of the pure crystals

Keynotes

- Stubborn constipation
- Inability to expel dung
- Hardening (induration) of tissues including the lymph nodes
- Weakening of the muscles
- Uneven, stumbling gait
- Paralysis
- Difficulty swallowing
- Oesophageal spasm

Modalities

WORSE/AGGRAVATED BY: Cold weather
BETTER/AMELIORATED BY: None listed

Remedy Interactions

INCOMPATIBLE WITH: Chamomilla, Nux vomica, Ipecac, aloe
CONSIDER ALSO: Alumina, aloe, Merc sol, Nux vom, Opium, Plumbum

Principal Equine Indications

- Impaction of the colon
- Grass sickness
- Muscle weakness
- Hind limb paralysis and weakness
- Chronically enlarged or hardened lymph nodes
- Choke

Alumina, Alum

COMMON NAME: Aluminium oxide, Aluminium oxydata
CLASSIFICATION: Mineral: Aluminiums
PREPARATION: By trituration

Keynotes

- Dry mucous membranes
- Dry skin
- Muscle weakness
- Ptosis
- Chronic conjunctivitis
- Contraction of the oesophagus
- Hard dry dung
- Great difficulty in passing dung, straining
- Weak bladder muscles
- Uneven gait
- Tenderness of soles
- Weakness and paralysis of the hind limbs

Modalities

WORSE/AGGRAVATED BY: In the morning, warmth of stable
BETTER/AMELIORATED BY: In the open air, evening, damp weather

Remedy Interactions

WORKS WELL WITH: Bryonia, Lachesis, Sulphur, Ferrum met
CONSIDER ALSO: Alumen, Bryonia, Graphites, Nux moschata, Opium, Plumbum

Principal Equine Indications

- Chronic conjunctivitis with thickening of the lids and sticky discharge
- Ptosis (drooping) of the eyelids
- Chapped or cracked skin with rough, dry scabs
- Chronic laminitis, especially where there is poor hoof quality
- Cracked, brittle or flaky hooves or horn
- Weakness of the hind limbs

- Paralysis of the bladder
- Impacted colic
- Cauda equina neuritis
- African horse sickness (respiratory form)
- Eqine protozoal myeloencephalitis
- Anhydrosis
- Hypothyroidism
- Choke

Ambra grisea

COMMON NAME: Ambergris, a secretion from the whale
CLASSIFICATION: Animal: Mammal
PREPARATION: By trituration or tincture

Keynotes

- Suited to thin nervous animals or elderly animals
- Impairment of functions generally
- Hypersensitivity
- Hysteria, excitability
- Desires to be alone, dislikes company
- Shyness
- Conditions arising from emotional shock
- Nymphomania
- One-sided conditions
- Loss of hair around the head area
- Itching around the female genital region
- Spasmodic cough, barking cough
- Increased reflexes

Modalities

WORSE/AGGRAVATED BY: Music, strangers, anything unusual, morning, warm room
BETTER/AMELIORATED BY: Gentle exercise, cold air, after eating

Remedy Interactions

WORKS WELL WITH: Lycopodium, Pulsatilla, Sepia, Sulphur
CONSIDER ALSO: Pulsatilla, Phosphorus, Ignatia, Nat mur, Ignatia, Baryta carb

Principal Equine Indications

- Nymphomania
- Excitability
- Spooking
- Fear of strangers or crowds
- Shyness
- Poor memory
- Ranula
- Vulval pruritis/itching
- Symptoms which suddenly change places
- As a general remedy for elderly animals

Ammonium carbonate, Ammon carb

COMMON NAME: Carbonate of Ammonia, Sal volatile
CLASSIFICATION: Mineral: Ammonias
PREPARATION: From a solution in distilled water

Keynotes

- Suited to lazy, slow, sluggish overweight animals
- Lack of strength and stamina
- Low vitality
- Flabby muscles
- Grumpy natured, dull and uninspiring animals
- Dislike of water and getting wet
- Affects the mucous membranes of the respiratory tract
- Cough with laboured noisy breathing
- Bubbly noises from the chest from an accumulation of mucus
- Fluid in the chest
- Wheezing, difficult breathing
- Emphysema
- Pneumonia
- Enlarged lymph nodes around the neck
- Renal (kidney) disease
- Abdominal pain from accumulation of gas

Modalities

WORSE/AGGRAVATED BY: Evening, in cold wet or stormy weather, 3–4am
BETTER/AMELIORATED BY: Dry weather

Remedy Interactions

WORKS WELL WITH: Belladonna, Bryonia, Phosphorus, Pulsatilla, Rhus tox, Sepia, Sulphur
INCOMPATIBLE WITH: Arnica, Hepar sulph, Lachesis
CONSIDER ALSO: Ant tart, Ars alb, Phosphorus

Principal Equine Indications

- Chronic bronchitis
- Respiratory catarrh
- Pneumonia in older horses

- Pulmonary oedema
- COPD
- Slow recovery after respiratory infections
- Weak constitution where symptoms fit
- Kidney failure (uraemia)
- Urolithiasis
- Flatulent colic

Anacardium, Anac

COMMON NAME: Marking nut, *Anacardium orientale*, (*Semecarpus anacardium*)
CLASSIFICATION: Plant: Anacardiaceae family
PREPARATION: Trituration of the nut using the layer between the shell and kernel

Keynotes

- Weak memory
- Forgetful
- Lack of confidence
- Suspicious
- Irritable or ill humoured
- Anxiety when ridden 'as if was being followed'
- Inactive bowel
- Intense itching of the skin
- Urticaria

Modalities

WORSE/AGGRAVATED BY: On first movement, mental activity
BETTER/AMELIORATED BY: Eating, massage

Remedy Interactions

CONSIDER ALSO: Rhus tox
WORKS WELL WITH: Lycopodium, Pulsatilla, Platina

Principal Equine Indications

- Behavioural problems associated with senility, dementia
- Lack of confidence
- Anxiety including anticipatory anxiety
- Constipation resulting from inactivity of the bowel
- Dermatitis with marked itching associated with irritability or short-tempered behaviour
- Stomach ulcers

Angustura vera

COMMON NAME: Bark of *Galipea cusparia*
CLASSIFICATION: Plant: Rutaceae family
PREPARATION: Trituration of the bark

Keynotes

- Main seat of action is on the musculo-skeletal system
- Bruising
- Stiffness, difficulty moving
- Cracking noises from joints
- Bone pain
- Bone degeneration

Modalities

WORSE/AGGRAVATED BY: Exertion
BETTER/AMELIORATED BY: None listed

Remedy Interactions

WORKS WELL WITH: Lycopodium, Ignatia, Sepia
CONSIDER ALSO: Ruta grav

Principal Equine Indications

- Arthritis, DJD, especially chronic cases with marked stiffness
- Stiff painful joints
- Bone spavin (especially)
- Joints that crack
- Stiffness of the neck
- Periostitis

Anthracinum

COMMON NAME: Anthrax poison
CLASSIFICATION: Animal: Mammal: Nosode
PREPARATION: From an alcoholic extract from the spleen taken from affected sheep

Keynotes

- Principal focus is on sepsis
- Foul smelling discharges
- Septic skin ulcers
- Boil-like eruptions on the skin
- Pustules
- Haemorrhage of dark blood

Modalities
WORSE/AGGRAVATED BY: None listed
BETTER/AMELIORATED BY: None listed

Remedy Interactions
WORKS WELL WITH: Arsenicum
CONSIDER ALSO: Pyrogen, Lachesis, Crotalus horr, Hippoz, Echinacea, Silica, Tarentula cubensis

Principal Equine Indications
- Septic skin infections
- Abscesses
- Cellulitis
- Myositis with decomposing muscle tissue
- Gangrene with gross sepsis
- Septicaemia with bleeding, toxaemia
- Fly strike
- Skin ulcers with foul discharges
- Oozing of dark, blackish blood from a wound or injury
- Snake bites
- Ulcerative lymphangitis
- Quitter
- Thrush
- Sole abscess, under-run sol

Antimonium crudum, Ant crud

CONSIDER ALSO: Black sulphide of Antimony, Antimony sulphide
CLASSIFICATION: Mineral
PREPARATION: By trituration

Keynotes
- Irritable nature
- Fretful
- Dislike of being touched
- Dislike of hot weather
- Red, itchy eyes with a sticky discharge
- Swelling of the eyelids
- Eczema with yellow crusts on the face
- Dermatitis with thick, pale-coloured hard scabs
- Eczema around the mouth
- Alternation of soft and hard dung
- Itching around the rectal area
- Warts
- Dung with mucus covering
- Brittle hooves
- Distorted hooves

Modalities
WORSE/AGGRAVATED BY: Evening, hot weather, heat, washing in cold water
BETTER/AMELIORATED BY: Open air, moist warm weather, from resting

Remedy Interactions
CONSIDER ALSO: Antimonium tartrate
WORKS WELL WITH: Pulsatilla, Merc sol, Sulphur

Principal Equine Indications
- Conjunctivitis with thick ropy discharge where the inner corners of the eyes are sore and the lids are sticky
- Blepharitis
- Chronic laminitis with pronounced laminitic rings
- Weak, deformed and brittle hooves, thickened distorted hooves
- Canker
- Keratoma
- Hyperkeratosis
- Dermatitis where there are thick honey-coloured scabs
- Mud fever
- Areas of hardened, thickened callous-like skin
- Photosensitisation
- Sarcoids
- Horse pox virus
- Hard horny skin growths, hard horn-like warts
- Diarrhoea from over-excitement
- Poor appetite with bloating of the abdomen

Antimonium tartaricum, Ant tart

COMMON NAME: Tartar emetic, tartrate of antimony and potash
CLASSIFICATION: Mineral: Antimonies
PREPARATION: By trituration

Keynotes
- Key action on the respiratory system and mucous membranes in particular
- Excess production of mucus
- Rattling mucus sounds in the trachea and chest

- Difficulty in coughing up mucus
- Difficulty breathing, laboured breathing, dyspnoea
- Neck extended to ease breathing
- Respiratory tract overloaded with catarrhal mucus
- Cough with difficult expectoration
- Spasmodic colic with much gas
- Drowsiness and weakness

Modalities

WORSE/AGGRAVATED BY: Evening, lying down, warmth, damp cold weather

BETTER/AMELIORATED BY: Extending neck, expectoration of mucus

Remedy Interactions

WORKS WELL WITH: Silica, Pulsatilla, Baryta carb, Ipecac, Sulphur

CONSIDER ALSO: Ipecac, Kali carb, Ammon carb, Stannum, Laurocerasus

Principal Equine Indications

- Respiratory infections
- Pneumonia especially severe cases
- Bronchopneumonia
- Emphysema
- Pulmonary oedema
- Rattling coughs with tough mucus present
- COPD
- Equine viral arteritis
- African horse sickness, respiratory and cardiac forms

Apis mellifica, Apis mel, Apis

COMMON NAME: The Honey bee, honey-bee venom

CLASSIFICATION: Animal: Insects

PREPARATION: Tincture of the whole bee or dilutions of the poison in alcohol

Keynotes

- Principal action is on cellular tissue leading to oedema especially the skin, mucous and serous membranes
- Swellings and puffiness
- Accumulation of fluid
- Inflammation with fluid production (effusion)
- Great sensitivity to touch
- Restlessness (from discomfort)
- Noisy and fidgety, whinnying, buzzing
- Jealousy
- Anger, short-tempered
- Hard to please
- Fright
- Rage and vexation
- Thirstless
- Swollen eyelids (may be everted)
- Photophobia
- Puffy conjunctival membranes
- Oedematous conjuctiva
- Keratitis
- Swelling of the throat and larynx
- Difficulty breathing, dyspnoea
- Swelling of genitalia
- Ovarian pains
- Nephritis with little urine output
- Urinary retention
- Swelling of limbs
- Swollen hot joints
- Hives, urticaria
- Burning red, inflamed skin
- Intense itching

Modalities

WORSE/AGGRAVATED BY: Heat in any form, touch, pressure, from covering up, late afternoon (4–5pm), after sleep

BETTER/AMELIORATED BY: Open air, uncovering, cold in any form, washing in cold water, motion

Remedy Interactions

WORKS WELL WITH: Nat mur (chronic), Baryta carb, Arnica, Arsenicum album, Sarsaparilla, Sulphur, Pulsatilla

INCOMPATIBLE WITH: Rhus tox, Phosphorus

CONSIDER ALSO: Vespa, Lachesis, Cantharis, Urtica urens, Rhus tox, Arsenicum album

Principal Equine Indications

- Peritonitis
- Hydrothorax
- Oedema, pulmonary oedema, laryngeal oedema
- Pharyngitis where the throat is swollen
- Ascites
- Pericarditis (to reduce oedema)
- Meningitis

- Allergic reactions, hives, urticarial swellings, anaphylaxis
- Allergic reactions to vaccines
- Reactions to insect bites
- Angioneurotic oedema
- Insect bites and stings
- Blistered skin
- Photosensitisation
- Cellulitis
- Lymphangitis
- Equine nodular skin disease
- Sweet itch
- Early stages of purpura haemorrhagica
- Acute, severe conjunctivitis with intensely swollen conjunctival membranes and eyelids
- Allergic conjunctivitis
- Keratitis with pronounced swelling of lids and conjunctival membranes
- Burns
- Filled legs
- Synovitis
- Acute joint pain with swelling, pain and heat
- Bog spavin
- Bursitis, capped hock, capped elbow, cunean bursitis
- Hygroma of the carpus
- Carpitis (acute)
- Tenosynovitis
- Thoroughpin
- Acute tendon injuries (to reduce swelling)
- Buttress foot
- Navicular syndrome
- Acute nephritis (acute renal failure)
- Urethritis
- Jealousy
- Marish behaviour
- Ovarian pain
- Cystic ovaries
- Acute mastitis
- Phimosis, paraphimosis, penile prolapse
- Hydrocele
- Acute leptospirosis
- African horse sickness (cardiac form)
- Equine viral arteritis
- Dourine
- Symptomatic treatment of poisoning

Apocynum cannabinum, Apoc cann

COMMON NAME: Black Indian hemp, American hemp
CLASSIFICATION: Plant: Apocynaceae family
PREPARATION: From whole fresh plant including the root

Keynotes

- Acts on cellular tissues increasing the production of fluid from mucous and serous membranes
- Oedema
- Heart murmurs
- Cyanosis
- Rapid and feeble pulse
- Thirsty
- Urinary retention
- Weak bladder
- Weak sphincters

Modalities

WORSE/AGGRAVATED BY: Cold weather
BETTER/AMELIORATED BY: Warmth

Remedy Interactions

CONSIDER ALSO: Apis, Arsenicum album, Phosphorus

Principal Equine Indications

- Ascites
- Oedema
- Hydrothorax
- Heart disease
- Urinary incontinence (from weak sphincter)
- Distension of the bladder arising from poor muscle tone
- To encourage urination
- Diabetes insipidus

Argentum metallicum, Arg met

COMMON NAME: Metallic silver, the element (ag)
CLASSIFICATION: Mineral: Metal: Argentums
PREPARATION: Trituration

Keynotes

- Acts on joints, bone, cartilage (especially), ligaments and tendons
- Tearing pains in the joints, tenderness

- Exostoses
- Atrophy (withering) of small blood vessels and consequent results

Modalities

WORSE/AGGRAVATED BY: Touch
BETTER/AMELIORATED BY: Open air

Remedy Interactions

WORKS WELL WITH: Alumina, platina, Calc carb, Pulsatilla
CONSIDER ALSO: Zinc, Palladium, Stannum, Selenium

Principal Equine Indications

- Arthritis (DJD) particularly of the hip joint, elbow and stifle
- Regeneration of damaged cartilage
- Chronic tendon and ligament injuries; injuries to connective tissue
- Navicular syndrome
- Angular limb deformities
- Osteochondrosis, OCD
- Chondromalacia of the patella
- Meniscal tears

Argentum nitricum, Arg nit

COMMON NAME: Silver nitrate, Lunar caustic
CLASSIFICATION: Mineral: Metal: Argentums
PREPARATION: Trituration

Keynotes

- Acts on the nervous system, both the brain and spinal cord
- Incoordination
- Trembling
- Irritates mucous membranes
- Muco-purulent discharges
- Flatulence and gas build up, distension
- Colic
- Ulceration of the stomach
- Watery dung with gas and mucus
- Damages red blood cells
- Impulsive behaviour
- Dislike uncertainty
- Anxiety
- Inclination to rush everything
- Swelling of the inner corner of the eye
- Photophobia
- Profuse purulent eye discharge
- Marked conjunctival swelling
- Eyelids thickened and swollen
- Clouding of the cornea
- Corneal ulceration
- Inflammation of the throat
- Thick mucous (catarrh) in the throat
- Unsteady uneven gait
- Weakness of the hind limbs

Modalities

WORSE/AGGRAVATED BY: Warmth in any form, at night, after eating, during oestrus, from stress
BETTER/AMELIORATED BY: Fresh air, cold weather

Remedy Interactions

INCOMPATIBLE WITH: Vespa
WORKS WELL WITH: Bryonia, Causticum, Lycopodium, Calc carb, Gelsemium, Nat mur, Pulsatilla, Sepia
CONSIDER ALSO: Argentum metallicum, Agaricus, Phosphorus, Zinc, Lycopodium

Principal Equine Indications

- Anticipatory anxiety especially with digestive symptoms
- Diarrhoea from travelling, excitement, anxiety
- Irrational fears
- Claustrophobia (does not like being trapped)
- Impulsive, unpredictable behaviour
- Dislike of being left alone
- Mental strain
- Gastric ulceration (stomach ulcers), duodenal ulceration
- Colitis or diarrhoea particularly if induced by stress
- Flatulent colic especially if induced by stress, anxiety, claustrophobia
- Weakness and incoordination of the hind limbs
- Severe conjunctivitis with a foul, yellowish, thick irritating, purulent discharge and photophobia
- Swelling and soreness of the inner corners of the eye
- Blepharitis
- Corneal ulceration
- Blood vessel invasion of cornea
- Keratitis
- Corneal opacity

- Fly worry
- Equine viral arteritis (eye symptoms)
- Anaemia
- Laryngitis
- Urethritis
- Testicular degeneration

Aristolochia cymbifera (Milhomens)

COMMON NAME: Brazilian Snake root
CLASSIFICATION: Plant: Angiosperm family
PREPARATION: From a tincture of the flowers

Keynotes

- Back pain
- Stiff legs
- Pain in the achilles tendon

Modalities

WORSE/AGGRAVATED BY: None listed
BETTER/AMELIORATED BY: None listed

Remedy Interactions – None listed

Principal Equine Indications

- Long-standing tendon inflammation

Arnica, Arn

CONSIDER ALSO: Leopard's bane, *Arnica montana*
CLASSIFICATION: Plant: Asteraceae (Compositae) family
PREPARATION: From the fresh whole plant or from the root

Keynotes

- Injuries of any kind, mental and physical
- Effects of overuse or over-exertion
- Special focus on soft tissues of the body, especially muscles
- Affinity for blood vessels
- Haemorrhages in any area
- Blood (venous) stasis
- Thrombosis
- Sepsis and abscesses
- Fear of being touched
- Unable to get comfortable when lying on hard surfaces
- Lies down on the right side in preference to the left side of the body
- Low pain threshold
- Weakness of the heart, heart enlargement (hypertrophy)

Modalities

WORSE/AGGRAVATED BY: Touch, at rest, great exertion, damp cold weather
BETTER/AMELIORATED BY: Lying down, gentle motion

Remedy Interactions

WORKS WELL WITH: Aconite, Hypericum, Rhus tox, Ipecac, Calc carb, Natrum sulph
CONSIDER ALSO: Bellis perennis, Hamamelis, Spigelia (chronic), Baptisia, Echinaea, Pyrogen, Ruta, Rhus tox

Principal Equine Indications

- As general first aid remedy
- Wounds of any type
- Shock both physical and mental
- The effects of past injuries, however remote
- Muscle, ligament or muscle injuries
- Strains, sprains, stiffness
- Effects of over-use, especially if muscular
- Eye injuries
- During and after foaling
- Routine use pre- and post-surgery to minimise trauma and to speed healing
- Haemorrhage, including post-operative bleeding, injuries which bleed
- Epistaxis (nosebleed)
- Bruising and tissue swelling
- Haematomas
- Contusions
- Concussion
- Abscesses, especially those which do not come to a head or following injury
- Sepsis or infection where the skin is a blue black colour
- Support of the heart muscle in older animals
- Splints
- Sore shins
- Ulcerative lymphangitis
- Navicular syndrome
- Overreach injuries
- Bruising of the sole
- Corns

- Traumatic laminitis
- Burns and scalds
- Excessive panting
- Localised vaccination reactions

Arsenicum album

(see Constitutional Remedies)

Arsenicum iodatum, Ars iod

COMMON NAME: Iodide of Arsenic
CLASSIFICATION: Mineral: Arsenicums
PREPARATION: Trituration

Keynotes

- Discharges that irritate the skin and mucous membranes
- Red, swollen angry looking mucous membranes
- Rhinitis with thin watery discharge
- Irritation of the end of the nose with sneezing
- Chronic thick yellow catarrh
- Mild hacking cough
- Dry scaly skin
- Itching

Modalities

WORSE/AGGRAVATED BY: Cold wind, exertion
BETTER/AMELIORATED BY: Warmth

Remedy Interactions

WORKS WELL WITH: Phosphorus, Kali iod
CONSIDER ALSO: Arsenicum album, Kali bich, Kali iod, Lachesis, Sulphur

Principal Equine Indications

- Equine flu
- To assist recovery after flu, pneumonia or other respiratory infection
- Bronchopneumonia
- Chronic bronchitis
- Chronic pneumonia
- Rhinitis
- COPD, RAO
- Headshaking
- Sweet itch
- Dandruff
- Post-viral syndrome (Equine ME)

Arundo

COMMON NAME: Reed, *Arundo mauritanica*
CLASSIFICATION: Plant, Poaceae (Gramineae) family
PREPARATION: From tincture of the root sprouts

Keynotes

- Catarrh
- Itching of the nostrils and roof of the mouth
- Itching of the conjunctival membranes

Modalities

WORSE/AGGRAVATED BY: None listed
BETTER/AMELIORATED BY: None listed

Remedy Interactions

CONSIDER ALSO: Arsenicum album, Allium cepa, Sabadilla, Wyethia

Principal Equine Indications

- Headshaking
- Allergic rhinitis
- Itching of the eyes

Asafoetida

COMMON NAME: Stinkasand gum
CLASSIFICATION: Plant: Apiaceae (Umbelliferae) family
PREPARATION: From tincture of the gum

Keynotes

- Symptoms closely related to the digestive system
- Flatulence
- Distension of the abdomen
- Gurgling noises in the abdomen
- Regurgitation of fluid
- Spasmodic contraction of the oesophagus
- Degeneration of bone
- Periosteal pain
- Inflammation inside the eye, iritis
- Corneal ulceration
- Destruction of the nasal bones
- Great distension of the udder from milk
- Lack of milk in mares with foals

Modalities

WORSE/AGGRAVATED BY: After eating
BETTER/AMELIORATED BY: In the open air

Remedy Interactions

WORKS WELL WITH: Causticum, Pulsatilla
CONSIDER ALSO: Ipecac, Aurum, Arg nit

Principal Equine Indications

- Guttural pouch mycosis
- Choke
- Flatulent or tympanic colic
- Iritis
- Periodic ophthalmia
- Periosteitis, periosteal reactions
- Periosteal pain
- Splints
- Sore shins
- Sesamoiditis
- Quittor
- Sole abscess (with watery pus)
- Abscesses with watery pus
- To dry up milk in mares without foals where the udder is greatly distended
- Lack of milk production in mares with foals

Aurum metallicum, Aurum met

COMMON NAME: Metallic gold
CLASSIFICATION: Mineral: Aurums: Metal: Polycrest
PREPARATION: By trituration

Keynotes

- Attacks the blood, glands and bone
- Mental depression, despondency
- Hard working, driven
- Suppresses anger
- Oversensitive to noise
- Destruction of tissues
- Exostoses
- Bone pain
- Tearing pains in the joints
- Weakening or destruction of bone
- Photophobia
- Pains in the bones around the eyes
- Inflammation of the cornea with blood vessel invasion
- Inflammation of the nose
- Destruction of the nasal bones
- Foul smelling nasal discharge
- Pain and swelling in the testicles
- Testicular atrophy

Modalities

WORSE/AGGRAVATED BY: Cold weather, becoming cold, at night
BETTER/AMELIORATED BY: Movement, riding, outside in the fresh air, summer, warm air

Remedy Interactions

WORKS WELL WITH: Sulphur, Symphytum
CONSIDER ALSO: Asafoetida, Kali iod, Merc sol, Mezerium, Nitric acid, Phosphorus, Syphilinum

Principal Equine Indications

- Arthritis/DJD accompanied by advanced bone degeneration
- Exostoses with joint enlargement
- Bone spavin
- Pedal osteitis
- Advanced cases of navicular syndrome
- Soreness around the eyes and orbit
- Keratitis accompanied by photophobia
- Pannus, corneal vascularisation
- Chronic rhinitis with destruction of the nasal bones and with a foul discharge
- Orchitis
- Testicular atrophy/underdeveloped testicles
- Rigs
- Depression/dullness, sadness
- Guttural pouch mycosis
- Mercury poisoning

Bacillinum

COMMON NAME: Tuberculous lung
CLASSIFICATION: Animal: Human: Nosode
PREPARATION: From a maceration of tuberculous lung

Keynotes

- Principal focus is in the respiratory system
- Elderly animals with respiratory diseases
- Chronic catarrh
- Thick catarrh causing difficulty breathing
- Expectorated material is foul

- Poor circulation to the lungs
- Cough
- Recurrent respiratory infections
- Ringworm
- Eczema of the eyelids

Modalities

WORSE/AGGRAVATED BY: At night, early morning, cold air

BETTER/AMELIORATED BY: Warmth

Remedy Interactions

WORKS WELL WITH: Calc phos, Kali carb, Kali iod, Hydrastis, Lachesis, Psorinum

Principal Equine Indications

- Ringworm
- Pneumonia, especially severe or non-responsive cases
- Bronchopneumonia
- Chronic hacking type cough
- COPD, RAO
- Failure to respond to other indicated respiratory remedies
- Recurrent respiratory infections
- Eczema around the eyelids

Badiaga

COMMON NAME: Freshwater sponge

CLASSIFICATION: Animal: Sea creature

PREPARATION: Trituration of the dried sponge

Keynotes

- Sore muscles
- Swollen glands
- Dandruff, scaling
- Cough with much mucus expelled
- Asthmatic breathing
- Neck pain

Modalities

WORSE/AGGRAVATED BY: Cold, motion

BETTER/AMELIORATED BY: Warmth

Remedy Interactions

CONSIDER ALSO: Merc sol, Spongia

Principal Equine Indications

- Seborrhoeic dermatitis of the head region with dandruff
- COPD with a profuse watery nasal discharge
- Sore muscles, especially the back and neck muscles
- Stiff neck

Balsamum peruvianum

COMMON NAME: Balsam of Peru, Peruvian balsam, *Myroxylon pereirae*

CLASSIFICATION: Plant: Fabiaceae (Leguminosae) family

PREPARATION: From a tincture of the balsam obtained from the stems of the plant

Keynotes

- Acts on the respiratory system
- Bronchial catarrh
- Foul expectorated mucus
- Noisy breathing
- COPD, RAO

Modalities

WORSE/AGGRAVATED BY: None listed

BETTER/AMELIORATED BY: None listed

Remedy Interactions – None listed

Principal Equine Indications

- Loose bronchial coughs
- Nasal and bronchial catarrh that is creamy/yellowish in nature

Baptisia

COMMON NAME: Wild indigo, *Baptisia tinctoria*

CLASSIFICATION: Plant: Fabiaceae (Leguminosa) family

PREPARATION: From the fresh root and its bark

Keynotes

- Fever (low fever)
- Symptoms appear less rapidly compared with Aconite or Belladonna
- Septic conditions of the blood
- Septicaemic conditions
- Prostration, stupor

- Offensive secretions including breath, dung, urine
- Mental confusion or state of delirium during fever
- Besotted appearance, slow
- Constriction of the oesophagus
- Inflammation of the throat with dark red membranes, ulceration
- Only able to swallow liquid
- Watery dark, blood tinged, foul smelling diarrhoea

Modalities

WORSE/AGGRAVATED BY: Warm, humid conditions, cold wind

BETTER/AMELIORATED BY: None listed

Remedy Interactions

CONSIDER ALSO: Echinacea, Gelsemium, Bryonia, Rhus tox, Arnica, Pyrogen, Crot horr

WORKS WELL WITH: Arsenicum album

Principal Equine Indications

- Fever accompanied by prostration, drowsiness or stupor
- Septicaemia
- Viral infections including Equine flu
- Endometritis
- Acute putrid or foul diarrhoea
- Enteritis accompanied by fever
- Salmonella infection (Salmonellosis)
- Abortion
- Laminitis with a toxic focus
- Vesicular stomatitis virus
- Potomac horse fever
- Choke

Baryta carbonica, Baryta carb

COMMON NAME: Barium carbonate

CLASSIFICATION: Mineral: Barytas: Polycrest

PREPARATION: Trituration

Keynotes

- Focuses on the extremes of life; young foals and veteran horses
- Slow, delayed development
- Shyness
- Memory loss, senile changes
- Lack of confidence
- Degeneration and weakening of blood vessels
- Blood vessel rupture
- Swollen lymph nodes
- Recurrent respiratory infections
- Weak, dry cough with mucus
- Weak spine
- Stiffness of the back
- Pain in the soles

Modalities

WORSE/AGGRAVATED BY: Cold air, damp weather, feeding

BETTER/AMELIORATED BY: In the open air, warmth, movement

Remedy Interactions

WORKS WELL WITH: Dulcamara, Silica, Psorinum

INCOMPATIBLE WITH: Calc carb

Principal Equine Indications

- Foals that are slow to develop
- Slow learners
- Fear of strangers
- Rigs or cryptochids (undecended testicles)
- Ailments associated with old age, muscle weakness
- Loss of mental agility
- General muscular weakness and trembling as a result of ageing
- Frequent desire to lie down
- Chronically enlarged lymph nodes around the neck (may cause difficulty breathing)
- Cystic skin masses, fatty lumps especially near the neck area
- Chronic low-grade laminitis in veteran horses
- Illness arising after the use of steroids
- Chronic coughs in older horses
- Aneurysm
- Prevention of thromboembolic colic
- Choke

Baryta muriatica, Baryta mur

COMMON NAME: Barium chloride

CLASSIFICATION: Mineral

PREPARATION: Trituration

Keynotes

- Conditions of older horses, mental and physical

- Stiff joints and muscles from overuse
- Nymphomania
- Hypersexuality in the stallion
- Weakness following respiratory infections
- Bronchial catarrh in older horses
- Rattling mucus
- Convulsions

Modalities

WORSE/AGGRAVATED BY: Wet weather
BETTER/AMELIORATED BY: None listed

Remedy Interactions

CONSIDER ALSO: Senega, Baryta carb

Principal Equine Indications

- Chronic cough with lymph node enlargement
- Bronchial catarrh in older animals
- Nymphomania
- Aneurysm
- As general support for older horses

Belladonna, Bell

COMMON NAME: Deadly nightshade, *Atropa belladonna*
CLASSIFICATION: Plant: Solanaceae family: Polycrest
PREPARATION: From the whole plant when it is just about to flower

Keynotes

- Conditions of acute onset
- Important remedy especially for fever and congestion
- Red-hot burning skin, radiates heat, redness
- Dilated pupils
- Throbbing
- Bounding, rapid pulse
- Acts on the nervous system, notably causing excitement, hallucinations, delirium
- Action on the glands including the mammary glands
- Fury, anger, rage, violence
- Excitement
- Desire to escape or run off
- Senses very acute, over-sensitivity of senses, to light, noise and motion
- Convulsions, twitching
- Bright red conjunctival membranes, photophobia
- Grinding of teeth
- Dry throat, swallowing difficult
- Red swollen throat
- Frequent swallowing
- Tender, distended abdomen
- Dry cough with pain in the larynx
- Rapid heart rate
- Swollen, inflamed shiny joints
- Abscesses with pain and redness
- Fever with no thirst

Modalities

WORSE/AGGRAVATED BY: At 3pm, touch, draughts, lying on painful side
BETTER/AMELIORATED BY: Resting

Remedy Interactions

WORKS WELL WITH: Calc carb (chronic), Chamomilla, Hepar sulph, Nat mur
CONSIDER ALSO: Stramonium, Hyoscyamus, Capsicum, Dulcamara

Principal Equine Indications

- Fever of acute onset with no thirst, dilated pupils, throbbing, rapid pulse, heat
- Early stages of many infectious diseases
- Sepsis with fever
- Viral infections with high temperature
- Bronchitis or pneumonia with a high fever
- Acute mastitis
- Peritonitis
- Toxic metritis
- Abscesses including sole abscesses with great heat in the foot
- Acute joint pain, joint sepsis, septic arthritis
- Red swollen shiny inflamed joints
- Acute laminitis (in conjunction with Aconite)
- Colic, severe with great pain
- Acute diarrhoea or colitis where remedy symptoms agree
- Heat exhaustion/heatstroke
- Excessive panting
- Meningitis, neuritis
- Epilepsy/convulsions with violent convulsive limb movements
- Early stages of tetanus
- Behavioural issues – ill tempered animals,

delirium
- Anger, irritability with tendency to bite or kick
- Acute uveitis, periodic ophthalmia
- Tyzzers disease
- Strangles (with a high fever)
- Acute azoturia
- Acute and severe back pain with much local heat
- Photosensitisation
- Headshaking

Bellis perennis, Bellis

COMMON NAME: The daisy, 'Wound-wort' or 'Bruise-wort'
CLASSIFICATION: Plant: Asteraceae (Compositae) family
PREPARATION: From tincture of the whole fresh plant

Keynotes
- Acts especially on the muscles and the muscular fibres of blood vessels
- Sore muscles
- Sore joints
- Venous congestion due to injury
- Small boils or pustules on the skin

Modalities
WORSE/AGGRAVATED BY: On the left side, warmth of stable, before storms, cold bathing
BETTER/AMELIORATED BY: Continued motion, local application of cold compress

Remedy Interactions
CONSIDER ALSO: Arnica, Calendula, Hypericum, Arsenicum album, Hamamelis, Ledum

Principal Equine Indications
- Injuries to muscles
- Injury to the deeper tissues
- Effects or consequences of over-exertion and resulting lameness
- Trauma especially to the pelvic region and lower back
- Bruises especially deep tissue bruising
- Bruising of the sole
- Sprains
- Post surgery to assist recovery
- Soreness or bruising of the walls of the abdomen especially after surgery or injury
- Nerve injuries
- Obdurator paralysis
- During foaling
- Bursitis caused by repeated trauma
- Hygroma of the carpus (knee)
- Trochanteric bursitis
- Capped hock
- Azoturia, tying up

Benzoicum acidum, Benz ac

COMMON NAME: Benzoic acid
CLASSIFICATION: Mineral: Carbon series
PREPARATION: From gum benzoin by sublimation or aromatic hydrocarbons from tincture or trituration

Keynotes
- Principal action is on the urinary system
- Dark-coloured, pungent smelling urine, ammoniacal smell
- Dribbling of urine
- Pain over the region of the kidneys
- Cracking of joints
- Red, swollen joints
- Stiffness in the back legs

Modalities
WORSE/AGGRAVATED BY: Motion
BETTER/AMELIORATED BY: Profuse urination

Remedy Interactions
WORKS WELL WITH: Berberis vulgaris, Solidago

Principal Equine Indications
- Cystitis with or without urinary incontinence
- Chronic renal failure with pungent urine
- Arthritis, DJD
- Joints that crack with or without deformity
- Bone spavin
- Stifle or knee pain
- Pain originating in the Achilles tendon
- Azoturia/tying up

Berberis vulgaris

COMMON NAME: Barberry
CLASSIFICATION: Plant: Berberidaceae family

PREPARATION: From tincture of the root bark

Keynotes

- Rapidly changing symptoms which move from place to place or change in character
- Important remedy for liver and urinary problems
- Pain in the kidney region
- Inflammation of the kidneys
- Blood in the urine
- Urine containing sediment and mucus
- Burning pain in the urethra
- Constipation due to underlying liver problems
- Acts on the venous system leading to engorgement in the pelvic region
- Back pain
- Arthritic symptoms
- Pains in the foreleg, lower hind limb, shoulder and smaller joints (metacarpus, metatasus)
- Pain under the hooves
- Dermatitis involving the lower limbs

Modalities

WORSE/AGGRAVATED BY: Motion
BETTER/AMELIORATED BY: None listed

Remedy Interactions

WORKS WELL WITH: Lycopodium, Bryonia, Kali bich, Rhus tox, Sulphur

Principal Equine Indications

- Lumbar and sacral back pain, spasm of the back muscles
- Sluggish kidney function
- Pain in the kidney region
- Chronic kidney disease
- As a drainage remedy for the urinary system (to remove toxins)
- As a drainage remedy for the skin (in conjunction with Petroleum)
- Chronic cystitis
- Haematuria (blood in the urine)
- Urolithiasis (gravel in the urine, bladder stones)
- Liver disease, jaundice
- Constipation originating from liver problems
- Azoturia/tying up
- Chronic laminitis
- Arthritis/DJD/stiffness especially involving the knee, hock, fetlock, pastern and coffin joints

Beryllium metallicum

COMMON NAME: Beryllium
CLASSIFICATION: Mineral: Metal
PREPARATION: Trituration

Keynotes

- Gradual weight loss (emaciation) with fever
- Frequent need to swallow
- Pain in the lower back
- Nodosities on the bones of the lower leg
- Difficulty breathing with a deep painful cough
- Weepy skin eruptions
- Nodules in the skin
- Skin growths

Modalities

WORSE/AGGRAVATED BY: Heat, exercise, movement
BETTER/AMELIORATED BY: Cold air

Remedy Interactions

CONSIDER ALSO: Bryonia

Principal Equine Indications

- Sarcoids
- Skin nodules
- Cysts
- Bony changes in the lower back (lumbar area)
- Ringbone

Blatta orientalis

COMMON NAME: Indian cockroach
CLASSIFICATION: Animal: Insects
PREPARATION: By trituration of the live insect

Keynotes

- Key remedy for asthmatic symptoms
- Bronchitis
- Cough with difficulty breathing
- Production of pus-like mucus

Modalities

WORSE/AGGRAVATED BY: Wet, rainy weather
BETTER/AMELIORATED BY: None listed

Remedy Interactions – None listed

Principal Equine Indications
- COPD where there is wheezing, bronchial involvement and a cough, especially where Arsenicum album fails to act
- In low potency for chronic cases
- High potency for acute cases

Borax

COMMON NAME: Sodium borate, sodium biborate
CLASSIFICATION: Mineral: Carbon series
PREPARATION: Trituration and subsequent solution in distilled water

Keynotes
- Irritates the gastrointestinal system
- Causes salivation and diarrhoea
- Ulceration of mucous membranes
- Fear of movement in a downward direction
- Anxious, nervous, easily frightened
- Reactive to sudden noises, even the slightest noise
- Inflammation of the eyelids
- Lids roll inwards
- Ulcers in the mouth with salivation
- Diarrhoea with mucus
- White uterine discharge with vulval irritation or eczema
- Scabs and sores around the nostrils
- Dermatitis around the lower limbs with unhealthy skin and matted hair

Modalities
WORSE/AGGRAVATED BY: Downward movement, noise, warm weather, after oestrus
BETTER/AMELIORATED BY: In the evening, cold weather

Remedy Interactions
CONSIDER ALSO: Calc carb, Bryonia, Nux vomica, Kali bich, Pulsatilla, Phosphorus, Graphites

Principal Equine Indications
- Anxiety, fear and general nervousness where there is an oversensitivity to noise
- Fear of sudden noises
- Dislike of crowds and crowded areas
- Fear of downward movement
- Seasickness, airsickness
- Poor travellers (upset by the movement of the horsebox)
- Mild entropion (rolling in of the eyelids)
- Mud fever
- Horse pox virus
- Contagious equine metritis (CEM)
- Coital exanthema
- Mouth ulcers

Bothrops lanciolatus

COMMON NAME: Yellow viper
CLASSIFICATION: Animal: Reptiles: Snakes: Crotalidae family
PREPARATION: From a solution of the venom in glycerine

Keynotes
- Issues related to the blood
- Thrombosis
- Haemorrhage
- Swollen lymphatic vessels
- Sepsis
- Pulmonary (lung) congestion
- Dark discoloration of the skin
- Paralysis of single limbs

Modalities
WORSE/AGGRAVATED BY: On the right side
BETTER/AMELIORATED BY: None listed

Remedy Interactions
CONSIDER ALSO: Lachesis, Crot horr

Principal Equine Indications
- Haemorrhage into the retina and associated blindness
- Haemorrhage of dark, fluid blood
- Blood clots
- Purpura haemorrhagica
- Difficulty breathing due to congestion of the lungs
- Septic states
- Lymphangitis
- Snake bites
- Gangrene (especially where the deeper tissues are involved)
- Iliac thrombosis

- Verminous aneurysm
- Thromboembolic colic
- Paralysis of a single leg
- Variocele

Botulinum

COMMON NAME: Botulinus toxin, toxin of bacillus botulinium, *Clostridium botulinum*
CLASSIFICATION: Animal: Bacteria: Nosode
PREPARATION: From the toxin

Keynotes
- Dropping of the eyelids (ptosis)
- Difficult breathing
- Swallowing difficult
- Incoordination (ataxia)
- Constipation

Modalities
WORSE/AGGRAVATED BY: None listed
BETTER/AMELIORATED BY: None listed

Remedy Interactions – None listed

Principal Equine Indications
- Shaker foal syndrome
- Forage poisoning
- Botulism
- Ptosis

Bovista

COMMON NAME: Puffball, Warted puffball, *Lycoperdon bovista*
CLASSIFICATION: Plant: Fungi: Lycoperdaceae family
PREPARATION: By trituration

Keynotes
- Has a particular action on the skin and circulation
- Eczema or dermatitis with irritation
- Urticaria (affected areas pit under pressure)
- Moist eczema
- Crusting
- Haemorrhage
- Uterine bleeding
- Cystic ovaries

Modalities
WORSE/AGGRAVATED BY: Early morning, hot weather, getting warm
BETTER/AMELIORATED BY: Cold applications

Remedy Interactions
WORKS WELL WITH: Calc carb, Rhus tox, Sepia
CONSIDER ALSO: Cicuta

Principal Equine Indications
- Eczema around the mouth and nose area
- Eczema/dermatitis affecting the head area generally
- Urticaria with pitting
- Chronic urticaria
- Angioneurotic oedema
- Moist eczema/dermatitis progressing to thick crusts
- Eczema around the head region
- Allergy based itching of the skin (self trauma leads to bleeding)
- Insect bites and stings
- Sweet itch
- Mud fever
- Cystic ovaries
- Joint swelling (where a fracture is involved)
- Purpura haemorrhagica
- Lymphangitis
- Capped elbow, capped hock
- Bog spavin
- Hygroma of the carpus (knee)
- Trochanteric bursitis
- Thoroughpin

Bromium

COMMON NAME: Bromine
CLASSIFICATION: Mineral: Element
PREPARATION: From a solution in distilled water

Keynotes
- Acts on the respiratory system especially the larynx and trachea
- Dry spasmodic cough with rattling mucus in the trachea
- Difficult breathing
- Asthma
- Enlarged lymph nodes hard to the touch

- Conditions arising from becoming over heated
- Swelling of the testicles
- Ovarian swelling

Modalities

WORSE/AGGRAVATED BY: Evening until midnight, entering warm stable, warm damp weather, cold air, at rest
BETTER/AMELIORATED BY: Motion, exercise

Remedy Interactions

WORKS WELL WITH: Argentum nitricum, Kali carb
CONSIDER ALSO: Conium, Spongia, Iodum, Silica, Calc fluor

Principal Equine Indications

- Parotitis, enlarged lymph nodes
- Inflammation of the ovaries
- Dry spasmodic cough, difficulty breathing
- COPD
- Conditions arising from becoming overheated

Bryonia, Bry

COMMON NAME: Wild hops, White bryony, *Bryonia alba*
CLASSIFICATION: Plant: Cucurbitaceae family: Polycrest
PREPARATION: From tincture of the root before flowering

Keynotes

- Acts on serous and synovial membranes
- Swollen joints
- Muscle pain, rheumatic like pains
- Stitching and tearing pains
- Dry mucous membranes
- Irritability, short tempered
- Thirst
- Dryness
- Hard, dry dung
- Swollen, painful udder
- Important focus on the respiratory system
- Dry hacking cough
- Tracheal irritation
- Difficult, laboured breathing
- Shallow breathing
- Periodic deep breaths
- Back pain
- Greasy skin and hair
- Desire to avoid movement

Modalities

WORSE/AGGRAVATED BY: Warmth and motion especially, in the morning, hot weather, exertion, touch, cold winds
BETTER/AMELIORATED BY: Lying on the painful side or area (pressure on the affected region affords relief by immobilising the area), cold, resting, wet weather

Remedy Interactions

INCOMPATIBLE WITH: Calc carb
WORKS WELL WITH: Alumina (chronic), Rhus tox, Kali carb, Nat mur (chronic but less so than Alumina)
Consider also Drosera, Phosphorus, Spigelia, Stannum, Sticta, Rumex

Principal Equine Indications

- Pneumonia, pleuropneumonia and other respiratory infections including Equine flu
- Pleurisy
- Hacking, dry painful coughs
- Tracheitis
- Pericarditis
- Constipation
- Impacted colic with great thirst
- Diarrhoea from hot weather
- Peritonitis
- Synovitis especially chronic cases
- Arthritis/DJD where symptoms agree with the remedy picture
- Swollen painful joints
- Sporadic lymphangitis
- Acute ligament strains
- Tenosynovitis
- Carpitis
- Sore shins
- Thoroughpin where there is lameness
- Bone spavin
- Navicular syndrome
- Bog spavin
- Back pain which is worse on movement, neck pain
- Acute laminitis
- Azoturia, tying up
- Mastitis
- To dry up excessive milk production
- Lyme disease
- Fever of slow onset, horse unwilling to move

Bufo

COMMON NAME: Poison of the Toad, *Bufo rana*
CLASSIFICATION: Animal: Amphibians
PREPARATION: From solution of the poison (expressed from cutaneous glands) in rectified spirit

Keynotes

- Acts principally on the skin and nervous system as well as the lymphatic system
- Epilepsy
- Impotence
- Pemphigus
- Muscle cramps
- Ataxia
- Hard nodules in the udder
- Pustules on the skin leading to blisters
- Dry skin which is rough
- Inclination to nip suddenly
- Stupid dull appearance and attitude
- Fearful of crowds
- Upset by bright lights

Modalities

WORSE/AGGRAVATED BY: None listed
BETTER/AMELIORATED BY: None listed

Remedy Interactions

INCOMPATIBLE WITH: Lachesis, Senega
WORKS WELL WITH: Calc carb
CONSIDER ALSO: Baryta carb, Baryta mur, Graphites, Tuberculinum, Zinc

Principal Equine Indications

- Lymphangitis
- Hard nodules in the tissues of the udder
- Epilepsy
- Impotence in the stallion
- Pemphigus
- Cracked dry skin
- Nipping (as if in a childish manner)
- Neonatal maladjustment syndrome

Cactus grandiflorus, Cactus

COMMON NAME: Night blooming cereus
CLASSIFICATION: Plant: Cactaceae family
PREPARATION: From a tincture of young, tender stems and flowers collected in the summer

Keynotes

- Principal focus is on the heart and blood vessels
- Constrictions akin to those of an iron band
- Spasmodic pain
- Bleeding from the nose and lungs
- Constriction of the throat leading to suffocation
- Difficulty breathing
- Retention of urine
- Heart murmur due to valvular incompetence
- Irregular, intermittent and feeble pulse

Modalities

WORSE/AGGRAVATED BY: At night, at 11am and 11pm
BETTER/AMELIORATED BY: In the fresh air

Remedy Interactions

WORKS WELL WITH: Arsenicum album
CONSIDER ALSO: Digitalis, Spigelia, Convallaria, Kalmia, Latrodectus, Naja

Principal Equine Indications

- As a general heart tonic
- Endocarditis
- Heart murmurs, especially where the mitral valve is involved
- African horse sickness

Caladium

COMMON NAME: American Arum
CLASSIFICATION: Plant: Araceae family
PREPARATION: From the tincture of the whole fresh plant

Keynotes

- Itching of the skin
- Prone to sweating
- Attracts flies
- Bites of insects itch badly
- Itching around the genital area; the scrotum and vulva
- Impotency
- Dislike of motion
- Asthma with catarrh

Modalities

WORSE/AGGRAVATED BY: Motion
BETTER/AMELIORATED BY: Daytime

Remedy Interactions

WORKS WELL WITH: Nitric acid, Cantharis, Causticum, Sepia

Principal Equine Indications

- Sweet itch
- To reduce attraction to flies

Calcarea carbonica

(see Constitutional Remedies)

Calcaria fluorica, Calc fluor

COMMON NAME: Fluoride of lime, Fluor spar
CLASSIFICATION: Mineral: Calcareas
PREPARATION: By trituration

Keynotes

- Main focus is on bone and its nutrition
- Hard glands
- Cataracts
- Reduces the formation of adhesions, scar tissue and deposits of fibrin
- Hard swellings on the face and on the jaw bone
- Vascular tumours and bony tumours
- Chronic back pain
- Enlargement of the joints of the lower limbs
- Exostoses
- Hard masses in tendons and ligaments
- Synovitis
- Fissure and cracks in the skin
- Skin callouses
- Ulcers secreting thick yellow pus

Modalities

WORSE/AGGRAVATED BY: Resting, changes of weather
BETTER/AMELIORATED BY: Heat, warmth, covering up by a rug, movement

Remedy Interactions

CONSIDER ALSO: Conium, Lapis albus, Heckla lava, Ruta grav

Principal Equine Indications

- Hard (like stone, indurated) glands including hardened, enlarged lymph nodes or hard masses in the udder
- Lymphadenitis
- Parotitis
- Periostitis
- Bony tumours or bony masses
- Exostoses, bone spurs
- Bone degeneration
- Arthritis/DJD especially of the fetlock, pastern, coffin and stifle joints
- Bone spavin
- Pedal ostitis
- Navicular syndrome
- Sidebone
- Buttress foot
- Poor hoof quality
- White line disease
- Chronic laminitis
- Seedy toe
- Splints
- Ringbone
- Sesamoiditis
- Chrondromalacia of the patella
- Cracking joints
- Strains
- Synovitis, especially chronic cases
- Calcified deposits in tendons and ligaments
- Chronic lumbar back pain
- To reduce the chances of adhesions after surgery
- To reduce scar tissue or strictures
- Dissolution of blood clots
- To reduce deposits of fibrin
- Haematoma where resolution is slow
- Fibrotic myopathy (to prevent ossification)
- Cataracts
- Alopecia

Calcaria iodata, Calc iod

COMMON NAME: Iodide of lime
CLASSIFICATION: Mineral: Calcareas
PREPARATION: Trituration

Keynotes

- Enlarged glands
- Chronic cough

- Pneumonia
- Ringworm

Modalities

WORSE/AGGRAVATED BY: None listed
BETTER/AMELIORATED BY: None listed

Remedy Interactions – None listed

Principal Equine Indications

- Enlarged lymph nodes
- Ringworm
- Nodular growths

Calcarea phosphorica, Calc phos

COMMON NAME: Phosphate of lime, Calcium phosphate
CLASSIFICATION: Mineral: Calcareas
PREPARATION: Trituration

Keynotes

- Important tissue remedy
- Special affinity for bone
- Diseases of bone
- Bone development
- Non-union of fractures
- Anaemia
- Tendency to sweat easily
- Glandular enlargements
- Flatulence
- Pain in the abdomen after eating
- Soreness at the sacroiliac junction
- Stiffness with pains in the joints and bones

Modalities

WORSE/AGGRAVATED BY: Motion, change of weather, damp wet weather
BETTER/AMELIORATED BY: Resting

Remedy Interactions

WORKS WELL WITH: Ruta grav, Arsenicum album, Iodum, Merc sol, Sulphur, Hepar sulph
CONSIDER ALSO: Calc carb

Principal Equine Indications

- To assist bone development in young animals
- Where bone growth is too rapid
- Bone weakness
- To promote fracture healing, slow healing fractures
- Epiphysitis (physitis)
- Carpus valgus and carpus varus (angular limb deformities)
- Sacroiliac pain or discomfort
- Pedal osteitis
- Bone spavin
- Carpal tunnel syndrome
- Osteochondrosis, OCD
- Bone cysts
- Anaemia resulting from prolonged illness
- Anaemia in young foals
- Uterine inertia
- Eclampsis, hypocalcaemia

Calcaria sulphurica, Calc sulph

COMMON NAME: Sulphate of lime, sulphate of Calcium, Plaster of Paris
CLASSIFICATION: Mineral: Calcareas
PREPARATION: Trituration

Keynotes

- Suppuration (infection) where pus is present
- Lumpy, yellow, thick pus
- Thick yellow discharge from the eyes
- Clouding of the cornea
- Pustules on the skin with small crusts
- Cystic tumours
- Pus in the lungs
- Thick, yellow catarrh
- Unhealthy cuts and wounds discharging pus

Modalities

WORSE/AGGRAVATED BY: Change of weather
BETTER/AMELIORATED BY: In the open air

Remedy Interactions

CONSIDER ALSO: Calendula, Hepar sulph, Silica, Kali mur, Nat sulph

Principal Equine Indications

- Abscesses with thick yellow pus including chronic cases
- Sole abscess, under-run sole
- Canker

- Gravel
- Fistulae, sinuses
- Discharging sinuses
- Conjunctivitis with a thick yellow discharge
- Empyema, sinus empyema, guttural pouch empyema
- Coughs with thick yellow catarrh
- Skin infections, bacterial folliculitis
- Strangles where discharging
- Coital exanthema
- Epizootic lymphangitis
- Equine viral papular dermatitis
- Pyometria

Calendula officinalis, Calendula

COMMON NAME: Marigold
CLASSIFICATION: Plant: Asteraceae (Compositae) family
PREPARATION: From a tincture of the leaves and flowers

Keynotes

- Key remedy for promoting healing
- Pain out of proportion to the injury
- Eye injuries with subsequent infection
- Haemostatic (stops bleeding) when applied locally

Modalities

WORSE/AGGRAVATED BY: Damp weather
BETTER/AMELIORATED BY: None listed

Remedy Interactions

WORKS WELL WITH: Hepar sulph, Arnica

Principal Equine Indications

- To promote healing in any situation including mucosal surfaces
- Open wounds, lacerations, excoriation of the skin
- Suppurating wounds
- Ulcers, pressure sores
- To encourage granulation
- Proud flesh
- Scald and burns
- Quittor
- Corneal injuries

Camphor, Camphora

COMMON NAME: Camphor
CLASSIFICATION: Plant: Lauraeae family
PREPARATION: From a solution of the gum in rectified spirit

Keynotes

- Important remedy for collapse
- Body icy cold, temperature subnormal
- Little strength
- Pulse weak and feeble
- Eyes staring
- Pupils dilated
- Wants to be uncovered
- Shock
- Violent epileptic convulsions
- Profuse diarrhoea with collapse and coldness
- Difficulty breathing, almost as if suffocating
- Cracking in joints

Modalities

WORSE/AGGRAVATED BY: Motion, at night, cold air
BETTER/AMELIORATED BY: Warmth

Remedy Interactions

WORKS WELL WITH: Cantharis
CONSIDER ALSO: Arsenicum album. Carbo veg, Veratrum album

Principal Equine Indications

- Shock
- Post-surgical shock
- Anaphylaxis
- Severe diarrhoea with collapse, weakness and prostration
- Viral infections leading to a state of collapse or exhaustion
- Salmonellosis
- Potomac horse fever

Cannabis sativa

COMMON NAME: American hemp
CLASSIFICATION: Plant: Cannabinaceae family
PREPARATION: From a tincture of both male and female flowering tops

Keynotes

- Focuses on the urinary system, genital tract and respiratory system
- Great tiredness as if from over-exertion
- Corneal opacity
- Cystitis with urinary retention, urge to urinate
- Phimosis
- Over-excited sexually
- Inflammation of the penis and prepuce
- Wheezing, rattling respiration
- Cough with green mucus
- Mucus in the trachea
- Dislocation of the patella going uphill

Modalities

WORSE/AGGRAVATED BY: Going uphill
BETTER/AMELIORATED BY: Resting quietly

Remedy Interactions

WORKS WELL WITH: Belladonna, Hyoscyamus, Lycopodium, Nux vom, Opium, Pulsatilla, Rhus tox
CONSIDER ALSO: Cannabis indica, Cantharis, Nux moschata, Opium, Veratrum album

Principal Equine Indications

- Corneal opacity, cloudiness of the cornea
- Urethra discharges in the stallion
- Phimosis
- Patella luxation when ridden uphill

Cantharis, Canth

COMMON NAME: Spanish fly, *Cantharis vesicator*
CLASSIFICATION: Animal: Insects
PREPARATION: From trituration of the whole insect

Keynotes

- Acts on the urinary and reproductive organs
- Acute, severe inflammation of the urinary tract
- Blood and mucus in the urine
- Severe urging to urinate
- Frequent urination
- Nephritis
- Irritation of the gastrointestinal tract
- Peritonitis
- State of delirium
- Sexual mania
- Whinnying
- Inflammation of the throat
- Tongue covered in vesicles
- Burning in the mouth, pharynx, throat and oesophagus
- Thick sticky mucus in the throat
- Difficulty drinking
- Mucus-covered dung with blood and straining
- Hypersexuality in both sexes
- Retention of the placenta
- Metritis
- Pleurisy
- Pericarditis
- Dermatitis and eczema with vesicles, raw patches or pustules
- Gangrene
- Burns and scalds

Modalities

WORSE/AGGRAVATED BY: From touch, urinating, drinking water
BETTER/AMELIORATED BY: By rubbing

Remedy Interactions

WORKS WELL WITH: Apis, Camphor, Argentum nitricum, Kali bich, Merc corr, Sepia, Terebinthina, Pulsatilla
CONSIDER ALSO: Apis mel, Arsenicum album, Merc corr, Nux vomica, Sarsaparilla

Principal Equine Indications

- Acute cystitis
- Nephritis, acute renal (kidney) failure
- Pyelonephritris
- Urethritis
- Acute skin inflammation
- Blistered skin
- Pemphigus
- Photosensitisation
- Burns and scalds
- Effects of insect bites
- Horse pox virus
- St John's Wort poisoning
- Hypersexuality, nymphomania, satyriasis
- Peritonitis
- Pericarditis
- Pleurisy
- Retained placenta
- False rigs
- Spermatorrhoea

- Priapism
- Scrotal dermatitis
- Severe inflammation of the mouth and tongue
- Acute salmonellosis
- Acute leptospirosis

Capsicum

COMMON NAME: Cayenne pepper, *Capsicum annuum*
CLASSIFICATION: Plant: Solanaceae family
PREPARATION: From a tincture of the dried pods

Keynotes

- Acts on the mucous membranes producing inflammation and suppuration
- General state of weakness, lacking energy, exhausted and worn out
- Lack of reaction, lazy
- Homesickness
- Chilly, need covering up
- Inflammation at the back of the throat
- Stomatitis
- Dung with mucus or blood
- Straining to pass dung
- Cystitis with straining
- Testicular atrophy

Modalities

WORSE/AGGRAVATED BY: Open air, being uncovered
BETTER/AMELIORATED BY: From warmth, having a rug on

Remedy Interactions

WORKS WELL WITH: Belladonna, Lycopodium, Pulsatilla, Silica, Nat mur
CONSIDER ALSO: Antimonium crudum, Calc carb, Cantharis, Ferrum met, Graphites

Principal Equine Indications

- Change of stable, 'homesickness'
- Worn out (with old age) animals as a tonic
- Pharyngitis
- Testicular atrophy
- Coccidiosis
- Acute salmonellosis
- Vesicular stomatitis virus

Carbo animalis

COMMON NAME: Animal charcoal
CLASSIFICATION: Mineral: Carbons
PREPARATION: From trituration of charred ox hide and then solution in distilled water

Keynotes

- Suited to older horses
- Helps recovery after long illnesses
- Depressed
- Sluggish circulation
- Weak digestion
- Flatulence
- Hardened, swollen lymph nodes in the neck
- Weak hocks

Modalities

WORSE/AGGRAVATED BY: Cold air
BETTER/AMELIORATED BY: Warmth

Remedy Interactions

WORKS WELL WITH: Calc phos

Principal Equine Indications

- General debility in old horses, especially where the digestion is weak or circulation poor
- Assists recovery after prolonged illness
- Pleurisy, in the later stages

Carbo vegetabilis, Carbo veg

COMMON NAME: Vegetable charcoal
CLASSIFICATION: Mineral: Carbons: Polycrest
PREPARATION: By trituration

Keynotes

- Suited to slow, lazy, sluggish animals
- Overweight
- Symptoms tend to be chronic
- Chilly, feels cold to the touch
- Poor circulation, weak pulse, venous stasis
- Lack of oxygen
- Symptoms resulting from fluid loss
- Collapse
- Lifelessness
- Desire for air
- Debility

- Flatulence
- Abdominal distension
- Slow digestion
- Colic
- Cough with mucus in the chest, wheezing
- Pneumonia (long-standing)
- Bleeding from the lungs
- Cold skin
- Falling out of hair
- Gangrene
- Haemorrhage of dark blood that does not clot

Modalities

WORSE/AGGRAVATED BY: Evening, at night, cold, warm damp weather, in the open air
BETTER/AMELIORATED BY: From release of gas, fresh air (especially fanning)

Remedy Interactions

WORKS WELL WITH: Kali carb, Drosera, Arsenicum album, Lachesis, Phosphorus
CONSIDER ALSO: China, Veratrum album, Lycopodium, Ammon carb, Graphites, Lycopodium, Sepia

Principal Equine Indications

- The 'corpse reviver'
- Collapse
- Near to death cases
- Severe shock, trembling
- Septicaemia, toxaemia
- Circulatory collapse, cyanosis
- Fluid loss (hypovolaemia)
- Pneumonia with great difficulty breathing
- Neglected pneumonia cases
- Air hunger
- Flatulent colic
- Gangrene
- Poor resistance to infection
- Lowered vitality
- Weakened digestion
- Severe offensive diarrhoea with collapse
- Acute salmonellosis
- Hair loss in elderly run down horses
- Haemorrhage of dark, oozing blood, patient collapsed
- Myositis with muscle gangrene
- White line disease
- Severe cases of laminitis
- Alopecia (hair loss) in debilitated animals

Carbolicum acidum

COMMON NAME: Phenol, carbolic acid
CLASSIFICATION: Mineral: Carbons
PREPARATION: From a solution in rectified spirit

Keynotes

- A destructive remedy
- State of stupor, disinclination to work
- Acts on the central nervous system (CNS)
- Paralysis
- Foul discharges
- Ulcerations on the inside of the mouth
- Back of the throat red
- Flatulence
- Post-partum fever
- Uterine inflammation
- Ulcerated burns

Modalities

WORSE/AGGRAVATED BY: From jarring
BETTER/AMELIORATED BY: None listed

Remedy Interactions

CONSIDER ALSO: Colchicum, Kreosotum, Sepia, Tabacum

Principal Equine Indications

- Weakness of the hind limbs with general depression and languor
- Severe ulcerated burns, scalding
- Ulceration of the inside of the mouth

Carcinosin, Carc

COMMON NAME: Breast carcinoma
CLASSIFICATION: Animal: Nosode
PREPARATION: From diseased epithelial tissue

Keynotes

- Important remedy with a wide sphere of action especially psychologically
- Like Phosphorus without all the fears
- Sense of responsibility
- Enduring, will carry on until they would drop

- Self-sacrificial
- Perfectionist
- Rebellious nature
- Overly sensitive to noises, general atmosphere, local surroundings
- Obsessional behaviour
- Suppressed emotions including grief and anger
- Sympathetic, sensitive to other humans and animals
- Sensitive to reprimand
- Affectionate, craves affection
- Anticipatory fears
- Chronic tiredness
- Cancer generally

Modalities

WORSE/AGGRAVATED BY: None listed
BETTER/AMELIORATED BY: None listed

Remedy Interactions

CONSIDER ALSO: Sepia (acute), Nat mur, Thuja, Silica, Tuberculinum, Phosphorus, Staphysagria

Principal Equine Indications

- History of repeated illness especially when younger
- Vaccinosis
- Equine ME
- Lyme disease
- Chronic fatigue
- Behavioural problems
- Anticipatory anxiety
- Illness arising from grief or sadness, pining
- Sarcoids
- Melanoma
- Skin cysts
- Slow-healing skin wounds
- Diabetes mellitus
- Cancer support
- Heavy worm burdens in young foals

Carduus marianus, Carduus

COMMON NAME: St Mary's thistle, Silybum
CLASSIFICATION: Plant: Asteraceae (Compositae) family
PREPARATION: From tincture or trituration of the seeds

Keynotes

- Key liver remedy
- Jaundice
- Cirrhosis
- Pain in the liver
- Congested portal system
- Ascites due to liver disease
- Bleeding associated with liver disease
- Hard dung
- Pain in the hip joints

Modalities

WORSE/AGGRAVATED BY: None listed
BETTER/AMELIORATED BY: None listed

Remedy Interactions

CONSIDER ALSO: Chelidonium, Taraxacum, Nux vomica, Lycopodium, Phosphorus

Principal Equine Indications

- As a liver tonic
- Liver disease generally, particularly chronic cases
- Liver enlargement
- Cirrhosis, jaundice
- Drainage of liver toxins
- Hyperlipaemia
- Cushing's disease (liver support)
- Supportive treatment in poisoning
- Ragwort poisoning
- Ascites
- Stiffness in the hips

Castor equi

COMMON NAME: Rudimentary thumbnail of the horse
CLASSIFICATION: Animal: Mammals
PREPARATION: Trituration of scales

Keynotes

- Acts on the nails, teats and bone
- Skin thickening
- Cracked and ulcerated teats
- Painful teats
- Warts

Modalities

WORSE/AGGRAVATED BY: None listed
BETTER/AMELIORATED BY: None listed

Remedy Interactions

CONSIDER ALSO: Graphites, Silica, Nitric acid

Principal Equine Indications

- Sore or cracked teats or nipples
- Brittle hooves
- To help improve the quality of horn
- Thickened areas of skin
- Warts around the head area and on the udder

Caulophyllum, Caul

COMMON NAME: Blue cohosh, Squaw root
CLASSIFICATION: Plant: Berberidaceae family
PREPARATION: From tincture or trituration of the root

Keynotes

- Main focus is on the female reproductive system and smaller joints
- Lack of tone in the uterus
- Abortion and threatened abortion
- Uterine discharge
- Pain and stiffness in the smaller joints of the body
- Arthritis of the smaller joints

Modalities

WORSE/AGGRAVATED BY: Open air, during pregnancy
BETTER/AMELIORATED BY: None listed

Remedy Interactions

CONSIDER ALSO: Gelsemium, Pulsatilla, Actea rac, Causticum, Sabina, Sepia, Viburnum opulus

Principal Equine Indications

- During the latter stages of pregnancy to encourage an easy foaling
- To help during foaling and encourage contractions
- Uterine atony
- During pregnancy to regulate gestation
- To reduce the risk of abortion including in cases of EHV-1
- Retained placenta
- Pyometria with a dark brown discharge, endometritis
- Arthritis and stiffness of the smaller joints; knee, hock, fetlock, pastern and coffin
- Carpitis
- Carpal tunnel syndrome
- Chronic laminitis

Causticum, Caust

COMMON NAME: Potassium hydrate, tinctura acris sine Kali, *Causticum hahnemanni*
CLASSIFICATION: Mineral: Causticums: Polycrest
PREPARATION: From distillation of a mixture of slaked lime and potassium sulphate

Keynotes

- An important remedy for arthritis, paralysis and rheumatic like symptoms
- Pain in muscular and fibrous tissue
- Restlessness at night due to pain in bone and in joints
- Deformed joints
- Gradual loss of muscular strength leading to paralysis
- Contracture of tendons
- Paralysis of the vocal cords, tongue, face, bladder and limbs
- Conditions arising after long-standing grief
- Warts
- Sore skin folds
- Dry cough
- Cataracts
- Corneal ulceration

Modalities

WORSE/AGGRAVATED BY: In clear fine weather, cold wind, dry weather
BETTER/AMELIORATED BY: Damp wet weather, warmth

Remedy Interactions

WORKS WELL WITH: Calc carb, Carbo veg, Arsenicum album, Cuprum, Ignatia, Pulsatilla, Rhus tox, Sepia
CONSIDER ALSO: Calc phos, Gelsemium, Kali bich, Phosphorus, Rhus tox, Sepia, Tuberculinum
INCOMPATIBLE WITH: Phosphorus

Principal Equine Indications

- Ptosis (drooping of the eyelids)
- Roaring, laryngeal hemiplegia
- Paralysis of the ear flap (neural paralysis)
- Facial paralysis
- Partial paralysis of the rectum

- Weakness or paralysis of the bladder, incontinence
- Cystitis due to urinary retention
- Weakness or paralysis of the limbs
- Ataxia
- Nerve paralysis following infectious diseases
- Cauda equina neuritis
- Sweeny
- Radial paralysis
- Stringhalt with laryngeal paralysis
- EHV-1-neurological symptoms
- Recovery from viral encephalitis
- Equine protazoal myeloencephalitis
- Uterine inertia during foaling
- Arthritis and DJD where the modalities agree
- General stiffness including the neck
- Bony distortion of the joints
- Bone spavin
- Contraction (shortening) of tendons
- Unsteady or uneven gait involving the front legs
- Weak hock joints
- Carpal tunnel syndrome
- Curb
- Large, sore bleeding warts, pedunculated or jagged warts
- Rough or jagged growths on the eyelids
- Burns that are slow to heal
- Gangrene arising from old burns or deep ulcers
- Excoriation of the skin
- Aural plaques
- Wounds or scars that keep reopening
- Chronic bronchitic cough (in elderly animals)
- Hard dry cough with difficult expectoration
- Cataracts
- Shaker foal syndrome
- Grief and pining

Ceanothus

COMMON NAME: New Jersey tea, Red root, *Ceanothus americanus*
CLASSIFICATION: Plant: Rhamnaaceae family
PREPARATION: From tincture of the fresh leaves

Keynotes

- Acts on the spleen
- Anaemia arising from liver disease
- Chronic bronchitis
- Haemostat

Modalities

WORSE/AGGRAVATED BY: Motion, cold weather
BETTER/AMELIORATED BY: Warm weather

Remedy Interactions

WORKS WELL WITH: Berberis vulgaris, Conium, Nat mur

Principal Equine Indications

- Splenic enlargement
- Anaemia where the liver is involved
- Equine infectious anaemia (supportive remedy)

Cenchris contortrix

COMMON NAME: Copperhead snake, *Ancistrodon contortrix*
CLASSIFICATION: Animal: Snake: Pit viper
PREPARATION: From a solution of the venom

Keynotes

- A deep acting remedy
- Symptoms tend to be right-sided
- Changes in mood
- Easily irritated
- Apt to kick or bite
- Suspicious
- Jealousy
- Nymphomania
- Ovarian pain
- Dislike of tight fitting tack
- Swelling around the eyes
- Chains of small nodules in the skin following the lymphatic vessels

Modalities

WORSE/AGGRAVATED BY: On the right side, after rest, on waking
BETTER/AMELIORATED BY: None listed

Remedy Interactions

CONSIDER ALSO: Lachesis

Principal Equine Indications

- Jealousy
- Nymphomania

- Right-sided ovarian pain
- Equine nodular skin disease

Chamomilla, Cham

COMMON NAME: German chamomile
CLASSIFICATION: Plant: Asteraceae (Compositae) family
PREPARATION: From tincture of the whole fresh plant

Keynotes

- Principal focus is on the nervous system
- Mental and emotional problems
- Sensitive and irritable
- Over-excitability
- Restlessness with whinnying
- Impatience
- Intolerance
- Spiteful
- Anger
- Thirsty
- Hot and sweaty
- Extreme (unbearable) pain
- Swelling of the salivary glands
- Conditions arising during eruption of teeth
- Distension of the abdomen
- Flatulent colic with profuse sweating
- Green, watery dung
- Stiff neck muscles
- Lower back pain
- Severe joint pain

Modalities

WORSE/AGGRAVATED BY: Heat, anger, in the open air, wind, at night, being touched or looked at
BETTER/AMELIORATED BY: Warm wet weather, from sweating

Remedy Interactions

WORKS WELL WITH: Belladonna, Calc carb, Mag carb, Pulsatilla
CONSIDER ALSO: Nux vomica, Staphysagria, Colocynthis, Calc phos

Principal Equine Indications

- Pain and intolerance of pain
- Post-operative pain
- Tooth pain
- Severe joint pain with irritability and restlessness
- Neck pain or stiffness
- Back pain especially from kissing spines
- Anger (and conditions arising from) and irritability
- Restlessness, difficult to calm
- Excitability
- Parotitis
- Flatulent colic
- Watery green diarrhoea

Chelidonium majus, Chel

COMMON NAME: Greater celandine, *Chelidonium majus*
CLASSIFICATION: Plant: Papaveraceae family
PREPARATION: From tincture of the whole fresh plant at the time of flowering

Keynotes

- An important liver remedy
- Jaundice
- Liver enlargement
- Yellow sclera
- Conjunctivitis with excessive tear production
- Pain around the eyes
- Sluggish digestion
- Constipation
- Alteration of diarrhoea and hard dung
- Pain under the blade (the caudal angle) of the scapula
- Stiffness of the neck
- Pain in the limbs
- Painful knees/metacarpal bones
- Rheumatic type pain in the hips
- Paresis (weakness) of the hind limbs, muscle weakness
- Flapping of the alae nasae (not linked with breathing)
- Right-sided pneumonia
- Lethargy, drowsy
- Tendency to bully
- Domineering character
- Conditions brought on by change of weather

Modalities

WORSE/AGGRAVATED BY: Motion, changes of weather, 4am and 4pm, right side, touch
BETTER/AMELIORATED BY: Warm feed, eating, from pressure

Remedy Interactions

WORKS WELL WITH: Lycopodium, Bryonia, Arsenicum album, Ledum, Sulphur
CONSIDER ALSO: Bryonia, Lycopodium, Merc sol, Opium, Sanguinaria

Principal Equine Indications

- Liver disease
- Hepatitis
- Jaundice
- Ragwort poisoning
- For general liver support
- Lethargy
- General muscular stiffness including the neck
- Pain and discomfort in the knee joints
- Sore hip joints
- DJD, arthritis especially of the right shoulder joint
- Carpitis
- Tying up (prevention)
- Photosensitisation (where there is liver disease)
- Poisoning-liver support

Chenopodium anthelminticum

COMMON NAME: Jerusalem oak
CLASSIFICATION: Plant: Chenopodiaceae family
PREPARATION: From tincture of the fresh plant

Keynotes

- Pain in the shoulder blade
- Yellow foaming urine
- Acts against worms

Modalities

WORSE/AGGRAVATED BY: None listed
BETTER/AMELIORATED BY: None listed

Remedy Interactions – None listed

Principal Equine Indications

- In the treatment of worms

Chimaphila umbellata

COMMON NAME: Pipsissewa, Prince's pine, Ground holly
CLASSIFICATION: Plant: Ericaceae family
PREPARATION: From a tincture of the root and leaves or from the fresh plant in flower

Keynotes

- Acts on the kidneys, genital and urinary tract, lymphatic glands and udder
- Cataracts
- Chronic cystitis with mucus, blood and sediment in the urine
- Strains before urination
- Sugar present in the urine
- Atrophy of the udder
- Tumours in the udder with milk production

Modalities

WORSE/AGGRAVATED BY: Damp weather, on the left side
BETTER/AMELIORATED BY: None listed

Remedy Interactions

CONSIDER ALSO: Conium, Copaiva, Medorrhinum, Pareira brava, Sulphur, Thuja

Principal Equine Indications

- Nephritis
- Chronic cystitis
- Sediment in the urine
- Diabetes
- Atrophy (shrinking) of the udder

China *see* Cinchona officinalis

Chininum arsenicosum, Chin ars

COMMON NAME: Quinine arsenate
CLASSIFICATION: Mineral
PREPARATION: By trituration

Keynotes

- Tiredness and weakness
- Asthma-type symptoms
- Poor appetite

Modalities

WORSE/AGGRAVATED BY: None listed
BETTER/AMELIORATED BY: None listed

Remedy Interactions – None listed

Principal Equine Indications
- As a general tonic after illness
- Poor appetite accompanied by weakness
- Equine infectious anaemia

Chininum sulphuricum, Chin sulph

COMMON NAME: Quinine sulphate
CLASSIFICATION: Mineral
PREPARATION: By trituration

Keynotes
- Acute joint pain
- Nephritis
- A decrease in red blood cells and haemoglobin
- Blood and albumen in the urine
- Pain and sensitivity of the tips of the spinal vertebrae
- Itching, redness and pustules of the skin

Modalities
WORSE/AGGRAVATED BY: None listed
BETTER/AMELIORATED BY: None listed

Remedy Interactions
CONSIDER ALSO: China, Phosphorus, Cedron, Salicylicum acid and TNT

Principal Equine Indications
- Supportive treatment in anaemia
- Urolithiasis (gravel in the urine)
- Spinal discomfort
- Haemolytic anaemia

Chionanthus

COMMON NAME: Fringe tree, *Chionanthus virginica*
CLASSIFICATION: Plant: Oleaceae family
PREPARATION: Tincture of the bark

Keynotes
- Acts on the liver principally
- Jaundice
- Liver enlargement
- Enlargement of the spleen
- Diabetes
- Listlessness
- Yellow conjunctiva
- Constipation
- Poor appetite
- Diseases of the pancreas
- Dark urine containing sugar

Modalities
WORSE/AGGRAVATED BY: None listed
BETTER/AMELIORATED BY: None listed

Remedy Interactions
CONSIDER ALSO: Cinchona, Chelidonium, Carduus, Podophyllum, Iris vers

Principal Equine Indications
- Liver disease
- Jaundice
- Pancreatic disease
- Diabetes mellitus

Cicuta virosa

COMMON NAME: Water hemlock, Cow bane
CLASSIFICATION: Plant: Apiaceae (Umbelliferae) family
PREPARATION: From a tincture of the root gathered at flowering

Keynotes
- Acts on the nervous system
- Spasms, cramps
- Tetanic-like movements
- Convulsions, epilepsy
- Head, neck and spine bent back in spasm, arching
- Head turned to one side
- Vertigo
- State of delirium, whinnying
- Meningitis
- Pupils dilated
- Eyes appear to stare
- Strabismus
- Thick, yellow scabs on the face and at the corners of the mouth
- Eats indigestible objects

Modalities
WORSE/AGGRAVATED BY: From touch, jarring or sudden movement, concussion, smoke
BETTER/AMELIORATED BY: Warmth

Remedy Interactions

CONSIDER ALSO: Hypericum, Hyoscyamus, Belladonna, Nux vomica

Principal Equine Indications

- Epilepsy, convulsions
- The effects of concussion
- Tetanus
- Opisthotonus spasm or cramping of the neck muscles
- Meningitis
- Myelitis
- Neonatal maladjustment syndrome (NMS)
- Poisoning where symptoms match
- Eczema around the face and mouth

Cimicifuga racemosa, Cimic or Actaea racemosa, Actea rac

COMMON NAME: Black snake root, Black cohosh
CLASSIFICATION: Plant: Ranunculaceae family
PREPARATION: From the root

Keynotes

- Main action is on the nervous system, muscles and female reproductive system
- Muscular stiffness with restlessness
- Muscles ache
- Sore muscles
- Chorea
- Jerking of the limbs
- Stiffness originating in the Achilles tendon
- Fear of travelling in an enclosed space, tries to escape
- Ovarian pain
- Irregular cycles
- Pain around the pelvic area
- Lumbo-sacral pain
- Stiffness in the back and neck
- Contraction of the muscles in the back
- Nervous and anxious, easily excited
- Well built

Modalities

WORSE/AGGRAVATED BY: Touch, at night, evening, during oestrus, motion, cold
BETTER/AMELIORATED BY: Rest, warmth, eating

Remedy Interactions

WORKS WELL WITH: Cuprum
CONSIDER ALSO: Bryonia, Pulsatilla, Caulophyllum, Lilium tigrinum, Actea spic

Principal Equine Indications

- Back pain
- Muscular spasm of the back or neck muscles
- Stiffness originating in the neck
- Muscular soreness and stiffness especially with restlessness
- Tying up, azoturia
- Lumbo-sacral pain
- Mareish behaviour
- Abortion (as possible preventative in 1x potency)
- Disordered oestrus cycle
- Delayed ovulation
- Ovarian pain
- Ovarian inflammation
- Foaling, to dilate cervix
- Poor or weak uterine contractions
- Claustrophobia in horseboxes

Cina

COMMON NAME: Wormseed, *Cina maritima, Artemisia maritima*
CLASSIFICATION: Plant: Asteracea (Compositae) family
PREPARATION: From the unexpanded flower heads

Keynotes

- Often suited to younger animals
- Principal action is on the digestive system
- Intestinal irritation
- Worms
- Irritability
- Short-tempered, ill-humoured
- Dislike of being touched
- Variable appetite
- Grinding of the teeth
- Dilated pupils
- Itching and rubbing of the ears
- Itching of the nose causing rubbing
- Spasmodic coughs
- Hungry
- Bloated abdomen
- Itching around the anus

- Twitching of the limbs
- Convulsions during the night

Modalities

WORSE/AGGRAVATED BY: At night, in the sun, summer
BETTER/AMELIORATED BY: Moving around

Remedy Interactions

CONSIDER ALSO: Chenopodium, Teucrium marum, Kamala, Chamomilla, Natrum phos

Principal Equine Indications

- Worms and conditions resulting from worms, diarrhoea from worms
- Anal irritation
- Epilepsy
- Colic with abdominal distension
- Stringhalt
- Headshaking

Cinchona officinalis, China, Chin

COMMON NAME: Peruvian bark
CLASSIFICATION: Plant: Rubiaceae family: Polycrest
PREPARATION: From a tincture of the dried bark

Keynotes

- Conditions arising from loss of fluids – excessive sweating, diarrhoea, haemorrhage
- Passive, slow haemorrhage
- Debility
- Anaemia
- Eyes look hollow
- Post-operative pains from gas build-up
- Apathy
- Violent sneezing with no discharge
- Suffocative catarrh
- Rattling in the chest
- Bleeding from the lungs
- Irregular heartbeat
- Sluggish digestion
- Flatulence
- Colic
- Liver enlarged, jaundice
- Pains in the limbs and joints
- Skin very sensitive to touch
- Profuse sweating

Modalities

WORSE/AGGRAVATED BY: The slightest touch, draughts of air, loss of fluids, at night, after feeding
BETTER/AMELIORATED BY: Hard pressure, open air, warmth

Remedy Interactions

WORKS WELL WITH: Calc phos, Ferrum metallicum, Arsenicum album, Carbo veg
CONSIDER ALSO: Ignatia, Natrum mur, Lycopodium, Nux vomica

Principal Equine Indications

- Dehydration
- Effects of haemorrhage
- Steady haemorrhage over a prolonged period of time
- Debility from any cause, including from viral infections, but especially from fluid loss
- Watery diarrhoea leading to collapse
- Foal diarrhoea (from milk)
- Flatulent colic
- Tympanic colic
- Post-operative gas build-up in the bowels
- Catarrh build-up in the chest
- EIPH
- Anaemia especially blood loss anaemia
- To cleanse the liver
- Moist gangrene
- Equine infectious anaemia
- Potomac horse fever
- Heat stroke
- Excessive panting
- Conditions which have a cyclical, recurrent nature

Cineraria

COMMON NAME: Dusty miller
CLASSIFICATION: Plant: Asteraceae (Compositae) family
PREPARATION: From tincture of the fresh wild plant gathered just before the flower buds open

Keynotes

- Used externally
- Acts on the eyes
- Cataracts – age related
- Cataracts arising from trauma to the eye

- Corneal opacities, ulcers

Modalities

WORSE/AGGRAVATED BY: None listed
BETTER/AMELIORATED BY: None listed

Remedy Interactions

CONSIDER ALSO: Phosphorus, Causticum, Silica, Calc fluor

Principal Equine Indications

- Cataracts, especially those arising after eye trauma
- Corneal opacity
- Eye injuries

Cinnabaris

COMMON NAME: Mercuric sulphide, Red sulphide of mercury
CLASSIFICATION: Mineral: Mercury series
PREPARATION: By trituration

Keynotes

- Pain around the eye and orbit region
- Conjunctivitis where the whole eye is red and painful
- Ulcers in the throat and mouth
- Swollen prepuce
- Bleeding warts on the prepuce

Modalities

WORSE/AGGRAVATED BY: Summer, at night
BETTER/AMELIORATED BY: Open air, rest

Remedy Interactions

CONSIDER ALSO: Thuja, Nitric acid, Natrum sulph, Merc sol

Principal Equine Indications

- Intense redness of the whole eye, severe conjunctivitis
- Sarcoids, especially on the prepuce
- Bleeding sarcoids
- Melanoma especially if ulcerated
- Phimosis
- Smegma

Cistus canadensis

COMMON NAME: Rock rose, Ice plant, Frost-weed
CLASSIFICATION: Plant: Cistaceae family
PREPARATION: From a tincture of the whole plant

Keynotes

- Has an affinity for glands and throat region
- Enlarged lymph nodes
- Hard lumps in the udder
- Mastitis
- Infected wounds and bites
- Lupus
- Skin ulcers

Modalities

WORSE/AGGRAVATED BY: On exposure to cold air, excitement
BETTER/AMELIORATED BY: From feeding

Remedy Interactions

CONSIDER ALSO: Conium, Calc fluor, Bufo, Calc carb, Silica

Principal Equine Indications

- Parotitis, parotiditis
- Enlarged, hardened lymph nodes, especially around the neck region
- Skin masses appearing in the neck area
- Mastitis with hard masses in the udder

Clematis erecta

COMMON NAME: Virgin's bower
CLASSIFICATION: Plant: Ranunculaceae family
PREPARATION: From a tincture of the leaves and stems

Keynotes

- Acts on the skin, glands, urinary and genital tracts
- Emaciation
- Chronic blepharitis
- Iritis
- Hardening of the testicles
- Scrotal swelling
- Inflammation of the testicles
- Violent erections
- Inability to pass urine
- Urine passed drop by drop
- Red burning skin, itching

Modalities

WORSE/AGGRAVATED BY: At night, warmth of stable, washing down with cold water, new moon
BETTER/AMELIORATED BY: In the open air

Remedy Interactions

WORKS WELL WITH: Silica
CONSIDER ALSO: Argentum metallicum, Cantharis, Medorrhinum, Pulsatilla, Rhododendron, Rhus tox

Principal Equine Indications

- Urethral strictures
- Itching and irritation around the genital region
- Orchitis
- Prolonged erections
- Rigs or cryptorchids
- Chronic blepharitis

Cobaltum

COMMON NAME: Cobalt
CLASSIFICATION: Mineral: Metal: Element
PREPARATION: By trituration

Keynotes

- Bone pain
- Back pain
- Pain in the knee joints
- Weak stifle joints

Modalities

WORSE/AGGRAVATED BY: None listed
BETTER/AMELIORATED BY: None listed

Remedy Interactions – None listed

Principal Equine Indications

- Lower back pain especially in the sacral region
- Knee pain
- Weak stifle joints

Cocculus

COMMON NAME: Indian cockle, *Cocculus indicus*
CLASSIFICATION: Plant: Menispermaceae family
PREPARATION: From a tincture of the powdered seeds which contain the poison, picrotoxin

Keynotes

- Spasms and weakness (paresis) originating in the cerebrum
- Contractions of the limbs and body
- Cramping of the jaw muscles
- Paralysis of the facial nerve
- Paralysis of the muscles of the throat preventing swallowing
- Contracted pupils
- Conditions worse from travelling
- Distension of the abdomen
- Choking in the upper oesophagus
- Pain in the middle of the back
- Pain in the shoulder and elbow region
- One-sided paralysis
- Cracking from stifle joints
- Weakness of the lower limbs

Modalities

WORSE/AGGRAVATED BY: Travel (in a vehicle), loss of sleep, touch, noise, emotional upset, jarring, heat of the sun
BETTER/AMELIORATED BY: None listed

Remedy Interactions

WORKS WELL WITH: Petroleum
INCOMPATIBLE WITH: Causticum, Nux vomica
CONSIDER ALSO: Petroleum, Tabacum, Picric acid, Ignatia, Nat mur, Gelsemium

Principal Equine Indications

- 'Travel sickness', seasickness
- Epilepsy and convulsions
- Loss of balance
- Meningitis
- Facial paralysis
- Myositis of the jaw muscles
- Weak stifle joints with cracking
- Weakness of the back legs
- Cauda equina neuritis
- Equine protozoal myeloencephalitis
- Grass sickness

Coccus cacti

COMMON NAME: Cochineal
CLASSIFICATION: Animal: Insects: Hemiptera
PREPARATION: From a tincture or trituration of the

bodies of the dried female insects

Keynotes

- Sensation of a foreign body in the eye
- Thick mucus in the throat
- Suffocating, spasmodic cough with thick white mucus
- Chronic bronchitis
- Stones or gravel in the urine
- Blood in the urine
- Dark-coloured urine

Modalities

WORSE/AGGRAVATED BY: Left side, after sleep, touch, exertion
BETTER/AMELIORATED BY: Riding

Remedy Interactions

CONSIDER ALSO: Cantharis, Sarsaparilla, Kali bich, Apis, Phosphorus

Principal Equine Indications

- Urinary gravel
- Chronic bronchitis
- Accumulation of thick mucus in the throat
- Eye discomfort evidenced by repeated rubbing

Coffea cruda

COMMON NAME: Unroasted coffee
CLASSIFICATION: Plant: Rubiaciae family
PREPARATION: From tincture of the raw berries

Keynotes

- General stimulation
- Nervous agitation, restlessness
- Mentally active
- Heightened sensitivity
- Conditions arising from fatigue, fear and fright
- Neuralgia
- Crural (femoral nerve) neuralgia
- Intolerance of pain
- Sleeplessness

Modalities

WORSE/AGGRAVATED BY: Emotional stimulation, narcotic drugs, strong odours, noise, cold, at night
BETTER/AMELIORATED BY: Warmth, resting, sleep

Remedy Interactions

INCOMPATIBLE WITH: Cantharis, Causticum, Cocculus, Ignatia, Nat mur, Sepia, Theridion

Principal Equine Indications

- Neuritis
- Intolerance of pain
- Neuralgic pain
- Post-operative pain
- Agitation and restlessness, excitability
- Oversensitivity to noise
- Nymphomania
- Ill effects of long journeys

Colchicum, Colch

COMMON NAME: Meadow saffron, *Colchicum autumnale*
CLASSIFICATION: Plant: Lilliaceae family
PREPARATION: From a tincture of the bulb dug up in the spring

Keynotes

- Main action is on muscles, periosteum and synovial membranes
- Affected areas are red, hot and swollen
- Tearing pains
- Collapse and prostration
- Acute and severe symptoms
- Increased thirst
- Flatulence
- Increased salivation
- Abdominal distension
- Increased gut sounds
- Colon distended
- Distension of the right lower area of the abdomen
- Ascites
- Jelly-like mucus in the dung
- Dysentery-like symptoms
- Watery diarrhoea with abdominal distension
- Straining to pass dung
- Dark-coloured urine
- Pains in the limbs, especially knee joints
- Stiff joints, rheumatic-like symptoms
- Swelling of the limbs
- Pain in the lumbo-sacral region

Modalities

WORSE/AGGRAVATED BY: Sundown to sunrise, movement, motion

BETTER/AMELIORATED BY: Warmth, lying down quietly

Remedy Interactions

WORKS WELL WITH: Lycopodium, Arsenicum album, Spigelia

CONSIDER ALSO: Carbo veg, Arsenicum album, Veratrum album, Bryonia, Berberis vulgaris, Lycopodium

Principal Equine Indications

- Important remedy for tympanic colic with rumbling and abdominal distension
- Dysenteric-like diarrhoea
- Diarrhoea composed of mucus
- Colitis X, Clostridial entertoxaemia
- Acute salmonellosis
- Swelling and stiffness of the joints
- Synovitis
- Painful joints, sensitive to the least touch or movement
- Acute renal (kidney) failure

Colocynthis, Coloc

COMMON NAME: Bitter cucumber, Bitter apple, *Citrullus colocynthis*

CLASSIFICATION: Plant: Cucurbitaceae family

PREPARATION: From tincture of the pulp of the fruit

Keynotes

- Action is focused on the abdomen and head (neuralgia)
- Intense sudden onset abdominal pain better for arching the back
- Pain comes in waves
- Irritable, angry, indignant
- Cramping and twitching in muscles
- Purging
- Dysenteric-like yellowish dung with mucus
- Ovarian pain
- Cystic ovaries
- Contraction of muscles
- Limbs drawn up together
- Cramping pain in the hip joints
- Luxation of the hip joints
- Shortening of tendons

Modalities

WORSE/AGGRAVATED BY: Anger, feeding

BETTER/AMELIORATED BY: Arching of the back, (bending double), hard pressure, warmth, movement

Remedy Interactions

WORKS WELL WITH: Staphysagria, Chamomilla, Merc sol, Causticum, Kali carb

CONSIDER ALSO: Bryonia, Elaterium, Causticum, Mag phos

Principal Equine Indications

- Spasmodic colic
- Colic from drinking cold water
- Hip pain
- Stringhalt
- Shivering
- Cystic ovaries
- Ovarian pain (causing arching of the back)
- Severe diarrhoea with abdominal cramping or colic
- Potomac horse fever

Conium

COMMON NAME: Poison hemlock, *Conium maculatum*

CLASSIFICATION: Plant: Apiaceae (Umbelliferae) family

PREPARATION: From tincture of the fresh flowering plant

Keynotes

- Has an affinity for the endings of motor nerves and nerve ganglia
- Ascending paralysis and stiffness
- Awkward gait
- Trembling
- Age-related changes, weakness
- Tumours and enlarged glands
- Depressed, lack of interest
- Vertigo
- Photophobia (induced by the slightest corneal damage)
- Excessive lachrymation
- Weakness of eye muscles
- Keratitis (inflammation of the cornea)
- Enlargement of the liver
- Chronic jaundice

- Urging to pass dung
- Difficulty in passing urine (stops and starts)
- Increased sexual desire in the stallion
- Effects of sexual repression
- Hard, shrunken udder
- Inflammation of the ovaries
- Dry cough
- Paralysis of the respiratory muscles
- Laboured breathing on the least exercise
- Pain in the lumbo-sacral region or between the shoulders
- Pain in the tail (coccydinia)
- Heavy, tired hind limbs
- Paralysis or weakness of the hind limbs
- Muscular weakness

Modalities

WORSE/AGGRAVATED BY: Before or during oestrus, exertion

BETTER/AMELIORATED BY: Motion, pressure

Remedy Interactions

WORKS WELL WITH: Arnica, Arsenicum album, Calc carb, Lycopodium, Nux vomica, Phosphorus, Pulsatilla

Principal Equine Indications

- Progressive and slow paralysis
- Weakness of the hind limbs
- Wobbler syndrome
- Cauda equina neuritis
- Crural paralysis
- Muscle weakness
- Loss of balance
- Paralysis and weakness of the hind limbs
- Paralysis or weakness of the bladder
- Dribbling of urine
- Keratitis with severe photophobia
- Corneal ulceration with phtophobia
- Enlarged, hardened lymph nodes
- Small hardened tumours cancerous lymph nodes
- Nodular type sarcoids
- As a general remedy for aged horses
- Mastitis (where hard nodules are present in the gland)
- Viral infections where there are neurological symptoms
- EHV-1, African horse sickness, dourine, Equine protozoal myeloencephalitis
- Symptomatic treatment of poisoning

Convallaria

COMMON NAME: Lily of the valley, *Convallaria majalis*

CLASSIFICATION: Plant: Liliaceae family

PREPARATION: From the whole plant

Keynotes

- An important heart remedy
- Increases the energy of the heartbeat
- Rapid and irregular pulse
- Heart enlargement
- Venous stasis
- Pulmonary (lung) congestion
- Difficulty breathing (dyspnoea) when ridden
- Ascites
- Endocarditis

Modalities

WORSE/AGGRAVATED BY: In a warm stable

BETTER/AMELIORATED BY: In the open air

Remedy Interactions

CONSIDER ALSO: Digitalis, Crataegus, Cactus

Principal Equine Indications

- Heart weakness with sluggish circulation and/or rapid irregular pulse
- Enlargement of the heart
- Lesions of the heart valves
- Endocarditis
- Ascites
- Lung congestion

Copaiva

COMMON NAME: Balsam of Copaiva, *Copaifera officinalis*

CLASSIFICATION: Plant: Fabiaceae (Leguminosae) family

PREPARATION: From tincture of the balsam

Keynotes

- Acts on mucous membranes especially the urinary and respiratory tracts
- Nasal catarrh with sore nostrils
- Bronchial catarrh

- Painful urination
- Frequent desire to urinate
- Colitis with mucus
- Allergic skin reactions, hives

Modalities

WORSE/AGGRAVATED BY: None listed
BETTER/AMELIORATED BY: None listed

Remedy Interactions

CONSIDER ALSO: Cantharis, Apis, Vespa, Sepia

Principal Equine Indications

- Cystitis
- Urticaria, hives
- Bronchial catarrh

Crataegus

COMMON NAME: Hawthorn berries, *Crataegus oxyacantha*
CLASSIFICATION: Plant: Rosaceae family
PREPARATION: From a tincture of the ripe berries

Keynotes

- A tonic to the heart acting on the heart muscle
- Increases the number and strength of the heartbeats
- Chronic heart disease with weakness
- Heart failure
- Heart enlargement
- Valvular heart murmurs
- Myocarditis
- Fluid retention
- Difficulty breathing on least exercise
- Cold extremities (limbs)
- Diabetes
- Anaemia

Modalities

WORSE/AGGRAVATED BY: Warm stable
BETTER/AMELIORATED BY: Fresh air, rest

Remedy Interactions

CONSIDER ALSO: Strophanthus, Digitalis, Cactus, Convallaria, Prunus

Principal Equine Indications

- Navicular syndrome
- Chronic laminitis
- Heart disease (as a general tonic)
- Heart failure and associated symptoms
- Heart murmurs where the pulse is feeble
- Myocarditis
- As a general heart tonic for aged horses
- Equine infectious anaemia (cardiac support)

Crocus sativa

COMMON NAME: Saffron, *Crocus sativus*
CLASSIFICATION: Plant: Iridaceae family
PREPARATION: From a tincture of dried stigmas or young fresh shoots

Keynotes

- Associated with haemorrhage of blood that is black, thick and clots as long strings
- Dilation of the pupils
- Slow reaction of pupils to light
- Retinal arteries occluded by blood clots
- Glaucoma
- Nosebleed
- Wheezy cough
- Constipation
- Risk of abortion
- Uterine bleeding of dark stringy blood
- Spasmodic muscular contractions
- Twitching of single sets of muscles
- Weakness in the back legs

Modalities

WORSE/AGGRAVATED BY: Lying down, hot weather, warm stable, in the morning
BETTER/AMELIORATED BY: In the open air

Remedy Interactions

WORKS WELL WITH: China, Nux vomica, Pulsatilla, Sulphur
CONSIDER ALSO: Platina, Sabina, Ipecac, Lachesis, Zincum metallicum

Principal Equine Indications

- Haemorrhage of dark, black, stringy blood
- Uterine haemorrhage
- Abortion

- Glaucoma

Crotalus horridus, Crot horr

COMMON NAME: The Rattlesnake of North America
CLASSIFICATION: Animal: Reptiles: Snakes: Crotalidae family
PREPARATION: From a solution of the venom in glycerine

Keynotes

- Has an action on the blood
- Haemorrhage of dark fluid blood that does not clot
- Decomposition of the blood
- Jaundice and cirrhosis of the liver
- Septic states
- Talkative
- Suspicious nature
- Dictatorial
- Desire to escape
- Intraocular haemorrhage
- Retinal haemorrhage
- Nosebleed
- Dark red swollen throat
- Oesophageal spasm
- Intolerance of tight-fitting tack
- Bleeding from the bowel of darkened blood
- Prolonged oestrus
- Uterine haemorrhage
- Post-partum fever
- Fever with haemorrhage
- Septicaemia
- Lymphangitis
- Discoloration and swelling of the skin
- Purpura haemorrhagica
- Abscesses
- Sepsis of the skin

Modalities

WORSE/AGGRAVATED BY: On the right side, open air, evening and morning, springtime, damp and wet weather
BETTER/AMELIORATED BY: Rest, motion

Remedy Interactions

WORKS WELL WITH: Arnica, Belladonna, Lycopodium, Nux vomica, Pulsatilla, Rhus tox, Stramonium
INCOMPATIBLE WITH: Lachesis, Psorinum
CONSIDER ALSO: Lachesis, Bothrops, Naja, Elaps

Principal Equine Indications

- Haemorrhage of dark, almost black, fluid blood that does not clot easily
- Absorption of intraocular haemorrhage
- Uterine haemorrhage
- Blood loss anaemia
- Sepsis and septic states
- Septicaemia, toxaemia
- Post-partum fever
- Abscesses and other skin infections where there is skin discoloration
- Septic skin wounds
- Purpura haemorrhagica
- Lymphangitis
- Warfarin poisoning
- Haematomas, especially recurring haematomas
- Snake and insect bites or stings
- Equine viral arteritis
- Coccidiosis
- Ill effects of vaccination

Croton tiglium, Crot tig

COMMON NAME: Croton seed oil
CLASSIFICATION: Plant: Euphorbiaceae family
PREPARATION: From a tincture of the oil from the seeds

Keynotes

- Acts as a purgative and skin irritant
- Diarrhoea with sudden evacuation
- Watery dung
- Straining and urging
- Gurgling noises from the bowel
- Intense itching of the skin
- Pustular eruptions especially on the face and in the genital area
- Oozing vesicles

Modalities

WORSE/AGGRAVATED BY: Eating or drinking, in the summer, touch, night, morning
BETTER/AMELIORATED BY: Sleep

Remedy Interactions

WORKS WELL WITH: Rhus tox

CONSIDER ALSO: Elaterium, Veratrum album, Colchicum, Gambogia, Rhus tox

Principal Equine Indications

- Watery diarrhoea forcibly evaluated with urging and with mucus
- Eczema or dermatitis with intense itching, especially on the face, and in the genital region, especially the scrotum
- Equine rotavirus infection

Cuprum metallicum, Cuprum met

COMMON NAME: Copper
CLASSIFICATION: Mineral: Element
PREPARATION: Trituration

Keynotes

- Key action in treating spasms, cramping, convulsions and epilepsy
- Symptoms tend to appear in ends of limbs first
- Symptoms appear periodically and in groups
- Tonic and clonic spasms
- Chorea (involuntary movements of the limbs)
- Spasm and constriction of the chest
- Jerking and twitching of the muscles of the limbs
- Muscular cramp
- Eyeballs rotated upwards
- Jaw contracted
- Foam seen around the mouth
- Severe colic
- Abdomen tender to touch
- Black-coloured dung
- Resentful
- Intuitive
- Sudden explosive behavioural episodes
- Conditions arising from suppressed emotions or conditions

Modalities

WORSE/AGGRAVATED BY: Before oestrus, evening, night, new moon
BETTER/AMELIORATED BY: Drinking cold water, sweating

Remedy Interactions

WORKS WELL WITH: Calc carb, Iodum, Arsenicum album
CONSIDER ALSO: Belladonna, Stramonium, Cicuta, Strychnine, Colocynthis, Dioscorea

Principal Equine Indications

- Muscle spasms, jerking and cramps
- Epilepsy and convulsions
- Azoturia
- Stringhalt
- Shivering
- Spasmodic colic with intermittent violent spasms
- Intussusception
- Diarrhoea with colic or cramping
- Eclampsia, hypocalcaemia
- Equine protozoal myeloencephalitis
- Tying up (prevention)
- Osteochondrosis, OCD (in low potency)
- Deep-seated grief

Curare

COMMON NAME: Arrow poison, *Curare woorari*
CLASSIFICATION: Plant: Loganiaceae family
PREPARATION: From dilution of the poison mixed with alcohol

Keynotes

- Affects the muscles and brain
- Causes muscular paralysis
- No loss of sensation or consciousness
- Respiratory muscles paralysed
- Diminished reflexes
- Diabetes
- Can be vicious or wicked
- Prone to chase people

Modalities

WORSE/AGGRAVATED BY: Damp weather, cold weather or wind, 2am, right side of the body
BETTER/AMELIORATED BY: None listed

Remedy Interactions

WORKS WELL WITH: Arnica, Belladonna
CONSIDER ALSO: Baryta carb, Nux vomica, Conium, Plumbum

Principal Equine Indications

- Total or complete paralysis of any area
- Muscular paralysis
- Facial paralysis

- Sweeny, radial paralysis, crural paralysis
- Weak limbs
- Trembling limbs
- Legs give way
- Debility in elderly horses
- Tetanus
- Equine ME, post-viral syndrome
- Debility in aged horses

Cyclamen

COMMON NAME: Sow-bread, *Cyclamen europaeum*
CLASSIFICATION: Plant: Primulaceae family
PREPARATION: From a tincture of the root gathered in spring

Keynotes
- Affects the gastrointestinal tract and the genitourinary tract
- Post-partum haemorrhage
- Swelling of the udder with milk production following oestrus
- Purging of the bowel
- Periosteal pains

Modalities
WORSE/AGGRAVATED BY: In the open air, evening
BETTER/AMELIORATED BY: After oestrus, moving around, warmth of stable

Remedy Interactions
WORKS WELL WITH: Phosphorus, Pulsatilla. Rhus tox, Sepia, Sulphur
CONSIDER ALSO: Pulsatilla, Sepia, Nat mur

Principal Equine Indications
- To dry up milk in non-pregnant mares

Digitalis

COMMON NAME: Foxglove, *Digitalis purpurea*
CLASSIFICATION: Plant: Scrophulariaceae family
PREPARATION: From a tincture of the leaves of the plant during its second year of growth

Keynotes
- Key heart remedy
- Irregular and weak pulse
- Irregular heartbeat
- Valvular incompetence
- Slow pulse
- Weak heart muscle
- Heart enlargement
- Cyanosis
- Collapse
- Liver enlargement
- Jaundice with heart disease
- Oedema and ascites

Modalities
WORSE/AGGRAVATED BY: Motion, least movement, night
BETTER/AMELIORATED BY: In the fresh air

Remedy Interactions
INCOMPATIBLE WITH: China, Strophanthus
CONSIDER ALSO: Crataegus, Apocynum cannabinum, Convallaria, Cactus, Lachesis, Spigelia

Principal Equine Indications
- Heart weakness
- Irregular and slow pulse
- Heart arrhythmias, irregular heartbeat
- Atrial fibrillation
- Mitral valve disease
- Oedema and ascites
- Filled legs where the problem is circulatory
- Lung congestion
- Cyanosis
- Myocarditis
- Cardiac support during illness

Dioscorea

COMMON NAME: Wild yam, *Dioscorea villosa*
CLASSIFICATION: Plant: Dioscoreaceae family
PREPARATION: From tincture of the fresh root

Keynotes
- A remedy for pain and spasm
- Flatulent colic
- Weak digestion
- Flatulence
- Rumbling noises from the abdomen
- Back pain
- Stiff joints
- Weak hooves

Modalities

WORSE/AGGRAVATED BY: During the evening, at night, lying down, arching of the back
BETTER/AMELIORATED BY: Moving around, stretching out, in the fresh air

Remedy Interactions

CONSIDER ALSO: Colocynthis, Bryonia, Nux vomica, Chamomilla, Belladonna, Mag phos

Principal Equine Indications

- Flatulent colic

Drosera

COMMON NAME: Round-leaved Sundew, *Drosera rotundifolia*
CLASSIFICATION: Plant: Droseraceae family
PREPARATION: From a tincture of the fresh plant

Keynotes

- Principal action is on the respiratory tract
- Associations with the lymphatic system, serous membranes, long bones and vertebrae
- Spasmodic dry cough
- Episodes of coughing follow each other rapidly
- Choking and difficulty breathing during coughing bouts
- Yellow catarrh
- Inflammation of the larynx
- Sensitive larynx-palpation induces coughing
- Inflammation of the pleura
- Asthmatic symptoms
- Pains in the hip joint

Modalities

WORSE/AGGRAVATED BY: Towards evening, after midnight, lying down, warmth
BETTER/AMELIORATED BY: Open air, at a gentle walk

Remedy Interactions

WORKS WELL WITH: Nux vomica, Calc carb, Pulsatilla, Carbo veg, Sulphur

Principal Equine Indications

- Spasmodic dry coughs
- 'Barking' type coughs
- Dry repetitive coughs
- Pleurisy
- Pneumonia
- Tracheitis
- Laryngitis
- Absorption of scar tissue

Dulcamara, Dulc

COMMON NAME: Woody nightshade, Bitter-sweet, *Solanum dulcamara*
CLASSIFICATION: Plant: Solanaceae family
PREPARATION: From a tincture of the fresh green stems and leaves gathered before flowering

Keynotes

- Acts on the skin, glands, mucous membranes and digestive system
- Rheumatic-type symptoms
- Paralysis of single areas
- Conditions arising at the end of summer with hot days and cold nights
- Problems caused by damp conditions
- Eczema with thick dark coloured crusts on the head
- Thick yellow mucus from the nose or from the eyes
- Colic induced by cold weather
- Slimy green dung
- Coughs in cold wet weather
- Excessive secretion of mucus
- Cough after exercise
- Stiffness in the neck and middle of the back
- Paralysis
- Itching of the skin in cold wet weather
- Vesicles
- Urticaria
- Moist eruptions on the face, in the genital region and lower limbs
- Large smooth warts, flat smooth warts

Modalities

WORSE/AGGRAVATED BY: Cold, damp, wet weather, at night, early autumn
BETTER/AMELIORATED BY: Moving around, warmth

Remedy Interactions

WORKS WELL WITH: Baryta carb, Bryonia, Calc carb, Lycopodium, Sepia, Rhus tox

INCOMPATIBLE WITH: Belladonna, Lachesis
CONSIDER ALSO: Rhus tox, Calc carb, Kali carb, Silica

Principal Equine Indications

- Conditions arising from exposure to wet, damp, getting wet and cold weather
- Conditions arising in the early autumn
- Stiffness alternating with skin symptoms
- Stiffness worse in damp weather, especially in the autumn
- Back pain worse in damp weather
- Rainscald
- Mange (symptomatic)
- Large flat, smooth warts
- Colic triggered by damp cold weather or by getting wet
- Moist skin eruption
- Skin conditions with thick yellow or brown crusts
- Mud fever
- Aural plaques

Echinacea

COMMON NAME: Purple coneflower, *Echinacea angustifolia*
CLASSIFICATION: Plant: Asteraceae (Compositae) family
PREPARATION: From tincture of the whole fresh plant

Keynotes

- Infections
- Toxaemia
- Septic conditions, septicaemia
- Gangrene
- Post-partum fever with foul discharge
- Snakebites
- Insect stings
- Ulcerated throat
- General weakness and drowsiness

Modalities

WORSE/AGGRAVATED BY: In the evening
BETTER/AMELIORATED BY: Resting

Remedy Interactions

CONSIDER ALSO: Baptisia, Cenchris contortrix, Arnica, Lachesis, Hepar sulph, Calendula

Principal Equine Indications

- Support for the immune system
- Toxaemia and septicaemia
- Viral and bacterial infections
- Infected wounds
- Skin infections
- Gangrene
- Metritis
- Pyometria
- Insect and snakebites
- Equine ME (post-viral syndrome)
- Cushing's disease (immune system support)

Eel serum, Serum anguillar ichthyotoxin

COMMON NAME: Eel serum
CLASSIFICATION: Animal: Fish
PREPARATION: By dissolving in water/alcohol and subsequent succussion

Keynotes

- Toxic action on the blood
- Urine contains protein
- Haematuria, blood in the urine
- Poor urine output

Modalities

WORSE/AGGRAVATED BY: None listed
BETTER/AMELIORATED BY: None listed

Remedy Interactions – None listed

Principal Equine Indications

- Acute renal (kidney) failure, acute nephritis
- Proteinuria (protein in the urine)

Elaterium, Elat

COMMON NAME: Squirting cucumber, *Ecballium elaterium*
CLASSIFICATION: Plant: Cucurbitaceae family
PREPARATION: From a tincture of the unripe fruit

Keynotes

- Profuse watery diarrhoea that gushes out
- Squirting diarrhoea
- Explosive diarrhoea
- Promotes opening of abscesses

- Drains fluid from waterlogged tissues
- Nodules around joints

Modalities

WORSE/AGGRAVATED BY: Damp weather, standing in damp conditions
BETTER/AMELIORATED BY: None listed

Remedy Interactions

CONSIDER ALSO: Croton tig, Gambogia

Principal Equine Indications

- Explosive, forceful, watery 'squirty' diarrhoea
- Green frothy diarrhoea
- Equine rotavirus infection
- Urticarial skin plaques

Equisetum

COMMON NAME: Scouring Rush, *Equisetum hyemale*
CLASSIFICATION: Plant: Ferns: Equisetaceae family
PREPARATION: From tincture of the fresh chopped and pulped plant

Keynotes

- Main action is on the bladder
- Difficulty urinating
- Leaking of urine, incontinence
- Involuntary urination
- Urge to pass urine with pain at the end of urination
- Pain in the kidneys and lower back (lumbar region)
- Albumen, mucus and sediment in the urine

Modalities

WORSE/AGGRAVATED BY: Right side, movement, touch, pressure
BETTER/AMELIORATED BY: In the afternoon, from resting

Remedy Interactions

WORKS WELL WITH: Silica
CONSIDER ALSO: Cantharis, Hydrangea, Apis, Nux vomica, Sarsaparilla

Principal Equine Indications

- Chronic cystitis
- Nephritis
- Incontinence

Erechthites

COMMON NAME: Fire-weed, *Erechthites hieracifolia*
CLASSIFICATION: Plant: Asteraceae (Compositae) family
PREPARATION: From tincture of the whole fresh plant

Keynotes

- A remedy for haemorrhage from any area especially the lungs
- Epistaxis, nosebleed
- Rapid pulse

Modalities

WORSE/AGGRAVATED BY: None listed
BETTER/AMELIORATED BY: None listed

Remedy Interactions

CONSIDER ALSO: Erigeron, Millefolium, Phosphorus, Ipecac, Ficus

Principal Equine Indications

- EIPH with rapid heart beat and bounding pulse

Erigeron

COMMON NAME: Fleabane, *Erigeron canadense*
CLASSIFICATION: Plant: Asteraceae (Compositae) family
PREPARATION: From tincture of the fresh plant in bloom

Keynotes

- A remedy for haemorrhage and congestion
- Haemorrhage of bright red blood which comes in gushes
- Affinity for the bladder and uterus
- Uterine prolapse

Modalities

WORSE/AGGRAVATED BY: Movement, rainy weather
BETTER/AMELIORATED BY: Rest

Remedy Interactions

CONSIDER ALSO: Ipecac, Arnica Hamamelis, Millefolium, Sabina, Secale, Ustilago

Principal Equine Indications
- Haemorrhages of bright red blood
- Persistent bleeding from the bladder
- Bleeding from the uterus
- Bleeding from the umbilical stump in foals

Eucalyptus globulus

COMMON NAME: Blue gum tree, Fever tree
CLASSIFICATION: Plant: Myrtaceae family
PREPARATION: From a tincture of the fresh leaves

Keynotes
- Acts on catarrhal states
- Viral respiratory infections
- Stuffed up nose
- Chronic catarrh, muco-purulent catarrh
- Asthma-like symptoms
- White thick mucus
- Bronchitis
- Emphysema
- Relapsing fevers
- State of exhaustion and toxaemia
- Sluggish digestion
- Flatulence
- Acute diarrhoea
- Bloody diarrhoea
- Acute nephritis with pus in the urine
- Haematuria (blood in the urine)
- Nodular swellings over the metacarpal and metatarsal joints

Modalities
WORSE/AGGRAVATED BY: None listed
BETTER/AMELIORATED BY: None listed

Remedy Interactions
CONSIDER ALSO: Hydrastis, Kali sulph, Antimonium tartrate

Principal Equine Indications
- Upper and lower respiratory tract infections with much purulent catarrh
- Equine adenovirus or rhinovirus infection
- Acute nephritis (kidney failure)
- Pyelonephritis

Eupatorium perfolatum, Eupat perf

COMMON NAME: Boneset, Thoroughwort
CLASSIFICATION: Plant: Asteracea (Compositae) family
PREPARATION: From tincture of the whole plant

Keynotes
- Key remedy for bone pain including fractures
- Also acts on the digestive tract, liver and upper airways
- Pains in the head and eyes
- Viral respiratory infections
- Chronic cough with loose mucus
- Fever including fever of a recurrent or intermittent nature
- Backache
- Aching in the limbs
- Sore joints
- Inflammation of nodular joint swellings
- Puffy joints
- Greenish diarrhoea

Modalities
WORSE/AGGRAVATED BY: 7–9pm
BETTER/AMELIORATED BY: When stabled

Remedy Interactions
CONSIDER ALSO: Bryonia, Arnica, Chelidonium, Symphytum, Pyrogen, Nat mur, Nux vomica
WORKS WELL WITH: Nat mur, Sepia

Principal Equine Indications
- Equine influenza
- Bone pain
- Epiphysitis
- Sore shins
- Joint pain
- Synovitis
- Windgalls

Euphrasia

COMMON NAME: Eyebright, *Euphrasia officinalis*
CLASSIFICATION: Plant: Scrophulariaceae family
PREPARATION: From a tincture of the whole plant

Keynotes
- Principal action is on the eyes, especially the

conjunctival membranes
- Profuse tear production (lachrymation)
- Catarrhal problems of the eyes and nose
- Acrid tear production
- Eyes constantly water
- Thick discharge which inflames the skin
- Swelling of the lids
- Sticky mucus stuck to the cornea
- Corneal opacity
- Ptosis
- Bland nasal discharge
- Fluent discharge from the nose with coughing

Modalities

WORSE/AGGRAVATED BY: In the evening, when stabled, warmth, light

BETTER/AMELIORATED BY: In the dark

Remedy Interactions

WORKS WELL WITH: Aconite, Calc carb, Lycopodium, Merc sol, Phosphorus, Pulsatilla, Rhus tox, Silica, Sulphur

CONSIDER ALSO: Allium cepa, Arsenicum album, Gelsemium, Sabadilla, Kali bich

Principal Equine Indications

- Conjunctivitis in general
- Catarrhal conjunctivitis
- Corneal ulcers
- Corneal opacities
- Blepharitis
- Iritis
- Watery eyes
- Sticky eyelids
- Rhinitis
- Fly worry (around the eyes)

Fagopyrum

COMMON NAME: Buckwheat, *Fagopyrum esculentum*

CLASSIFICATION: Plant: Polygonaceae family

PREPARATION: From a tincture of the whole mature plant

Keynotes

- Itching of the skin
- Erythema (reddening of the skin)
- Red blotches, swollen areas of skin
- Itching of the eyes and ears
- Itching around the vulva
- Yellow uterine discharge
- Itching of the lower limbs

Modalities

WORSE/AGGRAVATED BY: In the afternoon (3–6pm), in bright sunlight, rubbing or scratching, warmth, riding

BETTER/AMELIORATED BY: Application of cold water, cool air

Remedy Interactions

CONSIDER ALSO: Rhus tox, Bovista, Urtica

Principal Equine Indications

- Sweet itch
- Headshaking
- Non-specific dermatitis and eczema
- Skin allergies
- Photosensitisation

Ferrum metallicum

COMMON NAME: Iron

CLASSIFICATION: Mineral: Metal: Ferrums: Element

PREPARATION: Trituration

Keynotes

- Suited to younger animals
- Anaemia
- Haemorrhage
- Pale mucous membranes
- Weak muscles
- Irritated by slight noises
- Excessive or poor appetite
- Dry dung
- Abortion
- Vaginal or rectal prolapse
- Dry spasmodic cough with difficulty breathing
- Haemorrhage into the lungs

Modalities

WORSE/AGGRAVATED BY: When sweating, vigorous exercise, cold weather, midnight

BETTER/AMELIORATED BY: Gentle, slow riding

Remedy Interactions

WORKS WELL WITH: Alumina, China, Aconite, Arnica, Lycopodium, Merc sol, Phosphorus

Principal Equine Indications

- Anaemia due to bone marrow suppression or iron deficiency
- Haemorrhage of blood that clots readily and which contains dark clots
- EIPH
- Recovery from autoimmune haemolytic anaemia
- Equine ME (post-viral syndrome)
- Equine infectious anaemia
- Marked over-sensitivity to noises
- Vaginal or rectal prolapse

Ferrum phosphoricum, Ferrum phos

COMMON NAME: Iron phosphate
CLASSIFICATION: Mineral: Ferrums
PREPARATION: Trituration

Keynotes

- Important fever remedy especially before catarrh or mucus appears
- Nervous, sensitive animals
- Respiratory problems
- Respiratory infections in young animals
- Anaemia
- Haemorrhage of bright red blood
- Ill effects of overheating by the sun
- Hyperaemia or congestion of blood in the retina
- Epistaxis (nosebleed)
- Inflammation at the back of the throat
- Ulceration of the throat
- Laryngitis
- Early peritonitis
- Incontinence especially when coughing
- Coughing up of blood
- Stiffness in the neck and shoulder region

Modalities

WORSE/AGGRAVATED BY: At night, 4–6am, touching or jarring, moving around, right-hand side
BETTER/AMELIORATED BY: Rest

Remedy Interactions

WORKS WELL WITH: Calc phos, Kali mur, Nat mur
CONSIDER ALSO: Aconite (pulse more forceful, patient restless or fearful), Belladonna (higher fever), Gelsemium (with weakness)

Principal Equine Indications

- Early stages of many fevers or infections
- Early stage of many respiratory infections before any mucus or catarrh appears
- Early stage of any respiratory infections where symptoms appear more slowly compared with Aconite
- Laryngitis, pharyngitis, bronchitis, pneumonia
- Strangles (early on)
- Profuse haemorrhage of bright red blood which clots readily
- Heat stroke
- EIPH

Ficus religiosa

COMMON NAME: Ashwathya
CLASSIFICATION: Plant: Moraceae family
PREPARATION: From tincture of the fresh leaves

Keynotes

- Haemorrhages of various kinds
- Difficulty breathing
- Coughing up of blood
- Warfarin poisoning

Modalities

WORSE/AGGRAVATED BY: None listed
BETTER/AMELIORATED BY: None listed

Remedy Interactions

CONSIDER ALSO: Millefolium, Phosphorus, Erigeron, Ipecac

Principal Equine Indications

- Prevention of EIPH in susceptible horses

Filix mas

COMMON NAME: Male fern, *Dryopteris filix-mas*
CLASSIFICATION: Plant: Filices family
PREPARATION: From tincture of the fresh root

Keynotes

- A remedy for worms

Modalities

WORSE/AGGRAVATED BY: None listed

BETTER/AMELIORATED BY: None listed

Remedy Interactions

CONSIDER ALSO: Cina, Granatum, Kamala

Principal Equine Indications

- Tapeworms and associated symptoms

Fluoricum acidum, Fluor ac, Acid fluor

COMMON NAME: Hydrofluoric acid
CLASSIFICATION: Mineral: Fluorines
PREPARATION: By distilling pure fine powdered fluorspar with sulphuric acid and triturating the powder which is produced

Keynotes

- Acts on the deeper tissues of the body resulting in ulceration and destruction
- Conditions relating to elderly animals
- Distended blood vessels
- Decay of the teeth
- Alopecia
- Chronic nasal catarrh
- Fistulae, including dental fistulae
- Swelling of the scrotum
- Nymphomania
- Inflammation of the fetlock, pastern and coffin joints
- Weak hooves
- Pain under the hooves
- Weakness or necrosis of bone
- Pigmented skin growths
- Abscesses
- Weak capillary vessels and veins

Modalities

WORSE/AGGRAVATED BY: Warmth, morning
BETTER/AMELIORATED BY: Cold, gentle exercise

Remedy Interactions

WORKS WELL WITH: Silica, Sulphur, Nitric acid, Graphites
CONSIDER ALSO: Calc fluor, Calc phos, Nitric acid, Pulsatilla, Sulphuric acidum

Principal Equine Indications

- Brittle, crumbling or weak hooves
- Chronic laminitis
- Pedal osteitis
- Seedy toe
- Buttress foot
- Exostoses
- Weak or necrotic bone especially of the jaw and long bones
- Fistulae: dental, rectal or lachrymal duct especially
- Chronic tooth abscesses
- Chronic sinuses or fistulae
- Weak teeth (poor enamel)
- Arthritis/DJD of fetlock, pastern or coffin joints with bony destruction
- Alopecia (hair loss) especially around the head
- Pigmented, smooth sarcoids
- Melanomas
- Scar tissue

Folliculinum

COMMON NAME: Oestrogen
CLASSIFICATION: Animal: Mammals: Humans: Sarcode
PREPARATION: From human ovarian tissue

Keynotes

- Predominantly a female remedy
- Anxious nature
- Fears being alone
- Confusion
- Changes in mood
- Prone to panic
- Behavioural changes prior to oestrus
- Hormonal imbalances
- Poor sperm counts
- Considered a 'grounding' remedy for mares

Modalities

WORSE/AGGRAVATED BY: Heat, noise, touch, rest
BETTER/AMELIORATED BY: Fresh air

Remedy Interactions

CONSIDER ALSO: Sepia, Pulsatilla, Carcinosin, Lachesis, Apis mel, Staphysagria

Principal Equine Indications

- Infertility problems
- Establishment of regular cycles including after the use of synthetic hormones
- Regulation or balancing of the oestrus cycles (7c)
- Promotion of the oestrus cycle (low potency 4x) where cycles are absent
- Retardation of the cycle (9c) where cycling is too frequent
- Ovarian cysts
- Low sperm count in the stallion
- Equine ME (post-viral syndrome)
- Poor bonding with foal
- Mareish behaviour, nymphomania
- Behavioural issues following severe trauma or abuse

Formica rufa

COMMON NAME: The red ant
CLASSIFICATION: Animal: Insects
PREPARATION: From crushed live ants

Keynotes

- Main action is on joints
- Arthritis and stiffness
- Pains cause restlessness
- Sudden stiffness
- Contracted joints
- Weak hind limbs
- Hip pain
- Chronic nephritis
- Blood and albumen in the urine
- Red burning and itching skin
- Nettle rash
- Lupus
- Polyps

Modalities

WORSE/AGGRAVATED BY: Cold, damp, motion, on right side
BETTER/AMELIORATED BY: Warmth, rubbing, pressure on affected area, being groomed

Remedy Interactions

WORKS WELL WITH: Chamomile
CONSIDER ALSO: Dulcamara, Bryonia, Arsenicum album, Urtica

Principal Equine Indications

- Arthritis/DJD especially where the back legs are involved
- Joint stiffness of sudden onset
- Wandering lameness
- Stiffness causing hind limb weakness
- Skin eruptions with itching
- Area of itching and burning skin
- Sweet itch

Fraxus americana

COMMON NAME: White Ash
CLASSIFICATION: Plant: Oleaceae family
PREPARATION: From a tincture of the bark

Keynotes

- Action focused on the female reproductive system, principally the uterus
- Uterine enlargement
- Prolapse of the uterus
- Watery uterine discharge

Modalities

WORSE/AGGRAVATED BY: None listed
BETTER/AMELIORATED BY: None listed

Remedy Interactions

CONSIDER ALSO: Sepia, Lilium tigrinum, Secale

Principal Equine Indications

- As a uterine tonic especially following prolapse
- Pyometria

Gambogia

COMMON NAME: Gummi gutti
CLASSIFICATION: Plant: Clusiaceae (Guttiferae) family
PREPARATION: From a tincture of the gum

Keynotes

- Acts on the digestive system
- Sudden diarrhoea with forceful evacuation
- Straining after passing diarrhoea
- Watery diarrhoea

Modalities

WORSE/AGGRAVATED BY: Evening, at night

BETTER/AMELIORATED BY: Motion

Remedy Interactions

CONSIDER ALSO: Aloe, Croton tig, Podophyllum

Principal Equine Indications

- Watery, forceful diarrhoea
- Sudden, acute watery diarrhoea preceded by straining
- Equine rotavirus infection

Gelsemium

COMMON NAME: Yellow jasmine, *Gelsemium sempervirens*
CLASSIFICATION: Plant: Loganiaceae family: Polycrest
PREPARATION: From tincture of the root bark

Keynotes

- Main action is on the nervous system
- Paralysis
- Dullness
- Trembling
- Apathy
- Heaviness
- Fear, fright
- Effects of excitement
- Influenza
- Heaviness of the eyelids
- Ptosis
- Pupils insensitive to light
- Deep inflammation of the eye
- Retinal detachment
- Glaucoma
- Twitching of the muscles of the face and eyelids
- Difficulty swallowing
- Paralysis of the muscles of the throat
- Thirstless
- Diarrhoea from excitement or fright
- Partial paralysis of the anal sphincter
- Profuse watery urine
- Partial paralysis of the bladder
- Slow breathing
- Slow pulse in older animals
- Back pain especially lumbar and sacral region
- Neck pain
- Tires easily on even slight exercise
- Trembling of the limbs
- Muscle weakness
- Incoordination, ataxia
- Fever slow onset with shivering

Modalities

WORSE/AGGRAVATED BY: Motion, least exercise, damp weather, fog, before a thunderstorm, excitement or fear, 10am
BETTER/AMELIORATED BY: Open air, cold air, sweating, urinating

Remedy Interactions

WORKS WELL WITH: Argentum Nitricum, Sepia, Apis, Cactus, Caulophyllum, Ipecac
CONSIDER ALSO: Phosphorus, Conium, Curare, Causticum, Belladonna, Ferrum phos, Aconite, Baptisia

Principal Equine Indications

- Fever of slow onset with weakness and shivering
- Fevers with accompanying lethargy or depression
- Anticipatory anxiety, 'nerves'
- Anticipatory diarrhoea or loose dung, diarrhoea from fright, shock, emotional excitement
- Effects of shock, fear or fright
- Equine flu and its consequences
- Viral infections involving the nervous system or with neurological signs
- EHV-1, African horse sickness, Equine protozoal myeloencephalitis
- Fevers with accompanying lethargy or depression
- Post-viral syndrome
- Radial, facial and obdurator paralysis
- Paralysis following illness
- Ptosis
- Sweeny especially where there is partial paralysis of the shoulder muscles
- Roaring, laryngeal hemiplegia
- Weakness or incoordination of the hind limbs, ataxia
- Wobbler syndrome
- Paralysis of the hind limbs
- Paralysis of the bladder
- Trembling of the limbs
- Partial or complete upward fixation of the patella
- Luxation of the patella
- Shaker foal syndrome
- Grass sickness

- Meconium retention
- Headshaking
- Heat stroke

Glonoine, Glonoinum

CONSIDER ALSO: Nitro-glycerine
CLASSIFICATION: Mineral: Organic compounds
PREPARATION: From dilutions in alcohol

Keynotes
- Lethargy
- Confusion
- Congestion of the brain from excess heat or cold, cerebral congestion
- Convulsions
- Meningitis
- Neuralgia of the head and face region
- Seasickness

Modalities
WORSE/AGGRAVATED BY: Heat of the sun or fire, left side
BETTER/AMELIORATED BY: Cool air

Remedy Interactions
WORKS WELL WITH: Belladonna
CONSIDER ALSO: Belladonna, Opium, Stramonium, Lachesis

Principal Equine Indications
- Heat stroke
- Conditions brought on by travelling in a warm confined area
- Effects or conditions caused by travelling by boat
- Headshaking (in excessive heat)

Gossypium

COMMON NAME: Cotton Plant, *Gossypium herbaceum*
CLASSIFICATION: Plant: Malvacea family
PREPARATION: From tincture of the fresh inner root bark

Keynotes
- Disturbed uterine function, disturbed pregnancy
- Abortion
- Irregular oestrus cycles
- Intermittent ovarian pain
- Retained placenta

Modalities
WORSE/AGGRAVATED BY: Motion
BETTER/AMELIORATED BY: Rest

Remedy Interactions
CONSIDER ALSO: Lilium tigrinum, Sabina, Secale, Pulsatilla, Ustilago

Principal Equine Indications
- Irregular oestrus cycles
- Ovarian pain which comes and goes periodically

Granatum

COMMON NAME: Pomegranate, *Punica granatum*
CLASSIFICATION: Plant: Lythraceae (Granateae) family
PREPARATION: From tincture or trituration of the root or bark

Keynotes
- Acts as a vermifuge for expelling tapeworms
- Poor digestion
- Loss of body condition

Modalities
WORSE/AGGRAVATED BY: None listed
BETTER/AMELIORATED BY: None listed

Remedy Interactions
CONSIDER ALSO: Cina, Teucrium marum

Principal Equine Indications
- In combination with other remedies to deter tapeworms

Graphites

(see Constitutional Remedies)

Gratiola

COMMON NAME: Hedge hyssop, *Gratiola officinalis*
CLASSIFICATION: Plant: Scrophulariaceae family
PREPARATION: From tincture of the fresh plant before flowering

Keynotes
- Suited to mares especially
- Nymphomania
- Main action is on the digestive system
- Abdominal distension
- Colic after feeding or at night
- Green watery diarrhoea forcibly expelled

Modalities
WORSE/AGGRAVATED BY: Drinking large amounts of water
BETTER/AMELIORATED BY: None listed

Remedy Interactions
CONSIDER ALSO: Gambogia, Lycopodium, Mag phos, Nux vomica

Principal Equine Indications
- Nymphomania
- Mild colic after drinking excess water
- Equine rotavirus infection

Guaiacum

COMMON NAME: Resin of Lignum Vitae, Gum guaiacum, *Guaiacum officinale*
CLASSIFICATION: Plant: Zygophyllaceae family
PREPARATION: From tincture of the gum resin

Keynotes
- A minor joint remedy
- Additional action on fibrous tissue
- Arthritis and rheumatic symptoms
- Contraction of the limbs
- Joints almost immovable
- Swollen joints with intolerance of pressure and heat
- Stiffness of the neck and shoulder regions
- Bad odour from the body
- Promotes suppuration of abscesses
- Pupils dilated
- Build-up of gas in the intestines

Modalities
WORSE/AGGRAVATED BY: Motion, heat, cold wet weather, pressure, touch, 6pm–4am
BETTER/AMELIORATED BY: None listed

Remedy Interactions
WORKS WELL WITH: Sepia, Merc sol, Sulphur, Causticum, Calc carb
CONSIDER ALSO: Rhus tox, Bryonia, Colocynthis, Rhododendron, Ledum

Principal Equine Indications
- Stiff joints especially where fibrosed
- Joints with a very restricted range of movement
- Stiffness of the shoulder region
- Arthritic joints with contracted muscles or tendons

Gunpowder

COMMON NAME: Black gunpowder
CLASSIFICATION: Mineral: Inorganic compounds: Carbons
PREPARATION: Trituration

Keynotes
- Conditions relating to sepsis
- Abscesses
- Bite wounds
- Infected cuts
- Blood poisoning
- Osteomyelitis

Modalities
WORSE/AGGRAVATED BY: None listed
BETTER/AMELIORATED BY: None listed

Remedy Interactions
WORKS WELL WITH: Hepar sulph, Thuja, Silica

Principal Equine Indications
- Septic skin infections
- Septic wounds
- Suppuration
- Fly strike
- Wounds that refuse to heal
- Prophylactic use in preventing wound infections
- Abscesses
- Osteomyelitis
- Splints where there is secondary infection

Hamamelis

COMMON NAME: Witch-hazel, *Hamamelis virginica*
CLASSIFICATION: Plant: Hamamelidaceae family
PREPARATION: From a tincture of the fresh bark and twigs

Keynotes

- Has an affinity with the venous circulation
- Relaxation of veins and engorgement
- Congestion and passive haemorrhage
- Soreness akin to bruising
- Weakness from blood loss
- Trauma to the eye
- Bloodshot eyes with inflamed blood vessels
- Nosebleed (epistaxis)
- Blood in urine (haematuria)
- Congestion of the ovaries with pain
- Uterine haemorrhage with abdominal soreness
- Orchitis, testicular pain
- Coughing up of blood (haemoptysis)
- Soreness of cervical vertebrae
- Severe lower back pain
- Sore muscles and joints
- Phlebitis (inflammation of veins)
- Traumatic inflammation of tissues
- Mechanical injuries
- Ecchymosis

Modalities

WORSE/AGGRAVATED BY: Warm moist air, exertion, in the open air
BETTER/AMELIORATED BY: None listed

Remedy Interactions

WORKS WELL WITH: Ferrum metallicum, Fluor ac, Arnica
CONSIDER ALSO: Arnica, Bellis, Calendula, Sulphuric acid

Principal Equine Indications

- Slow persistent haemorrhage of dark passive blood
- Haematomas
- Bruising including deep bruising
- Bruising of the sole
- Acute or severe tendon injuries, sprains or ruptures
- Muscle injuries
- Rupture of the peroneus tertius
- Bleeding from the rectum
- The effects of injury on soft tissues especially muscles, trauma
- Eye injuries
- To hasten absorption of intraocular clots
- Phlebitis
- Burns
- Ecchymotic haemorrhages, purpura haemorrhagica
- Muscular soreness
- Azoturia, tying up
- EIPH
- Passive nosebleeds
- Lower back pain
- Orchitis
- Variocele

Hekla lava, Heckla lava, Hecla

COMMON NAME: Volcanic ash from Mount Hecla
CLASSIFICATION: Mineral: Inorganic compounds
PREPARATION: By trituration

Keynotes

- Has an important action on bone
- Exostoses, bone spurs, arthritic nosodities
- Bony nosodities (small hard lumps)
- Weakness of bone
- Necrosis of bone
- Tumours, especially of bone
- Tooth abscesses
- Acts on the bones of the jaw
- Affects the lymphatic glands, especially of the neck

Modalities

WORSE/AGGRAVATED BY: None listed
BETTER/AMELIORATED BY: None listed

Remedy Interactions

CONSIDER ALSO: Silica, Phosphorus, Kali iod, Symphytum, Ruta grav, Mineral

Principal Equine Indications

- Conditions relating to bone in general
- Exostoses
- Bone necrosis and weakness

- Bone tumours, osteosarcoma
- Periostitis
- Osteitis
- Enlarged, hard lymph nodes especially in the cervical region
- Tooth abscess
- Tooth pain, neuralgia
- Chronic gingivitis
- Arthritis
- Splints
- Sore shins
- Osslets
- Sesamoiditis
- Ringbone
- Bone spavin
- Navicular syndrome
- Pedal osteitis
- Sidebone
- Buttress foot

Helleborus

COMMON NAME: Christmas rose, Snow rose, Black hellebore, *Helleborus niger*
CLASSIFICATION: Plant: Ranunculaceae family
PREPARATION: From the juice of the fresh root

Keynotes

- Affects the central nervous system, digestive system and kidneys
- Depression of the senses, indifference, stupor
- Trance-like appearance
- Withdrawn
- Muscular weakness
- Paralysis
- Manic behaviour
- Presses head against a wall
- Eyeballs roll upwards
- Dilated pupils
- Looks vacant
- Bad smell from the mouth
- Grinds teeth
- Salivation
- Distension of the bladder
- Hydrothorax
- Dropsical swelling of the skin
- Angio-neurotic oedema

Modalities

WORSE/AGGRAVATED BY: From evening until morning, 4–8pm, cool air, exertion, motion
BETTER/AMELIORATED BY: Warm air,

Remedy Interactions

WORKS WELL WITH: Zinc, Belladonna, Bryonia, Lycopodium, Nux vom, Pulsatilla, Sulphur
CONSIDER ALSO: Natrum sulph. Arnica, Alumina, Bryonia, Phosphorus

Principal Equine Indications

- Effects of concussion
- Brain damage
- Epilepsy
- Meningitis
- Ascites (dropsy)
- Hydrothorax (fluid in the chest)
- Neonatal maladjustment syndrome (NMS)
- Dementia
- Slow recovery after anaesthesia
- Viral infections with neurological symptoms

Helonias

COMMON NAME: Unicorn root, *Helonias dioica*
CLASSIFICATION: Plant: Melanthaceae family
PREPARATION: From tincture of the root

Keynotes

- Affects the lumbo-sacral area
- Uterine prolapse, especially after abortion
- Abortion
- Pain in the lower lumbar region
- Congestion of the kidneys
- Pain over the kidney region
- Diabetes mellitus and insipidus
- Sadness
- Better working
- Seasons too frequent
- Swelling of the udder with pain and tenderness
- Uterine discharge
- Itching of the vulval region
- Albumen in the urine

Modalities

WORSE/AGGRAVATED BY: Motion, touch
BETTER/AMELIORATED BY: Working, riding

Remedy Interactions

CONSIDER ALSO: Lilium tigrinum, Sepia, Murex, Sepia

Principal Equine Indications

- Lumbo-sacral pain
- Pain over the kidney area
- Diabetes mellitus
- Diabetes insipidus
- Uterine prolapse
- Abnormalities of the oestrus cycle
- Infertility
- Abortion (prevention) and subsequent problems such as exhaustion
- Pain in the udder

Hepar sulph

COMMON NAME: Calcium sulphide, Hepar sulph, Calcareum
CLASSIFICATION: Mineral: Calcareas: Polycrest
PREPARATION: Trituration of the ash prepared from burning the white interior of oyster shells with pure flowers of Sulphur

Keynotes

- Suppuration (infection) aborted by high potencies, promoted by low potencies
- Great sensitivity to least touch
- Least touch is painful
- Low pain threshold
- Catarrhal and purulent inflammation of mucous membranes
- Pus formation
- Irritability
- Sad and dejected
- Oversensitivity
- Feels the cold easily
- Corneal ulcers
- Iritis with pus in the anterior chamber
- Chemosis (swelling of the eyelids)
- Profuse ocular discharge
- Red and inflamed lids and eyes
- Ulcerated nose with catarrhal discharge
- Sneezing
- Pain in the throat with suppuration
- Liver abscess
- Weakness of the bladder, urine expelled slowly
- Moist eruptions near scrotum and inner side of leg
- Bloody uterine discharge
- Foul uterine discharge
- Dry, hoarse cough
- Rattling cough, choking
- Wheezing
- Skin eruptions, unhealthy skin
- Offensive smell from the skin
- Skin abscesses
- Suppurating skin eruptions
- Angio-neurotic oedema
- Cracks on the skin of the lower limbs
- Recurrent or chronic urticaria
- Sweats easily

Modalities

WORSE/AGGRAVATED BY: Touch, dry, cold winds, cool air, least draught, lying on painful side
BETTER/AMELIORATED BY: Damp weather, warmth, after feeding

Remedy Interactions

WORKS WELL WITH: Calendula, Aconite, Arnica, Belladonna, Lachesis, Mercury, Nitric acid, Silica, Iodum
CONSIDER ALSO: Graphites, Merc sol, Mezerium, Nitric acid, Nux vomica, Psorinum, Silica

Principal Equine Indications

- Purulent conditions with great sensitivity to touch
- Suppurative conditions including suppurating wounds
- Abscesses including internal abscesses and tooth abscesses
- Sinuses and fistulae
- Purulent conjunctivitis with sensitivity to light
- Iritis with pus formation in the anterior chamber of the eye
- Catarrhal pneumonia
- Sinusitis
- Guttural pouch empyema
- Liver abscesses
- Painful skin abscesses
- Foot abscesses, nail prick
- Skin infections, bacterial folliculitis, cellulitis
- Mud fever
- Fly strike
- Mastitis
- Sweet itch

- Urticaria
- Chronic angioneurotic oedema
- Bursitis
- Septic arthritis
- White line disease
- Thrush, canker, quitter, seedy toe, gravel
- Ulcerative lymphangitis
- Myositis (with pus)
- Lymphadenitis
- Pyelonephritis
- Pyometria
- Coital exanthema
- Navel ill
- Tyzzer's disease
- Strangles

Hippomanes

COMMON NAME: Meconium deposit from the amniotic fluid of a colt
CLASSIFICATION: Animal: Mammals: Sarcode
PREPARATION: Trituration

Keynotes
- Sudden pain in the knee (carpal) joint
- Weakness of the fetlock, pastern and coffin joints
- Involuntary movements of the lower limbs

Modalities
WORSE/AGGRAVATED BY: None listed
BETTER/AMELIORATED BY: None listed

Remedy Interactions
CONSIDER ALSO: Causticum

Principal Equine Indications
- Pain and stiffness in the knee (carpal) joint
- General weakness of the lower limbs

Hippozaenium, Ozeana

COMMON NAME: Mallein, Glanderin, Farcine, Glanders nosode
CLASSIFICATION: Animal: Mammal: Nosode
PREPARATION: Trituration of milk sugar saturated with the organism

Keynotes
- Abscesses
- Pustules
- Catarrhal conditions
- Glutinous or shiny discharges
- Foul nasal discharge
- Ulceration of the sinuses
- Asthma
- Bronchitis in old horses
- Cough with difficulty breathing
- Excessive mucus leading to difficult breathing
- Lymphatic swellings
- Nodules in the skin

Modalities
WORSE/AGGRAVATED BY: None listed
BETTER/AMELIORATED BY: None listed

Remedy Interactions
CONSIDER ALSO: Bacillinum, Kali bich

Principal Equine Indications
- Mud fever
- Foul smelling catarrh
- Guttural pouch empyema
- Chronic chest problems in elderly horses
- Glanders

Histamine

COMMON NAME: Histamine hydrochloride
CLASSIFICATION: Animal: Sarcode
PREPARATION: From histamine bi-chlorhydrate

Keynotes
- Allergy based problems
- Allergic reactions to vaccines
- Red itching spots on the skin
- Irritable nature, impatient
- Itching in the nose, throat, ears, vagina

Modalities
WORSE/AGGRAVATED BY: Movement, heat
BETTER/AMELIORATED BY: Draft of cold air

Remedy Interactions
CONSIDER ALSO: Apis mel, Arsenicum album

Principal Equine Indications
- Urticaria
- Sweet itch
- Itchy skin, skin allergies
- Allergic conjunctivitis
- Headshaking, especially in horses with an irritable nature
- Equine nodular skin disease

Hydrangea

COMMON NAME: *Hydrangea arborescens*, Seven barks
CLASSIFICATION: Plant: Hydrangeaceae family
PREPARATION: From a tincture of the fresh leaves and young shoots

Keynotes
- Influences the urinary system
- Special action on the bladder
- Gravel in the urine
- Inflammation of the urethra
- Frequent desire to pass urine
- Mucus in the urine
- Increased thirst

Modalities
WORSE/AGGRAVATED BY: None listed
BETTER/AMELIORATED BY: None listed

Remedy Interactions
CONSIDER ALSO: Lycopodium, Berberis, Chimaphilia, Urtica

Principal Equine Indications
- Urolithiasis (bladder stones, urinary calculi, gravel)
- Urinary incontinence
- Dribbling of urine
- Diabetes insipidus

Hydrastis

COMMON NAME: Golden seal, *Hydrastis canadensis*
CLASSIFICATION: Plant: Ranunculaceae family
PREPARATION: From tincture of the fresh root

Keynotes
- Acts on mucous membranes
- A remedy for thick, ropy yellow catarrh
- Acts especially in older animals particularly if debilitated
- Weak muscles and powers of digestion
- Emaciation
- Acts on the liver
- Jaundice
- Cancers especially where pain is involved
- Sinusitis
- Thick infected nasal discharge
- Watery nasal discharges that make the nostrils sore
- Yellow thick mucus in the throat region
- Dry harsh cough
- Bronchial catarrh with thick yellow mucus
- Lower lumbar back pain
- Purulent (infected) discharge from the womb
- Constipation
- Unhealthy skin

Modalities
WORSE/AGGRAVATED BY: At night, harsh dry wind, outside
BETTER/AMELIORATED BY: Resting

Remedy Interactions
CONSIDER ALSO: Pulsatilla, Kali bich, Kali sulph, Antimonium crudum, Merc sol

Principal Equine Indications
- Yellow thick catarrh
- Sinusitis
- Rhinitis
- Chronic bronchitis in elderly horses
- Weak digestion with debility
- Stomach ulcers
- Jaundice
- Endometritis
- Pyometria
- Strangles
- CEM

Hydrocyanicum acidum

COMMON NAME: Prussic acid, Hydrocyanic acid
CLASSIFICATION: Mineral
PREPARATION: From the pure acid in 2% aqueous solution

Keynotes
- Epilepsy and convulsions
- Jaws clenched in spasm
- Salivation, frothing at the mouth
- Collapse with respiratory failure
- Venous congestion of the lungs
- Cyanosis
- Paralysis
- Constriction of the larynx, feels suffocated
- Asthma
- Colic

Modalities
WORSE/AGGRAVATED BY: None listed
BETTER/AMELIORATED BY: None listed

Remedy Interactions – None listed

Principal Equine Indications
- Later stages of colic where the horse is collapsed
- Respiratory failure with cyanosis or frothing at the mouth
- Tetanus
- Epilepsy
- Poisoining (symptomatic treatment)

Hydrophobinum

(see Lyssin)

Hyoscyamus

COMMON NAME: Henbane, *Hyoscyamus niger*
CLASSIFICATION: Plant: Solanaceae family
PREPARATION: From tincture of the fresh plant

Keynotes
- Acts on the nervous system profoundly
- Signs of excitement and mania
- Agitation
- Quarrelsome nature
- Noisy whinnying
- Jealousy
- Suspicious
- Nymphomania
- Muscular twitching, chorea
- Spasms
- Cramps
- Stupor
- Epilepsy
- Meningitis
- Dilated pupils
- Strabismus
- Colic with abdominal distension
- Paralysis of the bladder
- Involuntary urination

Modalities
WORSE/AGGRAVATED BY: At night, during oestrus, after eating, lying down, touch, cold and cold air
BETTER/AMELIORATED BY: Warmth

Remedy Interactions
WORKS WELL WITH: Belladonna, Pulsatilla, Stramonium, Phosphorus, Nux vomica, Opium, Rhus tox
CONSIDER ALSO: Stramonium, Belladonna, Agaricus, Gelsemium, Mag phos

Principal Equine Indications
- Flatulent colic
- Convulsions, epilepsy
- Muscle spasms
- Viral infections characterized by neurological symptoms
- Equine protozoal myeloencephalitis
- Meningitis
- Jealousy
- Aggression
- Suspicious nature
- Mareish behaviour with marked aggression
- Nymphomania
- Neonatal maladjustment syndrome
- Headshaking
- Stringhalt
- Tetanus

Hypericum

COMMON NAME: St John's wort, *Hypericum perforatum*
CLASSIFICATION: Plant: Clusiaceae (Guttiferae) family
PREPARATION: From the whole fresh plant

Keynotes
- Important remedy for nerves
- Nerve injury especially to lower limbs and tail
- Damage to nerve endings

- Neuritis
- Excessive pain
- Helps relieve pain
- Puncture wounds
- Spasms following injury
- Jerking and twitching of muscles
- Muscle cramps
- Spinal injury or spinal concussion especially the coccygeal region
- Concussion
- Pain around the pelvic region
- Tetanus
- Asthma/COPD
- Effects of shock
- Tooth pain
- Lacerated wounds

Modalities

WORSE/AGGRAVATED BY: Cold air and damp fog, touch
BETTER/AMELIORATED BY: Bending of the head backwards

Remedy Interactions

CONSIDER ALSO: Aconite, Arnica, Bellis, Chamomilla, Staphysagria, Calendula, Ledum, Ruta, Rhus tox, Bellis

Principal Equine Indications

- Nerve and spinal injuries in general
- Nerve paralysis resulting from trauma
- Neuritis
- Post-operative pain including after dental work
- Tooth pain
- Pain following injury and fractures
- Lacerated wounds, excoriation of the skin
- Incised wounds
- Bite wounds, insect bites
- Photosensitisation
- Puncture wounds
- Nail prick
- Bruising of the sole (where lame)
- Laminitis
- Trauma
- Effects of fright or shock
- Eye injuries
- Concussion and its consequences including epilepsy
- Corneal laceration
- Cauda equina neuritis
- Tetanus and tetanus prevention (in combination with Ledum)
- Paralysis including spastic paralysis
- Lumbo-sacral pain and sensitivity
- COPD which is much worse in foggy weather

Ichthyolum

COMMON NAME: Ammonium ichthyol sulphonate, fossil fish deposits
CLASSIFICATION: Animal: Fish
PREPARATION: From a viscid liquid in solution obtained from fossilised fish remains

Keynotes

- Acts on the skin and mucous membranes
- Coughs in older animals
- Chronic stiffness
- Hives
- Itchy skin
- Scaly dermatitis

Modalities

WORSE/AGGRAVATED BY: None listed
BETTER/AMELIORATED BY: None listed

Remedy Interactions

CONSIDER ALSO: Petroleum, Sulphur

Principal Equine Indications

- Chronic urticaria
- Dermatitis
- Scaly, itchy skin especially where lice are involved
- Bronchitis in elderly horses

Ignatia

COMMON NAME: St Ignatius bean, *Ignatia amara*
CLASSIFICATION: Plant: Loganiaceae family: Polycrest
PREPARATION: From trituration of the seeds

Keynotes

- Important emotional remedy
- Predominantly (but not exclusively) female
- Heightened sensitivity of all the senses, over sensitive

- Hysteria
- Nervous disposition
- Easily excited
- Apprehension
- Effects of grief, worry and shock
- Variable mood
- Lack of emotion
- Sadness
- Silent brooding
- Clonic spasms, cramps
- Twitching of the muscles of the face and limbs
- Jerking of the limbs, chorea, tremors
- Inflammation of the tonsils
- Craves indigestible items
- Rumbling noises in the abdomen
- Colic
- Prolapse of the rectum
- Dung passed with difficulty
- Diarrhoea from fright
- Itching of the skin
- Excoriation of the skin around the mouth and vagina

Modalities

WORSE/AGGRAVATED BY: Morning, open air, after feeding
BETTER/AMELIORATED BY: Changing position, while feeding

Remedy Interactions

WORKS WELL WITH: Nat mur (chronic), Arsenicum album, Belladonna, Calc carb, Lycopodium, Pulsatilla, Rhus tox, Sepia, Zinc
INCOMPATIBLE WITH: Nux vomica, Tabacum, Coffea
CONSIDER ALSO: Kali phos, Sepia, Zinc

Principal Equine Indications

- Grief, especially acute grief
- Separation of foal and mare
- Pining
- Sadness
- Homesickness
- Hysterical behaviour
- Failure to accept the stallion (due to hysteria-like behaviour)
- Mood changes in mares
- Jealousy
- Jerking and spasms of limbs
- Epilepsy
- Stringhalt
- Mild colic following emotional shock
- Stereotypic behaviour or stable vices

Iodum

COMMON NAME: Iodine
CLASSIFICATION: Mineral: Iodines: Element
PREPARATION: From tincture

Keynotes

- Principally affects the metabolism
- Increased (rapid) metabolism
- Hyperthyroidism
- Hypothyroidism
- Marked intolerance of heat
- Loss of weight despite a good appetite
- Hungry and thirsty
- Eats all the time
- Anxious to eat
- Debility
- Emaciation, thin and underweight
- Acts on glands, the respiratory system, connective tissue and circulation
- Atrophy, wasting, withering
- Oedema
- Ecchymosis
- Haemorrhage
- Pneumonia with dry cough
- Pleural effusion
- Myocarditis
- Rapid heart rate
- Anxiety and restlessness
- Needs to be occupied
- Hurried
- Dilated pupils
- Salivation
- Pancreatic disease
- Testicular atrophy
- Irregular oestrus cycles
- Ovarian pain
- Inflamed painful joints
- Joint pain worse at night
- Hard lumps in the skin

Modalities

WORSE/AGGRAVATED BY: In warm enclosed areas, when

quiet, right side, damp or wet weather
BETTER/AMELIORATED BY: When ridden, in the open air

Remedy Interactions

WORKS WELL WITH: Lycopodium, Silica, Phosphorus, Calc carb, Calc phos, Merc sol, Pulsatilla
CONSIDER ALSO: Tuberculinum, Abrotanum, Nat mur, Phosphorus, Spongia, Fluor ac

Principal Equine Indications

- Overactive horses with a fiery nature
- Sudden unexplainable impulsive behavioral episodes
- Animals which are unable to focus their attention
- Stereotypic behaviour (needs to be occupied)
- General debility and wasting especially with a good appetite or diarrhoea
- Diarrhoea due to malabsorrption
- Muscle atrophy
- Hardened, indurated glands (lymph nodes)
- Shrinking of the udder – atrophy
- Ovarian dysfunction
- Testicular atrophy, degeneration
- Hydrocele
- Skin nodules – equine collagen necrosis/nodular skin disease
- Withered skin with seborrhoea
- Poor coat quality, dry listless hair
- Pancreatic disease and diabetes

Ipecacuanha

COMMON NAME: Ipecac root
CLASSIFICATION: Plant: Rubiaceae family
PREPARATION: From trituration of the dried root

Keynotes

- Irritates the chest and stomach
- Nausea and vomiting
- Haemorrhage of bright red blood, which appears in gushes
- Dysenteric diarrhoea with straining
- Frothy green dung
- Uterine haemorrhage
- Difficulty breathing
- Chest constricted – asthma
- Repeated sneezing
- Violent cough
- Chest full of mucus not relieved by coughing
- Bubbling noises in the chest
- Suffocative cough
- Bleeding from the lungs, haemoptysis
- Body stretched out stiff

Modalities

WORSE/AGGRAVATED BY: Periodically, moist warm air, lying down, touch, winter, moving around
BETTER/AMELIORATED BY: Rest, in the open air

Remedy Interactions

WORKS WELL WITH: Arsenicum album, Bryonia, Cuprum, Ignatia, Phosphorus, Antimonium tartrate, Nux vomica, Sepia, Pulsatilla, China
CONSIDER ALSO: Antimonium tartrate, Kali sulph, Lobelia, Tabacum, Sanguinaria

Principal Equine Indications

- Bronchitis, bronchopneumonia
- Pneumonia
- Emphysema
- COPD, RAO
- Difficulty breathing as if suffocating
- EIPH, epistaxis, nosebleed
- Haemorrhage of bright red blood that appears in sudden spurts
- Uterine haemorrhage
- Vaginal bleeding between oestrus periods
- Slimy green diarrhoea
- Watery diarrhoea containing shreds of bowel lining
- Coccidiosis

Iris versicolor

COMMON NAME: Blue flag
CLASSIFICATION: Plant: Iridaceae family
PREPARATION: From tincture of the fresh root collected in the spring

Keynotes

- Acts on the glands
- Thyroid, salivary glands, pancreas, mucous membranes of the gastrointestinal tract
- Increased salivation
- Poor appetite
- Tenderness over the liver region

- Flatulent colic
- Watery diarrhoea
- Constipation
- Irregular patches of eczema with scaling

Modalities

WORSE/AGGRAVATED BY: Evening, at night, from resting
BETTER/AMELIORATED BY: Motion

Remedy Interactions

CONSIDER ALSO: Ipecac, Podophyllum, Colchicum, Arsenicum album

Principal Equine Indications

- Pancreatic disease
- Diabetes mellitus
- Watery diarrhoea with abdominal pain
- To stimulate appetite after episodes of colic

Jatropha

COMMON NAME: Purging nut, Physic nut, *Jatropha curcas*
CLASSIFICATION: Plant: Euphorbiaceae family
PREPARATION: From tincture or trituration of the seeds

Keynotes

- A diarrhoea remedy
- Sudden 'urgent' diarrhoea
- Very watery profuse forceful diarrhoea
- Distended abdomen with gurgling noises (borborygmi)
- Muscle cramping
- Body chilled and feels cold

Modalities

WORSE/AGGRAVATED BY: In the morning, walking around
BETTER/AMELIORATED BY: None listed

Remedy Interactions

CONSIDER ALSO: Camphora, Veratrum album, Gambogia, Crot tig, Aloe

Principal Equine Indications

- Acute, profuse watery diarrhoea in foals
- Muscle cramps arising from diarrhoea
- Equine rotavirus infection

Juglans cinerea

COMMON NAME: Butternut
CLASSIFICATION: Plant: Juglandaceae family
PREPARATION: Trituration of the resin

Keynotes

- Eczema and dermatitis of the lower limbs and sacral region with irritation

Modalities

WORSE/AGGRAVATED BY: Becoming over heated
BETTER/AMELIORATED BY: None listed

Remedy Interactions

CONSIDER ALSO: Juglans regia

Principal Equine Indications

- Eczema and dermatitis of the lower limbs and sacral region with irritation

Juglans regia

COMMON NAME: Walnut
CLASSIFICATION: Plant: Juglandaceae family
PREPARATION: From a tincture of the leaves and rind of green fruit

Keynotes

- Eczema and dermatitis of the face
- Itching around the face, pustules

Modalities

WORSE/AGGRAVATED BY: None listed
BETTER/AMELIORATED BY: None listed

Remedy Interactions

CONSIDER ALSO: Rhus tox, Graphites, Juglans cinerea

Principal Equine Indications

- Eczema and dermatitis around the facial area

Kali arsenicum

COMMON NAME: Fowler's solution, Potassium arsenate
CLASSIFICATION: Mineral: Kali salt
PREPARATION: From arsenious acid and potassium carbonate

Keynotes

- Important minor skin remedy
- Intolerable itching
- Dry, scaly, poor-looking skin
- Flaking
- Chronic skin irritation
- Fissures and cracks in the skin in the joint flexures
- Skin cancer
- Malignant cancers
- Nodules under the skin

Modalities

WORSE/AGGRAVATED BY: Markedly from warmth
BETTER/AMELIORATED BY: Cooler weather

Remedy Interactions

CONSIDER ALSO: Arsenicum album

Principal Equine Indications

- Sweet itch (especially in combination with Sulph iod)
- Cracked and fissured skin
- Poor-looking withered skin in debilitated horses
- Sarcoids
- Equine nodular skin disease

Kali bich

COMMON NAME: Potassium bichromate, Bichromate of Potash
CLASSIFICATION: Mineral: Kali salt
PREPARATION: From a solution in distilled water

Keynotes

- Has a special affinity with mucous membranes
- Action especially focused on the respiratory and gastro-intestinal tracts
- Acts also on bone and fibrous tissue
- Liver cirrhosis
- General weakness
- Catarrh especially of the airways: nose, pharynx, larynx and bronchi
- Stringy, tough, thick, greenish, yellow catarrh
- Foul smell from the nose
- Perforation of the nasal septum
- Nose blocked
- Violent sneezing
- Coughing, expectoration of thick yellow mucus
- Swollen eyelids with a ropy yellow discharge
- Corneal ulcers with little or no pain or photophobia
- Iritis
- Bones around the head sensitive
- Throat red and inflamed
- Swollen parotid glands
- Ulceration of the stomach or intestines
- Diarrhoea with blood and straining
- Burning in the urethra
- Mucus in the urine
- Kidney congestion, nephritis
- Pyelitis, urine contains pus and blood
- Ulcers on the penis
- Yellow thick uterine discharge
- Wandering bone pains
- Pain, swelling, cracking and stiffness
- Swelling and pain in the achilles tendon
- Punched-out ulcers on the skin

Modalities

WORSE/AGGRAVATED BY: Touch, at rest, hot weather
BETTER/AMELIORATED BY: Open air, warmth, moving the affected part

Remedy Interactions

WORKS WELL WITH: Antimonium tartrate, Arsenicum album, Phosphorus, Psorinum, Sepia
INCOMPATIBLE WITH: Calc carb
CONSIDER ALSO: Hydrastis, Pulsatilla, Antimonum tartrate, Ipecac, Silica, Hippozaenium

Principal Equine Indications

- Respiratory conditions characterised by catarrh
- Rhinitis
- Sinusitis and sinus empyema
- Guttural pouch empyema
- Broncho-pneumonia
- Pneumonia
- Barking type cough with production of thick yellow stringy mucus
- Conjunctivitis with swelling of the lids and a thick yellow discharge
- Deep corneal ulceration with minimal pain, absence of photophobia (sensitivity to light)

- Iritis
- Keratitis
- Deep skin ulcers
- Stomach ulcers
- Lymphangitis
- Cellulitis
- Mud fever
- Bone pain and exostoses
- Thick yellow urethral discharges
- Strangles
- CEM

Kali bromatum, Kali brom

COMMON NAME: Potassium bromide, Bromide of Potash
CLASSIFICATION: Mineral: Kali salt
PREPARATION: By trituration

Keynotes

- Loss of mental ability
- Poor memory
- Dullness, somnolence
- Restlessness, delirium
- Psoriasis-like skin lesions
- Convulsions, epilepsy, especially with a new moon
- Green watery diarrhoea
- Impotence
- Heightened sexual urges
- Cystic ovarian tumours
- Pustules on the face
- Poor coordination

Modalities

WORSE/AGGRAVATED BY: At night, 2am, hot weather, summer, new moon
BETTER/AMELIORATED BY: None listed

Remedy Interactions

CONSIDER ALSO: Hyoscyamus, Stramonium, Zinc, Tarentula hisp, Kali carb, Conium, Opium

Principal Equine Indications

- Poor libido, impotency
- Nymphomania
- Hypersexuality in the stallion (satyriasis)
- Sleepy foal disease
- Bacterial folliculitis
- Skin cysts
- Restlessness due to worry
- Green watery diarrhoea

Kali carb

COMMON NAME: Potassium carbonate
CLASSIFICATION: Mineral: Kali salt: Polycrest
PREPARATION: From a solution in distilled water

Keynotes

- Generalised weakness
- Intolerance of cold weather
- Obese animals
- Abortion
- Foaling
- Back pain and weakness
- Muscle twitching
- Irritable nature
- Changeable mood
- Stubborn nature
- Swelling of the upper eyelids
- Thick, fluent yellow nasal discharge
- Crusted mucus around the nostrils, ulceration of the nostrils
- Flatulence
- Jaundice
- Abdominal distension, ascites
- Prolapse of the rectum
- Involuntary urination during coughing
- Conditions arising after foaling
- Hard dry cough, bronchitis, little expectoration
- Hydrothorax
- Weak back legs
- Heaviness in the back legs
- Pain in the stifle or hip joints
- Pains in the carpal (knee) joint
- Sensitivity of the sole of the hoof
- Dry skin with falling out of hair

Modalities

WORSE/AGGRAVATED BY: After mating, cold weather, 3am
BETTER/AMELIORATED BY: Warm weather, moving around, during the day

Remedy Interactions

WORKS WELL WITH: Carbo veg, Nux vomica, Phosphorus, Sepia, Nitric acid, Nat mur, Fluoric acid, Arsenicum album, Arsenicum iodatum, Lycopodium, Sulphur

CONSIDER ALSO: Causticum, Kali bich, Sepia, Apis, Phos ac

Principal Equine Indications

- To assist recovery from a state of general weakness
- In general conditions arising after foaling, especially weakness
- Abortion (prevention)
- Infertility in the mare
- Lower back pain with irritability and uneven gait
- Heaviness or weakness of the hind limbs
- Vague hip or stifle pain leading to uneven gait
- DJD of the stifle where exostoses are present
- Laminitis
- Hypothyroidism
- Ascites
- Hydrothorax
- Hard dry rattling cough
- Acute bronchopneumonia in young foals

Kali chlor

COMMON NAME: Potassium chlorate
CLASSIFICATION: Mineral: Kali salt
PREPARATION: From a solution in distilled water

Keynotes

- Has a destructive effect on the kidneys
- Nephritis
- Haematuria (blood in the urine)
- Stomatitis, ulceration within the mouth
- Salivation
- Facial paralysis
- Twitching of the muscles of the face and eyes
- Diarrhoea with greenish coloured mucus
- Jaundice

Modalities

WORSE/AGGRAVATED BY: None listed
BETTER/AMELIORATED BY: None listed

Remedy Interactions

CONSIDER ALSO: Kali mur, Kali bich, Causticum

Principal Equine Indications

- Acute and chronic kidney disease
- Facial paralysis
- Ulceration within the mouth with salivation
- Stomatitis
- Horse pox virus
- Vesicular stomatitis virus

Kali iod, Kali hydriodicum

COMMON NAME: Potassium iodide, Iodide of potassium
CLASSIFICATION: Mineral: Kali salt
PREPARATION: From a solution in distilled water

Keynotes

- Acts on fibrous tissue
- Swollen glands
- Purpura
- Watery, irritating (acrid) discharge from the eyes
- Lachrymation
- Red injected inflamed conjunctival membranes
- Iritis
- Keratitis with chemosis (watery swelling of the lids)
- Thin watery discharge from the nose
- Sneezing
- Hard (bony) lumps around the head and eyes
- Facial neuralgia (pain)
- Pulmonary oedema
- Greenish expectoration
- Pneumonia (with hepatisation)
- Meningitis
- Hydrothorax
- Bone pains
- Thickening of the periosteum
- Joint contraction and stiffness
- Fluid effusion into the stifle joints
- Purple spots on the legs
- Nodules on the skin with oedematous swellings

Modalities

WORSE/AGGRAVATED BY: In a warm stable, at night
BETTER/AMELIORATED BY: Open air, moving around

Remedy Interactions

WORKS WELL WITH: Nitric acid, Merc sol
CONSIDER ALSO: Iodum, Kali carb

Principal Equine Indications

- Bony masses around the area of the head and eyes
- Bony tumours
- Severe bone pain
- Joint pain especially where the periosteum is thickened
- Contracted joints
- DJD of the knee joint
- Sore shins
- Bone spavin
- Iritis, periodic ophthalmia
- Keratitis with marked opacity of the cornea
- Pneumonia with pulmonary oedema
- Fluid in the pleural cavity
- Respiratory infections with an irritating watery nasal discharge
- Swollen lymph nodes
- Arteritis
- Testicular degeneration
- Equine nodular skin disease
- EHV-1 (conjunctivitis)
- EVA
- Horse pox virus
- Equine viral papular dermatitis
- Epizootic lymphangitis

Kali mur, Kali muriaticum

COMMON NAME: Potassium chloride
CLASSIFICATION: Mineral: Kali salt
PREPARATION: From a solution in distilled water

Keynotes

- Action is mainly focused on catarrhal problems
- Coughs up thick, sticky white mucus
- Spasmodic coughing
- Rattling mucus in the bronchi
- Catarrh in the Eustachian tubes
- Greyish white secretions on mucous membranes
- Swollen glands
- Tonsillitis
- Corneal opacity
- Bloody diarrhoea with slimy mucus
- Dry white flaky scales on the skin
- Fibrinous exudation
- Tissue salt

Modalities

WORSE/AGGRAVATED BY: Motion
BETTER/AMELIORATED BY: None listed

Remedy Interactions

WORKS WELL WITH: Calc phos, Calc fluor, Calc sulph, Ferrum phos
CONSIDER ALSO: Kali chlor, Kali bich, Kali carb, Hydrastis, Pulsatilla, Bryonia

Principal Equine Indications

- Chronic catarrhal problems
- Coughing up of white sticky mucus
- Swollen lymph nodes associated with catarrhal conditions
- Catarrh of the guttural pouch or sinuses
- Guttural pouch empyema or tympany
- Corneal opacity (clouding)
- Persistent swelling of surgical incisions
- Excessive panting

Kali phosphoricum, Kali phos

COMMON NAME: Potassium phosphate
CLASSIFICATION: Mineral: Kali salt
PREPARATION: From a solution in distilled water

Keynotes

- Better suited to younger animals
- A remedy for nerves
- Prostration, weakness
- Anxiety
- Starts easily
- Irritability
- Shyness
- Affects (disturbs) the sympathetic nervous system
- Mental and physical depression
- Drooping of the eyelids
- Paralysis of the vocal cords
- Foul putrid diarrhoea especially after stress
- Dysenteric-like diarrhoea
- Urinary incontinence
- Delayed foaling (weak uterine contractions)
- Asthma

- Cough with yellow mucus
- Shortness of breath
- Gangrene

Modalities

WORSE/AGGRAVATED BY: Worrying, excitement, mental and physical effort, cold weather, early morning
BETTER/AMELIORATED BY: Warmth, resting, feeding

Remedy Interactions

CONSIDER ALSO: Phosphorus, Phos ac, other Potassium (Kali) salts

Principal Equine Indications

- Recovery from states of generalised weakness
- Debility
- Exhaustion during foaling
- COPD with coughing up of yellow mucus
- Conditions arising from prolonged emotional stress
- Nervous exhaustion
- Paralysis of the vocal cords

Kali sulphuricum, Kali sulph

COMMON NAME: Potassium sulphate
CLASSIFICATION: Mineral: Kali salt
PREPARATION: Trituration

Keynotes

- Influences the later stages of inflammation
- Yellow mucus and watery discharges
- Cough with yellow slimy catarrh
- Nose obstructed
- Inflammation of the nasal passages
- Rattling mucus in the chest
- Bronchitis
- Profuse scaling (dandruff) of the skin
- Scurfy skin
- Papules
- Seborrhoea
- Nettle rash
- Ringworm
- Slimy yellow preputial discharge
- Orchitis

Modalities

WORSE/AGGRAVATED BY: Evening, hot atmosphere
BETTER/AMELIORATED BY: Cool air, open air

Remedy Interactions

WORKS WELL WITH: Calc sulph, Calc carb, Hepar sulph, Pulsatilla, Rhus tox, Sepia, Silica, Sulphur
CONSIDER ALSO: Pulsatilla, Kali bich, Hydrastis, Calc sulph

Principal Equine Indications

- Broncho-pneumonia
- Bronchitis
- Expectoration of slimy yellow catarrh
- Nasal obstruction caused by yellow mucus
- Seborrhoea (greasy skin)
- Skin conditions accompanied by seborrhoea and scaling, dandruff
- Itchy skin rashes with scaling
- Sweet itch with thick scurfy area or scaling and greasy skin, seborrhoea
- Ringworm

Kalmia laterifolia, Kalmia

COMMON NAME: Mountain laurel, American laurel
CLASSIFICATION: Plant: Ericaceae family
PREPARATION: From tincture of the fresh leaves when the plant is in flower

Keynotes

- Check for a slow, weak pulse together with a stiff, stilted gait. The shoulder region may be especially stiff and pain in the lower back may also be apparent
- Has an important action on the heart
- Weak, slow pulse
- Tachycardia
- Palpitation with fibrillation
- Shortness of breath
- Rheumatic symptoms, stiffness
- Red, hot swollen joints
- Wandering pains in the limbs
- Shooting pains in joints
- Lower back pain
- Stiff gait
- Weakness and trembling of the hind limbs
- Nephritis with albumen in the urine

Modalities

WORSE/AGGRAVATED BY: Motion
BETTER/AMELIORATED BY: Eating, cloudy weather

Remedy Interactions

WORKS WELL WITH: Nux vomica, Spigelia, Lithium, Lycopodium, Pulsatilla
CONSIDER ALSO: Tabacum, Pulsatilla, Cactus, Digitalis, Spigelia

Principal Equine Indications

- Heart conditions where the pulse is weak and slow
- Endocarditis
- Stiffness and pain in the lower back and shoulders especially on the right
- Stiffness that changes position
- Stilted or generally stiff gait
- Acutely swollen painful joints
- Joints which 'crack'
- African Horse Sickness
- Lyme disease

Kamala

COMMON NAME: Kamala, *Croton coccineus*
CLASSIFICATION: Plant: Euphorbiacea family
PREPARATION: From tincture

Keynotes

- A remedy for tapeworms

Modalities

WORSE/AGGRAVATED BY: None listed
BETTER/AMELIORATED BY: None listed

Remedy Interactions

CONSIDER ALSO: Cina, Granatum, Filix mas

Principal Equine Indications

- In combination with other remedies for helping eliminate worms

Kreosotum

COMMON NAME: Creosote, Kreosote, Beechwood Kreosote
CLASSIFICATION: Plant
PREPARATION: From a distillate of wood tar containing phenols in rectified spirit

Keynotes

- Profuse haemorrhages from small wounds
- Ecchymosis
- Excoriating, offensive discharges
- Ulceration
- Cancers and related problems
- Gangrene
- Rapid decomposition of fluids
- Inflammation of the eyelids with redness and itching
- Decay of the teeth, crumbling away
- Spongy bleeding gums
- Bad odour from the mouth
- Offensive nasal catarrh
- Chronic catarrh in old horses
- Distended abdomen
- Dark brown foul diarrhoea with blood
- Offensive smelling urine
- Severe itching around the vulva
- Swelling of the lips of the vulva
- Yellow, green uterine discharge
- Incontinence
- Cough in the evening with foul expectoration
- Itching of the skin

Modalities

WORSE/AGGRAVATED BY: In the open air, cold, rest, lying down, after oestrus
BETTER/AMELIORATED BY: Warmth, moving around

Remedy Interactions

INCOMPATIBLE WITH: Carbo veg, China
WORKS WELL WITH: Sulphur, Arsenicum album, Calc carb, Kali carb, Lycopodium, Rhus tox, Sepia
CONSIDER ALSO: Carbo animalis, Graphites, Psorinum, Sepia, Tellurium

Principal Equine Indications

- Thrush
- Quittor
- White line disease
- Sole abscess, under-run sole
- Pyometria
- CEM
- Vulval dermatitis with swelling of the labia

- Gangrene
- Skin ulcers
- Chronic foul-smelling catarrh in old horses
- Persistent haemorrhage from small wounds
- Sarcoids and melanomas
- Decay of the teeth

Lac caninum

COMMON NAME: Bitch's milk, Dog's milk
CLASSIFICATION: Animal: Mammals
PREPARATION: From whole milk

Keynotes

- Focuses on the throat area and female reproductive system
- Throat sensitive to touch
- Membranous deposit at the back of the tongue
- Painful swallowing
- Swollen glands
- Stiff neck and tongue
- Pains that alternate from side to side, wandering pains
- Pains in the limbs and back that move location
- Symptoms which pass from right to left and back again
- General weakness and prostration
- Despondency
- Sudden bouts of anger
- Sociable animals, liking company
- Loyal
- Affectionate
- Protective of young, strong desire to nurture
- Highly strung mares
- Lack of confidence
- Desire to please
- Fear of dogs
- Mastitis, pain worse on least movement, jarring or touch
- Excessive milk production, increased flow of milk
- Dries up the secretion of milk
- Seasons too early
- Udder painful and swollen
- Skin cracks at the corners of the mouth and by the nostrils
- Increased salivation
- Cracking noises from the jaw

Modalities

WORSE/AGGRAVATED BY: At night, cold wind, motion, touch
BETTER/AMELIORATED BY: Warmth, rest

Remedy Interactions

CONSIDER ALSO: Lachesis, Argentum nitricum, Pulsatilla, Lyssin, Phosphorus

Principal Equine Indications

- Mastitis including traumatic mastitis
- To dry up excessive milk secretion
- Nymphomania
- Behavioural issues
- Lack of confidence
- Placid mares with occasional bouts of aggression
- Pharyngitis
- Wandering joint pains, shifting lameness
- Lyme disease

Lachesis

(see Constitutional Remedies)

Lachnantes

COMMON NAME: Spirit-weed, Red root, *Lachnanthes tinctoria*
CLASSIFICATION: Plant: Haemodoraceae family
PREPARATION: From tincture of the whole plant

Keynotes

- Symptoms linked with the neck
- Torticollis (wry neck, twisted neck)
- Neck drawn over to one side
- Rheumatic like symptoms of the neck area
- Pain and stiffness of the neck
- Sweats easily

Modalities

WORSE/AGGRAVATED BY: None listed
BETTER/AMELIORATED BY: None listed

Remedy Interactions

CONSIDER ALSO: Cicuta

Principal Equine Indications

- Stiffness and pain in the neck

- Torticollis, wry neck

Lacticum acidum

COMMON NAME: Lactic acid, Milk acid
CLASSIFICATION: Animal: Mammals: Humans
PREPARATION: By dilution

Keynotes
- Problems relating to the udder
- Rheumatic-like pain in the joints
- Swollen joints
- Muscle injuries
- Increased thirst

Modalities
WORSE/AGGRAVATED BY: Movement
BETTER/AMELIORATED BY: None listed

Remedy Interactions
WORKS WELL WITH: Psorinum
CONSIDER ALSO: Phos ac, Acetic acid, Uranium nitrate, Lac caninum

Principal Equine Indications
- Diabetes
- Pain or tenderness in the udder
- Generalised stiffness which is worse for movement
- Chronic periostitis, exostoses
- Painful muscle tears

Lapis albus

COMMON NAME: Silico-fluoride of calcium, Calcarea silico-fluorate, 'White stone'
CLASSIFICATION: Mineral: Calcium salt
PREPARATION: Trituration

Keynotes
- Acts on glands and connective tissue
- Hardening of the tissues of the udder
- Enlarged lymph nodes (which are pliable rather than stony hard to touch)
- Increased appetite, ravenous
- Suppurative ear infections
- Abscesses
- Cancers, specifically carcinoma
- Fibrous tumours which bleed
- Fatty masses, lipomas

Modalities
WORSE/AGGRAVATED BY: None listed
BETTER/AMELIORATED BY: None listed

Remedy Interactions
CONSIDER ALSO: Silica, Ars iod, Calc iod, Conium, Kali iod

Principal Equine Indications
- Chronically enlarged lymph nodes
- Hard masses within the udder
- Melanoma
- Sarcoids

Lathyrus

COMMON NAME: Chick pea, *Lathyrus sativus*
CLASSIFICATION: Plant: Fabiaceae (Leguminosae) family
PREPARATION: From tincture of the flowers or green pods

Keynotes
- Affects the spinal cord
- Increased reflexes which are incoordinated
- Paralysis of the lower limbs
- Spastic paralysis
- Slow recovery and weakness after viral infections
- Weak nerve power following illness
- Tottering, unsteady gait
- Spastic gait
- Legs appear rigid or stilted
- Cramping in the limbs
- Myelitis
- Wasting of the muscles of the lower limbs
- Stiffness of the lower limbs
- Drags the toe of the hoof along the floor
- Involuntary voiding of urine
- Difficulty swallowing
- Constipation, bowel has weak expulsive power

Modalities
WORSE/AGGRAVATED BY: None listed
BETTER/AMELIORATED BY: None listed

Remedy Interactions

CONSIDER ALSO: Oxytropis, Secale, Phosphorus, Gelsemium, Conium, Causticum, Alumina, Strychnine

Principal Equine Indications

- Roaring
- Paralysis of the hind limbs
- Spastic paralysis
- Weakness of the hind limbs
- Ataxia, uneven gait
- Wobbler syndrome
- Radial paralysis where there are early signs of recovery
- Poor spatial awareness
- Stringhalt
- Shivering
- Tying up, cramping of the muscles of the lower limbs
- Stiff gaited horses, muscular rigidity
- Weakness following viral infections especially where nerves are involved
- Post-viral paralysis
- Equine protozoal myeloencephalitis
- Urinary incontinence
- Grass sickness
- Constipation

Laurocerasus

COMMON NAME: Cherry-laural, *Cerasus laurocerasus*
CLASSIFICATION: Plant: Rosaceae family
PREPARATION: From a tincture of young leaves

Keynotes

- A remedy focused primarily on the respiratory system and heart
- Asphyxia in young animals
- Gasping for breath
- Cyanosis
- Difficulty breathing (dyspnoea)
- Distress on exercise
- Tickling cough
- Cardiac murmurs
- Feeble pulse
- Distorted hooves
- Poor circulation to the limbs and laminae especially
- Lack of reaction, low vitality

Modalities

WORSE/AGGRAVATED BY: None listed
BETTER/AMELIORATED BY: None listed

Remedy Interactions

WORKS WELL WITH: Belladonna, Phosphorus, Pulsatilla, Veratrum album
CONSIDER ALSO: Digitalis, Antimonium tartrate, Camphor, Secale, Ammonium carbonate, Prunus spinosa

Principal Equine Indications

- Pneumonia with cyanosis and dyspnoea in young foals
- In reviving collapsed or weakened animals of any age especially foals
- Stimulation of breathing in newborn foals, asphyxia
- Chronic laminitis in older horses where the hooves are distorted
- Heart murmurs where the mitral valve is involved
- Poor circulation especially where the mucous membranes are cyanosed

Lecithin, Lecithinum

COMMON NAME: Lecithin
CLASSIFICATION: Animal: Mammals
PREPARATION: From egg yolk and animal brain tissue

Keynotes

- Influences nutrition and the blood
- Increases the number of red blood cells and haemoglobin content
- Increases milk production and improves quality
- Convalescence in general
- Weakness, lack of energy
- Loss of weight

Modalities

WORSE/AGGRAVATED BY: None listed
BETTER/AMELIORATED BY: None listed

Remedy Interactions

CONSIDER ALSO: Phos ac, China

Principal Equine Indications

- Anaemia
- Debility
- Recovery from illness
- Poor milk production or milk quality

Ledum

COMMON NAME: Marsh tea, Wild rosemary, *Ledum palustre*
CLASSIFICATION: Plant: Ericaceae family
PREPARATION: From the whole fresh plant

Keynotes

- Important equine remedy
- Rheumatic and joint symptoms
- Twitching of muscles, tetanus
- Skin symptoms
- Pimple-like eruptions on the face, dermatitis involving the face
- Crusty lesions around the mouth
- Itching of the fetlock and pastern regions
- Antidote to insect bites
- Puncture wounds of any type
- Ecchymotic haemorrhages
- Prolonged discoloration of the skin after injuries
- Eye injuries, bloodshot eyes, contusion of the eye
- Haemorrhage into the eye or into the eyelids
- Contused wounds
- Cough with bloody mucus
- Difficulty breathing
- Bronchitis and emphysema
- Pains in the hoof
- Pains in the joints of the lower limbs, fetlock, pastern and coffin
- Cracking noises from the joints
- Swelling of the hock joint, weak hocks

Modalities

WORSE/AGGRAVATED BY: At night, from heat of the stable, warmth, movement, evening, at night, covering up
BETTER/AMELIORATED BY: Cold weather, cold applications or hosing

Remedy Interactions

WORKS WELL WITH: Aconite, Arnica, Belladonna, Bryonia, Nux vom, Pulsatilla, Sulphur
CONSIDER ALSO: Arnica, Bellis, Hamamelis, Ruta, Kalmia, Bryonia, Guaiacum, Pulsatilla, Rhus tox, Ruta

Principal Equine Indications

- Eye injuries in general
- Haemorrhage into the eye
- Corneal abrasions
- Arthritis/DJD especially of the fetlock, pastern, hock and coffin joints
- Hock problems/injuries, especially sprains
- Cracking joints
- Laminitis, especially chronic traumatic laminitis
- Navicular disease/syndrome
- Recurrent ligament strains
- Acute tendon injuries, sprains or rupture
- Chronic synovitis
- Thoroughpin
- Bog spavin
- Bone spavin
- Curb
- Over-reach injuries
- Nail prick
- Corns
- Quittor
- Physical skin reactions to vaccination
- Skin contusions, contused wounds
- Bruising, particularly of the sole
- Puncture wounds, gunshot wounds, snake, insect and animal bites
- Slow resolution and healing where there is bruising to the skin
- Effects of insect or snake bites and stings
- Sweet itch (prevention)
- Tetanus and tetanus prevention (in combination with Hypericum)
- Ticks and tick reactions
- Equine nodular skin disease
- Lyme disease
- Lice and associated symptoms
- Mites and associated irritation of the lower limbs
- EIPH

Lemna minor

COMMON NAME: Duckweed
CLASSIFICATION: Plant: Lemnaceae family
PREPARATION: From tincture of the whole fresh plant

Keynotes
- A remedy for catarrh
- Foul smell from the nose
- Mucopurulent discharge
- Nose obstructed
- Degenerative changes to the nasal membranes and tissues
- Nasal polyps

Modalities
WORSE/AGGRAVATED BY: Damp weather, in the rain
BETTER/AMELIORATED BY: None listed

Remedy Interactions
WORKS WELL WITH: Calc carb, Merc sol, Psorinum
CONSIDER ALSO: Teucrium marum, Thuja, Aurum, Kali bich, Symphytum

Principal Equine Indications
- Chronic foul smelling nasal catarrh
- Chronic rhinitis
- Guttural pouch empyema

Lespidiza

COMMON NAME: Lespidiza, *Lespidiza capitata*
CLASSIFICATION: Plant: Fabiaceae (Leguminosae) family
PREPARATION: From the whole plant

Keynotes
- Acts on the kidneys

Modalities
WORSE/AGGRAVATED BY: None listed
BETTER/AMELIORATED BY: None listed

Remedy Interactions – None listed

Principal Equine Indications
- Nephritis, renal (kidney) failure especially chronic cases

Liatris spicata

COMMON NAME: Colic root, Devil's bit
CLASSIFICATION: Plant: Asteraceae (Compositae) family
PREPARATION: From tincture of the powdered fresh root

Keynotes
- Stimulates the circulation
- Ascites/oedema due to liver, kidney or heart disease

Modalities
WORSE/AGGRAVATED BY: None listed
BETTER/AMELIORATED BY: None listed

Remedy Interactions – None listed

Principal Equine Indications
- Oedema due to liver, kidney or heart disease
- Filled legs

Lilium tigrinum, Lil tig

COMMON NAME: Tiger lily
CLASSIFICATION: Plant: Liliaceae family
PREPARATION: From tincture of the fresh stalk, leaves and flowers

Keynotes
- Acts principally on the organs of the pelvic cavity
- Problems relating to the uterus and ovaries
- Depressed and anxious
- Aggravated by consolation
- Inclined to kick out or bite
- Highly sexed, nymphomania
- Does not give in
- Hurried, fidgets around, sense of urgency
- Needs to be kept occupied
- Soreness in the abdomen
- Frequent voiding of urine
- Frequent desire to pass dung
- Diarrhoea with mucus and blood, straining
- Irregular and rapid pulse
- Disordered oestrus cycle, seasons too close together
- Prolapse of the uterus, uterus congested
- Ovarian pain
- Brown, foul uterine discharge
- Abortion
- Infertility
- Difficulty walking on uneven ground
- Back pain
- Rapid, irregular pulse

Modalities

WORSE/AGGRAVATED BY: Consolation, 5–8pm, warmth of stable
BETTER/AMELIORATED BY: Riding, physical exertion, in the open air

Remedy Interactions

CONSIDER ALSO: Murex, Sepia, Platina, Palladium, Helonias, Pulsatilla, Lachesis

Principal Equine Indications

- Mareish behaviour
- Anxious irritable behaviour
- Kicking and biting
- Ovarian pain and associated back pain
- Cystic ovaries
- Frequent urination associated with ovarian or uterine problems
- Uterine prolapse
- Pyometria
- Infertility
- Abortion
- Irregular oestrus cycles
- Mis-mothering

Lithium carbonicum

COMMON NAME: Lithium carbonate
CLASSIFICATION: Mineral: Lithium salt
PREPARATION: Trituration

Keynotes

- Acts on the heart and the joints
- Stomach pain
- Dislike of tight-fitting tack
- Straining to pass urine
- Chronic cystitis
- Cardiac pain
- General stiffness
- Joint pain and stiffness, especially affecting the lower limbs – knee, hock, fetlock, pastern and coffin joints
- Hard swellings around the joints – exostoses
- Itching around the joints
- Itchy skin eruptions with scaling

Modalities

WORSE/AGGRAVATED BY: Right side of the body, morning
BETTER/AMELIORATED BY: Movement

Remedy Interactions

CONSIDER ALSO: Lycopodium, Benzoic acid, Calc carb, Ledum, Kalmia

Principal Equine Indications

- Arthritis/DJD of the knee, hock fetlock, pastern and coffin joints where accompanied by exostoses
- Bone spavin
- Bony exostoses
- Stiffness of the shoulder joints and elbow

Lobelia inflata

COMMON NAME: Indian tobacco
CLASSIFICATION: Plant: Campanulaceae (Lobeliaceae) family
PREPARATION: From tincture of the fresh plant when flowering or trituration of the dried leaves

Keynotes

- Acts as a vaso-motor stimulant
- Impedes respiration
- Relaxation of muscles
- State of languor
- Acts on the stomach (nausea and vomiting)
- Increased secretion of gastric acid
- Flatulence
- Increased salivation
- Asthma
- Dyspnoea (difficulty breathing)
- Breathing difficulty after feeding
- Emphysema
- Suppressed discharges
- Jaundice

Modalities

WORSE/AGGRAVATED BY: Evening, at night, cold weather, right hand side, when ridden
BETTER/AMELIORATED BY: Afternoon, warmth

Remedy Interactions

CONSIDER ALSO: Tabacum, Arsenicum album, Antimonium tartrate, Ipecac, Kali arsenicum

Principal Equine Indications

- COPD especially acute cases
- Acute spasmodic constriction of the airways
- Wheezing and coughing
- Slow recovery after flu
- Gastric ulceration, hyperacidity

Luna

COMMON NAME: Rays of the moon, moonlight
CLASSIFICATION: Energy: Universal force: Stellar body
PREPARATION: From milk sugar exposed to the rays of the moon

Keynotes

- Associated with the female reproductive system
- Irregular oestrus cycles
- Poor development of the udder
- Infertility
- Rejection of young, irritable
- Mareish behaviour
- Dry flaky skin
- Poor concentration

Modalities

WORSE/AGGRAVATED BY: After sleep
BETTER/AMELIORATED BY: None listed

Remedy Interactions – None listed

Principal Equine Indications

- Irregular oestrus cycles
- Infertility
- Mareish behaviour
- Mismothering
- Lack of concentration

Lycopodium

(see Constitutional Remedies)

Lycopus virginicus

COMMON NAME: Bugleweed, Virginia horehound
CLASSIFICATION: Plant: Lamiaceae (Labiatae) family
PREPARATION: From a tincture of the fresh flowering plant

Keynotes

- Acts on the blood, heart and circulation
- Passive haemorrhage
- Reduces blood pressure
- Rapid heartbeat
- Weak, irregular pulse
- Cyanosis
- Dry cough
- Blood-stained expectoration
- Wheezing
- Hyperthyroidism
- Diabetes

Modalities

WORSE/AGGRAVATED BY: None listed
BETTER/AMELIORATED BY: None listed

Remedy Interactions

CONSIDER ALSO: Kalmia, Spigelia, Crataegus, Cactus, Digitalis, Laurocerasus, Prunus spinosa

Principal Equine Indications

- EIPH
- Rapid heartbeat with intermittent or weak pulse
- Pericarditis
- Diabetes

Lyssin, Hydrophobinum

COMMON NAME: Rabies virus, Rabies nosode
CLASSIFICATION: Animal: Mammals: Nosode
PREPARATION: From the saliva of a rapid dog

Keynotes

- A remedy for behavioural problems
- Fear of water
- Manic, wild behaviour
- Rage
- Occasionally violent (sudden bouts) but sorry afterwards
- Agoraphobia and claustrophobia
- All senses hypersensitive; overreacts
- Salivation
- Craves salt licks
- Bites and their effects
- Matted oily (greasy) coat and skin
- Epilepsy

Modalities

WORSE/AGGRAVATED BY: Noise or sight of running water, bright objects, travelling in a horsebox
BETTER/AMELIORATED BY: Gentle massage

Remedy Interactions

CONSIDER ALSO: Stramonium, Belladonna, Hyoscyamus, Anacardium, Pulsatilla

Principal Equine Indications

- Wide-ranging behavioural issues
- Sudden outbursts of rage or anger
- Horses that suddenly bite or kick
- Manic behaviour
- Hysteria-like behaviour during transportation
- Self-mutilation
- Obsessive behaviour
- Abandoned animals
- Horses that have been abused
- Effects of grief and sorrow
- Horses that have been isolated for great periods
- Over-reactivity due to heightened senses
- Over-reaction to noises and bright lights or shiny objects
- Epileptics fits triggered by bright light or water
- Headshaking especially in very bright sunlight
- Claustrophobic horses
- Fear of water
- Horses that are difficult to load into horseboxes, poor travellers
- Dog or snake bites
- Animals that have never been well since being injured or poisoned
- Priapism

Magnesia carbonica, Mag carb

COMMON NAME: Magnesium carbonate
CLASSIFICATION: Mineral: Magnesium salt
PREPARATION: Trituration

Keynotes

- Generally have a poor ability to assimilate food
- Emaciated, undernourished
- Spluttery green dung
- Oversensitive
- Restless
- Appear sad
- Starts easily if touched
- Feel the cold easily; need rugging up
- Pain from the teeth

Modalities

WORSE/AGGRAVATED BY: Change of temperature, cold weather, cold wind
BETTER/AMELIORATED BY: Warm weather, in the open air

Remedy Interactions

WORKS WELL WITH: Chamomilla, Causticum, Phosphorus, Pulsatilla, Sepia, Sulphur
CONSIDER ALSO: Mag phos

Principal Equine Indications

- Suited to undernourished foals especially
- Foals with diarrhoea especially while still feeding from the mare
- Poor doers generally due to weak digestive system
- Green watery diarrhoea, especially if colicky
- Worn out older mares
- Oversensitivity especially to sudden noises, gun shots
- Horses that start easily

Magnesia phosphorica, Mag phos

COMMON NAME: Magnesium phosphate, Phosphate of magnesia
CLASSIFICATION: Mineral: Magnesium salt
PREPARATION: Trituration

Keynotes

- Important antispasmodic remedy
- Muscle cramps
- Neuralgia
- Toothache
- Indigestion
- Flatulent colic better for arching the back
- Bloating of the abdomen
- Constant passing of gas while walking around
- Watering from the eyes, lachrymation
- Twitching of the eyelids
- Nystagmus
- Strabismus
- Ptosis (dropping of the eyelids)

- Ovarian pain
- Asthma
- Spasmodic cough
- Involuntary trembling of the front legs
- Twitching
- Tetanic-like spasms
- General muscular weakness

Modalities

WORSE/AGGRAVATED BY: Right side, cold, from touch, at night
BETTER/AMELIORATED BY: Warmth, arching the back, pressure, massage or rubbing

Remedy Interactions

WORKS WELL WITH: Tuberculinum
CONSIDER ALSO: Kali phos, Colocynthis, Dioscorea, Zincum metallicum, Chamomilla, Mag carb, Nux vomica

Principal Equine Indications

- Flatulent colic with severe pain
- Tympanic colic
- Tying up
- Stringhalt (less severe cases)
- Ptosis
- Neuralgic-like pain eg intercostal (rib) pain
- Tetanus
- Cramps and spasms of the limb muscles
- Eclampsia, hypocalcaemia
- Shivering
- Poisonings involving muscular twitching
- Urolithiasis

Magnesia sulphurica, Mag sulph

COMMON NAME: Epsom salts, Magnesium sulphate
CLASSIFICATION: Mineral: Magnesium salt
PREPARATION: Trituration

Keynotes

- Acts on the urinary system
- Intermittent, dribbling urination
- Urine with sediment present
- Diabetes with great thirst
- Muscle spasms

Modalities

WORSE/AGGRAVATED BY: None listed
BETTER/AMELIORATED BY: None listed

Remedy Interactions – None listed

Principal Equine Indications

- Urinary incontinence with intermittent dribbling of urine
- Muscle cramping or spasms

Malandrinum

COMMON NAME: From the conditional called grease in horses
CLASSIFICATION: Animal: Mammals: Nosode
PREPARATION: Trituration of milk sugar saturated with the organism

Keynotes

- Useful for conditions arising after vaccination
- Dry, harsh, rough, skin conditions with cracks and scaly material
- Greasy skin
- Impetigo

Modalities

WORSE/AGGRAVATED BY: None listed
BETTER/AMELIORATED BY: None listed

Remedy Interactions

CONSIDER ALSO: Thuja, Silica, Graphites, Castor equi, Hippozaenium, Hippomanes

Principal Equine Indications

- Ill effects of vaccination, vaccinosis
- Mud fever
- Impetigo
- Excessively greasy coat and skin, seborrhoea
- Supportive or preventative treatment following removal of a sarcoid, melanoma or other skin mass

Mancinella

COMMON NAME: Manganeel apple, *Hippomane mancinella*
CLASSIFICATION: Plant: Euphorbiaceae family
PREPARATION: From tincture of the fruit, bark and leaves

Keynotes
- Acts on the skin
- Skin conditions characterized by oozing of sticky secretions
- Crust formation
- Vesicles
- Intense inflammation of the skin, erythema (redness)
- Hair loss
- Skin blisters
- Pemphigus
- Fungus-like skin growths

Modalities
WORSE/AGGRAVATED BY: None listed
BETTER/AMELIORATED BY: None listed

Remedy Interactions
CONSIDER ALSO: Croton tig, Cantharis, Arsenicum, Graphites, Malandrinum, Pulsatilla, Merc sol

Principal Equine Indications
- Mud fever
- Moist eczema with thick overlying crusts
- Rainscald
- Sarcoids – verrucose type particularly

Manganum aceticum

COMMON NAME: Manganese acetate, Acetate of manganese
CLASSIFICATION: Mineral: Manganum salt
PREPARATION: From a solution in distilled water

Keynotes
- Acts on red blood cells and the nervous system especially as well as throat and larynx
- Destruction of red blood cells
- Exaggerated reflexes
- Muscle twitches
- Muscle cramps, stiff legs
- Staggering gait
- Falls forward
- Progressive paraplegia
- Fatty degeneration of the liver
- Cellulitis
- Inflammation of bone and of the joints
- Chronic arthritis, joints sore to touch, swollen
- Bone pain, inflammation of the periosteum
- Accumulation of mucus in the respiratory tract, difficult to loosen
- Chronic catarrh
- Laryngitis
- Cough worse in damp weather
- Coughing up of blood
- Suppuration (infection) of the skin around the joints

Modalities
WORSE/AGGRAVATED BY: Cold, wet weather, dampness, change of weather, at night
BETTER/AMELIORATED BY: In the open air, after lying down

Remedy Interactions
WORKS WELL WITH: Pulsatilla, Rhus tox, Sulphur
CONSIDER ALSO: Conium, Asafoetida, Merc sol, Ferrum, TNT

Principal Equine Indications
- Autoimmune haemolytic anaemia in the foal
- Anaemia
- Babesiasis
- Chronic arthritis/DJD with swollen painful joints, especially where there is frequent stumbling
- Periostitis
- Bone pain
- Cellulitis
- Lymphangitis
- Injuries to the skin local to the joints
- Progressive weakness of the hind limbs
- Accumulation of thick catarrh in the upper respiratory tract; chronic cough
- Chronic nasal discharges

Medorrhinum

COMMON NAME: Gonorrhoea nosode
CLASSIFICATION: Animal: Mammals: Humans: Nosode
PREPARATION: From the organism

Keynotes
- Indicated for chronic conditions
- Association with the sycotic miasm
- Chronic rheumatic type symptoms; stiffness
- Periostitis

- Thick yellow catarrh
- Nervous and restless nature
- Cautious (thinks someone is always just behind them)
- Appears hurried
- Need to be kept busy
- Cunning
- Greedy and thirsty
- Thin foul smelling uterine discharge
- Ovarian pain
- Ovarian cysts
- Impotency
- Urethritis
- Swelling of the joints of the lower limb, fetlock, pastern and coffin joints
- Painful soles
- Skin tumours and other growths

Modalities

WORSE/AGGRAVATED BY: From dawn to sunset, heat
BETTER/AMELIORATED BY: Damp weather, at the seaside

Remedy Interactions

WORKS WELL WITH: Sulphur, Thuja, Pulsatilla
CONSIDER ALSO: Anacardium, Baryta carb, Lachesis, Nat mur, Nat sulph, Nux vomica, Sulphur, Tuberculinum

Principal Equine Indications

- Chronic stiffness
- Chronic laminitis
- Chronic yellow catarrh
- Ovarian cysts
- Pyometra, endometritis
- CEM
- Impotency in the stallion
- Urethritis
- Smegma
- Fears especially of the dark
- Highly suspicious animals
- Lack of confidence
- Sarcoids and melanomas

Medusa

COMMON NAME: Jellyfish
CLASSIFICATION: Animal: Cnidaria family
PREPARATION: From tincture

Keynotes

- Oedematous conditions
- Angioneurotic oedema
- Puffiness of tissues
- Prickling sensation in the skin
- Vesicular eruptions
- Nettle rash
- Increases production of milk

Modalities

WORSE/AGGRAVATED BY: None listed
BETTER/AMELIORATED BY: None listed

Remedy Interactions

CONSIDER ALSO: Apis, Urtica, Murex

Principal Equine Indications

- Oedematous skin reactions
- Pitting oedema especially around the face and head region
- Allergic skin reactions
- Allergic reactions to vaccination
- Insect bites
- Filled or puffy legs
- Bursitis
- Itching of the skin
- Purpura haemorrhagica
- To increase the production of milk in the mare, agalactia (lack of milk)

Melilotus

COMMON NAME: Sweet clover, *Melilotus officinalis*
CLASSIFICATION: Plant: Fabiaceae (Leguminosae) family
PREPARATION: From tincture of the whole fresh flowering plant

Keynotes

- Special focus on haemorrhage and congestion
- Poor ability of the blood to clot
- Haemorrhage of bright red blood, particularly from the mouth or nose
- Nosebleed; epistaxis
- Bleeding from the lungs; haemoptysis
- Constipation
- Epilepsy from trauma to the head
- Ovarian pain

Modalities

WORSE/AGGRAVATED BY: Wet weather, changeable weather, approaching storm, movement, 4pm
BETTER/AMELIORATED BY: Rest

Remedy Interactions

CONSIDER ALSO: Ipecac, Millefolium, Erigeron, Phosphorus

Principal Equine Indications

- EIPH which fails to respond to other remedies
- Haematomas
- Subcutaneous bleeding
- Warfarin poisoning

Mercurius corrosivus, Merc corr

COMMON NAME: Corrosive sublimate of mercury, Mercuric chloride
CLASSIFICATION: Mineral: Mercury series
PREPARATION: By trituration

Keynotes

- Has a destructive effect on the kidneys
- Nephritis
- Inflammation of the urethra
- Swelling of the penis
- Albumen in the urine
- Straining to pass urine
- Urethral discharge (thick and green in colour)
- Affects the lower bowel causing straining (tenesmus)
- Slimy foul-smelling dung
- Dysentery
- Deep corneal ulcers
- Photophobia
- Increased lachrymation (tear production)
- Iritis
- Retinitis
- Swollen oedematous lids, excoriation of the lids
- Bone pain
- Increased salivation
- Inflammation of the gums
- Intensely inflamed throat
- Swallowing painful

Modalities

WORSE/AGGRAVATED BY: Evening, at night
BETTER/AMELIORATED BY: Resting

Remedy Interactions

COMMON NAME: Aurum, Kali iod, Lachesis, Nux vomica, Causticum

Principal Equine Indications

- Iritis
- Deep corneal ulcers
- Keratitis
- Conjunctivitis with excoriated lids and greenish discharge, photophobia
- Acute and chronic nephritis, renal failure
- Pyelonephritis
- Severe pharyngitis
- Paraphimosis
- Urethritis
- Dysenteric-like diarrhoea with severe straining
- Colitis X, Clostridial enterotoxaemia
- Intussception
- Periostitis

Mercurius cyanatus, Merc cyan

COMMON NAME: Cyanide of mercury, Mercuric cyanide
CLASSIFICATION: Mineral: Mercury series
PREPARATION: By trituration

Keynotes

- Has an effect similar to toxins produced by infectious organisms
- Acute infections
- Pneumonia
- Nephritis
- Haemorrhage of dark blood
- Cyanosis, imminent suffocation
- Twitching and jerking of muscles
- Mouth ulcers
- Increased salivation
- Swelling of the salivary glands
- Sore, ulcerated throat, very inflamed, redness
- Necrosis (decay) of the tissues of the throat
- Foul black diarrhoea, straining

Modalities

WORSE/AGGRAVATED BY: None listed
BETTER/AMELIORATED BY: None listed

Remedy Interactions

CONSIDER ALSO: Causticum, Hepar sulph, Kali bich, Phytolacca, Echinacea, Lachesis, Gelsemium

Principal Equine Indications

- States of sepsis (infection) especially where the throat and pharynx are involved
- Ulceration of the mouth, throat and tongue

Mercurius dulcis

COMMON NAME: Calomel, Subchloride of Mercury, Mercurous chloride
CLASSIFICATION: Mineral: Mercury series
PREPARATION: By trituration

Keynotes

- Inflammation of the ear canal and Eustacean canal
- Peritonitis
- Meningitis
- Cirrhosis of the liver
- Increased salivation
- Ulceration of the throat
- Dark green watery diarrhoea with straining
- Dysentery
- Flabby poor-looking skin

Modalities

WORSE/AGGRAVATED BY: None listed
BETTER/AMELIORATED BY: None listed

Remedy Interactions

CONSIDER ALSO: Kali mur, Kali bich, Merc sol, Merc corr

Principal Equine Indications

- Guttural pouch empyema
- Guttural pouch tympanitis
- Peritonitis
- Catarrh
- Meningitis
- Foul green diarrhoea

Mercurius, Mercurius solubilis (Hahnemanni), Merc sol, Mercurius vivus, Hydrargyrum

COMMON NAME: Mercury, quicksilver
CLASSIFICATION: Mineral: Mercury series: Polycrest
PREPARATION: By trituration

Keynotes

- Remedy of major importance
- Affects every organ of the body; has a destructive effect
- Affinity for the salivary glands, lymph nodes, mucous membranes and bone
- Foul offensive discharges
- Tendency for suppuration, abscesses
- Green, thin blood-streaked pus
- Slimy mucous membranes
- Stomatitis
- Increased salivation
- Spongy gums, bleeding
- Bad odour from the mouth
- Sweats easily
- Oily, greasy skin
- Moist sweaty skin
- Pustules, yellow brownish crusty lesion
- Suppuration
- Shallow skin ulcers
- Itching
- Tremors
- Exostoses
- Red, swollen eyelids with a foul greenish (burning) discharge
- Photophobia
- Iritis with pus in the anterior chamber of the eye
- Thick yellow discharge from the ear
- Raw and ulcerated nostrils
- Swelling of the nasal bones
- Yellow green foul smelling nasal discharge
- Frequent sneezing in the sunshine
- Throat sore, has to keep swallowing
- Ulcers in the throat and mouth
- Increased thirst
- Weak digestion
- Jaundice
- Bloody and slimy dung
- Ineffectual urging to pass dung
- Urging to pass urine

- Urethritis
- Ulcers on the penis
- Ovarian pain
- Green vaginal discharge
- Cough with yellow purulent mucus
- Trembling of the limbs
- Joint pains
- Swelling of the joints
- Periostitis

Modalities

WORSE/AGGRAVATED BY: At night (sunset to sunrise), wet damp weather, right side, warmth of stable or rug, extremes of hot and cold

BETTER/AMELIORATED BY: Rest

Remedy Interactions

INCOMPATIBLE WITH: Silica

WORKS WELL WITH: Aconite, Hepar sulph, Lachesis, Sulphur, Arsenicum album, Belladonna, Calc carb, Lycopodium, Nitric acid, Phosphorus, Pulsatilla, Rhus tox, Sepia

CONSIDER ALSO: Belladonna, Hepar sulph, Pulsatilla, Nux vomica

Principal Equine Indications

- Conjunctivitis characterised by a green discharge and red/sore looking eye
- Keratitis
- Iritis with pus in the anterior chamber (hypopyon)
- Corneal ulceration with marked photophobia
- Greenish, yellow foul catarrh
- Sinus empyema
- Pharyngitis (with swelling)
- Acute bronchopneumonia
- Ulcers internally (mouth and throat especially) and externally (skin)
- Infected sores around the mouth
- Parotitis (right-sided)
- Soft bleeding gums
- Tooth abscesses
- Lymphadenitis (enlarged lymph nodes)
- Urethritis with constant desire to pass urine
- Acute nephritis (renal failure)
- Cystitis
- Green preputial discharges
- Ulceration of the penis and prepuce
- Orchitis
- Phimosis and paraphimosis
- Smegma
- Coital exanthema
- Severe dysenteric-like diarrhoea with mucus and with straining
- Cystitis
- Bony degeneration with local swelling
- Exostoses
- Limb tremors
- Abscesses and suppuration generally where the discharge or pus is greenish in colour
- Moist sticky dermatitis
- Mud fever
- Thrush
- Ulcerative lymphangitis
- Mites (symptomatic treatment)
- Vesicular stomatitis virus
- Strangles
- Potomac Horse fever
- Coccidiosis
- Mercury poisoning
- Anaemia caused by suppression of bone marrow by toxins
- Emotionally unstable horses often appear hurried
- Horses that seem to urinate more than they drink
- Excessive sweating

Mezereum

COMMON NAME: Spurge olive, Mezereon, *Daphne mezereum*

CLASSIFICATION: Plant: Thymelaceae family

PREPARATION: From tincture of the fresh bark taken before the plant flowers

Keynotes

- Affects mainly the skin and bone
- Neuralgic pain especially around the face
- Bone pain
- Skin symptoms appearing after vaccination
- Thick leathery looking crusts on the skin with pus underneath
- Eczema with severe itching
- Skin ulcers with surrounding reddening of the skin
- Decay of the tooth roots
- Gastric ulceration
- Rectal prolapse
- Constriction of the anus

- Testicular enlargement
- Haematuria
- Neck and back pain
- Hip and stifle pain
- Inflammation of the long bones
- Exostoses
- Intolerant of touch

Modalities

WORSE/AGGRAVATED BY: Motion, at night, evening, touch, damp weather
BETTER/AMELIORATED BY: In the open air

Remedy Interactions

WORKS WELL WITH: Merc sol, Calc carb, Causticum, Lycopodium, Nitric acid. Nux vomica, Phosphorus, Pulsatilla
CONSIDER ALSO: Spigelia, Thuja, Arsenicum album, Merc sol

Principal Equine Indications

- For relief of pain after eye surgery
- Tooth pain
- Bone pain
- Exostoses
- Periostitis
- Pitryiasis
- Skin lesions with thick crusts overlying pus
- Skin lesions appearing after vaccination
- Mud fever
- Rain scald
- Skin ulcers
- Vaccinosis (vaccine reactions)

Millefolium

COMMON NAME: Yarrow, *Achillea millefolium*
CLASSIFICATION: Plant: Asteraceae (Compositae) family
PREPARATION: From tincture of the whole plant

Keynotes

- Bright red haemorrhage
- Injuries from falling
- Muscle strains
- Persistent high temperature
- Nosebleed (epistaxis)
- Haematuria (blood in the urine)
- Bleeding from the uterus
- Cough with expectoration of mucus with blood
- Bleeding from the lungs (haemoptysis)

Modalities

WORSE/AGGRAVATED BY: Exertion,
BETTER/AMELIORATED BY: None listed

Remedy Interactions

CONSIDER ALSO: Senecio aureus, Hamamelis, Ipecac, Aconite, Arnica, Ledum

Principal Equine Indications

- Haemorrhage of bright red blood from any area of the body generally
- Haemorrhage after trauma
- Epistaxis, nosebleed
- EIPH
- Haematuria (blood in the urine)
- Persistent bleeding from small skin wounds
- Warfarin poisoning
- Uterine haemorrhage
- Severe muscle strains
- Equine viral arteritis (EVA)
- Babesiasis

Moschus

COMMON NAME: Deer musk, *Moschus moschiferus*
CLASSIFICATION: Animal: Mammal
PREPARATION: Trituration of secretion from preputial follicles

Keynotes

- Helps with hysterical or nervous behaviour
- Sudden starting
- Anxiety
- Flatulence with abdominal distension
- Over-sexed male horses
- Nymphomania
- Diabetes
- Constriction of the larynx and trachea
- Difficulty in breathing
- Asthma caused by anxiety

Modalities

WORSE/AGGRAVATED BY: Cold
BETTER/AMELIORATED BY: In the open air

Remedy Interactions

CONSIDER ALSO: Nux moschata, Ignatia, Lilium tigrinum, Plumbum, Tarentula hisp

Principal Equine Indications

- Uncontrollable, hysterical type behaviour
- Epilepsy triggered by stress
- Sudden starting, jumpy behaviour
- Hypersexuality in the stallion
- Nymphomania
- COPD especially where anxiety features
- Diabetes

Murex

COMMON NAME: Purple fish, *Murex purpurea*
CLASSIFICATION: Animal: Molluscs: Gastropod
PREPARATION: Trituration of desiccated or fresh juice

Keynotes

- Main focus is on the female reproductive system
- Sexual urges easily excited
- Uterine pain
- Irregular oestrus cycles
- Uterine prolapse
- Chronic pyometria
- Depressed spirits

Modalities

WORSE/AGGRAVATED BY: Least touch, exertion, at night, after sleep
BETTER/AMELIORATED BY: Before oestrus

Remedy Interactions

CONSIDER ALSO: Sepia, Lilium tigrinum, Platina, Origanum, Secale, Pulsatilla

Principal Equine Indications

- Nymphomania, excessive sexual excitement
- Uterine prolapse
- Irregular oestrus cycles
- Stimulation of ovulation
- Ovarian cysts
- Over-sexed stallions
- False rigs

Muriaticum acidum

COMMON NAME: Hydrochloric acid, Muriatic acid
CLASSIFICATION: Mineral: Muriaticums
PREPARATION: From a solution in distilled water

Keynotes

- Affects the blood
- Sepsis with high fever with prostration
- Weakness, tottery gait
- Decomposition of fluids
- Haemorrhage from the nose
- Lips raw and cracked
- Tongue ulcerated
- Swollen and oedematous throat
- Anal itching
- Itching skin eruptions
- Skin ulcers on the limbs with a foul discharge

Modalities

WORSE/AGGRAVATED BY: Damp weather, before midnight, rest
BETTER/AMELIORATED BY: Warmth

Remedy Interactions

WORKS WELL WITH: Bryonia, Rhus tox, Merc sol, Pulsatilla, Sepia
CONSIDER ALSO: Phos ac, Arsenicum album, Baptisia, Gelsemium

Principal Equine Indications

- Ulcerative lymphangitis (to help heal the ulcers)
- Pressure sores, decubitus, skin ulcers
- Ulceration of the tongue, mouth and lips

Mygale lasidora

COMMON NAME: Black cuban spider, *Mygale lasiodora cubana*
CLASSIFICATION: Animal: Arachnids
PREPARATION: From a tincture of the living spider in alcohol

Keynotes

- States of delirium
- Restless and sad
- Facial muscles twitch
- Mouth and eyes open alternately

- Head jerks to one side
- Teeth grating
- Unsteady gait
- Tremors and twitching of the limbs
- Dragging of the limbs during riding
- Red streaks following the lymphatic vessels
- Increased sexual desire in the stallion

Modalities

WORSE/AGGRAVATED BY: In the morning, eating, at rest
BETTER/AMELIORATED BY: None listed

Remedy Interactions

CONSIDER ALSO: Agaricus, Ignatia, Stramonium, Tarentula hisp

Principal Equine Indications

- Cases of poisoning where twitching is a feature
- Chorea
- Inflammation of the lymphatic vessels in the limbs
- Lymphangitis
- Behavioural problems where the animal appears nervous and excitable

Myristica sebifera

COMMON NAME: Brazilian ucuba
CLASSIFICATION: Plant: Myristicaceae family
PREPARATION: Trituration of the gum

Keynotes

- Has antiseptic properties
- Inflammation of the skin, periosteum and connective tissue
- Infections arising from trauma
- Fistulas
- Infections involving the hoof
- An alternative to Silica or Hepar sulph

Modalities

WORSE/AGGRAVATED BY: None listed
BETTER/AMELIORATED BY: None listed

Remedy Interactions

CONSIDER ALSO: Silica, Calc sulph, Hepar sulph, Pyrogen

Principal Equine Indications

- Sepsis
- Suppurating skin infections especially around joints
- Periostitis
- Cellulitis
- Hoof abscesses
- Fistulae and sinuses
- White line disease
- Quittor
- Thrush
- Seedy toe
- Gravel
- Persistent abscesses

Naja

COMMON NAME: Cobra, *Naja tripudians*
CLASSIFICATION: Animal: Reptiles: Snakes: Elapidae family
PREPARATION: Trituration of milk sugar saturated with the venom

Keynotes

- Brooding nature, can appear sad
- Changeable moods
- Paralysis of the eye region, throat, lips
- Ptosis of the eyelids
- Staring eyes
- Pains in the head
- Oedema
- Dark-coloured, purple looking wounds
- Salivation
- Heart problems
- Endocarditis
- Heart damage after infection
- Low blood pressure
- Dry cough
- Left-sided ovarian pain

Modalities

WORSE/AGGRAVATED BY: Touch, at night, after sleep, exertion, motion, lying on the left side
BETTER/AMELIORATED BY: Gentle work in the open air, lying on the right side

Remedy Interactions

CONSIDER ALSO: Arsenicum album, Cactus, Lachesis, Spigelia, Digitalis, Crot horr

Principal Equine Indications

- Puncture wounds with a livid purple colour but minimal sepsis
- Ptosis of the eyelids
- Heart valve problems especially those resulting from infection
- Acute and chronic endocarditis
- Oedema
- Angio-neurotic oedema
- Left-sided ovarian pain
- Itching of scar tissue
- Broody, morose behaviour
- Fear of rain

Naphthaline

COMMON NAME: Tar camphor derived from coal tar
CLASSIFICATION: Mineral
PREPARATION: By trituration

Keynotes

- Affects the eye
- Retinal detachment
- Retinal infiltration, patchy deposits in the retina
- Corneal opacity
- Cataracts
- Asthma, dyspnoea
- Emphysema
- Bronchitis with thick mucus
- Marked sneezing
- Pyelonephritis

Modalities

WORSE/AGGRAVATED BY: None listed
BETTER/AMELIORATED BY: Open air

Remedy Interactions

CONSIDER ALSO: Arsenicum album, Sabadilla, Phosphorus, Drosera, Argentum nitricum

Principal Equine Indications

- Acute keratitis
- Corneal opacity and scarring
- Retinal detachment and degeneration
- Cataracts
- COPD with sneezing, difficulty breathing and thick mucus in the chest
- Pyelonephritis

Natrum Arsenicum, Nat ars

COMMON NAME: Sodium arsenate
CLASSIFICATION: Mineral: Sodium salt
PREPARATION: By trituration

Keynotes

- Nasal catarrh with thick yellow bland mucus
- Conjunctivitis with green or yellowish mucus
- Blepharitis
- Eyelids stuck together
- Eyes water in the wind
- Oedema around the eyes
- Asthma
- Cracking of the knee joints

Modalities

WORSE/AGGRAVATED BY: The wind, motion or exertion
BETTER/AMELIORATED BY: None listed

Remedy Interactions

CONSIDER ALSO: Kali carb, Apis, Arsenicum album, Nat mur, Nat sulph

Principal Equine Indications

- Catarrhal conjunctivitis with sticky mucus and swollen lids
- Gummy eyes where the lids stick together
- Blepharitis
- Watery eyes, worse in windy conditions
- In the later stages of respiratory infections to assist recovery

Natrum carbonicum, Nat carb

COMMON NAME: Sodium carbonate, 'soda'
CLASSIFICATION: Mineral: Sodium salt
PREPARATION: By trituration

Keynotes

- Anxiety during thunderstorms
- Slow comprehension
- Problems caused by summer heat
- Sunstroke, heat exhaustion
- Effects from drinking cold water when hot
- Nasal obstruction
- Catarrh
- Lots of mucus in the throat

- Weak digestion
- Diarrhoea from milk
- Yellow pulpy diarrhoea
- Weak hocks
- Old sprains
- Sweats easily

Modalities

WORSE/AGGRAVATED BY: Resting, heat of the summer, the sun, mental effort, thunderstorms, draughts, changes of weather
BETTER/AMELIORATED BY: Moving around, riding

Remedy Interactions

WORKS WELL WITH: Calc carb, Nux vomica, Pulsatilla, Sepia, Sulphur, Kali sulph
CONSIDER ALSO: Kali bich, Nat mur, Lycopodium, Silica, Staphysagria

Principal Equine Indications

- Heat stroke
- Heat exhaustion
- Diarrhoea in foals especially from milk
- Anxiety during thunderstorms
- Colic arising from drinking large amounts of cold water
- Weak or swollen hocks
- Chronic ligament strains
- Joint dislocations, luxations and subluxations

Natrum muriaticum

(see Constitutional Remedies)

Natrum phosphoricum, Nat phos

COMMON NAME: Sodium phosphate
CLASSIFICATION: Mineral: Sodium salt: Tissue salt
PREPARATION: By trituration

Keynotes

- Refined appearance but nervy personality
- Involved in fluid distribution
- Constituent of intracellular fluid
- Found in blood, muscles, nerve and brain cells
- Helps in the breakdown of lactic acid
- Conditions arising from a build-up of lactic acid
- Acidity
- Inflammation of the throat
- Colic
- Cracking of joints
- Synovial crepitation
- Rheumatic stiffness
- Jaundice
- Yellow creamy discharge from the eyes
- Whites of the eye dirty yellow in colour
- Thick yellow offensive mucus in the throat
- Itching around the hocks
- Hives

Modalities

WORSE/AGGRAVATED BY: Thunderstorm
BETTER/AMELIORATED BY: None listed

Remedy Interactions

CONSIDER ALSO: Calc carb, Urtica, Kali carb, Carcinosin, Benzoic acidum, Sulphur

Principal Equine Indications

- Conjunctivitis with a creamy yellow discharge
- Grating and cracking of the joints
- Persistent catarrh/mucus in the throat
- Prevention of gastric ulcers
- Possible prevention of azoturia/tying up
- Animals upset by thunderstorms

Natrum sulphuricum, Nat sulph

COMMON NAME: Sodium sulphate, Glauber's salt
CLASSIFICATION: Mineral: Sodium salt: Polycrest
PREPARATION: By trituration

Keynotes

- A remedy for liver problems
- Hepatitis, both acute and chronic
- Jaundice
- Liver region painful
- Conditions brought on by living in damp conditions
- Affected by rain, water in any other form
- Affected by the change from dry to wet weather
- Meningitis
- Injuries to the head, bangs, blows, concussion
- Thick yellow catarrh
- Photophobia
- Yellow conjunctival membranes
- Gassy colic

- Flatulence
- Yellow diarrhoea with flatulence
- Diabetes
- Growths on the penis
- Thick, green preputial discharge
- Breathing laboured during damp weather, asthma
- Rattling in the chest
- Cough with thick green mucus
- Pain in the hip joints
- Stiffness in stifle joints
- Cracking joints
- Warts
- Sycotic traits

Modalities

WORSE/AGGRAVATED BY: Change from wet to dry weather, 4–5am, damp environment, wet or humid weather, tight-fitting tack, rest

BETTER/AMELIORATED BY: Dry weather, pressure, changing position, open air

Remedy Interactions

WORKS WELL WITH: Nat mur, Thuja, Belladonna, Arsenicum album, Calc carb, Calc sulph, Sepia, Sulphur, Pulsatilla

CONSIDER ALSO: Nat mur, Sulphur, Nitric acid, Silica, Merc sol, Nux vomica, Chelidonium, Pulsatilla, Aurum, Medorrhinum

Principal Equine Indications

- Conditions arising from damp weather or damp conditions
- Acute and chronic hepatitis
- Jaundice
- Tenderness over the liver region
- Low-grade flatulent colic
- Head injuries or falls
- Effects of concussion including epilepsy
- Meningitis
- COPD, RAO, which is markedly bad in damp wet weather
- Urethritis
- Penile warts
- Warts near anal region or flaps of nostrils
- General stiffness in damp weather where the horse has to keep shifting position
- Inflammation around the coronary band

Nitricum acidum, Nit ac, Acid nit

COMMON NAME: Nitric acid, Aqua fortis

CLASSIFICATION: Mineral: Nitricums: Polycrest

PREPARATION: From a solution in distilled water

Keynotes

- Unforgiving, vindictive nature
- Suspicious
- Resentful
- Obstinate
- Malicious
- Feels threatened all the time
- Oversensitive to noises
- Chilly, feels the cold
- Acts especially where mucous membranes meet the skin – mouth, eyes, anal region and genital regions
- Sycosis
- Rough jagged bleeding warts
- Bleeding skin ulcers with raw flesh appearance
- Blisters and ulcers on the tongue, mouth, genital region
- Offensive discharges
- Bleeding from capillaries
- Corneal ulceration
- Sore bleeding nostrils
- Chronic, yellow nasal catarrh
- Soft spongy bleeding gums
- Eats indigestible things such as soil
- Pain in the rectum after passing dung
- Haemorrhage from the bowels
- Offensive dark urine
- Uterine haemorrhage
- Ulcers around the vulva

Modalities

WORSE/AGGRAVATED BY: During the evening, at night, cold weather, warm weather, touch, exertion,

BETTER/AMELIORATED BY: None listed

Remedy Interactions

WORKS WELL WITH: Calc carb, Pulsatilla, Sulphur, Thuja, Arsenicum album, Caladium, Lac caninum, Sepia

INCOMPATIBLE WITH: Lachesis, Nat mur

CONSIDER ALSO: Agaricus, Arsenicum album, Kali

carb, Kreosotum, Medorrhinum, Merc sol, Nux vomica

Principal Equine Indications

- Exuberant granulation, proud flesh
- Sarcoids
- Melanomas
- Bleeding warts or other skin growths
- Pedunculated warts
- Bleeding growths on the eyelid margins
- Bleeding skin ulcers
- Pemphigus
- Mouth ulcers
- Sores or dermatitis at the mucocutaneous junctions
- Ulcers or growths on the penis or sheath, especially if cauliflower-like
- Haemorrhage of bright red blood
- Capillary haemorrhage especially after curettage
- Corneal ulceration with near perforation of the cornea
- Fly worry leading to ulcerated skin around the eye
- Ulceration and blisters involving the mouth area, especially if viral
- Vesicular stomatitis virus
- Vaginal bleeding between oestrus periods
- Coital exanthema
- CEM
- Phimosis
- Offensive smegma
- Resentment, malicious or overly suspicious behaviour

Nux moschata

COMMON NAME: Nutmeg, *Myristica moschata*
CLASSIFICATION: Plant: Myristicaceae family
PREPARATION: From the powdered seeds

Keynotes

- Fainting due to heart problems
- Dry mucous membranes
- Behaves as if bewildered
- Paralysis of the bowels
- Gaseous distension of the bowel
- Unable to pass dung easily
- Oestrus at variable intervals
- Stiffness from exposure to wet and cold weather

Modalities

WORSE/AGGRAVATED BY: Cold, wet weather, motion, touch, oestrus
BETTER/AMELIORATED BY: Warm dry weather, covering with a rug

Remedy Interactions

WORKS WELL WITH: Lycopodium, Nux vomica, Pulsatilla, Rhus tox, Stramonium, Antimonium tartrate
CONSIDER ALSO: Nux vomica, Pulsatilla, Rhus tox, Ignatia, Gelsemium

Principal Equine Indications

- Mild cases of grass sickness
- Partial paralysis of the colon
- Tympanic colic with gaseous distension

Nux vomica

(see Constitutional Remedies)

Oenanthe crocata

COMMON NAME: Water dropwort, Hemlock dropwort
CLASSIFICATION: Plant: Apiaceae (Umbelliferae) family
PREPARATION: From tincture of the fresh root at the time of flowering

Keynotes

- Epilepsy worse during oestrus or pregnancy
- Eclampsia
- Convulsive-like twitching of the facial muscles
- Dilated pupils
- Foaming at the mouth
- Jaws locked
- Convulsive movements of the limbs
- Opisthotonus

Modalities

WORSE/AGGRAVATED BY: Drinking water
BETTER/AMELIORATED BY: None listed

Remedy Interactions

CONSIDER ALSO: Cicuta, Bufo, Causticum, Cuprum, Hyoscyamus

Principal Equine Indications
- Tetanus
- Opisthotonus
- Epilepsy especially where the facial muscles twitch predominantly

Oleander, Nerium odorum

COMMON NAME: Rose Laurel
CLASSIFICATION: Plant; Apocynaceae family
PREPARATION: From tincture of the leaves

Keynotes
- Acts on the skin, heart and nervous system
- Skin eruptions on the head
- Moist eczema near the ears
- Weakness of the hind limbs, paralysis
- Sensitive skin
- Itchy eruptions which ooze and bleed

Modalities
WORSE/AGGRAVATED BY: None listed
BETTER/AMELIORATED BY: None listed

Remedy Interactions
WORKS WELL WITH: Lycopodium, Nat mur, Pulsatilla, Rhus tox, Sepia
CONSIDER ALSO: Graphites, Merc sol, Psorinum, Sulphur, Petroleum

Principal Equine Indications
- Lice
- Moist, sticky eczema
- Skin chafing, sore skin, skin lesions caused by friction
- Mud fever
- Dermatitis affecting the head area

Opium

COMMON NAME: Latex of the Opium poppy, *Papaver somniferum*
CLASSIFICATION: Plant: Papaveraceae family
PREPARATION: From tincture of the gummy latex from the unripe capsule

Keynotes
- Insensibility of the nervous system
- Stupor and torpor
- Drowsiness
- Sluggishness
- Loss of consciousness
- Coma
- Lack of reaction
- Stertorous breathing
- Sweaty skin
- Pupils contracted
- Ptosis
- Facial twitching especially at the corners of the mouth
- Paralysed tongue
- Bloated tympanic abdomen
- Colic
- Severe constipation with absence of straining
- Spasmodic retention of dung in the colon
- Feeble urination
- Retention of urine
- Loss of bladder control, bladder paralysis
- Irregular oestrus cycles following a fright or accident
- Puerperal convulsions
- Opisthotonus; arching of the back
- Twitching of limbs
- Jerky movements of the limbs as if the flexor muscles were overreacting
- Sweaty skin

Modalities
WORSE/AGGRAVATED BY: During and after sleep, heat, sweating, fear or fright
BETTER/AMELIORATED BY: Walking around, cold air

Remedy Interactions
WORKS WELL WITH: Aconite, Alumina, Belladonna, Bryonia, Hyoscyamus, Nux vomica, Nux moschata, Antimonium tartrate, Phosphorus, Plumbum
CONSIDER ALSO: Gelsemium, Apis, Belladonna, Nux moschata, Nux vomica, Arnica, Baptisia

Principal Equine Indications
- Lack of reaction to indicated remedies
- Conditions arising as a result of shock or fright even if some time in the past
- Slow recovery from general anaesthesia
- State of coma
- Effects of concussion

- Tympanic colic
- Severe impacted colic
- Bowel stasis
- Grass sickness
- Constipation; retention of dung; lack of peristaltic movements
- Intussusception
- Bowel obstruction
- Meconium retention
- Urinary retention
- Bladder paralysis
- Stringhalt
- Jerky movements
- Tetanus
- Epilepsy especially when triggered by bright light
- Lead poisoning
- Sunstroke, heat exhaustion
- Shaker foal syndrome – later stages
- Neonatal maladjustment syndrome
- African horse sickness

Origanum

COMMON NAME: Sweet marjoram, *Origanum marjorana*
CLASSIFICATION: Plant: Lamiaceae (Labiatae) family
PREPARATION: From tincture of the whole fresh plant

Keynotes
- Aroused sexual impulses
- Hysterical behaviour

Modalities
WORSE/AGGRAVATED BY: None listed
BETTER/AMELIORATED BY: None listed

Remedy Interactions
CONSIDER ALSO: Platina, Valerian, Cantharis, Hyoscyamus, Murex, Ustilago

Principal Equine Indications
- Nymphomania
- Sudden impulses to run away

Osmium

COMMON NAME: Osmium the metal
CLASSIFICATION: Mineral: Metal: Element
PREPARATION: Trituration of the precipitated metal

Keynotes
- Acts on the respiratory system
- Tracheal pain
- Catarrh and cough with tough stringy mucus
- Glaucoma
- Eye pain with lachrymation (excess tear production)
- Conjunctivitis with photophobia
- Eczema of the lower limbs, itchy eruptions

Modalities
WORSE/AGGRAVATED BY: None listed
BETTER/AMELIORATED BY: None listed

Remedy Interactions
CONSIDER ALSO: Iridium, Selenium, Tellurium, Thallium, Platina, Palladium

Principal Equine Indications
- Glaucoma
- Conjunctivitis with excessive lachrymation and photophobia

Oxalicum acidum

COMMON NAME: Oxalic acid, Sorrel acid
CLASSIFICATION: Mineral
PREPARATION: Trituration

Keynotes
- Acts on the spinal cord
- Motor paralysis
- Limbs weak
- Myelitis
- Spasmodic breathing problems
- Constriction of the larynx and chest
- Vocal cord paralysis
- Dyspnoea
- Pain in the knee joints

Modalities
WORSE/AGGRAVATED BY: Left side, least touch, exercise
BETTER/AMELIORATED BY: After passing dung

Remedy Interactions – None listed
CONSIDER ALSO: Picric acid, Arsenicum album,

Argentum metallicum, Causticum

Principal Equine Indications
- Meningitis
- Myelitis
- Paralysis as a result of myelitis
- Hind limb paralysis or weakness of spinal origin

Oxytropis

COMMON NAME: Loco weed, rattle weed, *Oxytropis lamberti*
CLASSIFICATION: Plant: Fabiaceae (Leguminosae) family
PREPARATION: Tincture of the fresh plant

Keynotes
- Acts on the nervous system
- Walks backwards
- Paralysis
- Staggering gait
- Loss of coordination
- Relaxed sphincters
- Loss of reflexes
- Pupils contracted
- Nerves and muscles of the eye paralysed

Modalities
WORSE/AGGRAVATED BY: Alternate days
BETTER/AMELIORATED BY: After rest

Remedy Interactions
CONSIDER ALSO: Lathyrus, Oxalic acid

Principal Equine Indications
- Neurological problems relating to coordination and paralysis
- Nerve paralysis leading to loss of coordination, uneven gait or staggering
- Wobbler syndrome
- Cauda equina neuritis
- Equine protazoal myeloencephalitis
- Weak sphincters

Palladium

COMMON NAME: Palladium the metal
CLASSIFICATION: Mineral: Metal
PREPARATION: By trituration

Keynotes
- Acts on the female reproductive system especially the ovaries
- Inflammation of the ovaries
- Pain and swelling of the right ovary
- Uterine prolapse
- Pelvic peritonitis
- Irregular oestrus cycles
- Cystic ovaries
- Easily upset or offended
- Inclined to kick out or bite
- Egotistical

Modalities
WORSE/AGGRAVATED BY: Local pressure over the ovary
BETTER/AMELIORATED BY: Rest, sleep

Remedy Interactions
WORKS WELL WITH: Platina
CONSIDER ALSO: Iridium, Osmium and Platina (close allies); Apis, Graphites, Podophyllum and Platina (right-ovarian remedies); Argentum metallicum, Lachesis, Lilium tigrinum, Actea rac and Sulphur (left-ovarian remedies)

Principal Equine Indications
- Ovarian dysfunction
- Cystic ovaries especially on the right side
- Irregular cycles
- Uterine prolapse
- Pyometria
- Poor libido in the mare
- Ailments from wounded pride

Paraffin, Paraffinum

COMMON NAME: Purified paraffin
CLASSIFICATION: Mineral: Carbons
PREPARATION: Trituration

Keynotes
- Affects the bowels, spine and uterus
- Severe constipation
- Chronic constipation with straining to no effect
- Milky uterine discharge
- Painful nipples
- Spinal pain
- Burns

Modalities

WORSE/AGGRAVATED BY: None listed
BETTER/AMELIORATED BY: None listed

Remedy Interactions

CONSIDER ALSO: Naphthaline, Petroleum, Kreosotum, Sepia, Murex, Nat mur

Principal Equine Indications

- Constipation
- Bowel obstruction
- Mild impacted colic in foals
- Painful nipples

Pareira brava

COMMON NAME: Virgin Vine, Velvet Leaf
CLASSIFICATION: Plant: Menispermaceae family
PREPARATION: From the fresh root

Keynotes

- Acts on the urinary system
- Kidney pain
- Dark urine containing much blood and mucus
- Constant straining
- Dribbling of urine after urination
- Bladder painful and distended
- Inflammation of the urethra

Modalities

WORSE/AGGRAVATED BY: None listed
BETTER/AMELIORATED BY: None listed

Remedy Interactions

Consider also: Hydrangea, Berberis vulgaris, Sarsaparilla, Causticum, Chimaphila

Principal Equine Indications

- Urethral calculi - symptomatic treatment
- Urethritis

Petroleum

COMMON NAME: Crude rock oil, Coal oil, Rock spirit
CLASSIFICATION: Mineral: Carbons
PREPARATION: Trituration and tincture of the rectified oil

Keynotes

- Acts on the skin especially on the sebaceous and sweat glands
- Sticky moist eczema patches on the head or ears
- Skin cracked, rough, leathery or fissured, dirty looking
- Thick green skin crusts
- Red raw skin, bleeds easily
- Rubs skin until it bleeds
- Suppuration of the skin
- Sweaty with a strong odour
- Intertrigo
- Pressure sores
- Eczema on the eyelid margins
- Dry scurfy skin around the eyes
- Cracked skin around the eyes
- Blepharitis
- Catarrh
- Ulcerated and cracked nostrils
- Sore genital region
- Itchy sore nipples
- Symptoms are worse during the winter
- Conditions arising from transportation
- Long-term stomach and lung problems
- Chronic watery diarrhoea
- Dry cough (only at night)
- Chronic sprains
- Stiffness in the stifle joint
- Joints crack
- Greedy nature
- Irritable nature

Modalities

WORSE/AGGRAVATED BY: Dampness, before and during thunder, travelling in vehicles, winter
BETTER/AMELIORATED BY: Warm air, dry weather

Remedy Interactions

WORKS WELL WITH: Sepia, Calc carb, Lycopodium, Nux vomica, Pulsatilla, Silica, Sulphur
CONSIDER ALSO: Calc carb, Graphites, Mezerium, Psorinum, Rhus tox, Sepia, Sulphur

Principal Equine Indications

- Mud fever
- Sweet itch
- Thickened, leathery blackened areas of skin
- Hyperkeratosis

- Cracked skin
- Sore nipples
- Lice (symptomatic treatment)
- Chronic eczema with cracked, fissured or raw areas of skin
- Pressure sores
- Eczema of the ear flaps
- Moist or sticky eczema or dermatitis involving the face region or corners of the mouth
- Eczema of the eyelids and margins
- Eruptions and sores in the region of the coronary band
- Drainage of skin toxins (in conjunction with Berberis)
- Chronic stomach and lung problems
- Chronic diarrhoea
- Conditions arising during travel/transportation especially at sea
- Chronic tendon sprains
- Cracking joints
- Joint luxation or subluxation
- Injuries which are slow to heal
- Suppurating wounds or injuries

Phosphoricum acidum, Phos ac

COMMON NAME: Phosphoric acid
CLASSIFICATION: Mineral
PREPARATION: From dilution in distilled water

Keynotes

- Key remedy for debility
- Nervous or emotional exhaustion
- Listless, apathetic behaviour, indifference
- After-effects of acute illness
- Grief
- Intolerance of noise
- Fluid loss, dehydration
- Debilitating diarrhoea
- Watery diarrhoea, involuntary with gas
- Diabetes
- Frequent urination especially at night
- Inflammation of the periosteum
- Distension of the bowel with gas
- Lack of sexual power in the stallion
- Scrotal eczema
- Prepuce swollen
- Growths on the penis
- Debility in the nursing mare
- Limbs weak
- Pain in the joints, bones, periosteum
- Stumbles easily
- Falling out of hair
- Skin ulcers with pus

Modalities

WORSE/AGGRAVATED BY: Touch, evening, night, loss of fluids, wind, snow, exertion, sexual excess
BETTER/AMELIORATED BY: Short sleep, walking

Remedy Interactions

WORKS WELL WITH: China, Nux vomica, Rhus tox, Arsenicum album, Causticum, Lycopodium, Pulsatilla, Sepia, Sulphur, Calc phos, Ferrum phos, Kali phos, Natrum phos
CONSIDER ALSO: Ignatia, China, Nat mur

Principal Equine Indications

- Debility of any kind
- Dehydration and fluid loss
- Nervous or emotional exhaustion
- Effects of grief or shock
- Pining
- 'Homesickness'
- Diabetes mellitus
- Painless watery diarrhoea leading to dehydration
- Preputial or penile growths
- Impotence
- Osteomyelitis
- Sore shins in young horses in training
- Buttress foot (acute cases)
- Urolithiasis
- Alopecia where caused by debility
- Post-viral syndrome, Equine ME
- Effects of heat stroke

Phosphorus

(see Constitutional Remedies)

Physostigma

COMMON NAME: Calabar bean, *Physostigma venenosum*
CLASSIFICATION: Plant: Fabiaceae (Leguminosae) family
PREPARATION: Trituration of the bean

Keynotes
- Affects the nervous system and the eye
- Contraction of the pupils
- Ocular muscles twitch
- Glaucoma
- Excess production of tears, lachrymation
- Spasms of the face muscles
- Pain over the eyes
- Cerebrospinal meningitis
- Spinal irritation
- Tetanic-like rigidity
- Tetanic convulsions
- Muscle cramps
- Ataxia
- Weak pulse
- Heart beat pronounced

Modalities
WORSE/AGGRAVATED BY: Motion, riding, change of weather
BETTER/AMELIORATED BY: Cool air

Remedy Interactions
CONSIDER ALSO: Lathyrus, Oxytropis, Strychnine, Conium, Gelsemium, Ruta

Principal Equine Indications
- Glaucoma
- Eye injuries
- Ataxia
- Chorea
- Progressive loss of muscle on the hind limbs
- Paralysis of the hind limbs
- Tetanus – prevention of

Phytolacca

COMMON NAME: Poke root, *Phytolacca decandra*
CLASSIFICATION: Plant: Phytolaccaceae family
PREPARATION: From tincture of the root, ripe berries or fresh leaves

Keynotes
- Associated with the syphilitic miasm (anti-syphilitic)
- Important remedy for glands, restlessness, prostration and soreness
- Swelling of the glands with heat and inflammation
- Hardening and induration of glands
- Acts on fibrous, osseous (bony) and scar tissue, muscle sheaths and fasciae
- Bone pain
- Chronic rheumatic symptoms
- Inflammation of the throat, appears dark or bluish red
- Pain at the root of the tongue
- Swollen tonsils especially on the right
- Exhudation of thick, yellow mucus
- Difficulty swallowing
- Pharyngitis
- Swelling of the parotid gland, parotitis
- Tetanus
- Opithotonus
- Retarded dentition
- Dental problems, bleeding mouth, blisters, salivation, clenched jaws
- Increased lachrymation
- Mastitis with great sensitivity to touch, affected area hard to the touch
- Mammary tumours
- Mammary abscess
- Cracked and ulcerated nipples
- Increased flow of milk
- Right-sided ovarian pain
- Swelling of the testicles
- Dry hacking cough
- Lumbar back pain
- Pains in the right shoulder, stiffness
- Dry, shrivelled itchy skin, pustules
- Warts and other pigmented masses

Modalities
WORSE/AGGRAVATED BY: Getting wet, rain, exposure to damp cold weather, night, right side, motion
BETTER/AMELIORATED BY: Dry weather, warmth, resting

Remedy Interactions
WORKS WELL WITH: Silica, Symphytum
CONSIDER ALSO: Bryonia, Lac caninum, Calc carb, Rhus tox, Kali iod

Principal Equine Indications
- Stiffness of the neck
- Hardened or enlarged lymph nodes, lymphadenitis
- Pharyngitis

- Sore throat
- Parotitis
- Glossitis (inflammation of the tongue)
- Difficulty swallowing
- Adenovirus, Rhinovirus infections
- Strangles
- Mastitis
- Mammary abscess
- Hard masses with the mammary glands
- Cracked, painful or sore nipples
- Abnormal lactation
- Bone pain, diseased bone
- Periostitis
- Ligament or tendon injuries at point of insertion on the periostium
- Distal sesamoidean ligament strains
- Conditions associated with eruption of teeth
- Warts
- Smaller pigmented sarcoids

Picricum acidum

COMMON NAME: Picric acid, Trinitrophenol
CLASSIFICATION: Mineral: Carbons
PREPARATION: From solution in rectified spirit

Keynotes

- Degeneration of the spinal cord
- Paralysis
- Prostration and weakness
- Dementia
- Back pain
- Muscular debility
- Limbs tired and heavy
- Myelitis
- Uraemia with little output of urine
- Nephritis
- Sexual excitement
- Satyriasis, increased sexual desire
- Anaemia
- Chronic conjunctivitis with profuse thick yellow discharge

Modalities

WORSE/AGGRAVATED BY: Least exertion, mental effort, after sleep, wet weather, hot weather
BETTER/AMELIORATED BY: Cold air, cold water

Remedy Interactions

CONSIDER ALSO: Oxalic acid, Gelsemium, Phosphorus, Silica, Conium, Ustilago, Murex, Phos ac

Principal Equine Indications

- Locomotor ataxia, weakness of the hind limbs
- Spinal cord degeneration
- Myelitis
- Paralysis of acute onset
- Cauda equina neuritis
- Equine protozoal myeloencephalitis
- Debility and senility in aged horses
- Satyriasis (over-sexed male behaviour)

Pilocarpus microphyllus

COMMON NAME: Jaborandi, Pilocarpinum, Pilocarpine
CLASSIFICATION: Plant: Rutaceae family
PREPARATION: From a solution of the alkaloid in distilled water

Keynotes

- Glandular stimulant
- Induces sweating
- Increased salivation
- Increased tear production
- Increased bronchial secretions
- Cough with difficulty breathing
- Oedema of the lungs
- Constricted pupils
- Staring eyes

Modalities

WORSE/AGGRAVATED BY: None listed
BETTER/AMELIORATED BY: None listed

Remedy Interactions – None listed

Principal Equine Indications

- Excessive sweating
- Fluid (oedema) in the lungs
- Inflamed bronchial mucous membranes with thin watery mucus
- Salivation and parotitis

Pix liquida

COMMON NAME: Liquid tar, Pine tar
CLASSIFICATION: Plant based
PREPARATION: Tincture derived by distillation of coniferous wood

Keynotes

- Acts on mucous membranes and the skin
- Bronchial irritation after viral infection
- Scaly, itchy skin eruptions
- Cracked skin, bleeds when rubbed
- Alopecia, hair loss

Modalities

WORSE/AGGRAVATED BY: None listed
BETTER/AMELIORATED BY: None listed

Remedy Interactions

CONSIDER ALSO: Petroleum, Kreosotum

Principal Equine Indications

- Mud fever
- Dermatitis in the region of and above the heels and around the coronary band
- Chronic sweet itch
- Skin lesions characterised by severe itching with scaling and cracked or fissured skin
- Skin which bleeds when scratched
- Alopecia with skin irritation
- Chronic bronchitis
- Persistent cough as a result of an infection with any of the respiratory viruses

Platina

COMMON NAME: Platinum, Platinum metallicum
CLASSIFICATION: Mineral: Metal: Element
PREPARATION: Trituration

Keynotes

- Principally a female remedy
- Bay-coloured mares especially
- Arrogance, proud nature, egocentric, aloof, dignified
- Contemptuous
- Destructive
- Impulse to injure or kill
- Nymphomania
- Hysterical behaviour
- Depression
- Ovarian pain
- Irregular oestrus cycles
- Itching around the vulva
- Numb sensation in the limbs
- Syphilitic tendency

Modalities

WORSE/AGGRAVATED BY: Evening, night, standing around, touch, warmth of stable
BETTER/AMELIORATED BY: Outside on gentle rides

Remedy Interactions

WORKS WELL WITH: Palladium, Belladonna, Ignatia, Lycopodium, Pulsatilla, Rhus tox, Sepia
CONSIDER ALSO: Anacardium, Cuprum, Gratiola, Ignatia, Lillium tigrinum, Medorrhinum, Nux vomica, Plumbum, Stannum

Principal Equine Indications

- Rejection of foal
- Mismothering
- Nymphomania, mareish behaviour
- Haughty arrogant behaviour
- Mares with tendency to bite or kick
- Vexation (displeasure), contemptuous nature
- Anxious over trifles
- 'Silly' moods
- Irregular oestrus cycles
- Cystic ovaries
- Refusal to accept the stallion during breeding
- Spermatorrhoea

Plumbum metallicum

COMMON NAME: Lead
CLASSIFICATION: Mineral: Metal: Plumbums: Element
PREPARATION: Trituration

Keynotes

- Important remedy for paralysis and the nervous system in general
- Symptoms appear slowly and are progressive
- Neuritis
- Anaemia, pale mucous membranes
- Jaundice

- State of delirium
- Depression, impaired memory
- Coma
- Convulsions
- Pupils constricted
- Glaucoma
- Optic neuritis
- Muscle atrophy, muscle wasting
- Ataxia
- Paralysis and weakness of the hind limbs
- Paralysis of single muscles
- Paralysis of the tongue
- Cramping
- Muscle twitching, tingling, numbness, tremors
- Emaciation
- Sclerosis
- Acute and chronic nephritis
- Straining to pass urine
- Severe colic with arching of the back to ease the pain
- Bowel obstructed or impacted
- Intussusception
- Hernia
- Abdominal pain with a tucked-up abdomen
- Constipation with hard dung, urge to pass dung
- Constriction of the anus
- Loss of sexual power in the stallion
- Hardening of the mammary glands
- Abortion

Modalities

WORSE/AGGRAVATED BY: At night, motion, touch
BETTER/AMELIORATED BY: Massage, rubbing, hard pressure, exercise, rest, arching the back, stretching the limbs

Remedy Interactions

WORKS WELL WITH: Arsenicum album, Belladonna, Lycopodium, Merc sol, Phosphorus, Pulsatilla, Silica, Sulphur, Rhus tox, Thallium
CONSIDER ALSO: Opium, Nux vomica, Phosphorus, Picric acid, Alumina, Platina, Zinc

Principal Equine Indications

- Paralysis of various areas or individual muscles
- Loss of nerve function
- Radial paralysis, facial paralysis
- Sweeny with muscle wasting
- Crural paralysis
- Myelitis
- Muscle wasting weakness or paralysis of the hind limbs
- Ataxia, weakness of the hind limbs
- Cauda equina neuritis
- Impacted colic
- Obstruction of the bowel
- Grass sickness
- Difficulty swallowing, paralysis of the throat
- Constipation
- Acute and chronic kidney disease, nephritis
- Anaemia from bone marrow suppression
- Anaemia caused by poisoning or from kidney disease
- Depression of the bone marrow
- Jaundice
- Epilepsy
- Emaciation and weakness
- Infections with neurological symptoms, encephalitis
- Dourine
- Equine protozoal myeloencephalitis
- EHV-1 – neurological symptoms

Podophyllum

COMMON NAME: May apple, *Podophyllum peltatum*
CLASSIFICATION: Plant: Berberidaceae or Ranunculaceae family
PREPARATION: From the whole fresh plant, root or ripe fruit

Keynotes

- Acts on the digestive system and liver
- Gastroenteritis with colic-like pain
- Profuse watery dung with mucus like jelly
- Offensive diarrhoea
- Green watery diarrhoea, gushes out effortlessly
- Long-standing diarrhoea especially bad in the morning
- Rectal proplapse
- Alternation of diarrhoea and constipation
- Jaundice
- Rolling of the head from side to side
- Grinding of the teeth
- Increased thirst for large amounts
- Distended abdomen

- Right-sided ovarian pain
- Uterine prolapse

Modalities

WORSE/AGGRAVATED BY: Touch, motion, morning especially early morning, hot weather
BETTER/AMELIORATED BY: Rubbing, rest, open air

Remedy Interactions

WORKS WELL WITH: Ipecac, Nux vomica, Calc carb, Sulphur, Nat mur, Calc sulph
CONSIDER ALSO: Sulphur, Natrum sulph, Chamomilla, Veratrum album, Aloe, Arsenicum album, Gambogia

Principal Equine Indications

- Diarrhoea especially in foals
- Diarrhoea from dietary causes
- Diarrhoea with colic-like pain or teeth grinding
- Profuse watery green diarrhoea
- Chronic diarrhoea
- Equine rotavirus infection
- Uterine prolapse after foaling
- Rectal prolapse

Prunus spinosa

COMMON NAME: Blackthorn, sloe
CLASSIFICATION: Plant: Rosaceae family
PREPARATION: From a tincture of the buds before flowering

Keynotes

- Acts on the urinary system and head area
- Neuralgic pains in the head
- Choroiditis
- Ascites, oedema
- Sprains
- Rapid, furious heartbeat
- Straining to urinate
- Takes a long time to pass urine

Modalities

WORSE/AGGRAVATED BY: Touch, pressure, motion, night
BETTER/AMELIORATED BY: Rest

Remedy Interactions

CONSIDER ALSO: Crataegus, Laurocerasus

Principal Equine Indications

- Swelling, oedema of lower limbs
- Tendon or ligament sprains
- Glaucoma
- Opacity of the vitreous humor

Psorinum

COMMON NAME: Scabies, Scabies vesicle
CLASSIFICATION: Animal: Nosode
PREPARATION: Trituration

Keynotes

- Important remedy for skin conditions
- Conditions associated with the psoric miasm
- Very sensitive to cold weather, feels the cold easily, the 'chilly Sulphur'
- Dirty, smelly filthy skin
- Dry matted coat, lustreless, rough
- Intense itching, worse for covering up
- Skin eruptions in the bends of the joints, crusty eruptions
- Secretion of excess grease, seborrhoeic skin and coat
- Skin eruptions in the region of the hooves
- Sweats easily
- Sticky, weepy eczema on the head
- Discharges offensive
- State of debility
- Weakness after acute illness
- Lack of reaction; weakened immune system or when other remedies fail to work
- Sad and depressed
- Always hungry
- Eyes sticky, blepharitis
- Chronic conjunctivitis
- Cracks and scabs at the corner of the mouth
- Red raw sticky eczema with irritation affecting the ears
- Foul-smelling saliva
- Chronic catarrh
- Sticky mucus in the throat
- Foul-smelling dung with mucus and blood
- Udders swollen and painful
- Difficulty breathing with dry hard cough

Modalities

WORSE/AGGRAVATED BY: Change of weather, hot

sunshine, cold weather, cold draughts, riding
BETTER/AMELIORATED BY: Heat, warmth, from being covered by a rug (except skin symptoms), rest

Remedy Interactions
WORKS WELL WITH: Sulphur, Bacillinum (acute), Sepia, Tuberculinum
INCOMPATIBLE WITH: Lachesis, Conium
CONSIDER ALSO: Sulphur, Nat mur, Lycopodium, Graphites, Calc carb, Petroleum

Principal Equine Indications
- Conditions associated with psoric miasm
- Cases which fail to respond to indicated remedies or which only improve for a short time
- Hopeless cases
- Chronic skin problems, eczema, dermatitis
- Dry, lustreless, dull coat and skin especially with a musty smell
- Greasy, oily, seborrhoic skin, seborrhoea
- Severe itching, sweet itch
- Recurrent urticaria
- Mud fever and other skin conditions, including those around the hoof and coronary band area
- Moist sticky skin eruptions
- Poor hoof quality, cracked, dry flaking hooves
- Parasitic skin conditions, lice, mites
- Ringworm
- Debility
- To promote recovery after acute illness
- Chronic catarrh which has a foul odour
- Chronic conjunctivitis, blepharitis
- Intractable corneal ulcers
- Smegma (use constitutionally)
- Post-viral syndrome, Equine ME

Ptelea

COMMON NAME: Wafer ash, Hop tree, *Ptelea trifoliata*
CLASSIFICATION: Plant: Rutaceae family
PREPARATION: From a tincture of the bark or root

Keynotes
- Acts on the stomach and liver
- Excess salivation
- Liver swollen and sensitive to palpation

Modalities
WORSE/AGGRAVATED BY: Lying on the left side, not stable, after sleep, afternoon
BETTER/AMELIORATED BY: Morning, evening

Remedy Interactions
CONSIDER ALSO: Nux vomica, Chelidonium, Merc sol

Principal Equine Indications
- Hepatitis
- Jaundice
- Congestion of the liver
- As a liver drainage remedy, to drain away toxins

Pulsatilla

(see Constitutional Remedies)

Pyrogenium, Pyrogen

COMMON NAME: Artificial sepsin, Pyrexin, Rotten meat
CLASSIFICATION: Animal
PREPARATION: From a dilution of decomposed beef in water allowed to stand in the sun for two or three weeks

Keynotes
- Fever and sepsis, septic infections
- Localised or systemic sepsis
- Infected, pussy wounds
- Offensive discharges
- Anxiety, restlessness; has to keep moving to ease the symptoms
- Black foul-smelling diarrhoea
- Constipation with inertia of the bowel
- Palpitation of the heart
- Abnormally rapid pulse, not in proportion to the body temperature
- Thready, weak pulse

Modalities
WORSE/AGGRAVATED BY: Cold, damp weather
BETTER/AMELIORATED BY: Warmth, stretching, moving around

Remedy Interactions

WORKS WELL WITH: Bryonia, Arsenicum album, Lachesis, Rhus tox

CONSIDER ALSO: Echinacea, Carbo veg, Lachesis, Baptisia, Arsenicum album, Rhus tox, Opium, Plumbum, Tarentula cubensis, Anthracinum

Principal Equine Indications

- Septicaemia, toxaemia, sepsis with fever with marked sweating and shivering
- High fever where other remedies do not work
- High fever with sepsis
- Stubborn cases where indicated remedies fail to act
- Septic fevers with sweating and high temperature
- Severe cases of lymphangitis
- Infected, septic wounds especially involving the limbs
- Infected wounds arising from the smallest injury
- Foul-smelling wounds
- Recurrent sepsis or abscessation in a wound
- Fistulae especially involving bone
- Peritonitis
- Post-partum metritis
- Pyometria, toxic metritis
- Pneumonia
- After-effects of abortion
- Retention of the afterbirth
- Severe, foul diarrhoea expelled with no effort
- Severe diarrhoea or enteritis with septicaemia, colitis X
- Impaction of the bowel
- Grass sickness
- Chronic skin ulcers
- Navel ill
- Septic arthritis
- Quittor
- Sole abscess, under-run sole
- Laminitis with a septic focus
- Infected insect bites
- Nephritis, pyelonephritis
- Abscesses accompanied by a fever
- Myositis
- Equine flu
- Sleepy foal disease

Quercus robur

COMMON NAME: English oak
CLASSIFICATION: Plant: Corylaceae family
PREPARATION: From a tincture of acorns

Keynotes

- Helps with conditions related to the spleen
- Ascites
- Puffy lower eyelids
- Foul breath

Modalities

WORSE/AGGRAVATED BY: None listed
BETTER/AMELIORATED BY: None listed

Remedy Interactions – None listed

Principal Equine Indications

- Cushing's disease
- Enlargement of the spleen

Radium, Radium bromatum, Rad brom

COMMON NAME: Radium bromide
CLASSIFICATION: Mineral
PREPARATION: Trituration

Keynotes

- Weakness and debility
- Affects the joints
- Severe joint pain especially in the stifle and hock
- Pains in the fetlock, pastern and coffin joints
- Rheumatic-like symptoms
- Sore muscles
- Weak hooves
- Skin ulcers, skin growths
- Depressed nature, irritable
- Cramping pains in the bowel with rumbling noises, gassy
- Nephritis
- Pains in the neck especially in the cervical vertebrae worse with the head down
- Lumbar and sacral back pain relieved by movement
- Small pimples on the skin, itchy dermatitis

Modalities

WORSE/AGGRAVATED BY: On first getting up, warmth of rug, at night, early hours of the morning
BETTER/AMELIORATED BY: Continued movement, in the open air, sleep, pressure

Remedy Interactions

WORKS WELL WITH: Rhus tox
CONSIDER ALSO: Rhus tox, Sepia, Uranium, Arsenicum album

Principal Equine Indications

- Arthritis, DJD especially the stifles, lower limbs – fetlock, coffin, pastern joints, metacarpal (knee) and metatarsal (hock) joints, symptoms eased by movement
- Chronic joint pain especially with restlessness
- Sarcoids (especially those which are pigmented)
- Melanoma
- After radiotherapy, supportive treatment

Rhododendron

COMMON NAME: Snow rose, *Rhododendron chrysanthum*
CLASSIFICATION: Plant: Ericaceae family
PREPARATION: From a tincture of the fresh leaves

Keynotes

- Arthritic and rheumatic symptoms
- Swollen joints
- Stiff neck
- Pains in the shoulder, forelegs and knee (carpal) joints
- Bone pain
- Worse before a storm
- Tooth pain
- Swollen testicles

Modalities

WORSE/AGGRAVATED BY: Before a storm, thunder, night, near morning, for touch, rest, rough weather, easterly winds, wet cold weather
BETTER/AMELIORATED BY: Warmth, feeding, after the storm breaks, on starting to move, covering with a rug

Remedy Interactions

CONSIDER ALSO: Dulcamara, Rhus tox, Nat sulph, Ruta

Principal Equine Indications

- Swollen stiff joints, general stiffness
- Stiffness of the neck and shoulder region
- Lyme disease
- Orchitis
- Hydrocele
- Fear of thunderstorms

Rhus toxicodendron, Rhus tox

COMMON NAME: Poison ivy
CLASSIFICATION: Plant: Anacardaceae: Polycrest
PREPARATION: From a tincture of the fresh leaves picked just before flowering

Keynotes

- Key actions on the skin, and fibrous tissue generally including tendons, tendon sheaths, ligaments as well as joints, the genital area, glands, mucous membranes, nerves and spinal cord
- Pain and stiffness typically better for movement and warmth, worse for rest and wet, damp or cold weather
- Restlessness, has to keep moving to ease pain or stiffness
- Worse on moving initially but continued motion eases the symptoms
- Mental stiffness, sadness
- Anxious, fearful of what may happen, impatient
- Easily vexed
- Conditions arising from overuse or getting wet
- Condition arising after fright
- Sepsis, septicaemia, cellulitis
- Marked restlessness
- Better for a change of position
- Apprehensive at night
- Swollen, red, oedematous eyes, cellulitis around the eyes
- Eyelids stuck together (agglutinated)
- Pustular inflammation
- Photophobia with discharge of yellow pussy material
- Iritis
- Eye injuries
- Corneal ulceration
- Blood vessel invasion of the cornea
- Nose sore and ulcerated

- Sneezing after getting wet
- Face swollen, parotitis
- Facial neuralgia (pain)
- Swollen glands
- Corners of the mouth ulcerated
- Abdominal pain, colic better for arching the back
- Abdominal distention
- Bloody diarrhoea with mucus, dysentery
- Bloody urine
- Intense itching and swelling of scrotum
- Swollen vulva with itching
- Uterine prolapse
- Inflammation of the testes (orchitis)
- Dry cough
- Bleeding of bright red blood from the lungs after exertion
- Enlargement of the heart
- Back pain, stiffness worse for rest, eases on movement
- Swollen, inflamed joints
- Legs stiff, almost as if paralysed from cold weather
- Skin itches intensely
- Skin red and swollen, vesicles, urticaria, pemphigus, scaling

Modalities

WORSE/AGGRAVATED BY: Wet, cold weather, change of weather, autumn, winter, damp stabling, at time of initial movement, after rest, over-exertion, over-use, before a storm, after midnight, cloudy days, evening, night

BETTER/AMELIORATED BY: Continued motion, heat, warmth, rubbing or massage, open air, covering with a rug

Remedy Interactions

WORKS WELL WITH: Belladonna, Bryonia, Calc carb (chronic), Calc fluor, Calc phos, Causticum, Conium, Graphites, Nux vom, Lycopodium, Mag carb, Medorrhinum, Phosphorus, Pulsatilla, Sepia, Sulphur, Tuberculinum

INCOMPATIBLE WITH: Apis

CONSIDER ALSO: Arnica, Apis, Bryonia, Dulcamara, Causticum, Calc carb, Ruta grav

Principal Equine Indications

- Arthritis, DJD, lameness, stiffness where modalities agree
- Tendon, tendon sheath and ligament injuries, strains
- Muscle injuries, tears or strains especially the larger muscles of the body
- Myositis
- Back and neck pain, stiff neck
- Bone pain
- Bursitis
- Carpitis
- Suspensory ligament strains
- Bone spavin
- Curb
- Cunean bursitis
- Tying up, azoturia
- Conditions arising from getting wet, from damp, from over exertion
- Restlessness caused by pain, unable to stay in one place for too long
- Allergic conjunctivitis
- Orbital cellulitis
- Iritis
- Periodic ophthalmia
- Fly worry
- Conjunctivitis with swollen eyelids and yellow gummy discharge
- Corneal ulceration
- Parotitis
- EIPH
- Cellulitis
- Itching of the skin, urticaria
- Allergic skin conditions, rashes, erythema, (reddening), vesicular eruptions
- Effects of insect bites or stings
- Sweet itch
- Rainscald
- Hyperkeratosis
- Photosensitisation
- Mud fever
- Pemphigus
- Mites (symptomatic treatment)
- Orchitis
- Scrotal eczema, dermatitis
- Coital exanthema
- Smegma with local irritation
- Dermatitis, eczema of the vulva
- Eczema on the ear flaps
- Ulceration of the corners of the mouth
- Lymphangitis

- Watery mucoid diarrhoea
- Septicaemia, symptoms eased by sweating
- Loss of balance especially on first getting up
- Tongue ulcers
- Colic from getting wet through
- Yellow mushy diarrhoea
- Equine viral arteritis
- EHV-1 early stages

Rhus veneata

COMMON NAME: Poison elder, Poison sumach
CLASSIFICATION: Plant: Anacardiaceae family
PREPARATION: From tincture of the fresh leaves or stem

Keynotes

- Itching of the skin
- Vesicles
- Skin inflamed and dark red in colour

Modalities

WORSE/AGGRAVATED BY: Hot weather, in the morning
BETTER/AMELIORATED BY: None listed

Remedy Interactions

WORKS WELL WITH: Rhus tox

Principal Equine Indications

- Allergic skin reactions
- Intensely red inflamed irritated skin
- Eczema with vesiculation

Rumex crispus

COMMON NAME: Yellow dock, Curled dock
CLASSIFICATION: Plant: Polygonaceae family
PREPARATION: Tincture of the fresh root

Keynotes

- Tickling, dry cough
- Touching the throat induces coughing
- Breathing in cold air induces coughing
- Cough triggered by eating
- Laryngitis accompanied by a dry cough
- Marked mucous discharge from the nose
- Mucus in the trachea
- Intense itching of the skin especially of the lower limbs
- Urticaria
- Enlarged lymphatic vessels
- Chronic inflammation of the stomach
- Brown watery diarrhoea
- Anal irritation

Modalities

WORSE/AGGRAVATED BY: Evening, night, inhalation of cold air, left side of chest, being uncovered, touch, change of temperature, lying down, at a walk
BETTER/AMELIORATED BY: Warmth, heat

Remedy Interactions

CONSIDER ALSO: Bryonia, Sticta, Spongia, Phosphorus

Principal Equine Indications

- Dry teasing cough, triggered by cold air or by touching the larynx
- Dry spasmodic coughs
- Laryngeal catarrh
- Bronchial catarrh
- Nasal catarrh which is thin and runny with tickly, nervous cough
- Dermatitis of the lower limbs
- Enlarged lymphatic vessels

Ruta graveolens, Ruta grav

COMMON NAME: Rue, Bitterwort
CLASSIFICATION: Plant: Rutaceae family
PREPARATION: From tincture of the whole plant

Keynotes

- Specific action on bone, cartilage, tendons and tendon sheaths
- Injuries to bone
- Bruises
- Affinity for the smaller joints
- Exostoses (bony lumps)
- Tendon strains, sprains or injuries
- Contracted tendons
- Back pain eased by pressure
- Weak hind limbs, legs give way suddenly
- Stiffness and pain in the lower limbs eases on movement
- Weakness of the eye muscles
- Difficulty passing dung, straining
- Rectal prolapse

- Restlessness

Modalities

WORSE/AGGRAVATED BY: Rest, on first movement, over exertion, cold, damp, wet weather, going uphill, at night

BETTER/AMELIORATED BY: Continued movement, warmth, massage

Remedy Interactions

WORKS WELL WITH: Calc phos, Arnica, Symphytum, Calc carb, Causticum, Lycopodium, Pulsatilla, Sulphur, Silica

CONSIDER ALSO: Arnica, Rhus tox, Heckla lava, Silica, Causticum

Principal Equine Indications

- Arthritis, DJD especially of the hock, knee, fetlock, pastern and coffin joints
- Sprains and strains, desmitis
- Tendon strains and injuries, tendonitis especially the flexor tendons
- Weak tendons
- Ligament injuries, sprains, inflammation and tears
- Synovitis especially if chronic
- Suspensory ligament injuries
- Superior and inferior check ligament injuries/desmitis
- Sesamoiditis
- Distal sesamoidean ligament strains
- Constriction of the palmar annular ligament
- Rupture of the peroneus tertius
- Carpitis
- Carpal tunnel syndrome
- Bony enlargement, exostoses
- Bone spavin
- Osteochondrosis (OCD)
- Chondromalacia of the patella
- Meniscal tears
- Bruising, trauma to the periosteal layer of bone, periostitis
- Splints
- Sore shins
- Osslets
- Navicular syndrome
- Pedal ostitis
- Sidebone
- Buttress foot
- Fractures, prevention of non-union fractures
- Dislocations, luxations and sub-luxations
- Cartilage injuries
- Bursitis
- Cunean bursitis
- Trochanteric bursitis
- Capped hock
- Capped elbow (where the bone is bruised)
- Curb
- Sore back after spinal manipulation such as osteopathy
- Weak back, lower back pain

Sabadilla

COMMON NAME: Cevadilla seed, *Sabadilla officinarum*

CLASSIFICATION: Plant: Melanthaceae family

PREPARATION: From a tincture of the seeds

Keynotes

- Acts on the mucous membranes of the nose
- Watery, thin, irritant nasal discharge with violent sneezing
- Inflamed eyelids
- Increased tear production
- Sore throat with tough mucus
- Constant need to swallow
- Absence of thirst
- Inflammation under the hoof
- Deformed, thickened hooves
- Dry skin
- Nervous timid nature, easily startled, agitated

Modalities

WORSE/AGGRAVATED BY: Full moon, cold weather, cold air, drinking cold water, lying down

BETTER/AMELIORATED BY: When covered with a rug, warmth

Remedy Interactions

WORKS WELL WITH: Sepia, Bryonia, Arsenicum album, Mercury, Nux vomica, Thuja, Pulsatilla

Consider also; Allium cepa, Arsenicum album, Euphrasia, Pulsatilla, Sanguinaria, Urtica urens

Principal Equine Indications

- Allergic based respiratory problems characterised

by repeated sneezing and a watery nasal discharge
- Allergic based conjunctivitis with red eyes and watery discharge
- Rhinitis
- Headshaking
- Mild cases of COPD
- Catarrh of the throat
- Chronic laminitis where the hoof quality is poor

Sabal serrulata

COMMON NAME: Saw palmetto
CLASSIFICATION: Plant: Arecaceae (Palmaceae) family
PREPARATION: From tincture of the fresh ripe berries and seeds

Keynotes
- Acts on the genital and urinary tracts
- Sexual weakness
- Loss of sexual power
- Prostatic enlargement (unlikely in the horse)
- Epididymitis
- Underdeveloped mammary glands
- Shrinking of the mammary glands
- Ovaries painful and swollen
- Frequent desire to pass urine at night
- Urinary incontinence
- Weak bladder sphincter
- Chronic bronchitis

Modalities
WORSE/AGGRAVATED BY: Early morning, motion
BETTER/AMELIORATED BY: After sleep

Remedy Interactions
CONSIDER ALSO: Merc sol, Apis, Conium, Calc carb, Solidago, Digitalis

Principal Equine Indications
- Poor libido
- Poorly developed udders
- Ovarian pain
- Testicular degeneration

Sabina

COMMON NAME: Savine, *Juniperis sabina*
CLASSIFICATION: Plant: Cupressaceae family
PREPARATION: From tincture of the young fresh branch tops

Keynotes
- Acts on the uterus as well as serous and fibrous membranes
- Pain in the region of the pelvis from the sacrum to the pubis
- Lower back pain
- Arthritic joint pain
- Haemorrhage of fluid blood which clots together
- Abortion
- Increased sexual desire
- Foul uterine discharge
- Retention of the placenta
- Inflammation of the ovaries and uterus after abortion
- Intolerance to music
- Tympanic distension of the abdomen
- Constipation
- Urine containing blood with urging
- Inflammation of the bladder and urethra
- Pus-like preputial discharge
- Warty growths on the penis
- Painful prepuce
- Warts with itching
- Exuberant granulation
- Black marks on the skin

Modalities
WORSE/AGGRAVATED BY: Touch, pressure, moving about, warm air, night, music
BETTER/AMELIORATED BY: Open air, cold

Remedy Interactions
WORKS WELL WITH: Thuja, Arsenicum album, Belladonna, Rhus tox, Spongia
CONSIDER ALSO: Hamamelis, Thuja, Nitric acid, Secale, Caulophyllum, Millefolium, Platina, Crocus, Sepia

Principal Equine Indications
- Infertility in the mare
- Threatened abortion

- After-effects of abortion
- Retained placenta
- Endometritis, pyometria
- CEM
- Nymphomania
- Haemorrhage of fluid bright red blood which clots
- Uterine bleeding
- Post-partum haemorrhage
- Vaginal bleeding between oestrus periods
- Lack of uterine tone
- Phimosis
- Penile growths
- Smegma
- Warts, especially those which itch and bleed
- Sarcoids
- Melanomas
- Skin cysts
- Exuberant granulation

Salicylicum acidum

COMMON NAME: Salicylic acid
CLASSIFICATION: Mineral
PREPARATION: Trituration

Keynotes

- Rheumatic-like stiffness
- Swollen stifle joint
- Acute rheumatism
- Softening and necrosis of bone
- Weakness after viral respiratory infections
- Blood in the urine
- Retinal haemorrhage
- Hot and burning skin
- Urticaria
- Purpura

Modalities

WORSE/AGGRAVATED BY: Touch, motion, night, cold air
BETTER/AMELIORATED BY: Warm applications, dry heat

Remedy Interactions

CONSIDER ALSO: Phosphorus

Principal Equine Indications

- Joint stiffness
- Swollen painful joints, especially the stifle and elbow
- Arthritis especially of the knee, hock, stifle and elbow joints
- Purpura haemorrhagica

Sambucus nigra

COMMON NAME: Elder
CLASSIFICATION: Plant: Caprifoliaceae family
PREPARATION: From tincture of fresh leaves and flowers

Keynotes

- Main action is focused on the respiratory system
- Thick mucus in the larynx
- Suffocative cough or loose cough with mucus
- Asthmatic symptoms
- Filled legs
- Frequent urination
- Acute nephritis
- Sweating

Modalities

WORSE/AGGRAVATED BY: Rest, motion, midnight and after, dry cold air
BETTER/AMELIORATED BY: Covering with a rug

Remedy Interactions

WORKS WELL WITH: Belladonna, Conium, Nux vomica, Phosphorus, Rhus tox, Sepia
CONSIDER ALSO: Kali carb, Kali sulph, Lachesis, Lycopodium, Nux vomica

Principal Equine Indications

- COPD with thick, tacky catarrh and laboured breathing
- Foals with respiratory infections

Sanguinaria

COMMON NAME: Blood root, *Sanguinaria canadensis*
CLASSIFICATION: Plant: Papaveraceae family
PREPARATION: From tincture of the fresh root

Keynotes

- Acts on mucous membranes
- Dry mucous membranes, swollen and hot

- Pre-eminently a right-sided remedy
- Affects the circulation leading to congestion and redness
- Neuralgic pain in the head
- Offensive yellow nasal discharge
- Blood-tinged catarrh
- Nasal polyps
- Chronic rhinitis
- Polyps on the ears
- Swollen throat
- Ulceration of the mouth and throat
- Oedema of the larynx
- Cough with thick sticky mucus
- Spasmodic cough
- Chronic hacking cough
- Severe difficulty breathing
- Chest constricted
- Pneumonia
- Asthma
- Increased thirst
- Sensitivity to cold
- Stiffness in the right shoulder
- Burning sensation in the foot
- Red blotchy itchy skin eruptions

Modalities

WORSE/AGGRAVATED BY: Right side of the body, motion, touch, cold air, damp weather
BETTER/AMELIORATED BY: Sleep, lying on the left side

Remedy Interactions

WORKS WELL WITH: Antimonium tartrate, Phosphorus, Sarsaparilla
CONSIDER ALSO: Opium, Chelidonium Kali sulph, Sabadilla, Sulphur

Principal Equine Indications

- Spasmodic cough following viral infections
- Severe COPD with great difficulty breathing
- Acute right sided pneumonia
- Chronic allergic-based rhinitis
- Haemoptysis
- Pain in the right shoulder region
- Pain in the lower cervical region of the neck
- Bursitis of the shoulder joint
- Ear and nasal polyps

Sanicula

COMMON NAME: Water of Sanicula Springs, Ottawa Illinois USA
CLASSIFICATION: Mineral: Water
PREPARATION: Trituration of the evaporated salt

Keynotes

- Effects of downward motion or jarring
- Excoriation of the skin around the anus and perineum
- No desire until a there is a large accumulation of dung in the rectum then only partially expelled
- Offensive lesions of the feet
- Dirty brown, greasy skin
- Eczema with fissures
- Thick yellow pus
- Dislikes to be touched or looked at

Modalities

WORSE/AGGRAVATED BY: Motion, touch, travelling, descending
BETTER/AMELIORATED BY: Resting, fresh air, warmth

Remedy Interactions

Consider also: Borax, Nat mur, Calc carb, Chamomilla, Silica, Sulphur, Tuberculinum

Principal Equine Indications

- Mud fever
- Thrush
- Seborrhoea (with bad skin odour)
- Poor travellers (travel sickness)
- Weak colonic muscles; constipation
- Soreness of the skin of the perineum and anus
- Strains
- Effects of jarring
- Lumbar and sacral pain
- Wasting
- Where Silica fails to act

Sarsaparilla

COMMON NAME: Wild liquorice, Smilax
CLASSIFICATION: Plant: Smilaceae family
PREPARATION: Trituration and tincture of the root

Keynotes
- Urinary symptoms
- Bloody urine
- Urinary gravel
- Pain at the end of urination
- Dribbling of urine when standing still
- Bladder distended and painful
- Straining to pass urine
- Kidney pain
- Scrotal eczema
- Small retracted nipples
- Emaciated, shrivelled skin
- Itchy eruptions
- Skin cracked around the foot region
- Thickened hardened skin
- Warts
- Tearing pains in the limbs
- Pains in the small bones of the lower limbs
- Pain under the hooves

Modalities
WORSE/AGGRAVATED BY: Springtime, before oestrus, after urinating, at close of urination, motion, cold wet weather

BETTER/AMELIORATED BY: Rest, warmth

Remedy Interactions
WORKS WELL WITH: Hepar sulph, Phosphorus, Rhus tox, Sepia, Sulphur, Merc sol, Apis mel, Allium cepa

CONSIDER ALSO: Berberis, Equisetum, Thuja, Causticum, Lycopodium, Cantharis

Principal Equine Indications
- Chronic laminitis
- Mud fever with deep cracks/fissures in the skin with lameness
- Urinary incontinence, dribbling of urine while standing
- Cystitis
- Urolithiasis, gravel in the bladder
- Small warts with localized hair loss
- Small itchy skin eruptions with hair loss
- Cracked or fissured skin in older horses
- Vaccinosis

Scrophularia nodosa

COMMON NAME: Knotted figwort

CLASSIFICATION: Plant: Scrophulariaceae family

PREPARATION: From tincture of the whole fresh plant

Keynotes
- Enlarged glands
- Eczema of the ear
- Hard nodules in the udder
- Lupoid ulceration
- Skin growths

Modalities
WORSE/AGGRAVATED BY: None listed

BETTER/AMELIORATED BY: None listed

Remedy Interactions
CONSIDER ALSO: Conium, Carcinosin

Principal Equine Indications
- Enlarged lymph nodes, lymphadenitis
- Hard nodular masses in the udder
- Eczema along the ear margins
- Sarcoids

Scutellaria lateriflora

COMMON NAME: Skullcap, Mad dog weed

CLASSIFICATION: Plant: Lamiaceae (Labiatae) family

PREPARATION: From tincture of the fresh plant

Keynotes
- Acts on the central nervous system
- Nervous fear
- Chorea
- Muscle twitching, tremors
- Night-time restlessness

Modalities
WORSE/AGGRAVATED BY: Overwork

BETTER/AMELIORATED BY: Moving around in the open air, sleep

Remedy Interactions
CONSIDER ALSO: Agaricus

Principal Equine Indications

- Anxiety and restlessness especially at night
- Excitement
- Fear-based behavioural problems
- Chorea (involuntary movements)

Secale cornutum, Secale

COMMON NAME: Ergot of rye, *Claviceps purpurea*
CLASSIFICATION: Plant: Fungi
PREPARATION: From the fresh fungus

Keynotes

- Causes contraction of smooth muscles
- Reduction of blood supply to regions of the body especially the lower limbs
- Coldness
- Petechial haemorrhage
- Gangrene
- Emaciation
- Shrivelled skin
- Varicose ulcers
- Haemorrhage with oozing thin watery black blood
- Muscle twitching
- Epistaxis, nosebleed with dark blood
- Dilated pupils
- Cataract
- Sunken eyes
- Face distorted
- Ravenous appetite
- Increased thirst
- Bloody green dung
- Involuntary stools
- Paralysis of the bladder, urinary retention
- Urinary incontinence
- Brown-coloured uterine discharge
- Oozing of dark blood from the uterus between seasons
- Abortion
- Metritis
- Poor milk production
- Spinal irritation
- Ataxia, trembling, staggering gait
- Spasmodic movements
- Violent cramps
- Myelitis
- Impaired circulation to the limbs
- Pain under the hooves

Modalities

WORSE/AGGRAVATED BY: Heat, warm covering over the body, touch, night, before oestrus
BETTER/AMELIORATED BY: Cold, uncovering, massage, stretching out legs, open air, wet applications

Remedy Interactions

WORKS WELL WITH: Arsenicum album, Aconite, Belladonna, Merc sol, Pulsatilla, China, Thuja
CONSIDER ALSO: Hamamelis, Erigeron, Ustilago, Ferrum met, Lachesis, Phosphorus, Sabina

Principal Equine Indications

- Laminitis both acute and chronic cases
- Poor hoof quality
- Navicular syndrome
- Quittor
- Canker
- Constriction of the palmar annular ligament
- Tying up
- Shivering
- Haemorrhage of thin watery dark blood
- Recurrent or persistent haematomas
- Purpura
- Small wounds which persistently ooze dark blood
- Thrombosis, iliac thrombosis
- Gangrene
- Skin ulcers
- Paralysis of the bladder
- Ataxia
- Myelitis
- Threatened abortion
- Post-foaling haemorrhage
- Retained placenta
- Endometritis, pyometria, toxic metritis
- Bleeding between oestrus periods
- Penile prolapse
- Pressure sores, decubitus
- Emaciation, debility

Selenium

COMMON NAME: Selenium
CLASSIFICATION: Mineral: Element
PREPARATION: By trituration

Keynotes

- Debility especially after prolonged illness

- Effects of over-exertion
- Sadness
- Loss of hair, alopecia
- Transparent mucus
- Liver painful
- Involuntary dribbling of urine
- Loss of sexual drive
- Hydrocele
- Dry scaly skin
- Itching around the hock region, fetlock, pastern and coffin joints
- Seborrhoea

Modalities

WORSE/AGGRAVATED BY: Touch, pressure, motion, after sleep, mental effort, draught of air, open air, hot weather, sun

BETTER/AMELIORATED BY: Rest

Remedy Interactions

INCOMPATIBLE WITH: China

WORKS WELL WITH: Caladium, Natrum carb, Staphysagria, Sepia, Nux vomica

CONSIDER ALSO: Calendula, Nat mur, Phos ac, Picric acid, Sulphur

Principal Equine Indications

- Itchy eczema of the lower limbs especially around joints
- Alopecia, hair loss around the head or lower limbs
- Seborrhoea, greasy skin
- Mud fever
- Mange (symptomatic treatment)
- Low white cell count
- Hydrocele
- Poor libido, impotency
- Effects of over exertion

Senecio aureus

COMMON NAME: Golden ragwort

CLASSIFICATION: Plant: Asteraceae (Compositae) family

PREPARATION: From a tincture of the flowering plant

Keynotes

- Nephritis
- Bloody urine with mucus
- Kidney pain
- Lower back pain over the region of the kidneys
- Uterine prolapse
- Irregular cycles

Modalities

WORSE/AGGRAVATED BY: In the afternoon

BETTER/AMELIORATED BY: Onset of oestrus

Remedy Interactions

CONSIDER ALSO: Caulophyllum, Sepia,

Principal Equine Indications

- Anoestrus in young mares
- Infertility
- Ragwort poisoning
- Acute nephritis

Senega

COMMON NAME: Snakewort, *Polygala senega*

CLASSIFICATION: Plant: Polygalaceae family

PREPARATION: From tincture of the dried root

Keynotes

- Principally a remedy for catarrh/mucus
- Respiratory catarrh
- Laryngeal, tracheal and bronchial catarrh
- Rattling noises in the chest
- Catarrhal inflammation of the throat
- Cough ending in a sneeze
- Watery mucus from the nose
- Repeated coughing to raise tough, sticky mucus
- Pleural exudations
- Hydrothorax
- Partial paralysis of the vocal cords
- Blepharitis with crusty dry eyelids
- Eyes appear dry
- Muscular weakness of the eyes, weak vision
- Promotes absorption of lens fragments
- Corneal opacity
- Facial paralysis
- Mucus in the urine

Modalities

WORSE/AGGRAVATED BY: Morning, night, during rest, touch, warm stable

BETTER/AMELIORATED BY: Moving around in the open air, from sweating

Remedy Interactions

WORKS WELL WITH: Calc carb, Phosphorus, Lycopodium, Sulphur
CONSIDER ALSO: Ammonium carbonate, Calc carb, Phosphorus, Spongia, Coccus cacti, Kali bich, Bryonia, Causticum

Principal Equine Indications

- Chronic catarrhal problems especially in elderly horses
- Chronic coughs in older horses
- Repeated coughing to loosen tough sticky viscid catarrh
- Chronic bronchitis with shortness of breath
- COPD
- Chronic pneumonia
- Pleurisy
- Hydrothorax
- Catarrhal conjunctivitis, blepharitis
- Clouding of the cornea with a catarrhal discharge
- Facial paralysis (left side)

Sepia

(see Constitutional Remedies)

Silica, Silicea

(see Constitutional Remedies)

Solanum nigrum

COMMON NAME: Black nightshade
CLASSIFICATION: Plant: Solanaceae family
PREPARATION: From tincture of the fresh plant

Keynotes

- Mania
- Tetanic spasms
- Stiffness of the whole body
- Meningitis
- Repeated dilation and contraction of the pupils
- Hydrocephalus

Modalities

WORSE/AGGRAVATED BY: Touch, motion, moving the head, light, bright sunshine, morning
BETTER/AMELIORATED BY: None listed

Remedy Interactions

CONSIDER ALSO: Belladonna

Principal Equine Indications

- Manic behaviour
- Epilepsy
- Convulsions occurring during fever
- Meningitis
- Tetanus

Sol

COMMON NAME: Sunlight, rays of the sun
CLASSIFICATION: Energy: Universal force: Stellar body
PREPARATION: Milk sugar exposed to concentrated sunlight

Keynotes

- Headache from sunshine, head pains
- Photic headshaking
- Sensitivity to sunlight
- Assertive nature, impatient

Modalities

WORSE/AGGRAVATED BY: None listed
BETTER/AMELIORATED BY: None listed

Remedy Interactions

CONSIDER ALSO: Glonoine, Belladonna

Principal Equine Indications

- Headshaking (photic type)
- Photosensitisation
- Sunburn
- Sunstroke

Solidago virgaurea, Solidago virga

COMMON NAME: Golden rod
CLASSIFICATION: Plant: Asteraceae (Compositae) family
PREPARATION: From tincture of the whole fresh plant or flowers

Keynotes

- Kidney congestion/pain
- Kidney failure

- Difficulty in passing urine
- Urine with blood, sediment and mucus
- Clear offensive smelling urine
- Back pain over the kidney region
- Repeated sneezing with runny mucus
- Bronchitis with blood-flecked catarrh
- Redness of the eyes with a watery discharge

Modalities

WORSE/AGGRAVATED BY: None listed
BETTER/AMELIORATED BY: None listed

Remedy Interactions

CONSIDER ALSO: Hydrangea, Berberis vulgaris

Principal Equine Indications

- Kidney (renal) failure, especially where there is back pain
- Drainage of kidney toxins
- Back pain over the kidney region
- Difficulty passing urine
- Urolithiasis
- Cystitis
- Headshaking

Spigelia

COMMON NAME: Pink root, Wormgrass, *Spigelia anthelmia*
CLASSIFICATION: Plant: Loganiaceae family
PREPARATION: From a tincture of the dried herb

Keynotes

- Acts on the nervous system, heart, fibrous tissue and eyes
- Pain (neuralgia) of the fifth cranial nerve
- Head pain (severe) over the eye, forehead and face regions
- Focus on the cervical spine and nerves
- Pupils dilated
- Photophobia
- Deep pain in the eyes
- Chronic catarrh
- Palpitations
- Weak, irregular pulse
- Difficulty breathing, short of breath
- Pericarditis
- Fear of needles
- Low pain threshold

Modalities

WORSE/AGGRAVATED BY: Touch, noise, turning, motion, jarring, concussion, cold damp weather, draughts
BETTER/AMELIORATED BY: Rest, warmth

Remedy Interactions

WORKS WELL WITH: Spongia, Arnica, Digitalis, Kalmia
CONSIDER ALSO: Cactus, Cimicifugia, Arnica, Naja, Spongia, Aconite, Cedron

Principal Equine Indications

- Headshaking
- Eye pain, as if from a foreign body
- Glaucoma
- Neuralgic pain
- Pericarditis
- Bursitis, left side of the body
- Pain in the left shoulder joint
- Fear of vaccination/needles

Spongia tosta

COMMON NAME: Roasted sponge, Common sponge
CLASSIFICATION: Animal: Sea creatures: Coelenterata family
PREPARATION: From a solution in alcohol

Keynotes

- Acts on the respiratory system
- Airways dry
- Burning in the larynx
- Larynx sensitive to touch
- Dry, barking, hard cough better after eating or drinking
- Persistent dry cough
- Difficult breathing, laboured, dyspnoea with anxiety
- Bronchial catarrh
- Wheezing
- Asthmatic cough
- Profuse expectoration with suffocative symptoms
- Mucus or watery eye discharge
- Rapid heart beat with palpitation
- Damaged heart valves
- Heart enlargement

- Exhaustion after slight effort
- Swollen glands especially lymph nodes of the neck
- Swollen thyroid
- Swelling of the testicles and spermatic cord

Modalities

WORSE/AGGRAVATED BY: Going uphill, exercise, before midnight, during sleep, dry cold wind, palpation of the larynx

BETTER/AMELIORATED BY: Going downhill, warmth, eating or drinking

Remedy Interactions

WORKS WELL WITH: Aconite, Hepar sulph, Spigelia

CONSIDER ALSO: Iodum, Lachesis, Naja, Kalmia, Spigelia, Rumex, Phosphorus, Lycopus, Ledum, Kali sulph, Hepar sulph, Coccus cactii

Principal Equine Indications

- Hard, dry, barking cough triggered by palpation of the larynx
- Coughs accompanied by laboured breathing
- Laryngitis
- COPD with wheezing and thick mucus in the airways
- Hardened (indurated) enlarged lymph nodes
- Heart enlargement
- Distorted heart valves, heart murmurs where there is exercise intolerance
- Breathing difficulties arising from heart problems
- Pericarditis and subsequent symptoms
- Orchitis
- Epididymitis

Squilla maritima

COMMON NAME: Sea onion

CLASSIFICATION: Plant: Liliaceae family

PREPARATION: From the dried bulb

Keynotes

- Acts on the respiratory system and the heart
- Bronchopneumonia
- Chronic bronchitis
- Dyspnoea, difficulty breathing
- Short dry cough
- Exhausting cough with rattling mucus noises in the chest
- Sneezing with coughing
- Urine passed involuntarily while coughing
- Watery nasal discharge
- Cardiac stimulant
- Passing of great amounts of watery urine

Modalities

WORSE/AGGRAVATED BY: Motion

BETTER/AMELIORATED BY: Rest

Remedy Interactions

WORKS WELL WITH: Antimonium crudum, Arsenicum album, Ignatia, Nux vomica, Rhus tox, Silica

CONSIDER ALSO: Kali carb, Bryonia, Digitalis, Arsenicum album, Causticum, Pulsatilla

Principal Equine Indications

- Bronchopneumonia
- Dry cough with thick tacky mucus
- Chronic bronchitis in elderly horses
- Pleurisy
- To loosen sticky mucus
- As a cardiac support remedy
- Thrush

Stannum

COMMON NAME: Tin

CLASSIFICATION: Mineral: Metal: Stannums: Element

PREPARATION: By trituration of the pure metal

Keynotes

- Acts on the respiratory and nervous systems
- Sad and exhausted
- General debility, weakness from least exertion
- Chronic bronchitis with a mucopurulent discharge
- Thick tacky mucus in the throat, difficult to free up
- Green or lemon-coloured mucus coughed up
- Forcible cough
- Violent dry cough (induced by irritation)
- Paralytic weakness
- Spasms
- Spasmodic twitching

- Swollen hocks
- Legs suddenly give out
- Early oestrus
- Depressed before coming into oestrus
- Vaginal discharge with weakness

Modalities

WORSE/AGGRAVATED BY: Evening until midnight, 4–5am, touch, rest, lying down (especially on the right side), using vocal cords

BETTER/AMELIORATED BY: Open air, lying down, after coughing, expectoration, hard pressure, moving around

Remedy Interactions

WORKS WELL WITH: Pulsatilla, Causticum, Calc carb, Phosphorus, Selenium, Sulphur, Bacillinum

CONSIDER ALSO: Bacillinum, Tuberculinum, Causticum, Senega

Principal Equine Indications

- Cough with expectoration of green or yellow slimy mucus
- Cough with debility
- Cough or weakness following equine flu
- African horse sickness (respiratory form)
- Neuritis characterised by stumbling
- Weak back legs
- Epilepsy

Staphysagria

COMMON NAME: Stavesacre, *Delphinium staphisagria*

CLASSIFICATION: Plant: Ranunculaceae family: Polycrest

PREPARATION: By trituration of the seeds

Keynotes

- Irritable nature, impetuous
- Angry, aggressive
- Extremely sensitive
- Likes solitude
- Injuries to the cornea
- Acts on the teeth and periosteum
- Poor (crumbling) teeth
- Gum disease, bleeding
- Colic
- Abdominal pain
- Cystitis
- Urge to urinate
- Urethral irritation
- Eczema with thick scabs and itching which changes location
- Warts
- Exostoses associated with arthritic joints
- Inflammation of the pastern or coffin joints

Modalities

WORSE/AGGRAVATED BY: Anger, indignation, grief, fluid loss, dehydration, sexual excess, touching the affected area, drinking cold water, new moon

BETTER/AMELIORATED BY: Warmth, rest, after morning feed

Remedy Interactions

WORKS WELL WITH: Causticum, Colocynthis, Nux vomica, Pulsatilla, Rhus tox, Sulphur

CONSIDER ALSO: Ignatia, Phos ac, Nux vomica, Chamomilla, Thuja, Calendula, Pulsatilla, Nat mur, Silica

Principal Equine Indications

- Anger, irritability, short temper
- Grief with resentment
- Agitation
- Indignation
- Violent outbursts
- Conditions arising from physical or mental insult or from suppressed anger
- Nymphomania
- Aversion to the opposite sex
- False rigs
- Tissue damage especially cuts, lacerations and injuries from sharp objects
- Lacerations or stretching to sphincters
- After surgery involving sphincters
- Post-operative abdominal pain
- To assist healing of surgical incisions, incised wounds
- Compound factures
- Pain after tooth extraction
- Pain after abdominal surgery
- Flatulent or tympanic colic arising from anger, irritability, resentment, frustration
- Acute cystitis especially after intervention
- After bladder surgery to relieve discomfort
- Traumatic urethritis

- Eye injuries
- Corneal lacerations, injuries
- Blepharitis
- Eyelid growths
- Small nodular sarcoids
- Warts and other cauliflower-like growths, dry in texture and appearance
- Eczema with thick scabs especially around the head, ears and body
- Sweet itch with intense itching
- Mange
- To reduce the effect/severity of insect bites
- Ringbone

Sticta

COMMON NAME: Lungwort, *Sticta pulmonaria*
CLASSIFICATION: Plant: Lobariaceae (Lichens) family
PREPARATION: From tincture

Keynotes

- Focus on the respiratory system and joints
- Repeated sneezing
- Bronchial catarrh
- Dry hacking cough
- Tracheitis (inflammation of the trachea)
- Tickly cough
- Loosens mucus
- Watery nasal discharge with local scabbing
- Stiffness of the neck
- Pain in the right shoulder
- Swollen joints with severe pain or heat
- Stifle pain

Modalities

WORSE/AGGRAVATED BY: Sudden temperature changes, touch, motion, as the day advances, night (cough), coughing (which induces more coughing), lying down
BETTER/AMELIORATED BY: In the open air, flowing of discharges

Remedy Interactions

CONSIDER ALSO: Bacillinum, Drosera, Nux vomica, Kali bich, Lemna minor, Teucrium marum, Thuja

Principal Equine Indications

- Tracheitis
- Dry hacking coughs worse in the evening or at night
- Post-viral cough
- Allergic-based sneezing bouts
- Stifle pain
- Pain in the right shoulder
- Neck pain

Stramonium

COMMON NAME: Thorn-apple, Stink weed, Jimson weed, *Datura stramonium*
CLASSIFICATION: Plant: Solanaceae family
PREPARATION: From tincture of the fresh plant in flower and from the fruit

Keynotes

- Acts mainly on the brain; the central nervous system and cerebellum
- Staggering uneven gait
- Tendency to fall forwards
- Rhythmical, graceful limb movements
- Vocalisation
- Sees 'ghosts' or 'spirits'
- Rapid changes in mood
- State of delirium
- Marked excitement
- Terror
- Desire to escape
- Violence
- Dislikes solitude and darkness, fears being alone
- Bright light or glittering objects or water brings on spasms
- Dilated pupils
- Eyes staring and wide open
- Wild look in the eyes
- Strabismus
- Dribbling of saliva
- Difficulty swallowing due to spasms
- Chewing motion of jaws
- Increased thirst
- Epilepsy and convulsions
- Chorea, spasms
- Trembling
- Twitching of tendons
- Increased sweating
- Uterine bleeding

Modalities

WORSE/AGGRAVATED BY: In a dark room, when alone, bright shiny objects, after sleep, from swallowing, touch, motion, wind, cold, evening, at night, sun, drinking cold water

BETTER/AMELIORATED BY: Warmth, company, in daylight

Remedy Interactions

WORKS WELL WITH: Belladonna, Cuprum metallicum, Aconite, Bryonia, Hyoscyamus, Nux vomica

CONSIDER ALSO: Belladonna, Lachesis, Agaricus, Cuprum, Zinc, Hyoscyamus, Nux vomica, Lyssin, Magnesium carbonate (chronic), Anacardium, Opium

Principal Equine Indications

- Wild and excitable, uncontrollable behaviour
- Anger, violence
- Aggression
- Bouts of delirium
- Fear of the dark or of being alone
- Fear of anything new or unusual
- Sudden mood changes
- Reactions to bright, shiny objects or water
- Convulsions, epilepsy
- Deep-seated effects of past trauma or shock
- Effects of birth separation
- Muscle or tendon spasms
- Isolated twitching of muscle groups or tendons
- Chorea
- Meningitis
- Head injuries
- Oesophageal spasms
- Choke where there is marked excitement
- Nymphomania
- Heat stroke
- Tetanus
- Equine protozoal myeloencephalitis
- Shaker foal syndrome
- Sleepy foal disease
- Photic head shaking
- Loading problems due to excitability

Strontia, Strontium carbonicum

COMMON NAME: Strontium carbonate

CLASSIFICATION: Mineral: Metal: Strontiums

PREPARATION: By trituration

Keynotes

- Rheumatic-like pains
- Chronic strains
- Effects of haemorrhage
- Bone problems
- Shock
- Neuritis
- Burning and redness of the eyes
- Diarrhoea at night with straining
- Swelling of the hock
- Pain in the right shoulder
- Chronic spasms
- Very sensitive to cold

Modalities

WORSE/AGGRAVATED BY: Touch, rubbing, riding, first movement, evening, night, early morning (2–3am), changes of weather

BETTER/AMELIORATED BY: Warmth, covering up

Remedy Interactions

CONSIDER ALSO: Baryta carb, Arnica, Ruta grav, Silica, Carbo veg

Principal Equine Indications

- Hock sprains
- Swelling of the hock
- Fetlock injuries
- Chronic tendon sprains or ligament injuries
- Curb
- Joint luxations of subluxations
- Shivering
- Consequences of chronic haemorrhage
- Post-operative oozing of blood
- After-effects of surgery (shock, coldness, slow recovery)
- Bone weakness (especially the femur)

Strophanthus hispidus

COMMON NAME: Kombe seed

CLASSIFICATION: Plant: Apocynaceae family

PREPARATION: From a tincture of the seeds

Keynotes

- Acts on the heart slowing the pulse rate, increases systole
- Ascites

- Oedema
- Where the heart valves are damaged
- Weakness from blood loss
- Difficulty breathing, congestion of the lungs
- Hives
- Increased urination

Modalities

WORSE/AGGRAVATED BY: None listed
BETTER/AMELIORATED BY: None listed

Remedy Interactions – None listed

Principal Equine Indications

- As a cardiac tonic in older horses
- Cardiac support during illnesses such as Equine infectious anaemia
- To slow the pulse rate
- Where the pulse is weak or irregular
- Cardiac weakness
- Myocarditis
- Heart valve weakness
- Filled legs where the circulation is not good
- Oedema and ascites
- Congestion of the lungs
- Weakness following haemorrhage
- Chronic urticaria (hives)

Strychninum

COMMON NAME: Strychnine (an alkaloid of Nux vomica)
CLASSIFICATION: Plant: Loganiaceae family
PREPARATION: By trituration

Keynotes

- Stimulates the motor areas of the spinal cord
- Exaggerated reflexes
- Excitability of the spinal cord
- Heightened senses
- Muscle spasms
- Cramps
- Jerking, twitching and trembling
- Rapid breathing
- Stiff muscles in the face and neck
- Opisthotonus
- Tetanus
- Dilated pupils
- Twitching eyelids
- Difficulty swallowing, laryngeal spasm
- Abdominal pains
- Dung passed involuntarily during spasms
- Stubborn constipation
- Nymphomania
- Neck muscles stiff
- Back stiff

Modalities

WORSE/AGGRAVATED BY: Slightest touch, noise or movement, feeding
BETTER/AMELIORATED BY: Lying down

Remedy Interactions

CONSIDER ALSO: Nux vomica, Cicuta, Arnica, Hypericum, Ledum, Stramonium

Principal Equine Indications

- Stringhalt
- Shivering
- Tetanus, especially the earlier stages
- Jerking, twitching and trembling, especially if violent
- Opisthotonus
- Chorea
- Stringhalt
- Severe constipation
- Neck pain, stiffness, spasm of the neck and back muscles
- Nymphomania
- Poisoning symptomatic treatment
- Viral infections characterised by neurological symptoms

Sulphur

(see Constitutional Remedies)

Sulphur iodatum, Sulph iod

COMMON NAME: Iodide of sulphur
CLASSIFICATION: Mineral: Sulphurs
PREPARATION: By trituration

Keynotes

- To assist recovery from strangles
- Useful for severe skin problems that are slow to clear

- Sticky, moist eczema
- Eruptions over the face and on the lips

Modalities

WORSE/AGGRAVATED BY: None listed
BETTER/AMELIORATED BY: None listed

Remedy Interactions – None listed

Principal Equine Indications

- Obstinate skin infections
- Weeping, moist dermatitis
- Pustules and boils
- Eczema or dermatitis around the face and lips

Sulphuricum acidum, Sulph ac

COMMON NAME: Sulphuric acid, Vitriol
CLASSIFICATION: Mineral: Sulphurs
PREPARATION: By dilution in distilled water

Keynotes

- General debility
- Weakness
- Tremors, jerking of the limbs, cramping
- Hurried, impatient
- Gangene
- Bruising
- Ecchymotic haemorrhages
- Purpura haemorrhagica
- Intraocular haemorrhage
- Haemorrhage of dark, black, blood
- Bacterial skin infections
- Chemosis (great swelling) of the conjunctiva
- Bleeding gums
- Oozing moisture from the rectum

Modalities

WORSE/AGGRAVATED BY: Heat or cold in excess, late morning, evening, touch, open air
BETTER/AMELIORATED BY: Warmth, resting

Remedy Interactions

WORKS WELL WITH: Pulsatilla, Arnica, Bellis
CONSIDER ALSO: Arnica, Calendula, Ledum, Sepia, Calc carb, Phosphorus, Ruta, Conium

Principal Equine Indications

- The effects of trauma on the skin and eye
- Mechanical injuries
- Sprains, bruises (especially deep bruising) falls, trauma
- Bruising of the sole
- Corns
- Chafing of the skin
- Concussion
- Bruises with deeply coloured, livid skin
- Ecchymotic haemorrhages
- Purpura haemorrhagica
- Haemorrhage of dark black blood from any orifice
- Reabsorption of intraocular haemorrhage after trauma to the eye
- Gangrene
- Staphylococcal and Streptococcal skin infections especially where the skin becomes a livid colour
- Slow healing wounds
- Scar tissue which becomes infected and fails to heal
- Problems arising post-surgery
- Lead poisoning

Symphytum

COMMON NAME: Comfrey, Bone-set, Knitbone, *Symphytum officinale*
CLASSIFICATION: Plant: Boraginaceae family
PREPARATION: From tincture of the fresh plant

Keynotes

- Acts on bone encouraging the healing of fractures
- Penetrating wounds to bone and the periosteum
- Injuries to tendons
- Acts generally on joints
- Pain in the stifle joint
- Eye injuries especially blows, trauma to the eyes
- Stimulates the growth of epithelium on ulcerated surfaces

Modalities

WORSE/AGGRAVATED BY: Touch
BETTER/AMELIORATED BY: None listed

Remedy Interactions

WORKS WELL WITH: Arnica

CONSIDER ALSO: Calc phos, Arnica, Calendula, Silica, Ledum, Ruta grav, Rhus tox, Hypericum

Principal Equine Indications

- To assist healing of fractures
- Non-union fractures
- Injuries to bones and joints
- Injury to the periosteal layer of bone, periostitis, exostoses
- Splints
- Sore shins
- Pedal osteitis
- Chondromalacia of the patella
- Meniscal tears
- Degenerative joint disease (DJD), arthritis to augment other remedies
- Angular limb deformities in foals
- Tendon and ligament injuries, sprains
- Eye injuries especially from blunt objects
- Slow healing wounds
- To assist in healing mucosal surfaces

Syphilinum

COMMON NAME: Syphilitic virus, Lueticum

CLASSIFICATION: Animals: Mammals: Humans: Nosode

PREPARATION: Attenuation

Keynotes

- Affects bone, mucous membranes and nerves
- Tissue destruction
- Shifting pains
- Chronic skin eruptions
- Abscesses and recurrent abscesses
- Pemphigus
- Ulceration of mucous membranes
- Ulceration of the mouth, nose, skin and genital organs
- Inflammation of the cornea
- Corneal abrasion
- Photophobia
- Iritis
- Increased production of tears
- Swollen lids
- Ptosis (drooping of the lids)
- Decay of the teeth at the gum line
- Progressive destruction of the nasal bones (ozaena)
- Diseases of bone
- Pain in the shoulder joint
- Hard, knotted muscles
- Watery profuse uterine discharge
- Chronic COPD with wheezing and rattling
- Hard dry cough, worse at night
- Trachea (windpipe) sensitive to touch
- Emaciation

Modalities

WORSE/AGGRAVATED BY: Touch, motion, night, damp weather, extremes of temperature, seashore

BETTER/AMELIORATED BY: None listed

Remedy Interactions

CONSIDER ALSO: Aurum, Asafoetida, Kali iod, Merc sol, Nitric acid, Abrotanum, Iodum, Rhus tox

Principal Equine Indications

- Recurrent abscesses, especially deep abscesses
- Chronic rhinitis with bony destruction and foul, thick, nasal discharge
- Diseases of bone with bony degeneration/weakness
- Severe, unresponsive cases of COPD especially those which are worse in warm weather
- Corneal ulceration or abrasion
- Iritis
- Periodic ophthalmia
- Generalised stiffness worse in damp weather
- Chronic or obstinate vaginal discharges
- CEM
- Lyme disease
- Obsessive, repetitive behaviour
- Violent behaviour if opposed

Syzgium jambolanum

COMMON NAME: Jambol seeds, Jumbul

CLASSIFICATION: Plant: Myrtaceae family

PREPARATION: Trituration of the seeds

Keynotes

- Acts on the pancreas
- Diabetes mellitus
- Increased thirst, emaciation

Modalities

WORSE/AGGRAVATED BY: None listed
BETTER/AMELIORATED BY: None listed

Remedy Interactions

CONSIDER ALSO: Uranium nitrate, Phos ac, Phosphorus

Principal Equine Indications

- Diabetes mellitus
- Cushing's disease

Tabacum

COMMON NAME: Tobacco, *Nicotiana tabacum*
CLASSIFICATION: Plant: Solanaceae family
PREPARATION: From tincture of the fresh leaves collected before the flowers are developed

Keynotes

- Travel sickness
- Sweating linked with travelling
- Increased peristalsis
- Diarrhoea, watery in nature and sudden in appearance
- Atrophy of the optic nerve, poor sight

Modalities

WORSE/AGGRAVATED BY: Travel by any means, evening, extremes of heat and cold, being rugged up while travelling
BETTER/AMELIORATED BY: In the open air, uncovering, at rest, walking around gently

Remedy Interactions

WORKS WELL WITH: Opium, Carbo veg
CONSIDER ALSO: Petroleum, Cocculus, Gelsemium

Principal Equine Indications

- Conditions arising as a consequence of travelling
- Agitation, sweating
- Profuse diarrhoea

Taraxacum

COMMON NAME: Dandelion, *Taraxacum officinale*
CLASSIFICATION: Plant: Asteraceae (Compositae) family
PREPARATION: From tincture of the whole plant just before the flower is at its best

Keynotes

- Primarily a liver remedy
- Jaundice
- Gassy abdomen
- Debility
- Stifle pain eased by local pressure
- Restless limbs

Modalities

WORSE/AGGRAVATED BY: At night, resting
BETTER/AMELIORATED BY: Touch, motion, open air

Remedy Interactions

CONSIDER ALSO: Chelidonium, Carduus, Nux vomica, Phosphorus, Ptelia

Principal Equine Indications

- In the management of liver disease
- To drain toxins from the liver

Tarentula cubensis

COMMON NAME: Cuban spider
CLASSIFICATION: Animal: Arachnid family
PREPARATION: From tincture of the spiders

Keynotes

- Toxic and septic conditions
- Severe inflammation with pain and considerable swelling
- Purple or blue/black colour to affected areas
- Gangrene
- Abscesses especially those which are painful
- Itching around the genital region
- Spots and pimples on the skin
- Skin ulcers

Modalities

WORSE/AGGRAVATED BY: At night
BETTER/AMELIORATED BY: None listed

Remedy Interactions

CONSIDER ALSO: Pyrogen, Echinacea, Arsenicum album, Crot horr, Anthracinum, Belladonna, Apis, Hepar sulph

Principal Equine Indications

- Septicaemia, sepsis

- Toxaemia
- Painful acute abscesses where the skin is discoloured
- Inflammation accompanied by skin discoloration
- Bacterial skin infections where discomfort is evident
- Gangrene
- Fly strike
- Eczema or dermatitis of the genital area
- Snake bites
- Lymphangitis

Tarentula hispania

COMMON NAME: Spanish spider
CLASSIFICATION: Animal: Arachnid family
PREPARATION: From tincture of the spiders

Keynotes

- Acts on the nervous system
- Hypersensitivity
- Hysterical behaviour
- Wound up 'like a spring'
- Extreme restlessness
- Constant state of excitement
- Epilepsy
- Sexual excitement
- Sudden alteration of mood
- Cunning, secretive nature
- Destructive impulses
- Dislike of company but wants someone close by
- Sensitive to music
- Twitching, cramps and jerking of the limbs, chorea
- Weakness of the limbs

Modalities

WORSE/AGGRAVATED BY: Motion, noise, touch, bright lights, loud noises, night, after sleep
BETTER/AMELIORATED BY: In the open air, for music, rubbing affected area, warm water

Remedy Interactions

CONSIDER ALSO: Agaricus, Arsenicum album, Cuprum metallicum, Mag phos, Mygale, Stramonium, Belladonna

Principal Equine Indications

- States of excitement and hysteria
- Extreme agitation and restlessness
- Constant agitation
- Sudden mood changes
- Cunning nature
- Other behavioural problems; destructive behaviour
- Fear of being closed in or trapped
- Heightened sexuality in the stallion
- Nymphomania
- Muscle twitching, jerking of chorea in excitable animals
- Tying up in excitable horses

Tellurium

COMMON NAME: Tellurium
CLASSIFICATION: Mineral: Element
PREPARATION: By trituration of the precipitated element

Keynotes

- Affects the skin and spine
- Offensive discharges
- Pain about the sacral region
- Pain in the middle region of the spine
- Distortion and twitching of the left side of the face
- Inflamed thickened eyelids
- Conjunctivitis
- Cataracts following other eye problems/lesions
- Assist the reabsorption of infiltrations into the eye
- Eczema around the region of the ear
- Watery nasal discharge
- Contracted tendons
- Itching of the lower limbs
- Ringworm
- Circular patches of dermatitis

Modalities

WORSE/AGGRAVATED BY: At rest, night, morning, cold weather, friction/rubbing, chaffing, touch
BETTER/AMELIORATED BY: None listed

Remedy Interactions

CONSIDER ALSO: Bacillinum, Sepia, Natrum

muriaticum, Selenium, Graphites, Rhus tox

Principal Equine Indications
- Ringworm especially in areas of friction
- Eczema or dermatitis around the ear region and ear flaps
- Skin lesions affecting the lower limbs
- Circular patches of dermatitis or eczema
- Equine viral papular dermatitis
- Chronically inflamed thickened eyelids
- Entropion
- Cataracts developing after eye problems
- Pain over the sacral region of the back

Terebinthina

COMMON NAME: Turpentine, Oil of turpentine
CLASSIFICATION: Plant: Pinaceae family
PREPARATION: From a solution in rectified spirit

Keynotes
- Acts on bleeding mucous membranes
- Focus on the urinary system
- Inflammation of the kidneys with haemorrhage
- Acute renal (kidney) failure
- Uraemia
- Straining to pass bloody urine (haematuria)
- Urethritis
- Back pain in the region of the kidneys
- Stomatitis
- Abdominal distension
- Watery green diarrhoea with blood
- Haemorrhage from the bowels
- Haemorrhagic gastroenteritis
- Metritis
- Pustules, vesicles
- Erythema
- Urticaria
- Purpura haemorrhagica

Modalities
WORSE/AGGRAVATED BY: Touch, pressure, lying on left side, damp stabling, 1–3am
BETTER/AMELIORATED BY: Walking in the fresh air, motion

Remedy Interactions
WORKS WELL WITH: Antimonium tartrate, Merc sol, Merc corr
CONSIDER ALSO: Apis, Cantharis, Merc sol, Merc corr

Principal Equine Indications
- Cystitis with blood and straining to pass urine
- Acute renal failure
- Pyelonephritis
- Uraemia
- Acute Leptospirosis
- Haemorrhagic diarrhoea
- Purpura haemorrhagica

Teucrium marum

COMMON NAME: Cat thyme
CLASSIFICATION: Plant: Lamiaceae (Labiatae) family
PREPARATION: From tincture of the whole fresh plant

Keynotes
- Chronic nasal catarrh, sneezing
- Nose obstructed
- Nasal polyps
- Dry tickling cough with mucus production
- Pains in the horny part of the foot
- Infection in the horn
- Anal irritation, itching
- Roundworms
- Dry skin

Modalities
WORSE/AGGRAVATED BY: Touch, evening, at night, warmth, wet weather
BETTER/AMELIORATED BY: Moving around

Remedy Interactions
WORKS WELL WITH: China, Pulsatilla, Silica

Principal Equine Indications
- Chronic nasal catarrh with blockage of the nose
- Chronic laminitis with evidence of seedy toe, white line disease or gravel
- Anal irritation or itching
- Elimination of roundworms

Thallium

COMMON NAME: Thallium
CLASSIFICATION: Mineral: Metal

PREPARATION: By trituration

Keynotes
- Affects the endocrine glands especially the thyroid and adrenals
- Muscle wasting
- Tremors, trembling
- Ataxia
- Paralysis of the hind limbs
- Loss of hair (alopecia) after acute illness
- Polyneuritis
- Chronic myelitis

Modalities
WORSE/AGGRAVATED BY: None listed
BETTER/AMELIORATED BY: None listed

Remedy Interactions
CONSIDER ALSO: Plumbum, Phosphorus

Principal Equine Indications
- To assist or encourage the growth of hair
- Alopecia
- Equine viral papular dermatitis
- Neurological weakness of the hind limbs
- Paralysis of the hind limbs
- Trembling of the hind limbs
- Neuritis with hind limb weakness
- Ataxia (uncoordinated movements)
- Myelitis, especially chronic cases

Theridion

COMMON NAME: Orange spider, *Theridion curassavicum*
CLASSIFICATION: Animal: Arachnid family
PREPARATION: From a tincture of the living spider

Keynotes
- Sensitivity to noise
- Restlessness
- Travel sickness
- Diseases of bone

Modalities
WORSE/AGGRAVATED BY: Touch, travelling in a vehicle or boat, least noise, motion, night, cold, left side
BETTER/AMELIORATED BY: Warmth

Remedy Interactions
WORKS WELL WITH: Sulphur, Calc carb, Lycopodium
CONSIDER ALSO: Phosphorus, Borax, Cocculus, Tabacum, Petroleum

Principal Equine Indications
- Extreme anxiety/sensitivity to noises
- Sensitivity to vibrations
- Horses that travel badly in the horsebox
- Bad effects of travelling particularly by sea
- Degeneration of bone when other remedies fail to act

Thiosinaminum

COMMON NAME: Allyl sulphocarbamide, a derivative of mustard seed oil
CLASSIFICATION: Plant: Brassicaceae (Cruciferae) family
PREPARATION: By trituration of the crystals

Keynotes
- Dissolves scar tissue
- Strictures
- Adhesions
- Tumours
- Enlarged lymph nodes
- Lupus
- Ectropion (rolling in of the eyelids)
- Corneal opacity
- Cataracts

Modalities
WORSE/AGGRAVATED BY: None listed
BETTER/AMELIORATED BY: None listed

Remedy Interactions
CONSIDER ALSO: Silica, Graphites

Principal Equine Indications
- In the treatment/removal of scar tissue, adhesions
- Strictures
- Blockage or obstruction of the nasolachrymal duct
- Dissipation of blood clots
- Chronically enlarged lymph nodes
- Benign skin masses, skin nodules, sarcoids
- Equine nodular skin disease
- Alopecia
- Fibrotic myopathy

- Clouding of the corneal, cornea opacity
- Cataracts
- Lupus
- Ectropion

Thlaspi bursa pastoris

COMMON NAME: Shepherd's purse, *Capsella bursa pastoris*
CLASSIFICATION: Plant: Brassicaceae (Cruciferae) family
PREPARATION: From tincture of the fresh flowering plant

Keynotes

- A remedy for haemorrhage and bladder problems
- Uterine haemorrhage
- Epistaxis (nosebleed)
- Dark, offensive uterine discharge
- Increased frequency of urination
- Chronic cystitis
- Blood in the urine
- Gravel in the urine
- High level of phosphate in the urine
- Urethritis

Modalities

WORSE/AGGRAVATED BY: None listed
BETTER/AMELIORATED BY: None listed

Remedy Interactions

CONSIDER ALSO: Urtica, Hydrangea, Lycopodium, Sarsaparilla, Millefolium, Trillium, Sabina, Secale

Principal Equine Indications

- Uterine haemorrhage
- Haemorrhage post-abortion
- Metritis with a foul, blood discharge
- Epistaxis
- Acute and chronic cystitis
- Bloody urine (haematuria)
- Acute urethritis
- Urinary gravel, stones, sediment, calculi
- Difficulty passing urine
- Short-term relief of partial obstruction of the urethra by calculi
- Urethral calculi stones

Thuja occidentalis

COMMON NAME: Arbor vitae, the tree of life, *Thuja occidentalis*
CLASSIFICATION: Plant: Cupressaceae family: Polycrest
PREPARATION: From a tincture of the fresh green twigs

Keynotes

- Important anti-sycotic remedy
- Overreaction, hyperactivity
- Inflexibility, rigidity
- Key remedy for the ill-effects from vaccination
- Wide-acting remedy especially with regard to the skin
- Warts, growths, polyps, tumours and bleeding skin masses on both mucous membranes and the skin
- Tearing pains in muscles and joints which are worse for rest and in the damp and better in dry weather
- Conditions which are worse for moonlight
- Exhaustion and emaciation
- Left-sided symptoms
- Feels the cold
- Emotionally sensitive
- Iritis
- Eyelids stuck together with sticky discharge
- Masses growing on the eyelids
- Inflammation of the sclera
- Chronic nasal catarrh with thick green mucus
- Inside of nostrils ulcerated
- Decay of the teeth next to the gums
- Chronic watery diarrhoea, forcibly expelled
- Flatulence and abdominal distension
- Rumbling in the abdomen, colic
- Inflammation and swelling of the urethra
- Frequent urination
- Inflammation of the prepuce with discharge
- Vaginal region very sensitive
- Thick greenish uterine discharge
- Inflammation of the ovaries worse left side
- Odd gait as if limbs would not bend
- Muscle twitching, weakness and trembling
- Brittle horn, cracked, soft areas
- Dry scaly skin
- Dry hacking cough

Modalities

WORSE/AGGRAVATED BY: At night, being covered up,

3am, 3pm, early morning, cold damp air, rainy or stormy weather, water, after vaccination, left side, touch, motion (except joint symptoms), sun, bright light

BETTER/AMELIORATED BY: Dry weather, pressure, massage, sweating

Remedy Interactions

WORKS WELL WITH: Arsenicum album, Natrum sulph, Silica, Sabina, Medorrhinum, Nitric acid, Merc sol, Sulphur, Calc carb, Ignatia, Lycopodium, Pulsatilla

CONSIDER ALSO: Nitric acid, Medorrhinum, Lycopodium, Sepia, Natrum sulph, Antimonium tartrate, Rhus tox

Principal Equine Indications

- Ill-effects of vaccination, vaccinosis
- Conditions arising following vaccination
- Overreaction in any situation medically (i.e. from drugs or with symptoms) or psychologically (with behavioural changes)
- Obsessive behaviour
- Dislike of company, avoids strangers
- Inflexibility, animal with an inability to adapt to changes easily
- Warts, melanomas, sarcoids, skin growths, nodules, bleeding masses, cysts
- Eyelid growths
- Keratitis with minor corneal opacity
- Ranula
- Proud flesh, exuberant granulation
- Ovarian cysts
- CEM
- Testicular atrophy
- Smegma
- Penile or preputial warts
- Generalized stiffness worse in damp weather, eased by movement
- Severe lower back pain
- Stilted gait (as if limbs made of wood)
- Thoroughpin
- Canker
- Brittle hooves as a result of chronic laminitis
- Cauda equina neuritis (especially following vaccination)
- Chronic nasal catarrh with sore nostrils
- Guttural pouch infections, empyema
- Sinusitis, sinus empyema
- Urethral and vaginal discharges
- Chronic, intractable skin conditions
- Mud fever
- Sweet itch
- Rainscald
- Vitiligo
- Pemphigus
- Poor dry or brittle coat
- Stubborn cases of ringworm
- Prevention of tetanus
- Lyme disease
- Cushing's disease

Thyroidinum

COMMON NAME: Thyroidin

CLASSIFICATION: Animal: Sarcode

PREPARATION: Trituration of the fresh thyroid gland from sheep

Keynotes

- Anaemia
- Emaciation
- Muscle weakness
- Sweating
- Tachycardia
- Slow healing of fractures
- Obesity
- Hungry yet loses weight
- Irritable nature
- Oedema of the legs
- Dry cough
- Dry flaky skin
- Lupus
- Retention of the testes

Modalities

WORSE/AGGRAVATED BY: Exertion, cold

BETTER/AMELIORATED BY: Resting

Remedy Interactions

CONSIDER ALSO: Spongia, Calc carb, Nat mur, Iodum

Principal Equine Indications

- Alopecia
- Cushing's disease
- Obesity

- Emaciation and weakness with good appetite
- Rigs (possibly to allow the testes to descend)

Titanium

COMMON NAME: Titanium
CLASSIFICATION: Mineral: Metal
PREPARATION: Trituration

Keynotes

- Lupus
- Skin conditions
- Poor vision
- Premature ejaculation

Modalities

WORSE/AGGRAVATED BY: None listed
BETTER/AMELIORATED BY: None listed

Remedy Interactions – None listed

Principal Equine Indications

Premature ejaculation in the stallion

Trillium pendulum

COMMON NAME: White Beth-root, Birthroot, Lamb's quarter
CLASSIFICATION: Plant: Liliaceae family
PREPARATION: From a tincture of the fresh root

Keynotes

- Haemorrhage
- Uterine haemorrhage of bright red blood worse on the slightest movement
- Epistaxis (nosebleed)
- Coughing up of blood
- Abortion
- Chronic diarrhoea with mucus and blood

Modalities

WORSE/AGGRAVATED BY: Movement
BETTER/AMELIORATED BY: None listed

Remedy Interactions

WORKS WELL WITH: Calc phos
CONSIDER ALSO: Hamamelis, Secale, Ustilgao, Sanguinaria, Ipecac, Millefolium, Sabina

Principal Equine Indications

- Uterine haemorrhage of bright red blood
- Threatened abortion preceded by a bloody discharge
- EIPH
- Epistaxis
- Warfarin poisoning

TNT, Trinitrotoluene

COMMON NAME: TNT
CLASSIFICATION: Mineral
PREPARATION: By trituration (carefully)

Keynotes

- Has a destructive effect on red blood cells leading to anaemia and jaundice due to destruction of red blood cells
- Changes haemoglobin so that it cannot carry oxygen as well
- Breathlessness, fainting, fatigue, muscle cramps, cyanosis
- Tachycardia, bradycardia, intermittent pulse
- Averse to company
- Apathy, delerium, convulsions
- Dermatitis with reddening (erythema) of the skin
- Haemorrhage under the skin

Modalities

WORSE/AGGRAVATED BY: None listed
BETTER/AMELIORATED BY: None listed

Remedy Interactions

CONSIDER ALSO: Phosphorus, Arsenicum album, Plumbum, Manganum acetate, Chin sulph, Lycopodium

Principal Equine Indications

- Autoimmune haemolytic anaemia in newborn foals
- Anaemia with associated jaundice
- Equine infectious anaemia
- Babesiasis

Triticum

COMMON NAME: Couch-grass, *Agropyron repens*
CLASSIFICATION: Plant: Poaceae (Gramineae) family
PREPARATION: From tincture of the fresh plant

Keynotes
- Irritability of the bladder
- Frequent, difficult urination
- Pyelonephritis (pus in the kidney and in the urine)
- Urinary incontinence
- Ill-effects of vaccination

Modalities
WORSE/AGGRAVATED BY: None listed
BETTER/AMELIORATED BY: None listed

Remedy Interactions
CONSIDER ALSO: Thuja

Principal Equine Indications
- Urinary incontinence
- Pyelonephritis
- Ill-effects of vaccination

Tuberculinum

(see Constitutional Remedies)

Tylophora indica

COMMON NAME: Indian Ipecac
CLASSIFICATION: Plant: Apocyanaceae family
PREPARATION: From mother tincture

Keynotes
- Arthritis (DJD)

Modalities
WORSE/AGGRAVATED BY: Cold weather, exercise
BETTER/AMELIORATED BY: None listed

Remedy Interactions
CONSIDER ALSO: Calc fluor, Heckla lava, Ruta grav, Rhus tox

Principal Equine Indications
- Lameness originating from arthritic changes in the fetlock, pastern and coffin joints

Uranium nitricum

COMMON NAME: Uranium nitrate, Nitrate of uranium
CLASSIFICATION: Mineral
PREPARATION: Trituration

Keynotes
- Increased output of urine
- Excessive thirst
- Urinary incontinence
- Ravenous appetite
- Glucose in the urine
- Nephritis
- Burning in the urethra
- Liver degeneration
- Fluid retention
- Great emaciation, debility
- Gastric and duodenal ulcers
- Bloated abdomen

Modalities
WORSE/AGGRAVATED BY: None listed
BETTER/AMELIORATED BY: None listed

Remedy Interactions – None listed

Principal Equine Indications
- Diabetes mellitus
- Diabetes insipidus
- Gastric ulceration, including in foals

Urtica urens, Urtica

COMMON NAME: Stinging nettle
CLASSIFICATION: Plant: Urticaceae family
PREPARATION: From tincture of the fresh plant in flower

Keynotes
- Urticaria, hives, itching blotches
- Violent itching
- Erythema
- Burns and scalds
- Swollen scrotum
- Itching around the vulval region

- Gravel in the urine, urolithiasis, bladder stones
- Rheumatic-like stiffness
- Neuritis
- Diarrhoea with large amounts of mucus
- Affects secretion of milk
- Excessively swollen udder (with milk)
- Uterine haemorrhage

Modalities

WORSE/AGGRAVATED BY: Cold air, water, cool moist air, touch, marked exertion, after sleep
BETTER/AMELIORATED BY: Resting

Remedy Interactions

CONSIDER ALSO: Nat mur, Apis, Medusa, Rhus tox, Formica, Lycopodium, Pulsatilla

Principal Equine Indications

- Urticaria, hives
- Oedema of allergic origin
- Angioneurotic oedema
- Marked skin irritation, itching
- Erythema (reddening of the skin)
- Dermatitis and eczema with marked irritation
- Irritation of the scrotum and vulva
- Burns and scalds
- Photosensitisation
- Equine nodular skin disease
- Insect bites or stings
- Urinary stones, gravel, calculi (urolithiasis) treatment and prevention
- Reduces secretion of milk in low potency (6x)
- Agalactia (lack of milk); increases milk production in high potency (200c)
- Swollen udder (with milk)
- Uterine haemorrhage of bright red blood
- Dourine

Ustilago maydis

COMMON NAME: Corn-smut
CLASSIFICATION: Plant: Fungi
PREPARATION: Trituration

Keynotes

- Haemorrhage
- Uterine haemorrhage of bright red blood with clots
- Uterine problems, enlargement
- Post-partum haemorrhage
- Oozing of dark clotted blood
- Hypersexuality
- Ovarian pain and swelling
- Orchitis
- Muscular weakness
- Muscular contractions
- Alopecia, dry skin

Modalities

WORSE/AGGRAVATED BY: Touch, local pressure (over the ovaries), travelling
BETTER/AMELIORATED BY: None listed

Remedy Interactions

CONSIDER ALSO: Secale, Sepia, Lilium tigrinum, Lachesis, Caulophyllum, Hamamelis, Millefolium, Elaps

Principal Equine Indications

- Uterine haemorrhage of bright red blood
- Post-partum haemorrhage worse on slightest movement
- Hypersexuality in the stallion
- False rigs
- Left-sided ovarian pain
- Nymphomania
- Vaginal bleeding between periods
- Muco-purulent, dark coloured uterine discharges
- Alopecia (hair loss)

Uva ursi

COMMON NAME: Bearberry, *Arctostaphylos uva ursi*
CLASSIFICATION: Plant: Ericaceae family
PREPARATION: From the fresh leaves

Keynotes

- Acts on the urinary system
- Cystitis with urine containing blood
- Urination painful
- Urine containing blood, pus and mucus
- Chronic inflammation of the bladder
- Pyelonephritis

Modalities

WORSE/AGGRAVATED BY: None listed
BETTER/AMELIORATED BY: None listed

Remedy Interactions – None listed

Principal Equine Indications
- Pyelonephritis

Valeriana

COMMON NAME: Valerian, *Valeriana officinalis*
CLASSIFICATION: Plant: Valerianaceae family
PREPARATION: Using tincture of the fresh root

Keynotes
- Behavioural problems
- Hypersensitivity, hysterical behavioiur
- Irritability
- Bloated, distended abdomen
- Watery diarrhoea
- Colic after feeding, spasmodic pains
- Asthma induced by anxiety
- Jerking limbs

Modalities
WORSE/AGGRAVATED BY: Midday, before midnight, open air
BETTER/AMELIORATED BY: After sleeping or resting, after feeding

Remedy Interactions
CONSIDER ALSO: Ignatia, Nux vomica, Aconite, Lac caninum, Zincum metallicum

Principal Equine Indications
- Behavioural problems
- Irritability, short temper
- Over-sensitivity, hysterical behaviour
- Anxiety
- COPD brought on by anxiety
- Spasmodic or flatulent colic induced by stress

Vanadium

COMMON NAME: Vanadium
CLASSIFICATION: Mineral: Metal
PREPARATION: By trituration

Keynotes
- Wasting and emaciation
- Anaemia
- Raises levels of haemoglobin
- Stimulates the immune system
- A tonic to the digestive system
- Degeneration of blood vessels

Modalities
WORSE/AGGRAVATED BY: None listed
BETTER/AMELIORATED BY: None listed

Remedy Interactions
CONSIDER ALSO: Phosphorus, Arsenicum album, China, Phos ac

Principal Equine Indications
- Emaciation and debility
- Poor appetite, to improve appetite
- Anaemia
- To stimulate the immune system by stimulating the white blood cells
- Low red and/or white blood cell count
- Equine ME, post-viral syndrome

Veratrum album

COMMON NAME: White hellebore
CLASSIFICATION: Plant: Melanthiaceae (Liliaceae) family
PREPARATION: From tincture of the fresh root gathered in early June

Keynotes
- Symptoms in general are very pronounced and appear suddenly
- Collapse, body feels markedly cold, icy cold, prostration
- Cyanosis (blue colour to the lips and mucous membranes)
- Extreme weakness
- Rapid, feeble pulse, irregular
- Cramping in the muscles
- State of stupor, indifference
- Eyes turned upwards
- Eyes sunken
- Skin icy cold to the touch
- Manic behaviour
- Pain leading to delirium, vocalisation
- Increased thirst
- Abdominal pain, spasms, colic

- Watery diarrhoea evacuated with force
- Constipation with straining, lack of peristaltic movement
- Rattling of mucus in the chest
- Bronchii full of mucus
- Chronic bronchitis

Modalities

WORSE/AGGRAVATED BY: At night, wet cold weather, touch, motion, damp weather, change of weather
BETTER/AMELIORATED BY: Warmth, rest

Remedy Interactions

WORKS WELL WITH: Arnica, Arsenicum album, Carbo veg
CONSIDER ALSO: China, Phos ac, Arsenicum album, Camphora

Principal Equine Indications

- Surgical shock, collapse, cold skin, slow recovery
- Severe shock
- Severe, acute watery diarrhoea with collapse, purging, weakness and shock in foals
- Acute salmonellosis
- Colitis X, clostridial enterotoxaemia
- Dehydration
- Exhaustion
- Severe colic with collapse and feeble circulation
- Constipation with straining leading to collapse or exhaustion
- As a tonic for the heart where there is cyanosis and collapse
- Chronic bronchitis in older horses
- Behavioural problems; destructive, aggressive behaviour with kicking or biting
- Coprophagia (eating dung) in foals

Veratrum viride

COMMON NAME: White American Hellebore, Indian Poke
CLASSIFICATION: Plant: Melanthaceae family
PREPARATION: From tincture of the fresh root

Keynotes

- Fall in blood pressure
- Lung congestion with severe pneumonia
- Twitching and convulsions
- Prostration
- Effects of sunstroke
- Pneumonia
- Congestion of the brain
- Pupil dilation
- Meningitis
- Twitching of the facial muscles
- Spasm of the oesophagus
- Post partum fever
- Muscle and joint pain
- Thirsty

Modalities

WORSE/AGGRAVATED BY: Morning
BETTER/AMELIORATED BY: Massage, rubbing, eating

Remedy Interactions

CONSIDER ALSO: Belladonna, Baptisia, Gelsemium, Aconite, Glonoine

Principal Equine Indications

- Bronchitis
- Severe pneumonia
- Toxic metritis
- Acute laminitis especially toxic laminitis
- Meningitis
- Sunstroke
- Choke

Verbascum

COMMON NAME: Mullein
CLASSIFICATION: Plant: Scrophulariaceae family
PREPARATION: From tincture of the fresh fruit

Keynotes

- Acts on the respiratory system and fifth (trigeminal) cranial nerve
- Facial pain (neuralgia)
- Catarrh with night-time cough
- Constant dribbling of urine
- Stiff joints in the lower limbs

Modalities

WORSE/AGGRAVATED BY: Change of temperature, sneezing, eating, left side, touch, pressure
BETTER/AMELIORATED BY: Gentle motion

Remedy Interactions

CONSIDER ALSO: Spigelia, Mag phos, Causticum

Principal Equine Indications

- Neuralgic pain around the jaw region especially the joint
- Left-sided facial pain
- Headshaking
- Chronic dribbling of urine

Vespa crabro, Vespa

COMMON NAME: Wasp, Wasp venom
CLASSIFICATION: Animal: Insects
PREPARATION: From a tincture of the living insects

Keynotes

- Acts on the skin and female reproductive tract
- Swollen conjunctival membranes (chemosis)
- Swelling around the mouth and throat
- Erythema
- Intense itching of the skin
- Wheals, hives, oedema
- Left-sided ovarian pain

Modalities

WORSE/AGGRAVATED BY: Motion, feeding
BETTER/AMELIORATED BY: Cold applications

Remedy Interactions

CONSIDER ALSO: Apis, Medusa, Bovista, Urtica

Principal Equine Indications

- Allergic skin reactions
- Acute allergic conjunctivitis with chemosis
- Hives, swellings
- Angioneurotic oedema
- Effects of insect bites
- Itching and reddening of the skin
- Left-sided ovarian pain, cystic ovaries
- Phimosis, paraphimosis

Viburnum opulus

COMMON NAME: High Cranberry, Cramp bark
CLASSIFICATION: Plant: Caprifoliaceae family
PREPARATION: From tincture of the fresh plant

Keynotes

- Muscular cramps and cramp-like pain
- Focus on the female reproductive system
- Colic-like pain in the pelvic organs
- Prevention of abortion
- Congestion of the ovaries
- Aching or discomfort around the pelvic region
- Lower back pain
- Excoriating uterine discharge
- Sensitivity in the umbilical region

Modalities

WORSE/AGGRAVATED BY: Sudden movement or jarring, motion, at night, cold, before oestrus
BETTER/AMELIORATED BY: Pressure, rest, open air

Remedy Interactions

CONSIDER ALSO: Caulophyllum, Chamomilla, Sepia, Secale, Actea rac, Lilium tigrinum, Lachesis

Principal Equine Indications

- Lower back pain present just before and during oestrus
- Colic present during oestrus
- Ovarian pain or discomfort
- General muscular discomfort in mares in oestrus
- Prevention of abortion

Vinca minor

COMMON NAME: Lesser periwinkle
CLASSIFICATION: Plant: Apocynaceae family
PREPARATION: From the whole fresh plant

Keynotes

- Skin problems
- Moist eczema on the head, hair matted together
- Eruptions on the nose
- Red sore itchy patches of skin, worse from rubbing
- Great sensitivity of the skin to touch
- Pustules
- Passive uterine haemorrhage

Modalities

WORSE/AGGRAVATED BY: None listed
BETTER/AMELIORATED BY: None listed

Remedy Interactions

CONSIDER ALSO: Merc sol, Oleander, Staphysagria, Graphites

Principal Equine Indications

- Moist, sticky dermatitis or eczema
- Areas of sensitive, red, inflamed skin, especially where the condition has arisen as a result of rubbing
- Mud fever
- Rainscald
- Seborrhoea

Viola tricolor

COMMON NAME: Pansy, Heartsease
CLASSIFICATION: Plant: Violaceae family
PREPARATION: From tincture of the fresh flowering plant

Keynotes

- Impetigo
- Marked itching
- Skin eruptions over the head region
- Thick scabs exuding yellow pus
- Sycosis

Modalities

WORSE/AGGRAVATED BY: At night, winter
BETTER/AMELIORATED BY: None listed

Remedy Interactions

WORKS WELL WITH: Pulsatilla, Rhus tox, Sepia, Staphysagria, Vinca minor, Merc sol, Oleander
CONSIDER ALSO: Rhus tox

Principal Equine Indications

- Mud fever with thick scabs and pus
- Eczema or dermatitis around the head region
- Dry scabby skin lesion with yellow exudation
- Skin eruptions with thick hard, cracked scabs
- Bacterial folliculitis

Vipera

COMMON NAME: Common viper, *Vipera comminis*
CLASSIFICATION: Animal: Reptiles: Snakes: Viperidae family
PREPARATION: From the venom

Keynotes

- Inflammation of the veins with marked swelling
- Acute phlebitis
- Enlarged liver, jaundice
- Haematuria (blood in the urine)

Modalities

WORSE/AGGRAVATED BY: Touch
BETTER/AMELIORATED BY: None listed

Remedy Interactions

CONSIDER ALSO: Bothrops, Apis mel, Bufo, Crot horr

Principal Equine Indications

- Acute lymphangitis especially with marked swelling
- Iliac thrombosis
- Snake bites

Viscum album

COMMON NAME: Mistletoe[15]
CLASSIFICATION: Plant: Loranthaceae family
PREPARATION: From tincture of the ripe berries, bruised leaves or whole plant

Keynotes

- Chronic metritis
- Left-sided ovarian pain
- Retained placenta
- Enlargement of the heart
- Valvular damage
- Pulse small and weak
- Epilepsy, petit mal
- Chorea
- In cancer therapy[15]

Modalities

WORSE/AGGRAVATED BY: Winter, cold stormy weather, movement
BETTER/AMELIORATED BY: None listed

Remedy Interactions

CONSIDER ALSO: Belladonna, Stramonium, Plumbum

Principal Equine Indications

- Petit mal

- Muscle twitching, chorea
- Heart enlargement concomitant with valvular disease
- Sarcoids, melanomas and other masses, cancers

Wyethia

COMMON NAME: Poison weed, *Wyethia helenoides*
CLASSIFICATION: Plant: Asteraceae (Compositae) family
PREPARATION: From tincture of the root

Keynotes

- Pharyngitis (inflammation of the throat)
- Swallowing difficult
- Mouth very dry
- Itching in the nose
- Dry hacking cough
- COPD

Modalities

WORSE/AGGRAVATED BY: Out riding, exercise, afternoon
BETTER/AMELIORATED BY: None listed

Remedy Interactions

CONSIDER ALSO: Sanguinaria, Rumex, Sticta

Principal Equine Indications

- COPD where itching or rubbing of the nose is a prominent feature
- Dry hacking cough with inflammation of the throat and difficulty swallowing
- Pharyngitis
- Headshaking

Xanthoxylum

COMMON NAME: Prickly ash, *Xanthoxylum americanum*
CLASSIFICATION: Plant: Rutaceae family
PREPARATION: From tincture of the fresh bark

Keynotes

- Acts on the nervous system and on mucous membranes
- Paralysis
- Rheumatic-like stiffness
- Colic from overeating
- Ovarian pain worse on the left side
- Pain which radiates down the legs and through the back
- Left-sided paralysis originating from spinal problems
- Poor capillary circulation

Modalities

WORSE/AGGRAVATED BY: 4am in the morning
BETTER/AMELIORATED BY: Rest

Remedy Interactions

CONSIDER ALSO: Cimicifugia (Actea rac), Plumbum, Lachesis, Hypericum

Principal Equine Indications

- Nerve or spinal injuries
- Left-sided hind limb paralysis or weakness
- Left-sided ovarian pain with associated back pain
- Chronic laminitis

Zincum metallicum

COMMON NAME: Zinc
CLASSIFICATION: Mineral: Element: Metal: Zincums
PREPARATION: Trituration of the metal

Keynotes

- Important action on the nervous system
- Tissues worn out faster than repaired
- Animals that have been worked too hard
- Poor vitality
- Depression
- Weak memory
- Sensitive to noise, starts easily
- Often have a friendly nature
- Alternating moods
- Yielding
- Spinal problems
- Twitching, chorea, trembling
- Convulsions, epilepsy
- Rolls head from side to side
- Bores head into wall
- Ptosis
- Rolling of the eyes
- Conjunctiva inflamed
- Lids itchy and sore
- Lack of tear production

- Cracks at the corners of the lips
- Teeth loose, gums bleed
- Greedy, eats very quickly
- Colic with rumbling noises
- Abdominal distension, flatulent colic
- Involuntary urination while walking
- Constipation, dung is small and hard
- Swollen testicles
- Left-sided ovarian pain with notable restlessness
- Nymphomania
- Sore udder, sore nipples
- Spasmodic cough worse for eating
- Blood-tinged expectoration
- Asthma with bronchitis eased by coughing up mucus
- Back pain (in the lumbar region), reacts to the least touch
- Burning heat along the spine
- Hind limbs weak.
- Cannot keep feet still
- Sensitivity/discomfort in the sole/frog
- Itching around the thighs, stifle region and lower leg
- Anaemia, destruction of red blood cells

Modalities

WORSE/AGGRAVATED BY: During oestrus, touch, pressure, rubbing, scratching, when ridden, exertion, rest, 5–7pm, becoming overheated, warm stable, if secretions suppressed

BETTER/AMELIORATED BY: While eating, appearance of discharges or eruptions, after oestrus

Remedy Interactions

INCOMPATIBLE WITH: Nux vomica, Chamomilla

WORKS WELL WITH: Sepia, Sulphur, Pulsatilla, Ignatia, Belladonna, Calc phos

CONSIDER ALSO: Plumbum, Pulsatilla, Lycopodium, Argentum nitricum, Phosphorus, Agaricus

Principal Equine Indications

- Conditions linked to the nervous system
- Agitated nervy horses
- Lack of motor control
- Paralysis accompanied by muscular tremors
- Viral infections characterised by neurological symptoms
- Equine protozoal myeloencephalitis
- Symptomatic treatment of poisoning
- Trembling, twitching, spasms, chorea
- Shivering
- Restlessness, weakness
- After-effects of concussion
- Epilepsy, fits, convulsions especially petit mal type fits
- Meningitis
- Loss of balance with tendency to fall to the left
- Neonatal maladjustment syndrome in foals
- Over-sensitivity to noise
- Depressed nature, lack of vitality, forgetful
- Effects of being worked too hard
- Ptosis, drooping of the lower eyelid
- Dry, inflamed cornea, dry eye (absence of tear production)
- Conjunctivitis with red inflamed lids
- Flatulent colic especially recurrent cases
- Constipation
- Colic from overeating
- Grass sickness
- Lumbar back pain with great sensitivity to touch
- Cracking in joints
- Osteochondrosis, OCD
- Left-sided ovarian pain often with nymphomania
- Anaemia
- Autoimmune haemolytic anaemia in foals
- Agalactia (lack of milk)
- Post-viral syndrome, Equine ME

Minor and Rarely Used Remedies

The following section includes brief details of some of the minor remedies that are used occasionally in treating horses.

Ammonium phosphoricum, Ammon phos

COMMON NAME: Ammonium phosphate, Phosphate of Ammonia
CLASSIFICATION: Mineral

Principal Equine Indications

- Facial paralysis

Anilinum

COMMON NAME: Aniline, Amidobenzene, a product of coal tar
CLASSIFICATION: Mineral: Carbon series

Principal Equine Indications

- Haematuria (blood in the urine)
- Tumours of hte urinary tract

Arsenicum hydrogenisatum

COMMON NAME: Arseniuretted Hydrogen
CLASSIFICATION: Mineral

Principal Equine Indications

- Coital exanthema

Arum triphyllum

COMMON NAME: Jack in the Pulpit
CLASSIFICATION: Plant: Araceae family

Principal Equine Indications

- Headshaking

Astacas

COMMON NAME: Crawfish, *Astacas fluviatilis*
CLASSIFICATION: Animal: Crustacean

Principal Equine Indications

- Urticaria
- Intense itching over the whole body

Atropinum

COMMON NAME: Atropine sulphate
CLASSIFICATION: Plant: Solanaceae family

Principal Equine Indications

- Stomach ulcers

Bamboo gum

COMMON NAME: Bamboo gum
CLASSIFICATION: Plant: Poaceae family

Principal Equine Indications

- Arthritis, Degenerative joint disease (DJD)
- OCD

Cadmium sulphate

COMMON NAME: Cadmium sulphate
CLASSIFICATION: Mineral

Principal Equine Indications

- Facial paralysis
- Corneal opacity
- Choke, oesophageal constriction
- Nasal polyps

Cajuputum

COMMON NAME: Cajuput oil

CLASSIFICATION: Plant: Myrtaceae family

Principal Equine Indications
- Choke
- Oesophageal spasm

Calcarea silicata, Calc sil

COMMON NAME: Calcium silicate, Silicate of Lime
CLASSIFICATION: Mineral

Principal Equine Indications
- Epizootic lymphangitis

Caltha palustris

COMMON NAME: Cowslip
CLASSIFICATION: Plant: Ranunculaceae family

Principal Equine Indications
- Pemphigus especially around the coronary band

Chelone

COMMON NAME: Snakeshead, *Chelone glabra*
CLASSIFICATION: Plant: Scrofulariaceae family

Principal Equine Indications
- Worms

Chrysarobinum

COMMON NAME: Goa powder, *Andira araroba*
CLASSIFICATION: Plant: Asteracea (Compositae) family

Principal Equine Indications
- Ringworm

Condurango

COMMON NAME: Condor Plant
CLASSIFICATION: Plant: Ascleipadaceae family

Principal Equine Indications
- Choke
- Eczema with marked cracks at the corners of the mouth
- Eczema at muco-cutaneous junctions
- Lupus
- Ulcerated melanomas

Cortisone

COMMON NAME: Hydrocortisone, a steroid
CLASSIFICATION: Animal: Sarcode

Principal Equine Indications
- Cushing's disease

Dolichos

COMMON NAME: Cowhage, *Mucuna pruriens*
CLASSIFICATION: Plant: Fabiaceae (Leguminosae) family

Principal Equine Indications
- Intense itching of the skin
- Severe sweet itch especially around the mane and withers region

Elaps

COMMON NAME: Brazilian Coral Snake
CLASSIFICATION: Animal: Reptile: Snake

Principal Equine Indications
- Oesophageal spasm, choke
- Black discharges, bleeding of dark, black blood
- Photic headshaking in bright light
- Itching of the ears
- Offensive and voluminous discharge of black material from the ears
- Chronic laminitis
- Fear of the rain

Eupion

COMMON NAME: Wood tar
CLASSIFICATION: Plant: Hydrocarbon

Principal Equine Indications
- Sweating from the least exertion, excessive sweating
- Severe lower back pain

Homarus

COMMON NAME: Digestive fluid of the live lobster
CLASSIFICATION: Animal: Crustacean

Principal Equine Indications

- Bone spavin

Hydrocotyle

COMMON NAME: Indian Pennywort, *Centella asiatica*
CLASSIFICATION: Plant: Apiaceae (Umbelliferae) family

Principal Equine Indications

- Hyperkeratosis, thickening of the skin with severe scaling
- Intolerable itching of the skin where thickened with marked scaling
- Sweet itch
- Lupus

Insulin

COMMON NAME: Insulin
CLASSIFICATION: Animal: Hormone: Sarcode

Principal Equine Indications

- Diabetes mellitus
- Cushing's disease

Laburnum

COMMON NAME: Laburnum, *Cystisus laburnum*
CLASSIFICATION: Plant: Fabacae family

Principal Equine Indications

- Meningitis

Lutenising hormone releasing hormone

COMMON NAME: LHRH
CLASSIFICATION: Animal: Hormone: Sarcode

Principal Equine Indications

- Infertility with normal cycling

Mercurius sulphuricus

COMMON NAME: Yellow sulphate of mercury
CLASSIFICATION: Mineral: Mercury series

Principal Equine Indications

- Hydrothorax
- Chronic hepatitis
- Severe watery diarrhoea

Mineral

COMMON NAME: Vermiculite
CLASSIFICATION: Mineral

Principal Equine Indications

- Bone spavin (used in 6x potency)
- Ringbone
- Exostoses, bone spurs

Ocimum canum

COMMON NAME: Brazilian Alfavaca
CLASSIFICATION: Plant: Lamiaceae (Labiatae) family

Principal Equine Indications

- Pyelonephritis
- Kidney pain
- Gravel in the urine, urolithiasis

Ornithogalum umbellatum

COMMON NAME: Star of Bethlehem
CLASSIFICATION: Plant: Hyacinthaceae family

Principal Equine Indications

- Stomach ulcers

Onosmodium

COMMON NAME: False Gromwell
CLASSIFICATION: Plant: Boraginaceae family

Principal Equine Indications

- Sprains
- Enlargement of the retinal blood vessels
- Misjudgement of distances or jumps
- Poor coordination of the hindlimbs

- Equine protozoal myeloencephalitis, EPM

Osteoarthritic nosode

COMMON NAME: Arthritic bone
CLASSIFICATION: Animal: Nosode

Principal Equine Indications

- Arthritis, DJD

Passiflora

COMMON NAME: Passion flower
CLASSIFICATION: Passifloraceae family

Principal Equine Indications

- Tetanus
- Hysterical behaviour

Progesterone

COMMON NAME: Progesterone
CLASSIFICATION: Animal: Hormone: Sarcode

Principal Equine Indications

- Infertility with normal cycling

Ranunculus bulbosus

COMMON NAME: Buttercup
CLASSIFICATION: Plant: Ranunculaceae family

Principal Equine Indications

- Skin vesicles or skin blisters with intense itching especially around the nose
- Shoulder and lower neck pain
- Sarcoids
- Hard wart-like skin growths
- Adhesions after pleurisy

Ranunculus scleratus

COMMON NAME: Marsh Buttercup
CLASSIFICATION: Plant: Ranunculaceae family

Principal Equine Indications

- Pemphigus

Raphanus

COMMON NAME: Black Garden Radish
CLASSIFICATION: Plant: Brassicaceae (Cruciferae) family

Principal Equine Indications

- Tympanic colic
- To prevent build-up of gas in the intestine post-operatively

Salvia officinalis

COMMON NAME: Sage
CLASSIFICATION: Plant: Laminaceae (Labiatae) family

Principal Equine Indications

- Excessive sweating

Santoninum

COMMON NAME: Santonin
CLASSIFICATION: Plant: Asteraceae (Compositae) family

Principal Equine Indications

- Worms

Shark cartilage

COMMON NAME: Dried Shark Cartilage
CLASSIFICATION: Animal: Sarcode

Principal Equine Indications

- OCD
- Osteochrondrosis
- Degenerative joint disease (DJD), arthritis

Staphlococcal nosode

COMMON NAME: Staphylococcal bacteria
CLASSIFICATION: Nosode

Principal Equine Indications

- Skin infections
- Bacterial folliculitis

Stillingia

COMMON NAME: Queen's Root
CLASSIFICATION: Plant: Euphorbiaceae family

Principal Equine Indications

- Bone pain, especially of the lower limbs and back

Succinum

COMMON NAME: Amber, Fossil resin
CLASSIFICATION: Plant

Principal Equine Indications

- Fear of closed places
- Poor travellers

Tetanus nosode, Tetanotoxinium

COMMON NAME: Tetanus
CLASSIFICATION: Animal: Nosode

Principal Equine Indications

- Tetanus (to augment other remedies)

Upas tiente, Upas

COMMON NAME: Upas tree, *Strychnos tiente*
CLASSIFICATION: Plant: Loganiacea family

Principal Equine Indications

- Tetanus
- Tonic spasms

Viola odorata

COMMON NAME: Violet
CLASSIFICATION: Plant: Violaceae family

Principal Equine Indications

- Carpal tunnel syndrome
- Poor memory

The Bowel Nosodes

The word nosode has its roots in the Greek for disease but now denotes a remedy prepared from diseased material, either infected tissue or the associated organisms, often bacteria or viruses. Various nosodes are used in veterinary homeopathy, but the bowel nosodes comprise a small group of remedies prepared homeopathically from bacteria commonly found in the gut. A large proportion of the development of the bowel nosodes was carried out by Dr Edward Bach in the 1920s, the same Dr Bach that went on to develop the flower remedies a decade later. A Scottish doctor, John Paterson and his wife carried out further work on the bowel nosodes during the 1930s, 40s and 50s, adding additional observations and indications.

The Bowel and Bacteria

The bacteria comprising the bowel nosodes were originally cultured from the stools of human patients with chronic ill health, although the same bacteria are also found in healthy patients. Chronic disease appears to 'stress' patients leading to a change in the levels of bacteria in the bowel. This causes larger numbers of a particular type of bacteria to appear in the gut and stools. The particular organism that proliferates depends on the patients' symptom picture; patients with similar pictures tended to have abnormally large amounts of the same bacteria in their stools. With a correlation between symptoms of ill health and bacteria in the gut, it is possible to use the relevant bacteria in its homeopathic potentised form to help treat the appropriate symptom picture.

Although these remedies, known commonly as the bowel nosodes (or occasionally as the intestinal nosodes), were originally prepared from bacteria[16] found in human stools, their associated symptom pictures are clearly seen in animals including horses. This means that we can still use these remedies with definite advantage where the symptom picture is present. In addition to this, each individual bowel nosode is linked with a group of associated remedies.

Using the Bowel Nosodes

There are certain instances where the bowel nosodes can be used, particularly where there is a clear symptom picture corresponding to the nosode and no other remedy is clearly indicated. The matching symptom picture should include mental as well as physical symptoms. They can also be used:

- Where a case is not responding to current treatment
- Where the choice of remedy may lie between several remedies. If those remedies fall in the group of remedies associated with a particular nosode, there is an indication for using that bowel nosode
- Where an animal may have had a number of remedies over a period of time with varying degrees of failure and success

Choice of Potency

In general the **30c potency** should be used *twice daily for a few days,* the exact length of time determined by observing any change in symptoms. As deep-acting remedies they should not be repeated too frequently nor should they be used one after the other without a period of several weeks in between. Higher potencies can be used under professional guidance, where the mental symptoms of the remedy correspond exactly with the patient's mental symptoms. Here the 200c or 1M potency can be employed giving a few doses over four or five days only and not repeated for a period of two or three months.

Specific Bowel Nosodes and their Symptom Pictures

Of the 11 or so bowel nosodes, the following can be used in horses. Associated remedies are graded. Those in **bold** type have a close association with the nosode. Those in *italics* are less closely linked and those in plain type have the weakest association.

Morgan or Morgan Bach

Keynotes: Congestion

This nosode (which is further divided into two sub-groups) has an affinity for the skin and mucous membranes of the digestive tract, urinary tract and reproductive system. There is also an action on the liver.

(i) Morgan-Pure

The main focus of this remedy is on the skin. Symptoms to check for include itching, thickened, fissured or cracked skin (such as in mud fever), red raw patches of eczema, weeping eczema and dandruff-like scaling. All the skin symptoms are worse for heat. Other points of note include the mental symptoms of irritability, depression, fear of crowded areas and anxiety if left alone. Where the digestive system is concerned Morgan can help with symptoms of gut stasis (constipation), liver pain, liver congestion and jaundice. There are some specific actions on the locomotor system. Morgan is indicated in cases where there are arthritic changes affecting the spine and sacro-iliac joints, for shoulder pain (which eases on movement), where there is pain and swelling of the knee (carpal joint) and fetlock joints (front or hind legs), arthritis and swelling of the stifle with crepitus (grating noises in the joint) and cases of acute laminitis where there is marked heat and pain in the front feet.

Associated remedies

Sulphur, *Psorinum, Medorrhinum, Graphites,* Calc carb, Calc sulph, Petroleum, Sepia, Tuberculinum

(ii) Morgan-Gaertner

The focus here is on the urinary tract and digestive system. Behavioural symptoms to note include irritability, a short temper, impatience and nervous tension. There may also be a fear of crowded areas and of strangers. Of the digestive symptoms the keynote is flatulent colic especially where the colon is markedly distended. Morgan-Gaertner can also help with general flatulence, sluggish digestion and constipation where the dung is dry, as well as kidney pain, pyelonephritis and cystitis.

Associated remedies

Lycopodium, *Lachesis*, Chelidonium, Helleborus, Hepar sulph, Sanguinaria

Proteus-Bach

Keynotes: Nervous system

Proteus focuses on imbalances within both the peripheral and central nervous system and covers symptoms such as spasms, cramping and epilepsy. Illness arising as a consequence of prolonged stress or strain can also benefit from this remedy with symptoms appearing suddenly as an important guiding keynote. Behavioural problems covered include tendency to a fiery, explosive nature and sudden impulsive behaviour with anger and the possibility of kicking out or a bite. Horses needing Proteus often appear edgy with the autonomic nervous system working overtime; they are keyed up and ready to go and appear edgy with signs of fear or apprehension but may also appear stubborn at times. They are often loners and will not form close associations with other horses.

Along with behavioural indications, specific indications for Proteus include azoturia (tying up), epilepsy, stringhalt, shivering (shivers), gastric (stomach) ulcers arising from prolonged stress (where the symptoms appear without warning) and refractory cases of tetanus. Chronically thickened flexor tendons may also benefit as the remedy has the ability to reduce fibrous thickenings if given over a prolonged period of time. In this context it may also be of benefit in treating fibrotic myopathy, curb and stricture of the palmar annular ligament. Horses which are unduly sensitive to ultraviolet light may also respond, suggesting that Proteus is of use in treating cases of photosensitisation and sunburn. With the regard for the skin, Proteus is also one of the key remedies for treating cases of angioneurotic oedema and for alleviating eczema which occurs at the junctions where mucous membranes meet the skin, such as the lips and the vulval area. Proteus has an association with the adrenal glands and kidneys as well as the chloride ion, and hence is linked with many of the chloride group of remedies – the muriaticums.

Associated remedies
Natrum mur, Apis, Borax, Cuprum met, Ignatia, Secale, Acid mur, Ammon mur, Baryta mur, Calc mur, Kali mur, Mag mur.

Gaertner-Bach

Keynotes: Nutrition and digestion
The most striking feature of animals needing this remedy is that of emaciation or malnourishment and poorly developed muscles as a result of poor nutrition or digestive problems. They appear lean and slender with a poor conformation, although some horses may have a potbelly. As bright, sensitive, intelligent animals, they can appear ill at ease and restless; they have a need to know what is going on all the time. Prone to becoming excitable from time to time, they are always keen to do their best. They prefer company and will avoid being left alone where possible.

Indications include emaciation from any cause where the digestive system is involved, ranging from inadequate feeding, weak digestion, chronic diarrhoea or heavy worm burdens, as well as chronic Salmonellosis. Gaertner is one of the remedies to be considered after the use of antibiotics where the digestive system has been upset and has not returned to normal.

Associated remedies
Phosphorus, **Silica**, **Merc sol**, Calc fluor, Calc phos, Kali phos, Nat phos, Pulsatilla, Zinc phos

Dysentry Co Bach (Dys Co)

Keynotes: Nervous system, heart, digestion
The action of Dysentry Co covers such nervous symptoms as anticipatory anxiety, specific fears (such as of certain objects, of people or places), irrational fears, impatience, restlessness, insecurity, shyness and lack of confidence. Noise aggravates any problems and there is a tendency to become easily flustered and to display soft or sloppy dung before events brought on by anxiety.

Dys Co is a key remedy (along with Lycopodium) for anticipatory anxiety and will help relieve the tension which builds before performing in any important event, as well as helping horses that are difficult to load into horseboxes. Specific non-behavioural indications include gastric ulcers whose symptoms appear slowly over a period of time, back pain (which eases with movement), a tendency to flatulent colic (brought on by nervous tension), cardiac arrhythmias, cases of mud fever where Graphites fails to work and chronic laminitis where there are marked ridges or cracks on the hooves caused by poor circulation and nutrition to the laminae.

Associated remedies
Arsenicum album, Argentum nitricum, Kalmia, Anacardium, Tuberculinum, Veratrum album

Sycotic Co Paterson

Keynotes: Irritability, skin, mucous membranes
The behavioural symptoms linked with Sycotic Co are in many ways similar to those of Gaertner but the worries of the horse needing Sycotic Co are more hidden. These animals are nearly always fat, in direct contrast to the emaciated appearance of the horse requiring Gaertner. They are also easily irritated or tense and may kick out or bite suddenly without warning.

Any condition where yellow, green, thick catarrh is present can respond, suggesting the use of this remedy in chronic rhinitis, sinus infections and guttural pouch problems that fail to respond to other remedies. Cases of COPD can also respond where there is wheezing and coughing with production of thick, yellowish mucus. Cases of flu that are refractory to treatment may also be given Sycotic Co to encourage a speedy recovery. Skin symptoms are prominent with Sycotic Co, which is indicated in the treatment of warts, sarcoids and melanomas as well as allergic skin problems (such as sweet itch) where other remedies such as Rhus tox have not worked. It can also help with mud fever cases (especially where there are very deep cracks in the skin) that fail to resolve completely and in cases of equine nodular skin disease (allergic collagen necrosis) where the nodules fail to shrink away.

Further indications for this remedy include lumbo-sacral and sacro-iliac pain that eases with movement and warmth, DJD of the fetlock joints of the forelimb and chronic synovitis with distension of the affected joints. Sycotic Co is also useful in cases of a persistent urethral discharge (urethritis) in geldings or stallions where other remedies have not proved successful.

Associated remedies
Thuja, **Medorrhinum**, Nitric acid, Ant tart, Natrum sulph, Rhus tox, Bacillinum, Kali bich, Hydrastis, Lycopodium, Sepia

The Tissue Salts

The twelve biochemic tissue salts, sometimes referred to as cell or mineral salts, were first identified by Dr Schuessler and represent minerals that are found in the body. They are all required for normal cell or body function and support the body from both a physical and structural aspect. Imbalances in these minerals can lead to health problems or diseases which can benefit from taking the remedies to help restore the balance to the body once more.

The remedies are prescribed therapeutically in low potency homeopathic potency (6x) and are used either singly or in combination. The same remedies are frequently used in higher potency for other far ranging problems, as will be evident from looking at the Materia Medica or the rest of the book. The main difference that you will note, however, is in their mode of action. The tissue salts work in a homogenous way acting almost nutritionally in contrast to the heterogeneous or more diverse action of most homeopathic remedies which work energetically.

Dose: *The normal dose is four to eight tablets (depending on the size of the horse) three times daily*

Calc fluor 6x, Calcium fluoride

Keynote: Elasticity

Function

Helps with the elastic, connective tissue of the skin, muscles and blood vessels. Is a constituent of teeth enamel and bone.

Indications

- To encourage the return of elasticity to tissues
- Weak muscles
- Poor tooth enamel
- Cracked skin
- Tendon and ligament injuries
- Synovitis
- To strengthen bone
- Chronic joint inflammation
- Chronic sinus problems
- Sluggish circulation
- Chronic laminitis
- Bowel impaction resulting from lack of muscle power

Calc phos 6x, Calcium phosphate

Keynote: Nutrition

Function

- Helps in the formation of new blood cells
- Found in bone, teeth, connective tissue and in the digestive juices
- Promotes growth

Indications

- Bone weakness
- Fractures
- Muscle spasms
- Fatigue
- Debility
- Where there is poor assimilation of food or poor nutrition

- As a tonic after bowel surgery
- Anaemia (in combination with Ferrum phos)

Calc sulph 6x, Calcium sulphate

Keynote: Blood purifier

Function

- To purify the blood. Helps the liver in the removal or elimination of waste products.

Indications

- In general most skin problems where infection is evident
- Abscesses
- Ulcers in the mouth
- Slow or poor healing wounds
- Catarrh (in combination with Kali mur)
- Works well in combination with Kali mur and Nat sulph

Ferr Phos 6x, Ferrum phosphate, Iron phosphate

Keynote: First aid

Function

- Carries oxygen around the body and strengthens blood vessel walls.

Indications

- Respiratory infections including Equine flu
- Haemorrhage
- Anaemia
- Fevers especially with high temperature and a rapid pulse
- To reduce the intensity of fevers
- Pharyngitis or laryngitis
- Early stages of inflammation
- Muscle injuries, strains and sprains
- Poor appetite
- Effects of insect bites
- Poor coat, lack of shine
- Encourages the uptake and assimilation of iron

Kali Mur 6x, Kalium muriaticum, Potassium chloride

Keynote: Blood conditioner and glandular tonic

Function

- Blood conditioner and glandular tonic

Indications

- Respiratory problems including coughs and equine flu
- Catarrh and wheezing
- Bronchitis
- White-coloured discharges
- Swollen lymph nodes
- Can be alternated with Ferr Phos
- Works well with Calc sulph to clean the blood of toxins

Kali Phos 6x, Kalium phosphate, Potassium phosphate

Keynote: The nervous system

Function

- Supports the nervous system, present in brain cells and nerve tissue

Indications

- Stress, anxiety
- Mental and physical exhaustion
- Poor memory and concentration
- Despondency and iritability

Kali Sulph 6x, Kalium sulphate, Potassium sulphate

Keynote: The skin

Function

- Oxygenates the cells and tissues of the body
- Ensures health of the cells lining the mucous membranes and the cells of the skin

Indications

- Skin, hair, coat and hoof problems
- Catarrh
- Sticky glutinous discharges especially if yellowish or green
- Wandering lameness
- Ringworm
- Dandruff, skin scaling
- Can be used with Silica to treat brittle hooves and where the coat and hair is poor or sparse

Mag Phos 6x, Magnesium phosphate

Keynote: Nerves and pain

Function

- Anti-spasmodic, ensures proper muscle function
- Constituent of bone, teeth, nerves, blood cells

Recommended for

- Cramps, tying up, azoturia (in combination with Nat mur and Calc fluor)
- Back pain in mares in season
- Spasms
- Paralysis
- Relief from sharp pain
- Flatulence and flatulent colic
- Poor energy levels
- Nerve pain
- Urolithiasis (bladder stones or gravel)

Nat mur 6x, Natrum muriaticum, Sodium chloride, Common salt

Keynote: Water and fluid regulation

Function

- Regulates water metabolism
- Ensures hydration of the body tissues

Indications

- Dryness or excessive moisture in any area of the body
- Watery catarrh, rhinitis with a watery nasal discharge
- Dry itchy skin, sweet itch
- Fatigue
- Ascites, oedema, water retention
- Dry dung
- Emaciation

Nat phos 6x, Natrum phosphate, Sodium phosphate

Keynote: Digestion and acidity

Function

- To neutralise acid in the body
- Assists in the assimilation of fatty acids
- Helps to regulate the function of the liver.

Indications

- Stomach ulcers
- Colic
- Joint pain and stiffness
- Joint swelling
- Hyperlipaemia
- Jaundice

Nat sulph 6x, Natrum sulphate, Sodium sulphate

Keynote: Water/fluid regulation

Function

- To eliminate excess water and to help maintain the health of the liver

Indications

- Ascites
- Equine flu
- Liver problems including jaundice
- Hepatitis
- Digestive disturbances
- Joint stiffness

Silica 6x, Silicea, Silicon dioxide

Keynote: Tissue integrity and strength

Function

- Acts as a cleanser and detoxifier
- Present in blood, skin, hoof, hair, bones, connective tissue and mucous membranes.

Indications

- Abscesses, sinuses and fistulae
- Expulsion of foreign material from the body
- Any type of skin condition with pus or suppuration
- Cracked, brittle damaged hooves

Caution
Since one of the effects of Silica is to promote expulsion of foreign matter from the body, this remedy shouldn't be used for long periods in any animal with implanted material such as bone plates or screws.

Useful combinations for chronic conditions

Colic combination: **Calc phos, Mag phos, Nat sulph**

Cough combination: **Ferrum phos, Kali mur, Nat mur**

Poor coat or hooves combination: **Kali sulph, Nat mur, Silica**

Combination for skin problems: **Kali mur, Kali sulph, Silica**

Combination for debility: **Calc phos, Kali phos, Ferrum phos**

Headshaking combination: **Mag phos, Nat mur, Silica**

Glossary and Other Homeopathic Terms

Acute disease
An illness that appears quickly but which only lasts for a short period of time. There are several possible outcomes. Spontaneous recovery, recovery in response to treatment or failure to recover culminating in death.

Acute remedy
One used to treat acute symptoms or in an emergency situation, in contrast to a chronic remedy which might be used to treat a long-term problem. Acute remedies often have a shorter duration of action and may need to be repeated more frequently. There is a close association between some acute and chronic remedies, for example between Apis mel and Nat mur. Some of these relationships are given in the Materia Medica.

Aggravation
An increase in the severity or worsening of the symptoms. In homeopathic terms a short-lasting aggravation following a homeopathic prescription usually implies a favourable response to the remedy.

Allopathy
A system of medicine using therapeutic agents that have no direct relationship to the disease or symptoms in their effect.

Amelioration
An improvement or reduction in the severity of the patient's symptoms. This can be due to successful administration of a remedy or from other factors. For example a change in external temperature, change of season, the passing of dung or urine or a change in body position.

Antiopathy
A system of medicine using therapeutic agents to treat illness that have an action directly opposite to the effects of the underlying disease. For example the use of purgatives to treat impacted colic.

Antipathic
In relation to antiopathy, antagonistic to or in opposition to the symptoms of the disease.

Antipsoric
A term applied to a homeopathic remedy used to treat the clinical symptoms associated with the psoric miasm.

Antisycotic
A term applied to a homeopathic remedy use to treat the clinical symptoms associated with the sycotic miasm.

Antisyphilitic
A term applied to a homeopathic remedy used to treat the clinical symptoms associated with the syphilitic miasm.

Autonosode
A nosode prepared (homeopathically) from diseased material from the patient. For example, pus from an abscess or mucus from a nasal discharge.

Bowel nosodes
A group of homeopathic remedies prepared from culture of the bacteria in the stools of (human) patients showing specific disease traits that had improved with particular homeopathic remedies. Although remedies in their own right, they can be used to strengthen the effect of remedies in their own medicine group.

C potency
An abbreviation 'c' for the centesimal potency range sometimes denoted as 'cH' or 'C'.

Centesimal potency
Homeopathic preparations (remedies) produced by dilutions of 1 part in 100. More specifically 1 part of the previous dilution added to 99 drops of diluent. The number of dilution steps determines the potency and is represented by a number followed by the letter 'c' signifying the centesimal range. For example the 30c potency represents a dilution of 1 in 100 performed serially 30 times with succussion at each stage and represents a dilution of $1/10^{60}$ or concentration of 10^{-60}. The 'c' is often omitted so that, for example Arnica 30 is the same as Arnica 30c. In other European countries the 'c' is sometimes replaced by 'C' or 'cH' so that Arnica 30 would be Arnica C30 or 30cH.

Chronic disease
A disease which progresses gradually and which becomes established. The symptoms may become chronic with no periods of relief or may consist of a series of recurrent acute episodes.

Chronic remedy
A remedy used to treat long-term illness in contrast to the related acute remedy which might be used to treat symptoms which suddenly flare up in the same patient.

Cinchona, Cinchona bark
A source of quinine used to treat malaria. Hahnemann took repeated doses, following which he developed symptoms similar to the disease. It was from this experiment that he developed his Similia Principle – let like be cured by like.

Clinical picture
A collection of symptoms associated with an illness which includes particular, general and mental symptoms as applied to an individual patient.

Compatability
Applied to homeopathic remedies that can be used in combination with each other but with either no advantage or disadvantage to each other.

Concomitant symptoms
These are symptoms that are linked with other symptoms during an illness. For example, irritability in mares associated with the days leading up to oestrus or sweating associated with pain.

Constitutional prescribing
The use of a remedy prescribed on the patient's constitution in comparison to prescribing on the clinical symptoms alone.

Constitutional remedy
A remedy matched to the patient as a whole encompassing both psychological and physical characteristics. Exactly what constitutional remedies cover in their remit is greater than it would initially appear, including inherited traits, the effect of life events or reaction to external stimuli, lifestyle, diet and environment in contrast to the presenting symptoms of an illness which represents the way the body responds to disease.

D potency
An abbreviation for the decimal potency usually denoted by 'x'. In some countries the x is replaced by the letter D.

Decimal potency
Homeopathic preparations (remedies) produced by dilutions of 1 part in 10. More specifically 1 part of the previous dilution added to 9 drops of diluent. The number of dilution steps determines the potency and is represented by a number followed by the letter 'x' signifying the decimal range. For example the 6x potency represents a dilution of 1 in 10 performed serially 6 times with succussion at each stage, and represents a dilution of 1/1,000,000 or concentration of 10^{-6}. The 'x' is sometimes replaced by 'D' in other European countries so that, for example, Urtica 6x is the same as Urtica D6.

Dilution
A process or stage used in the manufacture of homeopathic remedies involving a reduction in the strength of a substance by adding diluent, usually a mixture of alcohol or water. This is performed using specific quantities of diluent added to either the stock solution of a remedy or the previous dilution

prior to succussion, to produce different potency ranges. The term dilution usually refers to liquids but where insoluble substances are involved, the first few stages of dilution are carried out by trituration using lactose as the diluent.

Disease
Fundamentally disease means disorder relating to one or more of the following: the tissues of the body, individual organs, the way in which they act or to a physiological system at an anatomical, cellular or biochemical level. Disease can also be viewed as a disturbance of the balance that exists between the vital force and the body.

Doctrine
Principles, which together, form the basis of both teaching and practice of a system of medicine such as homeopathy.

Dosage forms
These represent the ways in which remedies can be given to the patient. Most remedies are presented in one of the following ways:

- **Tablets** – lactose base – biconvex, white, hard
- **Tablets** – lactose base – soft (powdery) and crumbly
- **Pills, pillules and globules** – sucrose base – small hard balls – varying sizes
- **Coarse granules** – sucrose base – resembles sugar, free flowing
- **Powders** – lactose base – individually wrapped in white paper
- **Liquid potency** – water and alcohol base
- **Mother tincture** – strong water and alcohol extract of a remedy denoted by the symbol Ø

Drainage remedy
A remedy, usually given in low potency over a period of weeks, used to drain toxins from a particular organ system. For example, Petroleum is a drainage remedy used to drain toxins from the skin.

Dynamisation
The process by which the medicinal activity or medicinal power of a homeopathic remedy is harnessed. Involves serial dilution and succussion for substances which are soluble and initial trituration for insoluble substances to render them soluble, followed by serial dilution and succussion.

Exacerbation
Is said to occur when the patient's symptoms become worse or the signs associated with a disease increase in severity.

General symptoms
Symptoms applying to the patient as a whole in contrast to a specific area or system. Usually the reaction of the patient (as a whole) to factors such as temperature, weather, time of year, time of day, foods and external stimuli.

Hahnemann
Christian Friedrich Samuel Hahnemann (1755–1843). German doctor and founder of homeopathy. Founded the *Similia Principle,* published in 1796. Author of the *Organon,* published in 1810 and *Materia Medica Pura,* published between 1811 and 1821.

Herbal medicine
Often confused with homeopathy as both systems of medicine share plant-based source material. Herbal medicine often referred to as phytotherapy employs the use of medicinal plants in the form of alcoholic extracts (not to be confused with mother tinctures), teas, decoctions or dried plant material.

Hering's law or rule
A law formulated by a German doctor Constantin Hering (1800–1880), relating to the direction in which symptoms resolve (the direction of cure) as the patient's condition improves. Essentially symptoms improve:

- From above downward
- From inside to the outside
- From deeper organs to those which are more superficial

- From the mental level to the physical level
- From important organs to those which are less important
- From more recent symptoms to older symptoms i.e. symptoms disappear in reverse order to their appearance

Hippocrates
Philosopher and Greek physician (*c.* 460–377 BC). The 'Father of Medicine'. He noted that illness could be resolved by medicines that caused the same symptoms.

Homeopathic remedy
A medicine produced (prepared) by homeopathic principles in a specific dosage form and potency ready for administration to the patient.

Homeopathy
A system of medicine founded on the Similia Principle of 'like cures like' as developed by Samuel Hahnemann. The use of substances whose effect on healthy patients correspond to the symptoms associated with illness (or disease) of an individual patient.

Inimical
Incompatibility relating to a homeopathic remedy which interferes with the effect of another but does not directly antidote it.

Isopathy
The treatment of illness using remedies produced either from the causative agent itself (such as the E.coli bacterium or allergens such as rapeseed pollen) or from a substance produced by the disease (such as diarrhoea or pus).

Lactose
Milk sugar used in the production of tablets or powders as the base for delivering a homeopathic remedy to the patient. Lactose is also used a diluent in the process of trituration of insoluble remedies.

Layers of disease
This refers to disease patterns in chronic illness, superimposed on one another, each having a symptom picture of its own. Treatment using homeopathy can peel away each individual layer to reveal the next layer hidden underneath.

Life force
Also known as the vital force, this is the energy that gives life to living organisms. It is a concept that is recognised throughout many different world cultures by a variety of names such as *Qi* in Chinese medicine and *Prana* in Indian medicine.

LM potency
The term LM is derived from the Latin L (50) and M (1000) and is applied to a range of potencies with a dilution factor of 1/50,000. LM potencies are of special benefit to some patients as they are unlikely to cause aggravations and act at a deep level. They are usually administered in liquid form and use the 3c potency of the remedy as the base for the first dilution and succussion.

Local symptom
A symptom relating to a specific organ, body system or particular part of the body.

M potency
M denotes the millesimal potency and represents dilutions of 1 part in 1,000 or 1 part of the previous potency to 999 parts of diluent. They are normally made by a special method using the 3c potency of the remedy for the base for the first dilution and succussion.

Materia Medica
In homeopathy a textbook containing therapeutic details of remedies detailing their source, pathology (symptoms) relating to each body system, modalities and characteristics of the patient, together with their relationship (interaction) with other remedies. The information is gathered from provings and clinical experience in practice.

Mental symptoms
Psychological symptoms displayed by a patient. The symptoms may relate to the illness (problem) itself for example anxiety while travelling in a horsebox, fear of sudden noises or may relate to the animal in general i.e. excitable, jealous, obstinate, shy.

Miasm
Originally postulated by Hahnemann as a term to be applied to an infectious agent, but extended to relate to noxious vapours or atmospheres. More specifically, a miasm is an inherited trait within an individual or family to become ill in a particular way or to show a certain susceptibility to illness. Hahnemann attributed these traits to be the result of inheriting the effects of three diseases:

- Itch – Psora – underreaction
- Gonorrhoea – Sycosis – overreaction
- Syphilis – breakdown or destruction

Where these traits can be identified, specific remedies can be prescribed to help.

Modality
A factor which alters a symptom in terms of severity, degree or intensity. Includes factors such as ambient temperature, weather, season, effects of specific foods or specific actions such as eating, passing urine as well as emotions, movement, pressure, massage, the oestrus cycle and phase of the moon.

Mother tincture
This forms the starting material for the production of most remedies and is the liquid produced from a water and ethanol extraction of the source material. The exact extraction method used depends on the nature of the source material. Mother tinctures are often denoted by the symbol Ø, although the term MT is occasionally used.

Nosode
A homeopathic remedy produced from diseased material. This may be bacteria, viruses, diseased tissue, pus, mucus or any other type of discharge associated with the disease. Nosodes are used in the prevention and treatment of disease.

Organ affinity
The tendency for certain remedies to act upon or influence certain organs. For example Solidago influences the kidneys, Chelidonium the liver and Crataegus the heart.

Organon
Published works extending over six editions between 1810 and 1842 by Hahnemann stating the principles of homeopathy.

Particular symptom
Relates to symptoms linked with individual organs, organ systems or parts of the body.

Polycrest
Applied to a homeopathic remedy with a wide spectrum of uses or applications acting on nearly all or most parts of the body. Polycrests have a wide range of clinical uses and can be used in treating both acute and chronic conditions. Many are used as constitutional remedies.

Potency
Used to define the 'strength' or degree of medicinal 'power' of a homeopathic remedy produced by the process of potentisation.

Potency scales
Scales used to indicate the degree of potency of a homeopathic remedy. Often divided into the following arbitrary categories:

- **Low potency**
  Potencies below 12c or 24x
- **Medium potency**
  Potencies between 12c and 30c
- **High potency**
  Potencies above 30c

Potentisation
The term applied to the process developed by Hahnemann through which the medicinal power or potency of a remedy is released or can be increased. Potentisation involves both serial dilution and succussion. Dynamisation is often taken to mean the same as potentisation.

Proving
The administration to healthy volunteers of material doses, mother tincture or potency of a remedy in order to determine its medicinal uses which can be compiled into a Materia Medica. It can also be taken to mean the administration of a remedy to a patient

sufficient to lead to those symptoms of the remedy as listed in the Materia Medica, in effect a form of homeopathic overdosing.

Psoric miasm or Psora
One of three chronic miasms. Symptoms associated with or susceptibility to, a picture of disease linked originally with itching of the skin but now associated with lack of reaction or under-reaction of the body.

Recapitulation
The temporary resurgence or reappearance of old symptoms, often those which have been suppressed by conventional medicine. Usually taken to indicate good progress with a case.

Remedy
A colloquial term applied to a homeopathic medicine.

Remedy picture
Synonymous with the term drug picture. Comprises the characteristic features of a remedy as detailed in the Materia Medica listing all the noted mental, general and particular (local) symptoms along with the modalities and other notable points relating to the remedy.

Repertory
A book containing a cross reference of symptoms and their associated remedies which are graded to show the strength of the association between the remedy and the symptoms. A remedy with a strong association with a remedy will usually be shown in **bold** type. Where the link is less prominent the remedy will be in *italics* and those with the weakest association in plain type.

Repertorisation
The process of using a repertory to analyse a case to determine the most appropriate remedy by looking at the remedies whose Materia Medica best matches the clinical picture of the patient.

Rubric
A symptom in the repertory (with, where relevant, related details and categories) with a list or lists of graded remedies whose materia medica encompasses the symptom.

Sarcode
A homeopathic medicine produced from healthy tissue or from a specific organ.

Serial dilution
A process involved in the potentisation of a homeopathic remedy which involves a series of equal dilutions with succussion or trituration at each step.

Similia Principle
Principle whose basis is *Similia Similibus Curentur* and which states that a substance can be used to treat conditions whose symptoms correspond to those induced by taking the substance in a healthy person.

Similia Similibus Curentur
Latin phrase whose meaning is 'let like be cured by like', the basic principle on which homeopathy is based.

Simillimum
A term applied to the remedy whose symptom picture matches most closely the clinical symptoms of the patient or that remedy whose Materia Medica best matches the clinical symptoms of the patient.

Strange symptoms
Encompasses symptoms also described as rare and peculiar, signifying symptoms or signs that are unusual or uncommon. Such individual symptoms are extremely useful in determining the correct remedy as they can often point to a specific remedy.

Succussion
A step in the potentisation of a remedy involving vigorous shaking (with impact on a hard surface) at each stage of dilution.

Sucrose
Sugar used a dosage medium for homeopathic remedies.

Suppression
The treatment of a symptom or condition by palliative means using conventional medicine such

that the problem is relieved but not resolved. As a result of this the condition may remain hidden or may become active later as a more serious or deep-seated problem. Suppression can make the homeopathic treatment of a patient more complex.

Sycotic miasm or Sycosis
One of three chronic miasms. Symptoms associated with or susceptibility to, a picture of disease linked originally with gonorrhoea and figwarts but now associated with over-activity or overreaction of the body.

Symptom
A sign observed as the patient's reaction to disease that differs from those that are seen in normal health. Taken also to mean the signs noted in an illness that are expressed by the patient, seen by others or by the homeopath.

Symptom picture
A list of the features which correspond and describe the illness of a specific patient. Synonymous with clinical picture.

Syphilitic miasm
One of three chronic miasms. Symptoms associated with or susceptibility to, a picture of disease linked originally with the venereal disease syphilis characterised by destruction or breakdown of body tissues or a failure of the structure or function of the body.

Tincture
A solution comprising a solvent (usually alcohol and water in specific ratios) containing plant material which is used medicinally. Tinctures can be taken to mean homeopathic mother tincture use as the basis for a remedy or herbal tincture, a dosage form used by medicinal herbalists.

Trituration
Dilution of a solid or insoluble substance by grinding and the initial step in the production and potentisation of a homeopathic remedy produced from such material. Lactose is used as the diluent until such as stage is reached that the trituration can be dissolved in water to continue the manufacturing process by succussion.

Vaccinosis
A term applied to the symptoms produced as a result of an adverse reaction to a vaccination or the chronic health problems that can be attributed to vaccination.

Vital force
Synonymous with the term life force which is that force, energy or power which gives life to a living organism.

X potency
An abbreviation 'x' signifying the decimal potency of a remedy.

Notes

1 This is now the current accepted spelling, which omits the second 'o'. Older spellings, homoeopathy and homœopathy are still in occasional use and present in many older texts.

2 Allopathically prescribed medicines have no direct relationship to the patient's symptoms. Antibiotics are a good example.

3 Antipathic medicines work to oppose the patient's symptoms such as kaolin used in the treatment of diarrhoea.

4 Avogadro's number is approximately 6.022×10^{23} representing the number of molecules in a mole which (in chemistry) is the molecular weight of a substance expressed in grams.

5 With a great many homeopathic books detailing these interactions, there is some disparity between different authors on the relationship between individual remedies.

6 Often used in sequence: Sulphur first, then Calc carb followed by Lycopodium

7 Nux vomica and Pulsatilla are considered opposites

8 There are several Tuberculinums. This is the remedy most often prescribed when treating horses

9 Notifiable diseases. In the UK these are named in section 88 of the Animal Health Act 1981 or an order made under that Act including the Infectious Diseases of Horses Order 1987. Signs of any of the following diseases in horses must be reported to DEFRA. African Horse Sickness, Contagious Equine Metritis, Dourine, Epizootic Lymphangitis, Equine Viral Arteritis, Equine Viral Encephalomyelitis, Equine Infectious Anaemia, Glanders and Farcy, Rabies, Vesicular Stomatitis, West Nile Virus.

10 In the UK a code of practice exists on the prevention and control of EHV available from the Horserace Betting Levy Board.

11 In the UK a code of practice exists on the prevention and control of EVA available from the Horserace Betting Levy Board.

12 In the UK a code of practice exists on the prevention and control of CEM available from the Horserace Betting Levy Board.

13 In other parts of the world horses can be vaccinated against diseases other than influenza and tetanus. Conventional vaccines are available for Eastern Equine Encephalitis (EEE), Western Equine Encephalitis (WEE), Venezuelan Equine Encephalitis (VEE), Potomac Horse Fever, Rabies, West Nile Virus, Strangles, Rotavirus, EHV-1 and 4, Botulism and Equine Viral Arteritis.

14 A detailed materia medica is recommended to elaborate on the specific interactions of each remedy with others. The information supplied is general; however, you will almost certainly find inconsistencies between different authors. *The Dictionary of Practical Materia Medica* by Clarke is one of the most suitable books to help detail remedy relationships.

15 Mistletoe can be prescribed in conventional homeopathic potency and can be used as an anthroposophical preparation (Iscador, available from Weleda) for the specific treatment of cancers.

16 Specifically non-lactose fermenting bacteria. These are bacteria that are not able to use milk sugar as an energy source.

Further reading

General introduction

Boyd H, *Introduction to Homoeopathic Medicine,* 2nd edition, Beaconsfield (1989)

Homoeopathy. An Introduction and Guide to Homoeopathy, Wigmore Publications (2000)

Homoeopathy for Your Pets – An introduction and Guide to Homoeopathy for Your Pets, Wigmore Publications (2000)

Vithoulkas G, *The Science of Homeopathy,* Grove (1980)

Philosophy and principles

Hahnemann C F S, *Chronic Diseases, Their specific nature and Homoeopathic treatment,* Boericke & Tafel (1896)

Hahnemann C F S, *The Organon of Medicine* 6th edition, translated by Kunzli J, Naude & Pendleton (1842)

Hahnemann C F S, *Organon of the Medical Art* translated from *The Organon* 6th edition (1842) Birdcage Books (1996)

Kent J T, *Lectures on Homoeopathic Philosophy* 2nd edition, Ehrhart & Karl (1932)

Koehler G, *The Handbook of Homoeopathy,* Thorsens (1986)

Roberts H A, *The Principles and Art of Cure by Homeopathy,* B Jain India (1995)

Sankaren R, *The Spirit of Homoeopathy* 3rd edition, Homoeopathic Medical Publishers (1999)

Repertories

Boger C M, *Boenninghausen's Characteristics and Repertory,* B. Jain, India (2002)

Clarke J H, *A Clinical Repertory,* B. Jain, India (2003)

Kent J T, *Repertory of the Homoeopathic Materia Medica,* Homeopathic Book Service (1986)

Murphy R, *Homeopathic Medical Repertory,* Hahnemann Academy of North America (1993)

Schroyens F (ed), *Synthesis 9.1,* Homeopathic Book Publishers (2004)

Materia medica

Allen H C, *Keynotes of Leading Remedies,* Boericke & Tafel (1950)

Boericke W, *Materia Medica and Repertory,* B. Jain, India (1996)

Clarke J H, *Dictionary of Materia Medica* - in 3 volumes, 3rd edition (1991) Homeopathic Book Service

Coulter C, *Portraits of Homoeopathic Remedies* - in 3 volumes, Quality Medicine Publishing (1997)

Gibson D, *Studies of Homeopathic Remedies,* Beaconsfield (1987)

Macleod G, *A Veterinary Materia Medica and Clinical Repertory,* C W Daniel (1983)

Materia Medica Homoeopathica Veterinaria (currently only in German) Multi author, J. Millemann (Ed.) IAVH, Sonntag (2005)

Phatak S R, *Materia Medica of Homoeopathic Medicines,* Homeopathic Book Service (1982)

Tyler M L, *Homoeopathic Drug Pictures,* C W Daniel (1989)

Tyler M L, *Pointers to the Common Remedies,* B Jain India (1988)

Vermeulen F, *Concordant Materia Medica,* Emryss BV (1997)

Wallace, John *Remedy notes 1,* SrP (1999)

Wallace, John *Remedy notes 2,* SrP (2003)

Clinical books – homeopathy only

Horses only

Day C, *Homeopathy* Threshold Picture Guide (44), Kenilworth Press (2000)

Elliott M & Pinkus, *Horses and Homoeopathy, A Guide for Yard and Stable*, Ainsworths Homeopathic Pharmacy (1994)

Macleod G, *Treatment of Horses by Homeopathy* C W Daniel (1993)

Peker J & Issautier M N, *Homéopathie et Cheval*, Editions Boiron (2000)

Rakov M, *Soignez votre Cheval par L'Homéopathie*, Vigot (2000)

Other species

Biddis K, *Homoeopathy in Veterinary Practice*, C W Daniel (1987)

Day C, *The Homoeopathic Treatment of Small Animals* 3rd edition, C W Daniel (1995)

Day C, *Homoeopathic Treatment of Beef and Dairy Cattle*, Beaconsfield (1995)

Elliott M & Pinkus, *Homoeopathy, The Shepherd's Guide*, Ainsworths Homeopathic Pharmacy (1993)

Elliott M & Pinkus, *Homeopathy for a Healthier Cat*, Ainsworths Homeopathic Pharmacy (1999)

Elliott M & Pinkus *Dogs and Homeopathy - An Owner's Guide*, Ainsworths Homeopathic Pharmacy (1996)

Hansford P & Pinkus T, *The Herdsman's Introduction to Homeopathy* 2nd edition, Ainsworths Homeopathic Pharmacy (1998)

Hunter F, *Homoeopathic First Aid Treatment for Pets* 2nd edition, Thorsons (1988)

Hunter F & Kayne S, *People are Pets*, British Homeopathic Association (1997)

Hunter F, *Everyday Homeopathy for Animals*, Beaconsfield (2004)

Macleod G, *The Treatment of Cattle by Homeopathy*, C W Daniel (1981)

Macleod G, *Goats: Homoeopathic Remedies*, C W Daniel (1991)

Macleod G, *Cats: Homoeopathic Remedies*, C W Daniel (1990)

Macleod G, *Dogs: Homoeopathic Remedies*, C W Daniel (1983)

Macleod G, *Pigs: Homeopathic Approach to Treatment and Prevention of Diseases*, C W Daniel (1994)

Rush J, *The Handbook of Veterinary Homeopathy*, Boericke & Tafel (1911)

Saxton J G G and Gregory P, *Textbook of Veterinary Homeopathy*, Beaconsfield (2005)

Westerhuis, Atjo, *Your Dog and Homoeopathy*, Qualipet C Products & Education BV (2003)

Wolff H G, *Homoeopathic Medicine for Dogs*, C W Daniel (1998)

Wolff H G, *Your Healthy Cat*, North Atlantic Books (1991)

Clinical books – multi-therapy

Horses only

Brennan M L, *Complete Horse Care and Healing for Horses*, Kenilworth Press (2001)

Emich G, *Naturopathy for Horses*, J A Allen (1994)

Including other species

Schoen A and Wynn S G, *Complementary and Alternative Veterinary Medicine*, Mosby (1998)

Wynn S G & Marsden S, *Manual of Natural Veterinary Medicine*, Mosby (2003)

Useful Addresses

Suppliers List – Homeopathic Remedies

Homeopathic Pharmacies – UK

Ainsworths Homeopathic Pharmacy
36 New Cavendish Street
London W1M 7LH
tel: 0171 935 5330
fax: 0171 486 4313
website: www.ainsworths.com

Freeman's Homeopathic Pharmacy
18–20 Main Street
Busby
Glasgow G76 8DU
tel: 0141 644 4465
fax: 0141 644 5735
website: www.freemans.uk.com

Weleda (UK) Limited
Heanor Road
Ilkeston
Derbyshire DE7 8DR
tel: 0115 944 8200.
Freefax: 0800 132069
website: www.weleda.co.uk

Galen Homoeopathics
Lewell Mill
West Stafford
Dorchester
Dorset DT2 8AN
tel: 01305 263996
fax: 01305 250792

Nelsons Homeopathic Pharmacy
73 Duke Street
London W1K 5BY
tel: 020 7629 3118
email: pharmacy@nelsonbach.com

Helios Homoeopathy Ltd
89–97 Camden Road
Tunbridge Wells
Kent TN1 2QR
tel: 01892 537254/536393 (24 Hours)
fax: 01892 546850
email: pharmacy@helios.co.uk
website: www.helios.co.uk

Buxton & Grant
176 Whiteladies Road
Bristol BS8 2XU
tel: 0117 973 5025

E Gould & Son
14 Crowndale Road
London NW1 1TT
tel: 020 7387 1888
website: www.alternativepharmacy.co.uk

Dr Reckeweg (UK) Ltd
Dalton House
33 Leigh Road
West Houghton
Bolton BL5 2JE
tel: 01942 811444

Other UK Suppliers

Hilton Herbs Limited
Downclose Farm, North Perrott
Crewkerne
Somerset
TA18 7SH
tel: 01460 78300
fax: 01460 78302
website: www.hiltonherbs.com

USA

Boiron USA
Box 449
6 Campus Boulevard
Building A, Newtown Square
PA 19073
tel: 0800-Blu-Tube
website: www.boiron.com

Standard Homeopathic Co
PO Box 61067
210 West 131st Street
Los Angeles
CA 90061
tel: 0800 624 9659
website: www.hylands.com

Dolisos USA
3014 Rigel Avenue
Las Vegas
NV 89102
tel: 0800 365 4767
website: www.dolisosamerica.com

Heel Inc
11600 Cochiti S.E.
Albuquerque
NM 87123
tel: 0800 621 7644
website: www.heelusa.com

Weleda USA
175 North Route 9VV
Congers
NY 10920
tel: 0800 241 1030
website: www.weleda.com

Contacts

Homeopathic Veterinary Surgeons

United Kingdom

British Association of Homeopathic Veterinary Surgeons (BAHVS)
The Secretary, BAHVS
Chinham House
Stanford in the Vale
Faringdon
Oxon
SN7 8NQ
tel: 01367 710324
fax: 01367 718243
website: www.bahvs.com

United States of America

American Holistic Veterinary Medical Association (AHVMA)
2218 Old Emmorton Road
Bel Air
MD 21015
tel: 410-569-0795
fax: 410-569-2346
email: ahvma@verizon.net
website: www.ahvma.org

Academy of Veterinary Homeopathy
PO Box 9280
Wilmington
DE 19809
tel: 866 652 1590
website: www.theavh.org/members

Worldwide

International Association for Veterinary Homeopathy
website: www.iavh.at

General Information

British Homeopathic Association
Hahnemann House
29 Park Street West
Luton
LU1 3BE
tel: 0870 444 3950
fax: 0870 444 3960
email: info@trusthomeopathy.org
website: www.trusthomeopathy.org

BHA Book Service
20 Main Street
Busby
Glasgow
G76 8DU
tel: 0845 2255492
fax: 0845 2255493
email: orders@bhabooks.com
website: www.bhabooks.com

Horserace Betting Levy Board
52 Grosvenor Gardens
London
SW1W 0AU
tel: 0207 333 0043
fax: 0207 333 0041
email: hblb@hblb.org.uk

Computer Repertorisation Software

Miccant Ltd
Isis and Cara Software
tel: 0870 141 7053
website: www.miccant.com

Macrepertory
Kent Homeopathic Associates Inc.
tel: 0208 399 4291
www.kenthomeopathic.com

Radar
www.archibel.com/homeopathy/radar

Index

Ringworm 30
Echinacea 30
Bacillinum 30
Chrysarobinum 30.